ADVANCES IN

# Pharmacology and Chemotherapy

VOLUME 14

## ADVISORY BOARD

ADVANCES IN

# Pharmacology and Chemotherapy

EDITED BY

**Silvio Garattini**

*Istituto di Ricerche Farmacologiche "Mario Negri"*
*Milano, Italy*

**A. Goldin**

*National Cancer Institute*
*Bethesda, Maryland*

**F. Hawking**

*Commonwealth Institute of Helminthology*
*St. Albans, Herts., England*

**I. J. Kopin**

*National Institute of Mental Health*
*Bethesda, Maryland*

Consulting Editor

**R. J. Schnitzer**

*Mount Sinai School of Medicine*
*New York, New York*

VOLUME 14–1977

**ACADEMIC PRESS** New York San Francisco London

**A Subsidiary of Harcourt Brace Jovanovich, Publishers**

ACADEMIC PRESS, INC.
111 Fifth Avenue, New York, New York 10003

*United Kingdom Edition published by*
ACADEMIC PRESS, INC. (LONDON) LTD.
24/28 Oval Road, London NW1

LIBRARY OF CONGRESS CATALOG CARD NUMBER: 61-18298

ISBN 0-12-032914-X

PRINTED IN THE UNITED STATES OF AMERICA

# CONTENTS

CONTRIBUTORS TO THIS VOLUME . . . . . . . . . . . . . . . . ix

## Chemotherapy of Schistosomiasis mansoni

NAFTALE KATZ

I. Introduction . . . . . . . . . . . . . . . . . . . . . 2
II. Laboratory Maintenance of *Schistosoma mansoni* . . . . . . . . 5
III. Drug Testing *in Vitro* . . . . . . . . . . . . . . . . . 10
IV. Drug Testing *in Vivo* . . . . . . . . . . . . . . . . . 11
V. Preclinical Trials . . . . . . . . . . . . . . . . . . 15
VI. Clinical Trials . . . . . . . . . . . . . . . . . . . 16
VII. Antischistosomal Drugs in Clinical Use . . . . . . . . . . . 21
VIII. Compounds with Antischistosomal Activity . . . . . . . . . . 46
References . . . . . . . . . . . . . . . . . . . . . 55

## The Behavioral Toxicity of Monoamine Oxidase-Inhibiting Antidepressants

DENNIS L. MURPHY

I. Introduction . . . . . . . . . . . . . . . . . . . . . 72
II. Methods . . . . . . . . . . . . . . . . . . . . . . 75
III. Iproniazid-Related Adverse Behavioral Changes . . . . . . . . . 76
IV. Phenelzine-Related Adverse Behavioral Changes . . . . . . . . . 83
V. Tranylcypromine-Related Adverse Behavioral Changes . . . . . . 90
VI. Adverse Behavioral Changes Associated with Other Monoamine Oxidase-Inhibiting Antidepressants . . . . . . . . . . . . 90
VII. Comparison of Adverse Behavioral Effects during Monoamine Oxidase Inhibitor Treatment with Those during Treatment with Other Antidepressant Drugs . . . . . . . . . . . . . . . . 95
VIII. Behavioral Effects of Monoamine Oxidase-Inhibiting Drugs in Animals of Possible Relevance to Their Behavioral Toxicity in Man . . . . 97
IX. Biochemical Effects of Monoamine Oxidase-Inhibiting Drugs in Animals and Man of Possible Relevance to Their Behavioral Effects . . . . 97
X. Discussion and Conclusions . . . . . . . . . . . . . . . 98
References . . . . . . . . . . . . . . . . . . . . . 101

## Biology, Diagnosis, and Chemotherapeutic Management of Pancreatic Malignancy

JOHN S. MACDONALD, LAWRENCE WIDERLITE, AND PHILIP S. SCHEIN


I. Introduction . . . . . . . . . . 107
II. Adenocarcinoma of the Pancreas . . . . . . . . . . 108
III. Islet Cell Tumors . . . . . . . . . . 127
IV. Conclusion . . . . . . . . . . 136
References . . . . . . . . . . 137


## Mechanisms of Action of Immunopotentiating Agents in Cancer Therapy

WILNA A. WOODS


I. Introduction . . . . . . . . . . 143
II. Biological Stimulators . . . . . . . . . . 144
III. Chemical Stimulators . . . . . . . . . . 151
IV. Conclusions . . . . . . . . . . 154
References . . . . . . . . . . 155


## Persorption of Particles: Physiology and Pharmacology

GERHARD VOLKHEIMER


I. Introduction . . . . . . . . . . 163
II. Mechanism of Persorption . . . . . . . . . . 165
III. Determination of the Rate of Persorption . . . . . . . . . . 167
IV. Modification of Persorption Rates . . . . . . . . . . 175
V. Excretion of Persorbed Particles . . . . . . . . . . 178
VI. Breakdown of Persorbed Particles . . . . . . . . . . 182
VII. Discussion . . . . . . . . . . 184
VIII. Future Developments . . . . . . . . . . 186
IX. Conclusion . . . . . . . . . . 186
References . . . . . . . . . . 187


## Pharmacological Control of the Synthesis and Metabolism of Cyclic Nucleotides

BENJAMIN WEISS AND RICHARD FERTEL


I. Introduction . . . . . . . . . . 189
II. Adenylate Cyclase . . . . . . . . . . 191
III. Guanylate Cyclase . . . . . . . . . . 221
IV. Cyclic Nucleotide Phosphodiesterases . . . . . . . . . . 226
V. Transport of Cyclic AMP . . . . . . . . . . 262
VI. Inhibition of Action of Cyclic AMP . . . . . . . . . . 262
VII. Directions of Future Research in Pharmacological Control of Cyclic Nucleotides . . . . . . . . . . 263

VIII. Clinical Implications . . . . . . . . . . . . . . . . 264
IX. Concluding Remarks . . . . . . . . . . . . . . . . 265
References . . . . . . . . . . . . . . . . . . 266

## 5-Azacytidine—A New Anticancer Drug with Significant Activity in Acute Myeloblastic Leukemia

DANIEL D. VON HOFF AND MILAN SLAVIK

I. Introduction . . . . . . . . . . . . . . . . . . 285
II. Chemical and Physicochemical Properties . . . . . . . . . . 286
III. Biological Properties . . . . . . . . . . . . . . . . 288
IV. Modes of Action and Resistance . . . . . . . . . . . . 291
V. Experimental Activity . . . . . . . . . . . . . . . . 297
VI. Animal Toxicity . . . . . . . . . . . . . . . . . 300
VII. Drug Metabolism and Disposition . . . . . . . . . . . . 303
VIII. Clinical Studies . . . . . . . . . . . . . . . . . 309
IX. Summary and Conclusions . . . . . . . . . . . . . . 322
References . . . . . . . . . . . . . . . . . . 323

## Copper in Mammalian Reproduction

GERALD OSTER AND MIKLOS P. SALGO

I. Introduction . . . . . . . . . . . . . . . . . . 328
II. Copper Intrauterine Device . . . . . . . . . . . . . . 329
III. Hormonally Induced Changes in Copper Levels . . . . . . . . 357
IV. Copper Influences on Reproductive Hormones . . . . . . . . 362
V. Copper in Pregnancy . . . . . . . . . . . . . . . . 368
VI. Copper and Sperm . . . . . . . . . . . . . . . . 379
VII. Copper and the Neonate and Infant . . . . . . . . . . . 382
VIII. Copper Antagonists . . . . . . . . . . . . . . . . 388
IX. Copper in the Environment . . . . . . . . . . . . . . 391
References . . . . . . . . . . . . . . . . . . 393
Notes Added in Proof . . . . . . . . . . . . . . . . 409

SUBJECT INDEX . . . . . . . . . . . . . . . . . . 411

# CONTRIBUTORS TO THIS VOLUME

Numbers in parentheses indicate the pages on which the authors' contributions begin.

RICHARD FERTEL* (189), *Department of Pharmacology, Medical College of Pennsylvania, Philadelphia, Pennsylvania*

NAFTALE KATZ (1), *Centro de Pesquisas René Rachou, Instituto de Endemias Rurais, Fundação Oswaldo Cruz and Seção de Parasitoses da Prefeitura de Belo Horizonte, Minas Gerais, Brazil*

JOHN S. MACDONALD (107), *Division of Medical Oncology, Vincent T. Lombardi Cancer Research Center, Georgetown University, Washington, D. C.*

DENNIS L. MURPHY (71), *Section on Clinical Neuropharmacology, Laboratory of Clinical Science, National Institute of Mental Health, National Institutes of Health Clinical Center, Bethesda, Maryland*

GERALD OSTER (327), *Graduate School of Biological Science, Mount Sinai School of Medicine of the City University of New York, New York, New York*

MIKLOS P. SALGO† (327), *Department of Physiology and Biophysics, Mount Sinai School of Medicine of the City University of New York, New York, New York*

PHILIP S. SCHEIN (107), *Division of Medical Oncology, Vincent T. Lombardi Cancer Research Center, Georgetown University, Washington, D.C.*

MILAN SLAVIK (285), *Investigational Drug Branch, Division of Cancer Treatment, National Cancer Institute, National Institutes of Health, Bethesda, Maryland*

GERHARD VOLKHEIMER (163), *Bayerischer Platz 9, Berlin, West Germany*

* Present address: Department of Pharmacology, Ohio State University School of Medicine, Columbus, Ohio 43210.

† Present address: Physiological Laboratory, University of Cambridge, Cambridge, Great Britain.

DANIEL D. VON HOFF (285), *Investigational Drug Branch, Division of Cancer Treatment, National Cancer Institute, National Institutes of Health, Bethesda, Maryland*

BENJAMIN WEISS (189), *Department of Pharmacology, Medical College of Pennsylvania, Philadelphia, Pennsylvania*

LAWRENCE WIDERLITE (107), *Division of Medical Oncology, Vincent T. Lombardi Cancer Research Center, Georgetown University, Washington, D.C. and Gastroenterology Section, Veterans Hospital, Washington, D.C.*

WILNA A. WOODS* (143), *Virus and Disease Modification Section, Viral Biology Branch, National Cancer Institute, National Institutes of Health, Bethesda, Maryland*

* Present address: RNA Virus Studies Section, Collaborative Research Branch, National Cancer Institute, National Institutes of Health, Bethesda, Maryland.

# Chemotherapy of Schistosomiasis mansoni*

NAFTALE KATZ

*Centro de Pesquisas René Rachou*
*Instituto de Endemias Rurais*
*Fundação Oswaldo Cruz and Seção de Parasitoses da Prefeitura de Belo Horizonte*
*Minas Gerais, Brazil*

I. Introduction . . . . . . . . . . . . . . . . . . . . . 2
II. Laboratory Maintenance of *Schistosoma mansoni* . . . . . . . . 5
A. Culture of Snail Vector . . . . . . . . . . . . . . . 5
B. Infection of Snails . . . . . . . . . . . . . . . . 6
C. Infection of Laboratory Animals . . . . . . . . . . . 8
III. Drug Testing *in Vitro* . . . . . . . . . . . . . . . . 10
IV. Drug Testing *in Vivo* . . . . . . . . . . . . . . . . 11
V. Preclinical Trials . . . . . . . . . . . . . . . . . . 15
VI. Clinical Trials . . . . . . . . . . . . . . . . . . . 16
A. Trials in Hospital . . . . . . . . . . . . . . . . 16
B. Trials in Outpatient Clinic . . . . . . . . . . . . . 18
C. Trials in the Field . . . . . . . . . . . . . . . . 18
VII. Antischistosomal Drugs in Clinical Use . . . . . . . . . . . 21
A. Antimonials . . . . . . . . . . . . . . . . . . 21
B. Niridazole . . . . . . . . . . . . . . . . . . . 31
C. Lucanthone and Hycanthone . . . . . . . . . . . . . 36
D. Oxamniquine . . . . . . . . . . . . . . . . . . 42
VIII. Compounds with Antischistosomal Activity . . . . . . . . . . 46
A. Nitrofuran Derivatives . . . . . . . . . . . . . . 46
B. Thiazolines and Nitrothiazolines . . . . . . . . . . . 47
C. Arylazonaphthylamine Derivatives . . . . . . . . . . . 48
D. Thiophene Derivatives . . . . . . . . . . . . . . 48
E. Organophosphorus Compounds . . . . . . . . . . . . 49
F. Tubercidin . . . . . . . . . . . . . . . . . . . 50
G. SN 10,275 . . . . . . . . . . . . . . . . . . . 50
H. Amphotericin B . . . . . . . . . . . . . . . . . 50
I. S-201 . . . . . . . . . . . . . . . . . . . . . 51
J. A-16,612 . . . . . . . . . . . . . . . . . . . 51
K. RD-12,869 . . . . . . . . . . . . . . . . . . . 51
L. Tris(*p*-aminophenyl)carbonium Salts . . . . . . . . . . 52
M. *p*-Aminophenoxyalkane Derivatives . . . . . . . . . . 52
N. Dehydroemetine . . . . . . . . . . . . . . . . . 53
O. Other Active Compounds . . . . . . . . . . . . . . 53

* This review has been supported, in part, by the Conselho Nacional de Pesquisas, Brazil.

P. Egg Suppressants and Chemosterilants . . . . . . . . . . . 54
Q. Biological Agents and Materials . . . . . . . . . . . . . 55
References . . . . . . . . . . . . . . . . . . . 55

## I. Introduction

Schistosomiasis, a world-wide parasitic disease, affects more than 200 million people, about 70 million of them infected with *Schistosoma mansoni*.

Although the introduction of the first antischistosomal agent occurred more than five decades ago (Christopherson, 1918) and despite the efforts expended in the search for active compounds—according to Standen (1967) more than 250,000 chemical substances have already been tested—few drugs have qualified for clinical trial and can be considered as antischistosomal agents of proven value.*

The various prerequisites for an ideal antischistosomal agent have been discussed by Fairley (1951), Newsome (1962b), Friedheim (1967), Pellegrino and Katz (1968). With some modifications, they can be summarized as follows: (*1*) absence of side effects and toxicity in man; (*2*) high activity against the three main human schistosome infections; (*3*) efficient when given in a single dose or, at most, for 2 days; (*4*) equally effective by injection or by the oral route; (*5*) active against all stages of the schistosome in mammalian hosts; (*6*) chemically stable under common storage conditions; and (*7*) low priced. However, as has been pointed out by Newsome (1962b), this ideal drug represents an aim to be achieved and serves as a criterion for the evaluation of the results so far obtained and those yet to come. A less ambitious and more realistic approach to the problem of chemotherapy of schistosomiasis is to consider that three types of drugs are necessary; (*a*) prophylactic, to prevent infection; (*b*) suppressant, to prevent egg laying; and (*c*) curative, to kill all or most of the adult worms.

So far, the compounds routinely used in clinical treatment, namely, antimonials, hycanthone, niridazole, and oxamniquine fulfill only some of the prerequisites mentioned.

Three approaches have been followed in the search for new drugs for

* General reviews on chemotherapy of schistosomiasis have been published, among others, by Standen (1963), Lämmler (1968), Pellegrino and Katz (1968), Werbel (1970), Archer and Yarinsky (1972), Friedheim (1973), Katz and Pellegrino (1974a). A very extensive bibliography of the world literature about schistosomiasis, from 1852 to 1962, can be found in Warren and Newill (1967). The present review contains references up to and including 1975.

the chemotherapy of schistosomiasis: the empirical, the selective, and the biochemical.

The empirical approach consists of blind screening a large number of compounds from chemically unrelated groups. The substances are tested in a standardized way in the hope that one or more of them may display activity against the infection and be, therefore, useful as a chemical "lead." This is the most usual approach in large-scale experimental chemotherapy. Once the lead is in hand, the active group becomes the focus of the selective approach.

The selective approach is the biological investigation of compounds chemically related to those already known to have some antischistosomal activity. The principal aim is to increase activity and/or decrease toxicity through structure modifications of that parent compound. Two drugs, at least, have recently emerged from this approach: hycanthone, from Miracil D (Rosi *et al.,* 1965), and oxamniquine, from the mirasan series (Richards and Foster, 1969).

The biochemical approach [also called rational approach (Standen, 1967)] is based on the chemical differences between the metabolic pathways and enzymes in the *S. mansoni* worm and in its host. Theoretically, this would be the best approach, since the drug could interfere with some vital system in the worm, without exhibiting toxicity to the host. However, up to the present, too little is known of the parasite's biochemistry to permit such forecasting. During the last decades, basic studies of the biochemistry and physiology of schistosomes have been carried out, especially by Bueding and co-workers, Senft, and others. These papers will not be reviewed here, and those interested in further details may refer to the articles of Bueding *et al.* (1947, 1953), Bueding (1949, 1950, 1952, 1959, 1962, 1967, 1969), Bueding and Koletsky (1950), Bueding and Charms (1951), Bueding and Peters (1951), Mansour and Bueding (1953, 1954); Mansour *et al.* (1954), Bueding and MacKinnon (1955a,b), Bueding and Mansour (1957), Timms and Bueding (1959), Senft (1963, 1965, 1966), Barker *et al.* (1966), Fripp (1967a,b), Booth and Schulert (1968), Nimmo-Smith and Raison (1968), Bruce *et al.* (1969), Smith and Brooks (1969), Zussman *et al.* (1970), Bennet and Bueding (1971, 1973), Senft *et al.* (1972, 1973a,b). Although some of the metabolic pathways and enzymic systems of schistosomes are already known, and, as it has been shown, some schistosome enzymes are not identical with those of the mammalian hosts (Mansour and Bueding, 1953; Mansour *et al.,* 1954), more fundamental data are necessary before this biochemical approach can actually serve for designing new antischistosomal drugs.

The aforementioned approaches for screening antischistosomal candidates can be performed *in vitro, in vivo* or *in vivo/in vitro*. The *in vitro* test is handicapped by the fact that metabolism of the drug may be necessary to form an active transformation product. Moreover, there is no consistent correlation between *in vitro* and *in vivo* tests. For example, diaminodiphenoxyalkanes, which are highly active against *S. mansoni in vivo* (Raison and Standen, 1955; Hill, 1956), show low activity *in vitro,* whereas alkylenebisbenzylamines, highly active *in vitro* (Bueding and Penedo, 1957), display little efficacy *in vivo* (Standen, 1963). Hycanthone, the hydroxymethyl analog of Miracil D, is highly active against infection in different laboratory animals (Rosi *et al.* 1965; Berberian *et al.,* 1967a,b) but inactive *in vitro* (Archer and Yarinsky, 1972). Lack of correlation is also observed with glucosamine and naphthoquinones (Bueding *et al.,* 1947, 1954; Brener, 1960; Pellegrino *et al.,* 1962; Standen, 1963).

Nevertheless, *S. mansoni in vitro* cultures are very useful for investigating the mechanism of action of active compounds and, afterward, for selecting the best compounds of a series through *in vivo/in vitro* tests; finally, they can also be used as a biological measure of drug concentration in body fluids.

The *in vivo* tests, although the most useful and widely employed, present some disadvantages: they are time consuming, more expensive, and require previous experiments on several animal species and different types of assessment of drug activity. For routine *in vivo* screening, the common working model in use is the white mouse, as the host, and *S. mansoni*, as the infecting agent. However, Okpala (1959) and Berberian and Freele (1964) prefer the hamster as a primary host, and Petranyi (1969) and Lämmler and Petranyi (1971) use *Mastomys natalensis* (multimammate rat).

It must be pointed out that some schistosomicidal compounds have proved highly effective in mice, but showed no, or just moderate, activity in hamsters, monkeys, or man (Standen, 1963; Lämmler, 1964, 1968; Pellegrino and Katz, 1968; Katz and Pellegrino, 1974a).

As basic criteria in the search for new chemical leads, both suppressive and curative effects have been used. Although the former seem more sensitive, as measured by the oogram method (Pellegrino *et al.,* 1962; Pellegrino and Faria, 1965), the latter are, nevertheless, generally preferred (Standen, 1967). However, any drug found to interfere with egg laying (suppressive effect) will also be evaluated as a curative agent.

During the trials for antischistosomal drugs, the degree of maturity of the infection is very important. For example, thioxanthones, antimonials, *p*-aminophenoxyalkanes, mirasans, niridazole, and other compounds show different activity when administered to animals at different times, on the day of infection, 2–3 weeks later, or when the schistosomes are sexually mature (Kikuth and Gönnert, 1948; Watson *et al.,* 1948; Schubert, 1948c; Standen, 1955; Lämmler, 1958; Bruce *et al.,* 1962; Stohler and Frey, 1963, 1964a; Sadun *et al.,* 1966).

## II. Laboratory Maintenance of *Schistosoma mansoni*

Culture and infection of *Biomphalaria glabrata* snails, as well as infection of mice, hamsters, and monkeys will now be discussed as the main steps for the maintenance of *S. mansoni,* emphasizing in particular the routine methods employed in our laboratories for screening purposes and preclinical trials in schistosomiasis.

### A. Culture of Snail Vector

*Biomphalaria glabrata* is the most suitable snail for mass culture and for infection. It must be pointed out, however, that, as is true for several parasitic diseases, there will exist differences in the infectivity of various parasite strains and the susceptibility of the intermediate host species used. It has been clearly demonstrated that a snail serving as an intermediate host for a schistosome in one geographical area may be poorly susceptible or even refractory to infection with the same parasite from a different area (Vogel, 1942; Cram *et al.,* 1947; Files and Cram, 1949; Files, 1951; Newton, 1953; Paraense and Corrêa, 1963; Kagan and Geiger, 1965; Saoud, 1965).

As claimed by Kagan and Geiger (1965), the genetic constitution of the miracidium may be an important factor in determining its invasiveness. As a practical conclusion, for the maintenance of the parasite life cycle in the laboratory, snails and miracidia from the same endemic area are preferable.

*Biomphalaria glabrata* readily deposit their egg masses on shoots of *Ludwigia palustris* (Standen, 1951a) or on polyethylene plastic sheets (Olivier *et al.,* 1962) floating on the water surface. Snails kept in polyethylene bags, lay the egg masses on the inner surface of the bags (Pellegrino and Gonçalves, 1965).

In our laboratory, egg masses are obtained by floating pieces of polystyrene foam of about 10 × 15 cm in the aquaria. The snails prefer these to glass or vegetation. This method also makes handling very easy, since the pieces may be transferred to polyethylene containers, where the snails emerge. Newly hatched snails feed on the algal film that usually grows on the polystyrene foam or plastic sheets. A special food for fish is also dusted onto the water surface. After reaching the size of about 0.5 cm, the snails are transferred to an aquarium filled with dechlorinated and artificially aerated water. The bottom of each aquarium is covered with a layer of sand and sterilized earth.

Dechlorinated water from a cement-asbestos reservoir is distributed into the aquaria at the rate of about 10 liters/day per aquarium. Excess water is automatically drained through an overflow tube. Artificial aeration and illumination are provided for 8 hours a day. Each aquarium contains 30 liters of water which is adequate for about 200 snails. The snail room is maintained at 25–27°C. Fresh lettuce and commercial fish food are used for feeding the snails. Every 2 months, the snails are removed so that the aquarium may be cleaned.

*Daphnia* can be used for control of microflora and fauna (Berberian and Freele, 1964), whereas snail feces and decaying vegetable or food materials are removed by the oligochete *Tubifex* (Standen, 1963).

Optimal physical conditions for *B. glabrata* culture are pH 7.2–7.8; high oxygen tension; absence of chlorine, copper and, zinc from the water; calcium carbonate concentration of approximately 18 ppm; sodium–calcium ratio of 1:1; and temperature of 23°–28°C (Cowper, 1946; Michelson, 1961; Frank, 1963; Standen, 1963). It is very important to maintain low population density and avoid crowding if good survival and reproduction are to be obtained (Chernin and Michelson, 1957a,b).

Under optimal conditions, allowing 8–9 days incubation of the snail eggs, the egg-to-egg cycle can be completed in 1 month. The reproductive potential of *B. glabrata* is about 14,000 eggs (Ritchie *et al.*, 1963, 1966a). A system for mass-producing *B. glabrata* has been described by Rowan (1958) and Sandt *et al.* (1965).

Although lettuce is generally used for breeding the snails, other types of food and formulations have been proposed, such as calcium alginate (Standen, 1951a), further modified by Moore *et al.* (1953), and a diet consisting of a mixture of Cerophyl, wheat germ cereal, Glandex fish food, and powdered milk in a ratio of 4:2:2:1, respectively (Moore *et al.*, 1953; Etges and Ritchie, 1966).

### B. Infection of Snails

For the infection of *B. glabrata,* miracidia are easily obtained from eggs excreted with the feces, or retained in tissues (liver and intestine preferably) of mice and hamsters experimentally infected with *S. mansoni*. Three main methods are employed for separating the eggs: digestion, flotation, and sedimentation.

The digestion method was proposed for the isolation of schistosome eggs from tissues of infected animals (Bénex, 1960; Smithers, 1960; Browne and Thomas, 1963). According to Smithers (1960), trypsin digestion by itself fails to remove collagen fibers. Further treatment with pepsin is necessary to digest the collagen, leaving the eggs free from the host's tissues. A final washing by centrifugation can be utilized to remove most of the dead eggs in the supernatant.

Ritchie and Berrios-Duran (1961) developed an interesting method for recovering *S. mansoni* eggs from the liver and intestine of mice and hamsters or from their feces. This technique consists of introducing 2.0% saline through a porous stone at the bottom of a sidearm Erlenmeyer flask containing the suspension of eggs and tissue in 1.7% saline. The flow (70–100 ml/minute) is continued until the suspension in 1.7% saline is entirely displaced through the sidearm overflow. The eggs fall through the interface and collect at the bottom of the flask.

In our laboratories, Standen's method (1949, 1953) is used with slight modifications. Infected mice (or hamsters) are sacrificed, the gut removed, and its superficial layer scraped into a Waring Blendor; the liver is then added, and the whole is transformed into a paste with 0.9% saline. After passing through a wide-mesh stainless steel screen more saline is added to the paste, which is allowed to sediment in the dark at 4°C. Resuspension and decanting are repeated until a clear supernatant is obtained. The final sediment is suspended in water at 28° to 30°C and placed under a bright light. The eggs start hatching within 0.5 to 1 hour. During this procedure it is important to bear in mind that salinity, low temperature, and darkness represent inhibitory conditions, whereas fresh water, higher temperature, and illumination stimulate the hatching process (Maldonado and Acosta Matienzo, 1948; Maldonado *et al.*, 1950a,b; Standen, 1951b). The average life span of the free-living miracidium is from 5 to 6 hours. About 91% of the miracidia remain active 1 hour after hatching, but only 25% after 8 hours (Maldonado and Acosta Matienzo, 1948).

Techniques for miracidium concentration based on their positive phototropism and negative geotropism have been described (Stunkard, 1946; Chaia, 1956).

Individual and mass exposure of snails to miracidia are two methods used for *B. glabrata* infection. In the former, the snails are exposed to 10 miracidia each, in small glass containers with the minimum volume of water required for snail movement (Cram, 1947; Standen, 1952). In the latter, batches of 300 *B. glabrata* in 30-liter glass aquaria are exposed to about 5000 miracidia at a temperature of 27°C. High mortality of infected snails is observed 6–7 weeks after infection, coincidental with the emergence of large numbers of cercariae. The infected snails must be maintained at 26° to 28°C, since snails can lose their infection if they are kept at lower temperatures.

In experiments with the Belo Horizonte strain of *B. glabrata* and L. E. strain of miracidium (isolated by Pellegrino, 15 years ago in Belo Horizonte from an adult patient only once exposed to *S. mansoni* cercariae) and using the individual method of 10 miracidia for each snail, between 80–90% of the molluscs became infected, shedding large amounts of cercariae for several months.

For obtaining cercariae, 30–50 laboratory-infected *B. glabrata* are placed in a beaker with 150 ml dechlorinated water and left under an electric lamp for 2 to 3 hours. After removing the snails, the cercarial suspension is screened to retain snail feces and three 1-ml samples are counted after killing the cercariae with formalin. When only a small number of snails is used to obtain this cercarial suspension, the parasites have an unbalanced sex ratio.

## C. Infection of Laboratory Animals

### 1. *Mouse*

The white mouse, widely used in most laboratories for screening and preclinical trials, may be easily infected by *S. mansoni* cercariae by the intraperitoneal, subcutaneous, and percutaneous routes.

Although the intraperitoneal route has been used for routine chemotherapeutic work, it must be remembered that this is an unnatural way to infect and that part of the schistosomes will not migrate to the portal system, but will remain in the peritoneal cavity (Moore and Meleney, 1955), thus hindering the assessment of therapeutic drugs.

Two methods are used for the percutaneous route: (*a*) the wading method and (*b*) the tail-immersion method.

The wading method allows the cercariae to penetrate the animal's body. After letting the mice run about in a container with warm water to stimulate voidance of feces and urine, the animals are transferred to suitable-sized wide-mouthed glass jars provided with bung and ventilating shaft. The cercarial suspension is introduced through the vent by a spring-loaded syringe. After 20 minutes the mice are removed and dried off in warm wood-wool (Standen, 1949).

The tail-immersion method consists of immersing the tails of mice into tubes containing cercariae. Previously anesthetized mice, are exposed for 45 minutes, after which the mice are returned to their cages (Olivier and Stirewalt, 1952; Stirewalt and Bronson, 1955; Pellegrino and Katz,

1968). A small plastic cage was designed by Radke *et al.* (1971) making anesthesia unnecessary.

In our laboratories, as in Hoffman-La Roche and Ciba laboratories, the subcutaneous route of infection is preferred. The cercariae (100–120 per mouse) are inoculated with a syringe into the subcutaneous tissue of the animal's back. The mean percentage of adult schistosomes recovered has been about 20% with practically all infected mice.

For exposing mice to large amounts of cercariae, the subcutaneous route should be avoided because of the large volume of suspension to be injected. In this case, the percutaneous route, already described, is preferable, using the technique of Radke *et al.* (1971).

2. *Hamster*

By the intraperitoneal route, the worm yield has been inferior to 20% (Cram and Figgat, 1947; Moore *et al.,* 1949; Berberian and Freele, 1964), no worms having been found in the peritoneal cavity after 28 days of infection (Moore and Meleney, 1955). Percutaneous exposure through the shaved skin of hamsters induces a regular infection, the recovery of worms being about 30 to 40% (Cram and Figgat, 1947; Moore *et al.,* 1949; Faria and Pellegrino, 1963).

In our laboratories, cheek pouch infection is routinely employed (Pellegrino *et al.,* 1965a). The percentage of recovery has been 30–50% adult *S. mansoni* worms.

3. *Monkeys*

Rhesus monkeys (*Macaca mulatta*) have been commonly used in schistosomiasis mansoni preclinical trials (Kikuth and Gönnert, 1948; Hill, 1956, Bruce and Sadun, 1963, 1966; Thompson *et al.,* 1962, 1965; Campbell and Cuckler, 1963; Sadun *et al.,* 1966). The use of rhesus monkeys, however, is handicapped by their cost, by difficulty in handling, and by the self-limiting nature of the infection (Vogel 1949, 1958; Lichtenberg and Ritchie, 1961; Smithers and Terry, 1965; Ritchie *et al.,* 1966b; Foster and Broomfield, 1971).

Other genera of monkeys have also been used, namely, *Cercopithecus, Papio,* and *Cebus* (Oesterlin, 1934; Newsome, 1953, 1963; Luttermoser *et al.,* 1960; Meisenhelder and Thompson, 1963; Pellegrino *et al.,* 1966, 1967a,b; Katz *et al.,* 1967b; Pellegrino and Katz, 1969, 1972; Foster, 1973; Katz and Pellegrino 1974b,c).

In our laboratories, *Cebus apella macrocephalus,* a very good host for *S. mansoni* (Coelho and Magalhães Filho, 1953; Brener and Alvarenga,

1962), is the monkey used for preclinical trials. It presents the following advantages: (*a*) relatively low cost, (*b*) easy handling and maintenance, (*c*) high percentage of cercariae maturing into schistosomes (30–50%), (*d*) large numbers of *S. mansoni* eggs in the feces and rectal mucosa, (*e*) no tendency to self-cure (at least up to 3 years), and (*f*) good correlation of therapeutic response to drugs as compared with man (Pellegrino *et al.*, 1965b; Katz *et al.*, 1966b; Pellegrino and Katz, 1968; Katz and Pellegrino, 1974a,b).

Although *Cebus* monkeys can be infected by percutaneous, subcutaneous, and oral routes, the first is preferable to the two other methods since it permits a more regular infection and better worm yield. The cercariae (120–150 per animal) are applied for 30 minutes on the shaved skin of the monkey's abdomen, after immobilizing the animal in a metal holder.

Gerbils, cotton-rats, and multimammate rats have been occasionally used for chemotherapeutic studies in *S. mansoni* infections but presented no advantages over mice, hamsters, and monkeys.

## III. Drug Testing *in Vitro*

Culture of *S. mansoni in vitro* for drug testing or study of mechanisms of action can be performed in at least three different media.

Standen (1963) suggested the use of a culture medium having equal volumes of Tyrode's solution and horse or guinea pig serum with streptomycin and penicillin, its pH being 7.4. Five milliliters of this medium is aseptically transferred to a Carrel flask, and 500 units of streptomycin and 250 units of penicillin are added per flask. The flask is incubated at 37°C. The drug to be tested is dissolved in the minimum volume of Tyrode's solution, buffered as required, and then this same volume of medium is removed from each Carrel flask and replaced by the drug-containing aliquot to restore the original total volume. Two pairs of schistosomes are added to each flask and the incubation continued at 37°C. Worms in drug-free control cultures may survive for 2 to 3 weeks, but daily observations of the drug cultures, for 4 or 5 days, should be enough for conclusive evidence of their adverse effects on the schistosomes.

Lambert (1964) employed a medium having the following constituents: inactivated calf serum (30%), Hank's medium (50%), Difco 199 medium (20%), penicillin (100 μg/ml), streptomycin (40 μg/ml). The medium was buffered to pH 7.6 with sodium bicarbonate. Michaels (1969) used 90% Medium 199 and 10% calf serum in a base of Earle's balanced salt solution with 1.0 mg/ml of added glucose and final concentrations of 100 units of penicillin and 100 $\mu$g of streptomycin per milliliter (Michaels and Prata, 1968; Michaels, 1969).

The signs of damage to the worms are loss of ventral sucker function, alterations of the muscular activity pattern, inhibition of egg laying, immobilization, and finally death.

For accurate measurement of the worms movements, two instruments have been described (Brown *et al.,* 1973; Hillman and Senft, 1973). By using the instrument they described for measuring quantitatively and automatically *S. mansoni* body movements, Hillman and Senft (1973) and Hillman *et al.* (1974) were able to conclude that normal activity of the parasite could be represented by a complex of bursts of movement alternated with periods of lesser activity. Pentobarbital depresses activity, but catecholamines and cyclic nucleotides have no effect. Serotonin and 5-hydroxytryptophan stimulate movements. Carbamylcholine abolishes activity and its effects cannot be reversed by serotonin. Dihydroergotamine and methysergide have a stimulatory effect at some concentrations and a depressant effect at others. Senft and Hillman (1973) determined the effect of antimony tartrate, niridazole, and hycanthone on schistosome activity *in vitro*. Accurate dose–response curves were obtained. Antimony tartrate and niridazole suppress worm motility at doses from $10^{-3}$ to $10^{-5}$ $M$ concentration. Hycanthone decreases worm activity.

Although no promising drug has so far been discovered by way of *in vitro* tests, several aspects concerning schistosome biochemistry and physiology have been investigated, such as regeneration (Cheever and Weller, 1958), sperm formation (Clegg, 1959), and egg production (Robinson, 1960; Newsome, 1962a; Michaels, 1969; Michaels and Prata, 1968). Also, mechanism of action of schistosomicidal drugs, such as *p*-aminophenoxyalkanes (Standen, 1962), tris(*p*-aminophenyl)carbonium chloride or pamoate (TAC) (Bueding *et al.,* 1967), niridazole (Lambert, 1964), hycanthone (Archer and Yarinsky, 1972), and oxamniquine (Foster, 1973), have been investigated.

## IV. Drug Testing *in Vivo*

According to Stohler and Frey (1964a), three different types of drug action can be evaluated: (*a*) prophylactic—the drug is injected before infection to study the effect on subsequently injected cercariae; (*b*) protective—the drug is injected 1–38 days after infection to study its effect on immature schistosomes; and (*c*) therapeutic—the drug is injected at least 41 days after infection to study its effect on mature schistosomes.

The drug may be administered in single or 5-day doses, at different intervals before and after infection. For evaluation of drug activity, the animals are killed and examined 8–10 weeks after infection, using the following parameters: (*a*) mean number of living worms per animal; (*b*) distribution of worms within the hepatic portal system; (*c*) presence of dead worms; (*d*) percentage of animals in untreated controls is assigned the value of 100% and the corresponding mean number in the treated group is expressed as a percentage of the controls (Stohler and Frey, 1964a).

Radke *et al.* (1971) developed a mouse mortality test system for mass screening of prophylactic drugs. Albino mice exposed to 2750 ± 250 cercariae will present a 100% mortality rate within 25 ± 5 days. The compounds were administered in single doses, 2 days after cercarial exposure, to 5 mice per test, at a dosage of 640 and 1920 mg/kg. The percentage of survival among treated mice gave a measure of the degree of the drug's antischistosomal activity.

Jewsbury (1972) used a quantitative technique for schistosomiasis chemoprophylaxis in both mice and hamsters. This approach consisted of two stages. In the first one, four experimental groups were treated, respectively, with one-quarter, one-eighth, one-sixteenth, and one-thirty-second part of the drug mean lethal dose ($LD_{50}$) for 4 consecutive days. This inital treatment was conducted immediately before infection. Post-mortem examinations were carried out on the twenty-ninth day of infection. The degree of protection relative to the controls was calculated, and from these data the compound's effective dose ($ED_{10}$, $ED_{25}$, and $ED_{90}$) values were determined. The ratio of $LD_{50}/ED_{50}$ was determined with the aid of a log/probit scale. The second stage consisted in the administration of the $ED_{50}$, for 4 consecutive days, to six groups of animals treated, respectively, on days 0–3, 7–10, 14–17, 21–25, 29–33, and 35–38. The degree of protection compared with the controls was determined for each group 42 days after infection (Jewsbury, 1972).

For chemoprophylactic tests, Pereira *et al.* (1974) suggest the use of schistosomula in the peritoneal cavity of mice intraperitoneally infected with *S. mansoni* cercariae. Drugs were administered for 5 consecutive days at the daily dose of about one-fifth of the $LD_{50}$. The animals were sacrificed 8 days after the beginning of treatment. Schistosomula recovered through peritoneal washing with saline were counted under a dissecting microscope. In nontreated controls the number of recovered larvae was about 30% of the injected cercariae.

For assessment of antischistosomal activity in primary drug screening, the working model "*S. mansoni*-mouse" has been widely used. The most important criteria in such a model for the evaluation of drug activity are enumerated in the following.

1. Reduction in the number of eggs. With the technique of Kikuth and Gönnert (1948), the assessment of activity is mainly based on the decrease or complete cessation of egg passing by treated mice. Stool examination (by concentration and hatching methods) is carried out twice weekly, for 3 weeks after treatment. Dosing is started 48 days after exposure to *S. mansoni* cercariae, when eggs are regularly present in the feces.

In experimental chemotherapy of schistosomiasis, the evaluation of activity based on the search for excreted eggs has also been extensively used with hamsters (Bueding *et al.*, 1953; Newsome, 1963) as well as with several primate species (El Ayadi, 1947; Luttermoser *et al.*, 1960; Elslager *et al.*, 1961; Bruce *et al.*, 1962; Bruce and Sadun, 1966; Sadun *et al.*, 1966).

According to Schwink's (1955) technique, female mice are sacrified 3 weeks after the beginning of treatment. The intestines of treated and control mice are digested in 5% NaOH for 5 to 6 hours. Egg counts, made on the residues, showed an inverse correlation between the number of eggs and the size of the drug dose used.

With the method of Brener *et al.* (1956), the schistosome granulomas formed around the eggs accumulated in the liver are separated, counted, and their number compared with that found in untreated mice (Pellegrino and Brener, 1956; Brener, 1957; Brener and Chiari, 1957).

2. Increase in the survival time of treated mice. Luttermoser's technique (1954) provides that mice previously exposed to cercarial concentrations (22–25 *S. mansoni* cercariae per gram body weight), lethal to young animals within 6 to 8 weeks, are given early treatment (maximum tolerated dose) with the compounds under test. The increase of the survival time of treated animals compared with that of untreated controls will indicate the drug antischistosomal activity. This criterion was used by Okpala (1959) for assessing drug activity in experimentally infected hamsters.

3. Hepatic shift of schistosomes. Schubert's technique (1948a,b) and its modification by Standen (1953, 1963) are based on the fact that active drugs interfere with the distribution of schistosomes within the hepatic portal system. Normally, in mice and hamsters with mature infection, 60–70% of worms are located in the mesenteric veins, 20–30% in the portal vein, and 0–20% in the liver.

Although this technique is widely used and provides reliable results, constant correlation with schistosomicidal activity could not be observed. In fact, mature worms can shift to the liver after administration of glucosamine (Abdallah *et al.,* 1959), dimercaprol (Khayyal, 1965b) as well as anesthetics (Dickerson, 1965; Khayyal, 1965a).

4. Reduction in worm burden. This criterion is of fundamental importance for the assessment of antischistosomal activity and for a sound quantitative evaluation of active compounds belonging to the same or different chemical group (Watson *et al.,* 1948; Raison and Standen, 1955; Brener and Pellegrino, 1958; Luttermoser, 1959; Thompson *et al.,* 1962, 1965; Campbell and Cuckler, 1963; Stohler and Frey, 1963, 1964a; Lambert and Stauffer, 1964; Bruce and Sadun, 1966; Berberian *et al.,* 1967a,b; Foster, 1973).

5. Oogram changes. Studies on *S. mansoni* oviposition demonstrated that when eggs are laid they are still immature and that a period of about 6 days is needed for the embryo to develop (Gönnert, 1955a; Prata, 1957; Pellegrino *et al.,* 1962). It is assumed that oviposition constitutes a continuous process, at least during a certain period after worm migration to the mesenteric veins and that, shortly after egg laying has begun, the intestinal wall contains a large number of eggs.

Based on Prata's (1957) findings from clinical trials through rectal biopsies, Pellegrino *et al.* (1962) adapted the oogram method for use in the screening of drugs. When mice infected with *S. mansoni* are treated with active drugs, a progressive change in the number of eggs and in the percentage of viable eggs in the different stages (from first to fourth stages as well as in mature eggs) takes place. This change is brought about by the interruption of oviposition in the intestinal wall and by the maturation of viable eggs already there. Accordingly, the percentage of mature eggs increases progressively after the administration of effective compounds (Pellegrino *et al.,* 1962; Pellegrino and Faria, 1964, 1965; Brener, 1965).

The oogram method proved very helpful for the study of relapse (Pellegrino *et al.,* 1963) as well as for the detection of drug activity on schistosome eggs (Hill *et al.,* 1966; Monteiro *et al.,* 1968).

6. Other criteria for assessing therapeutic activity. Besides the criteria already discussed, other observations may be of value for assessing drug activity in schistosomiasis: separation of coupled schistosomes, opacity and depigmentation of worms, and gross morphological alterations involving diminution in size, absence of intrauterine eggs, atrophy of the ovary, vitellaria, and testes, decrease of pigment deposited in the liver, presence of worms ensheathed in inflammatory tissues, etc. (Bang and Hairston, 1946; Kikuth and Gönnert, 1948; Standen, 1953, 1955; Gönnert, 1955b; Hill, 1956; Brener and Pellegrino, 1958; Lambert, 1967;

Sadun *et al.,* 1966; Striebel and Kradolfer, 1966; Bueding *et al.,* 1967; Bourgeois and Bueding, 1971).

It must be remarked that, although for screening purposes the use of a single host and of a single criterion may be adequate, the final evaluation of a promising drug must be based on experimental work carried out in different laboratory animals and using multiple criteria for assessing antischistosomal activities.

## V. Preclinical Trials

Compounds found active in screening tests are further tested in mice, hamsters and monkeys, experimentally infected with *S. mansoni.*

At this point when comparing different drugs, it is imperative to use quantitative criteria of assessment. Accordingly, the methods described in the screening procedures can now be used quantitatively. Therapeutic indexes based on toxicity data ($LD_{50}$) and on the dose that clears 50–90% of infected animals have been widely employed (Schubert *et al.,* 1949; Hill, 1956; Collins *et al.,* 1959; Brener, 1960, 1962; Berberian and Freele, 1964; Rosi *et al.,* 1965, 1967; Berberian *et al.,* 1967a,b; Foster, 1973). Also, the $LD_{50}$ and the dose producing oogram alterations in 50% of the animals ($OD_{50}$) have been proposed by Pellegrino and Faria (1965).

The assessment of drug activity in *Cebus* monkeys can be made through repeated mucosal curettages performed at different periods after treatment. Using a stainless-steel curette, four fragments of the *Cebus* monkeys rectal mucosa are normally obtained weighing together about 30 mg, and consisting solely of the mucosa and muscularis mucosae. Rectal snips, tightly pressed between slide and cover slip are examined under the microscope, all schistosome elements being counted and classified. The assessment of drug activity is based on the gradual disappearance of viable eggs in the rectal snips (Pellegrino *et al.,* 1965b). By weighing the rectal fragments obtained by mucosal curettage and counting all schistosome elements, the number of eggs per gram of tissue is then calculated. This quantitative approach (Katz *et al.,* 1966b) permits the classification of drugs as active, inactive, and partially active (Katz and Pellegrino, 1974b).

It must be pointed out that the curettage technique cannot be employed with *Cercopithecus* monkeys, since very few eggs are found in the rectal snips of this animal (Foster *et al.,* 1971b).

Although the systematic use of mice, hamsters, and monkeys in preclinical studies can provide considerable amounts of informative data for a tentative forecast of possible efficacy in clinical trials, it must be pointed out that whether an antischistosomal agent be fully or partially active or even totally ineffective will depend on the absorption, metabolism, and retention of that particular compound in a particular host (Berberian *et al.,* 1967a; Katz *et al.,* 1967b; Rosi *et al.,* 1967).

## VI. Clinical Trials

Whereas preclinical studies of newly screened schistosomicidal drugs are standardized and fairly rapidly performed (Standen, 1963; Pellegrino and Katz, 1968), the passage to the clinical phase, is difficult, slow, and greatly handicapped by the lack of rigid well-defined criteria regarding procedure.

Well-conducted preclinical studies allow us to foresee, with great probability, the results that can be obtained in clinical treatment, especially those related with the drug's antiparasitic activity.

When starting clinical trials, the following items concerning the compound to be used must be known: (*a*) physical and chemical properties (purity, stability, etc.); (*b*) pharmacology and tolerability by various animal species; (*c*) pharmacology, tolerability, and counterindication in volunteers. These indispensable data being available, the clinical trials may be carried out in the following order (WHO, 1966): first phase—trials in hospital; second phase—trials in outpatient clinic; third phase—trials in the field.

### A. Trials in Hospital

The candidates for treatment, after careful selection, must be taken as inpatients and informed about the new drug still under experiment. The schedules for drug administration are then determined (formulation, dose, duration of treatment, etc.). After therapy, the drug activity will be assessed and its effects on the organs and systems of the human body (as well as any other local or general repercussions of treatment) investigated.

The following norms are indicated for the selection of patients.

a. The schistosome infection must be parasitologically confirmed through quantitative feces examination and/or rectal biopsy. Patients with infection of high or medium intensity are chosen.

b. The patients should not be allowed to have contact with foci of infection after treatment, at least until performance of the last control examinations. In areas of high endemicity, this problem may be avoided by conducting the experiments on prisoners, students in a boarding school, etc.

c. Individuals whose last contact with infested waters occurred less than 1 year before should be excluded. Recent infections have proved more resistant to treatment (Tonelli and Neves, 1966; Katz, 1971; Oliveira *et al.*, 1971). Nevertheless, when studying drugs for prophylactic action or to be used against immature forms of the worm, this norm may be disregarded.

d. Male patients from 18 to 45 years of age ought to have preference over other candidates, because the performance of complementary examinations is usually more difficult in women and children. For example, the activity of a drug may be different in women during the age of reproduction (El-Abdin *et al.*, 1974), and menstruation may complicate clinical analyses. In children some schistosomicidal agents have proved less effective (Newsome, 1962c; Jordan, 1966; Katz *et al.*, 1966a). Nevertheless, for a complete study of the drug's action, women and children should be treated in the second phase of the trials.

e. The selected patients should present the hepatointestinal form of the disease, but must be physically healthy otherwise. Thus, the investigator should exclude individuals presenting serious conditions in vital organs such as heart, lungs, kidneys, and liver; systemic diseases (arterial hypertension, collagenoses, diabetes, etc.); fever, anemia, or marked degree of undernourishment; pregnancy; or advanced forms of schistosomiasis (hepatosplenic, pulmonary with cardiac involvement, etc.).

f. Patients who have not yet been submitted to specific therapy should be given priority.

For the assessment of drug toxicity, the patients should be clinically examined several times a day, and the following data recorded: temperature, pulse, arterial pressure, and body weight or any other sign or symptom observed during and/or after treatment.

The following complementary examinations will be routinely performed: hemogram, urinalysis, hepatic function tests (bilirubin, transaminases, and alkaline phosphatase), blood urea as well as electrocardiogram. These examinations will be conducted before and at different intervals after treatment (1 and 7 days; 2 and 4 months).

The data from laboratory animals and chemical similarity to other compounds already studied will indicate further complementary examinations, such as spermogram, electroencephalogram, and renal function tests. Immediate control must be used for evaluation of drug activity.

## B. Trials in Outpatient Clinic

After determining the most adequate schedule regarding clinical pharmacology and therapeutic acitivity of the drug, the second phase of the trial must be started. A large number of patients is then to be treated not necessarily with hospitalization. At this stage, the same criteria as previously used for the selection of candidates should be applied, except that women and children, now have to be included. The complementary examinations to be performed will be restricted to those suggested by the data obtained. Late control will be used for the assessment of drug therapy.

It is advisable that the compound under investigation be distributed to several researchers for clinical trials in different geographical regions, attention being called to counterindications, possible alterations observed in laboratory test results, side effects, toxicity, etc.

After treatment of a large number of patients, the therapeutic schedules, the tolerance of the drug, etc., ought to be reevaluated.

## C. Trials in the Field

This last phase should be performed, only when a large amount of data has been obtained, sufficient to provide quite dependable information about the drug's action and after treatment of thousands of patients. Specific treatment must always be preceded by careful clinical examination and complementary tests (i.e., those considered absolutely necessary). Only a drug exhibiting high tolerability and very low toxicity can be considered for mass treatment.

For assessment of therapy, parasitological methods are the most important, although serological ones have also been used.

Three parasitological methods have been employed: feces examination, the hatching test, and rectal biopsy.

Until recently, qualitative techniques, such as sedimentation in water (Hofman *et al.,* 1934) and Merthiolate-iodine-formaldehyde concentration (MIFC) (Blagg *et al.,* 1955), were used for assessing the therapeutic effect of schistosomicidal drugs through stool examination. More recently, however, quantitative techniques have been recommended (Jordan and Randall, 1962; Bell, 1963; WHO, 1966; Katz, 1972).

The first quantitative stool examinations were performed during epidemiological studies using a dilution method (Stoll and Hausheer, 1926; Scott, 1942a,b).

The Bell technique (1963), which is favored in some African countries and in St. Lucia, consists in diluting the stool 10 times in water, and afterward 1 ml of this suspension is filtered successively through nylon screens with 500-μm mesh, and then 350-μm mesh, onto a filter paper. The paper is then submerged in satured ninhydrin solution. After drying, the filter paper is cut and examined under the microscope. The stained *S. mansoni* eggs are counted and, by multiplying by 10 the number of eggs per gram of feces is obtained.

Barbosa's technique (1969) is a quantitative version of the sedimentation in water method (Hoffman *et al.*, 1934).

More recently, the cellophane thick-smear technique (Kato, 1960) has been widely used with good results. Kato's technique was evaluated by Martin and Beaver (1968), Chaia *et al.* (1968), and Katz *et al.* (1970a). This technique has a sensitivity of 20 eggs per gram of feces (Katz *et al.*, 1970a).

Katz *et al.* (1972) reported a simple device for adapting Kato's quantitative technique to field studies or situations in which an analytical balance is not available. It consists of using a 1.37-mm thick card with a 6-mm diameter hole in it. After screening the feces through a stainless-steel sieve (150 μm), the disposable card is placed on a slide and the hole filled with the material. After covering the feces with a cellophane cover slip previously kept at least for 24 hours in a special solution (100 ml of water, 100 ml of glycerin, and 1 ml of a 3% aqueous solution of malachite green), the slide is inverted and pressed down. The preparations are kept at room temperature for 1 to 2 hours and then examined under the microscope. After counting the eggs in each slide, the number of eggs per gram of feces may be calculated since the weight of the sample examined with this standardized card is about 44 mg. This quantitative method is very useful for therapeutical control and survey of schistosomiasis because of its reliability, low cost, and easy performance (Katz *et al.*, 1972; Coura and Conceição, 1974).

The hatching test has not been sufficiently investigated in *S. mansoni* (Standen, 1951b; De Carneri, 1958), but it has been widely used in African countries, where *Schistosoma haematobium* predominates. This method has to be used if the investigator wishes to know if the eggs are viable.

Zicker *et al.* (1974) made a comparison between stool examination using Kato's quantitative technique (Katz *et al.*, 1972) and the hatching test in 1046 patients. The stool examination revealed 86.8% and the hatching test 89.3% cases of infection. However, the results with both techniques agreed only in 75.0% of the patients with *S. mansoni*. In 341 patients treated with a known antischistosomal drug, 58 were positive, by both techniques, 4 being negative by the hatching and 3 by the stool examination.

Rectal biopsy has proved quite reliable for parasitological diagnosis of schistosomiasis mansoni since its introduction by Ottolina and Atencio (1943). After Prata's excellent thesis (1957), the oogram technique performed in rectal snips obtained by biopsy has been largely employed for the therapeutic evaluation of schistosomicidal agents. The determination of the oogram in rectal snips 1 week after the end of treatment provides rapid and exact data about the oviposition of the worms (Prata, 1957; Cunha *et al.,* 1963). By weighing the rectal snips and then calculating the number of eggs per gram of tissue, Cançado *et al.* (1965) and Cunha and Carvalho (1966) developed a quantitative tool for the assessment of schistosomicidal drugs.

Different opinions exist regarding the relative value of stool examinations and rectal biopsy for finding *S. mansoni* eggs in patients. For example, Jesus and Hernandez-Morales (1959) concluded that rectal biopsy was superior to stool examination. Meira (1951) showed that the percentage of positive cases depended on the clinical form of schistosomiasis, and Prata (1957) demonstrated that 10 stool examinations revealed twice as many relapse cases than a single rectal biopsy.

The possibility of using the periovular reaction in the assessment of cure of schistosomiasis has been suggested by a series of investigations performed in Puerto Rico (Oliver-Gonzalez *et al.,* 1955; Rodriguez Molina *et al.,* 1959, 1962). Periovular reactions performed with patient's sera, after specific treatment, begin to decrease in intensity between day 60 and day 120, becoming negative, in most cases, after 6 months.

An interesting finding was that there is an increase in the precipitation lines detected by the immunodiffusion technique in patients treated with schistosomicidal drugs (Dodin *et al,* 1966; Gentilini *et al.,* 1967; Silva *et al.,* 1971). This method can differentiate drugs that just inhibit *S. mansoni* egg-laying from those that display real schistosomicidal activity. Other serological tests did not prove valid for evaluation of drug activity (Kagan and Pellegrino, 1961).

When starting clinical trials with a new drug, both immediate and late control must be considered. Immediate control is performed within 1 month after the end of treatment, and quantitative stool examinations or rectal biopsy can be used. Before beginning of therapy, an oogram must be performed from the rectal snips and repeated 1 or 2 weeks after the end of therapy. With active compounds, immature eggs will disappear (Prata, 1957). According to the results obtained, the oogram may be repeated 3–4 weeks later, so as to detect any slow activity of the drug or to find out whether interruption of oviposition still persists (Katz *et al.,* 1968a). The qualitative oogram is suitable to find out whether a compound is active or inactive. The quantitative oogram should be preferred since it detects drugs or schedules that destroy totally or just part of the worm population (Cançado *et al.*, 1965; Cunha and Carvalho, 1966). Stool examinations for immediate control must be performed at least 2 weeks after treatment using quantitative techniques. The mere presence of mature eggs does not indicate failure of treatment; more important is the decrease of the number of *S. mansoni* eggs in the feces (Katz, 1972).

Late control is best performed by means of 6 feces examinations after treatment. The first three tests should be done, respectively, after the first, the second, and the third months, and the remaining three at any time during the fourth to sixth months. Also, rectal biopsy involving examination of four fragments may be performed in the sixth month. It is interesting to point out that, after 1 year of treatment, some patients living in an area where schistosomiasis did not exist and who presented negative stool examinations even on late control, subsequently started to eliminate viable eggs in the feces (Brumpt *et al.*, 1968). Nevertheless, 6 months of follow-up seems to be a good average period for parasitological control (WHO, 1966).

It is believed that in man, dead eggs may remain in the intestinal wall for several months, even up to 2 years, and, therefore, be occasionally found in the feces or biopsy snips from cured patients (Prata, 1957).

## VII. Antischistosomal Drugs in Clinical Use

Drugs that are routinely used for clinical treatment of *S. mansoni* infection are limited to antimonial compounds, niridazole, hycanthone, and, more recently, oxamniquine. In African countries and mainland China, antimonials have been favored for some decades. Actually, in those countries there must be millions of people treated with antimonial derivatives. Niridazole has also been widely used in Africa, some thousands of patients having already been treated. Hycanthone, introduced into clinical medicine a few years ago, has been administered to more than 1 million schistosome patients in Africa and South America, whereas oxamniquine, which came onto the market in Brazil only in 1975, has been used in a few thousand cases.

One must keep in mind that, although the progress in schistosomiasis mansoni chemotherapy has been rewarding in the last decade, the need for less toxic drugs still persists.

### A. Antimonials

After the introduction, by Christopherson (1918), of tartar emetic as a drug active against *S. haematobium* infection in man, more than 10,000 antimony compounds have been synthesized and tested against the three main types of schistosome infections in man (Friedheim, 1973). Only the trivalent antimonials, and not the pentavalent ones, are active in schistosomiasis. Also, antimony–oxygen and antimony–sulfur compounds, but not antimony–carbon compounds, are active in schistosome infections.

The toxicity and the side effects produced by the different trivalent antimonial compounds are rather similar: coughing, vomiting, gastrointestinal disturbance, skin rashes, arthralgia, and myalgia. Liver and heart may be affected, and fatal cases have occurred.

It has been suggested that the toxicity of an organic antimonial is related to the fraction of ionized antimony in equilibrium with the undissociated species (Werbel, 1970; Friedheim, 1973). Toxicity increases with the degree of dissociation in aqueous solution and is depressed by an excess of complexant (Friedheim, 1973). Other important factors influencing toxic and therapeutic effects are the absorption and elimination rates of the antimonial compounds by the host and the sensitivity of the parasite's phosphofructokinase enzyme (Bueding, 1967). In fact, antimony potassium tartrate is rather more toxic to cardiac muscle than antimony sodium tartrate, and they both are more toxic than trivalent sodium antimony gluconate, stibophen, or lithium antimony thiomalate (Standen, 1963). However, according to Abdallah and Saif (1964), introduction of stibophen (Fuadin) in Egypt led to a marked increase in the occurrence of sudden death as compared with that from tartar emetic applications.

It must be pointed out that with antimonials, as with other antischistosomal drugs, the results obtained in laboratory animals cannot always be extrapolated to humans. In fact, mice need much more antimonial than man to be cured.

Much effort has been made to decrease the toxicity and/or increase the activity of trivalent antimonials. Liang *et al.* (1957a,b) used dimercaptans in conjunction with tartar emetic in mice and rabbits infected with *S. japonicum*. Although these compounds reduced toxicity, they also reduced activity. Dimercaprol, by itself, induces an hepatic shift of worms, which lasts as long as that produced by tartar emetic. Nevertheless, it does not seem to influence significantly the action of tartar emetic on the worms (Khayyal, 1965b). Luttermoser (1959) was able to increase the activity of tartar emetic in mice infected with *S. mansoni* by including glycerol, which prevented premature dissociation of tartar emetic but did not decrease its toxicity. Ercoli (1967, 1968) made up a preparation containing 1 mole potassium antimonyl tartrate to 3.4–4.5 moles dimethylcysteine (penicillamine) (NAP) and claimed this compound to be less toxic to animals than the same amount of antimony in the form of tartar emetic, while only slightly reducing its therapeutic activity toward schistosomes. Similar results were reported by Friedheim (1967) and Khayyal *et al.* (1967, 1973) when penicillamine and potassium antimonyltartrate (PAT) were simultaneously administered. Tarrant *et al.* (1971) found, however, that penicillamine in doses sufficient for reducing the acute toxicity of PAT also reduces its activity.

Pedrique *et al.* (1970), in a rural area of Venezuela, treated 108 patients with a schedule of daily intramuscular injections (400 mg of NAP: sodium antimony dimethylcysteine tartrate) for 5 days. In all patients but 4, treatment was completed and 94% of the treated patients were considered cured. Similar results were obtained by Morales and Oliver-Gonzalez (1972) in Puerto Rico.

Katz and Pellegrino (1974c) treated 5 patients with NAP (4 mg/kg/day) for 5 days. To 1 patient, the drug was administered for only 1 day because of bradycardia increase (52–38 heart beats). All other patients presented T-wave alterations but no cure was observed. Another patient was treated with 8 mg/kg/day for 4 consecutive days. The side effects were nausea, anorexia, vomiting, abdominal pain, and headache. After the fourth injection, the patient developed precordial pain and his ECG tracing showed subendocardial ischemia. Ten days later, the patient's ECG was back to normal (Katz and Pellegrino, 1974c). A.D. Coutinho (personal communication) treated in Recife, Brazil, 26 patients with daily intramuscular doses of 400 mg of NAP for 5 days. A high frequency of cardiovascular side effects and the sudden death of 2 patients were observed.

Thompson *et al.* (1965) have shown that the association of tris(*p*-aminophenyl)carbonium (TAC) salts and certain antimonials proved more effective against *S. mansoni* than could be expected from the simple addition of their activities. Waitz *et al.* (1965) demonstrated that this additive or synergistic effect of the two drugs against schistosomes is not due to higher or longer sustained levels of antimony in the blood and tissues.

Stohler and Frey (1964a) reported that, in mice and hamsters, antimony dimercaptosuccinic acid injected in olive oil suspension had higher prophylactic and therapeutic effects against *S. mansoni* than the sodium salt in water. This may be related to the fact that the acid form, in oil, produces higher and longer-lasting antimony levels than the sodium salt in water (Browne and Schulert, 1963; Thommen *et al.*, 1964). This finding was also observed in rhesus monkeys (Bruce and Sadun, 1966). Farid *et al.* (1965) performed a clinical trial with TWSb in the free-acid form in oil in 4 patients who were treated with 6 mg/kg in 5 intramuscular injections, given twice weekly. The i.m. injections were not unduly painful, no local abscess formation being observed. No radical cures were observed, only a marked reduction in the excretion of *S. haematobium* eggs. Katz (1965) treated 4 *S. mansoni* patients using a similar schedule, and 2 of them presented abscess formation whereas the other 2 showed an induration that persisted for 2 to 4 weeks, all patients having complained of intense, severe pain at the site of injection.

Other attempts for prolonging drug action have been carried out on mice, using tartar emetic absorbed into a resin (Zeng and Lu, 1965) and Astiban in silicone rubber capsules (Powers, 1965). When the latter formulation was intraperitoneally implanted in mice, 5 days prior to infection with *S. mansoni* cercariae, a 90% worm reduction was observed 60 days later.

As was quoted by Standen (1963) and Werbel (1970), a large effort for developing more efficient antimonial agents through structural modifications has been made in mainland China, but no significant clinical advantage have been obtained up to now. These facts can be found in several publications of Chinese researchers, such as in Chu *et al.* (1957a,b), "National Chinese Schistosomiasis Research Committee" (1959a,b), Hsiao and Lo (1962), Huang and Chen (1963), and Lu *et al.* (1965).

More recently, in Egypt, Shoeb *et al.* (1970) described new antimonylbenzothiazole derivatives of which at least one was claimed to be very promising, since its $LD_{50}$ in mice was 3 times higher than that of tartar emetic. This compound is in clinical trial.

Luttermoser and De Witt (1961) found that, when mice on a deficient semisynthetic diet were treated with stibophen, the drug was 4–16 times more effective as regards the elimination of schistosomes than in those on crude commercial ration. Bell (1964) reported that, in humans, the sodium salt of TWSb was significantly more efficient in nonvegetarians than in vegetarian patients.

Good results were obtained by Friedheim and De Jongh (1959), Friedheim *et al.* (1959), Salem and El Sherif (1961), Davis (1961) using monthly TWSb injections in *S. haematobium* infections. In an attempt to diminish the compound's side effects and toxicity, Davis (1961) and Rodrigues da Silva *et al.* (1964) tried this monthly schedule against *S. mansoni*. Although the tolerance was good, the therapeutic action proved practically nonexistent.

The action of trivalent antimonial drugs has been studied *in vivo* and *in vitro*. In laboratory animals and in humans, a single dose was sufficient to paralyze the worms and to prolong their subsequent shift to the liver for 30 minutes to 2 hours after drug administration. Death of the worms was achieved by repeated doses (Standen, 1953; Luttermoser, 1954; Stohler and Frey, 1964b; Khayyal, 1964; Goldsmith *et al.*, 1967). The activity of these drugs seems to depend on the concentration of antimony in the worms. Female worms are more susceptible to antimony compounds than males, probably because the female schistosomes retain higher levels of antimony (Browne and Schulert, 1963, 1964; Khayyal, 1964, 1969; Molokhia and Smith, 1969). The drug tends to concentrate in the testicles and ovaries (Fraga de Azevedo *et al.*, 1966).

Besides inducing hepatic shift and cessation of egg-laying (Kikuth and Gönnert, 1948; Pellegrino *et al.*, 1962), the antimonials also affect the miracidium inside mature eggs, thus interfering with its viability and infectivity (Friedheim and De Jongh, 1959; Salem and El Sherif, 1961).

When treatment with antimonials was performed at the time of cercarial exposure or a few days after, these drugs exerted a schistosomistatic action, that is, they delayed the development of schistosomula into adult worms (Ercoli and Payares, 1974).

Schubert (1948c) demonstrated that different trivalent antimonial compounds, including Fuadin and tartar emetic, were able to reduce the number of developing worms and to protect a significant number of mice from infection when these compounds were administered for 5 consecutive days immediately after exposure to *S. mansoni* cercariae. Sodium antimony dimercaptosuccinate was used in mice and monkeys infected with *S. mansoni* (Bruce *et al.*, 1962). A marked reduction in the number of worms was obtained when the compound was administered to mice, on successive days, either from the seventh day before, until the twenty-seventh day after, exposure. When treatment began on the fourteenth or twenty-first day after infection, only a small reduction in worm burden was observed. In monkeys the drug showed higher prophylactic activity (Bruce *et al.*, 1962). When, however, the five doses of sodium antimony dimercaptosuccinate were given on alternate days, beginning 2 days before exposure, the prophylactic activity of the drug in monkeys was less pronounced (Bruce and Sadun, 1963).

This prophylactic and protective activity of sodium antimony dimercaptosuccinate against recently penetrated cercariae and young schistosomes has also been described by Stohler and Frey (1963). These authors demonstrated that in mice, tartar emetic was active only against mature worms, whereas, in hamsters, the action of this drug surpassed that of sodium antimony dimercaptosuccinate in immature infections.

In mice and hamsters, neither sodium antimony dimercaptosuccinate, suspended in olive oil, nor TWSb, suspended in water, showed higher prophylactic activity than an aqueous solution of its sodium salt. Nevertheless, when the acid was suspended in oil, its prophylactic activity increased about 10 times. This increase in prophylactic and also protective activity may be due to the slow absorption of the drug from the site of injection (Stohler and Frey, 1964a). Similar results were obtained in rhesus monkeys by Bruce and Sadun (1966).

Adult *S. mansoni* consume, in a single hour, an amount of glucose equivalent to about one-fifth of their dry weight. The worms depend, for their major source of energy, on the anaerobic metabolism of carbohydrate into lactic acid through the Embden-Meyerhof glycolysis pathway (Bueding, 1950; Bueding and Peters, 1951; Bueding and Mansour, 1957). In *S. mansoni*, phosphofructokinase (PFK) catalyzes the phosphorylation of fructose-6-phosphate (F-6-P) by ATP leading to the formation of fructose-1,6-diphosphate (FDP) and ADP. The selective inhibition of *S. mansoni* PFK by trivalent antimonials is responsible for the chemotherapeutic activity of these compounds (Mansour and Bueding, 1954; Bueding and Mansour, 1957; Bueding, 1962, 1967). The inhibition of PFK by the antimonial drugs is reversible both in worm extracts and in live worms, the reversal of the inhibition coinciding with worm recovery and remigration to the mesenteric veins (WHO, 1966).

After parenteral administration of antimonial compounds by the intravenous or intramuscular route, high but transient blood levels are found. Antimonials present high affinity to blood cells and tissues, in particular to liver and kidneys (Brady *et al.*, 1945; Molokhia and Smith, 1969). Antimony accumulates in body tissues after multiple-dose therapy. In fact, more than 100 days after the discontinuation of tartar emetic injections, antimony is still present in the feces in man (Lippincott *et al.*, 1947). In mice, hamsters, and humans, trivalent antimonials are excreted by the bowel and by the kidney (Gellhorn *et al.*, 1946, 1947; Otto *et al.*, 1947; Otto and Maren, 1950; Thommen *et al.*, 1964).

The following trivalent antimonials are used in current clinical practice: potassium (PAT) or sodium antimonyltartrate (SAT); sodium antimony biscatecholdisulfonate; lithium antimony thiomalate; sodium antimony gluconate; and sodium antimony dimercaptosuccinate.

### 1. *Tartar Emetic and SAT*

Potassium antimonyltartrate (Fig. 1), the first antischistosomal agent, and SAT have been widely used in Egypt and China. The mode of administration has been limited to intravenous injections, since it is corrosive to tissues and presents intense emetic effect when orally administered. The claim of Mao *et al.* (1959) that tartar emetic can be

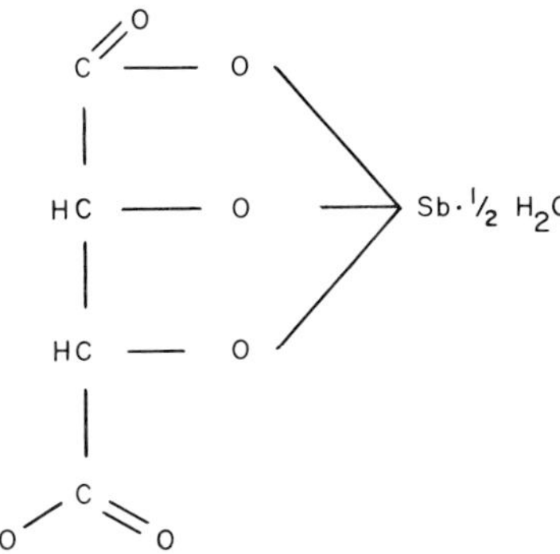


FIG. 1. Chemical structure of potassium antimonyltartrate.

used orally, with good results, was not confirmed by Forsyth and Simpson (1961). A detailed discussion about different schedules using these drugs (namely, intensive or semiintensive schemes) can be found in Dias (1949). After a critical review of the data on intensive treatment (1–2 days) of Alves (1945), of Alves and Blair (1946), and of Halawani (1946) and based on his own experience, Dias (1949) precludes its use because of severe side effects and frequent fatal results.

In 1921, Lasbrey and Coleman treated 1000 patients with tartar emetic and had 1% lethality. Lampe (1926), after treating 326 patients, had 6 (1.8%) fatal cases. Other authors related fatalities after tartar emetic or SAT administration (Walker, 1928; Khalil, 1931; Bittencourt, 1937; Mainzer and Krause, 1940; Alves and Blair, 1946; Dias, 1949; Abdallah and Saif, 1964). In the autopsied cases in Brazil, the pathological picture responsible for death was seen to be intense heart lesion—*fragmentatio cordis* (Dias, 1949).

In the Endemic Diseases Unit in Egypt, tartar emetic has been used for mass treatment for over 40 years. The drug, as a 6% solution, is administered in twelve doses, twice weekly, for a period of 4 weeks. Although side effects, such as cough, nausea, anorexia, vomiting, and myalgia are common, accidents of sudden death during treatment were estimated to occur in 2.8 per million treated individuals (Halawani, 1964; Friedheim, 1973).

Percentages of cure from schistosomiasis in humans varied, with the different authors, from 27.7 to 100% (Alves, 1946; Alves and Blair, 1946, 1947; Rodrigues da Silva, 1948, 1958; Dias, 1949; Dias *et al.*, 1952).

Egyptian investigators have tried spaced doses of tartar emetic, i.e., weekly or twice weekly administration of the standard course of twelve 120-mg intravenous doses. The weekly scheme produced a rate of about

50% cure and 50% uncompleted courses. The twice weekly course (6 weeks) was well tolerated, all 176 *S. mansoni* patients were considered cured (Abdallah, 1964).

2. *Stibophen*

Sodium antimony bis(pyrocatechol-3,5-sodium disulfonate) (stibophen, Hoechst 615, Fouadin, Neoantimosan, Fuadin, Repodral, Fantorin) (Fig. 2) was first introduced in 1929, by Khalil. Two of its characteristics were considered a progress in antimonial chemotherapy: the possibility of it being used by intramuscular injection and the shorter time of application (less than 3 weeks) (Khalil and Betache, 1930).

The schedule more commonly used was to start with 1 ml on the first day and, then, increase the doses up to 5 ml, this maximum daily dose being maintained until completing 15 5-ml injections.

Attempts to shorten the course of stibophen administration to 48 hours were also tried (Dias, 1949), but the cure rates obtained were about 40%. In different places in Brazil, another schedule of treatment with stibophen (1 ml solution per kilogram, divided into twelve daily injections) was tried but presented a great discrepancy in the percentages of cure—from 3 to 80.9% (Rodrigues da Silva, 1958).

In Egypt, from 1953 to 1955, when stibophen was used for mass treatment, a marked increase in the occurrence of sudden death during administration of the compound was reported (Abdallah and Saif, 1964). The fatalities were due to intravascular hemolysis with the formation of sulf- and methemoglobinemia with renal failure (Halawani *et al.*, 1955; Abdallah and Saif, 1964).

More than 2 million patients were treated with stibophen before its use was abandoned due to fatal cases (35 per 1 million treated patients), in 1961, by the Bilharzia Authorities of Egypt (Friedheim, 1973). Also, the National Schistosomiasis Research Committee of China (1959a,b), after observations on the treatment of *S. japonicum* infections, reported stibophen to be, not less toxic, but less active than tartar emetic.

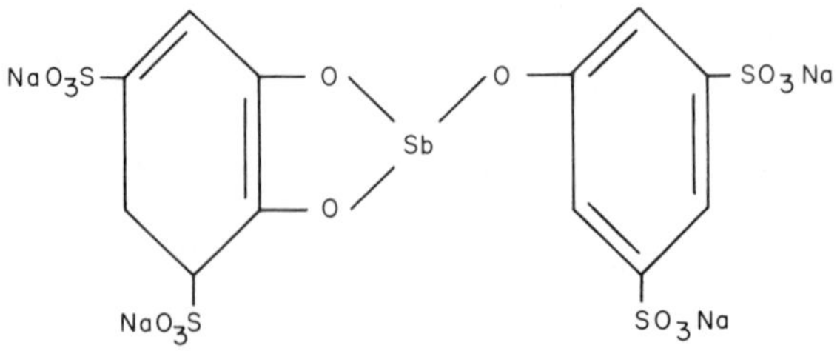

FIG. 2. Chemical structure of stibophen.

### 3. *Lithium Antimony Thiomalate*

The drug (Thiomalate, Anthiomaline) (Fig. 3) is usually administered intramuscularly. It may, however, be used intravenously, although the latter route may induce fever after each injection (Rodrigues da Silva, 1958). It is given on alternate days, starting with 1.0 ml of 6% solution and gradually increasing to 4.0 ml per day, until 35–40 ml has been administered.

Rodrigues Molina *et al.* (1950) followed up 30 *S. mansoni* patients who were treated with ten 3 ml doses on alternate days, and they obtained 66.6% cure. Dias (1949), with 24- and 48-hour, courses using 0.30 and 0.45 ml/kg, respectively, achieved about 50% cure in *S. mansoni* patients.

### 4. *Sodium Antimony Gluconate*

For this drug (TSAG, Triostam), the schedule of treatment is 2.5–3.3 mg/kg/day, for 6 days, by intravenous injection of a 6% solution in distilled water. The side effects observed were similar to those induced by other antimonial salts. Preliminary clinical trials with TSAG were performed by Erfan and Talaat (1950) and Watson and Pingle (1950). One death was reported in Brazil after the fifth injection of an intensive course completed in 1½ days (Rodrigues da Silva, 1958). The cure rates were about 50% with the schedule used, namely, 15 mg/kg in 2 days and 20 mg/kg in 6 to 8 days (Rodrigues da Silva and Dias, 1957).

### 5. *Stibocaptate*

Antimony dimercaptosuccinate (sodium or potassium antimony dimercaptosuccinate, stibocaptate, TWSb, Astiban) (Fig. 4) is a complex formed by trivalent antimony and *meso*-2,3-dimercaptosuccinic acid. It was synthesized and isolated in 1952 as the free acid, and as the lithium, sodium, potassium, magnesium, diethylamine, methylglucamine, etc., salts by Friedheim in 1973. The first studies were performed with the potassium salt and, from 1960 on, with the sodium salt.

In mice, the TWSb $LD_{50}$ is 50 times lower than that of tartar emetic (Friedheim *et al.*, 1954).

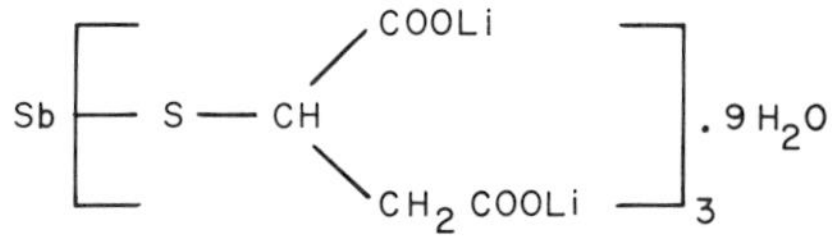


FIG. 3. Chemical structure of lithium antimony thiomalate.

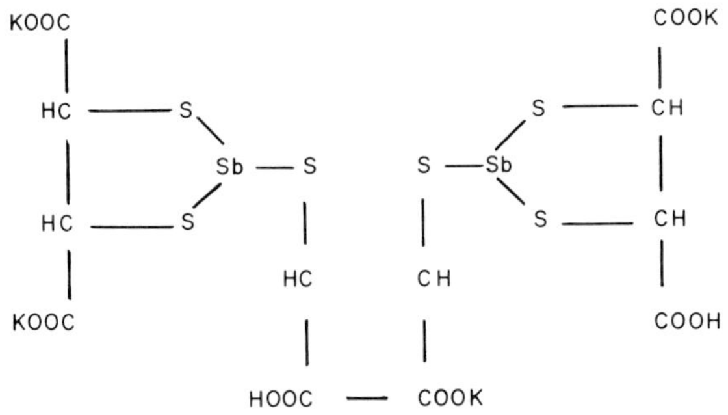

```
KOOC                                                   COOK
  |                                                      |
 HC ——— S                              S ——— CH
          \                           /          |
           Sb — S           S —Sb               |
          /                           \          |
 HC ——— S         |         |          S ——— CH
  |                HC        CH                   |
KOOC               |         |                   COOH
                HOOC  —  COOK
```

FIG. 4. Chemical structure of stibocaptate.

As with the other antimonial salts, different schedules were employed in clinical trials; the two usually followed were (*a*) 5 daily intramuscular injections with single doses of 8–10 mg/kg and (*b*) 5 injections at weekly intervals.

In Brazil, Friedheim *et al.* (1954) reported observations on hundreds of *S. mansoni* cases treated under different TWSb schedules. The most common side effects were anorexia, nausea, vomiting, "bitter mouth," abdominal discomfort, skin rashes, myalgia, etc. In 58 patients, treatment involving a 1–3 day, intensive intravenous TWSb regimen, with doses totalling 1.1–2.3 gm, produced 91% cure. Prata (1956) administered 2.0 gm, divided into 6 intravenous injections, within 36 hours, to 58 patients and obtained 55% cure. When the dose was 2.4 gm, applied in 6 daily intramuscular injections, the cure rate was 68%.

In Egypt, Nagaty and Rifaat (1960) obtained 100% cure, and Salem *et al.* (1961) 82%. Farid *et al.* (1967) administered TWSb to 17 Egyptian *S. mansoni* patients at a dosage of 8 mg/kg per dose, i.m., twice weekly, in a total of 5 injections. Using quantitative evaluation 3 months after treatment, they considered only 29% cured, but an 88.4% reduction in egg excretion had been obtained. In 15 patients treated with daily intravenous injections of Astiban, Abdallah and Saif (1964) observed signs and symptoms of intolerance, including severe prostration, nausea, vomiting, tachycardia, myalgia, chest oppression, and rise in temperature. With daily intramuscular injections, 26 patients (out of 50) could not complete the course of 5 injections, due to side effects and toxic reactions. Of the remaining 24 patients who completed the course of treatment, 1 died unexpectedly, 10 hours after the last injection, due to sudden cardiac arrest. Necropsy was not performed. The patients tolerated treatment well with twice-weekly or once-weekly doses the therapeutic results being around 90% (Abdallah and Saif, 1964).

In Uganda, Rosanelli and Price (1963) used TWSb (0.4 gm/day, on 5 successive days, i.m.) in Africans and Europeans infected with *S. mansoni*. Four months or more after treatment, no living eggs were found in the stools of 6 (out of 21) Africans and 15 (out of 16) Europeans. The reason for such difference in the results could not be accounted for. Nausea, vomiting, joint pains, and skin rash were observed in both groups. In all cases, electrocardiograms showed changes in the T waves, such as depression or reversion and/or prolongation of Q-Te.

Experimental studies have shown that antimony increases capillary permeability (especially in the splanchnic area), that pulmonary stagnation and greater permeability of lung capillaries increase the resistance to the right heart which causes dilatation of the heart (Anrep *et al.*, 1941), and that the action of antimony on the cardiac muscle is mainly effected through disruption in the structure of sarcoplasm (Dias, 1949; Badran, 1966). Nevertheless, 20 cardiac patients (mitral stenosis and/or insufficiency, tricuspid regurgitation, aortic insufficiency, cor pulmonale, etc.) treated with 50 mg/kg TWSb, divided into 5 i.m. injections applied once a week, did not present untoward effects on the heart as judged by electrocardiograms and X-ray examinations performed before and after treatment (Badran and Abdallah, 1967).

The principal handicaps to the use of antimonial compounds in *S. mansoni* infections are the long courses necessary (since intensive courses are very dangerous) and the toxic effects observed, the worst being that on the heart, not infrequently, leading to sudden death. Finally, as was pointed out by Werbel (1970), the inherent disadvantages of this class of compounds make it unlikely that any of these drugs will be the answer to control of schistosomiasis by mass chemotherapy.

## B. Niridazole

A nitrothiazole derivative, niridazole [1-(5-nitro-2-thiazolyl)-2-imidazolidone, nitrothiamidazole, CIBA 32,644-Ba, Ambilhar] (Fig. 5) was synthesized at CIBA laboratories by Wilhelm and Schmidt. It was first

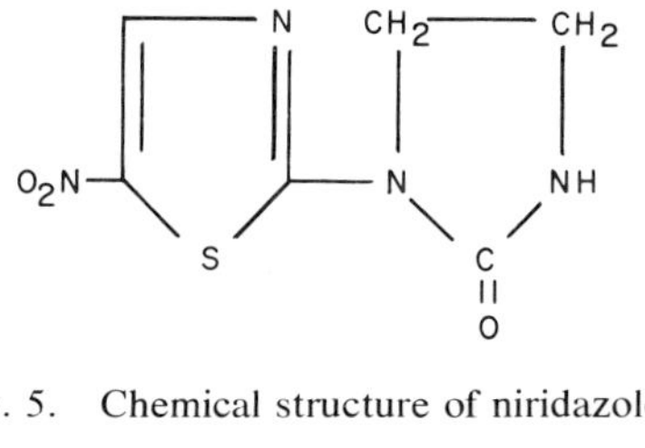

N $CH_2$ $CH_2$
$O_2N$ N NH
S C
O

Fig. 5. Chemical structure of niridazole.

evaluated by Lambert and co-workers (Lambert and Stauffer, 1964; Lambert *et al.*, 1964; Lambert, 1964). These authors reported niridazole to be active *in vitro* and in *in vivo–in vitro* tests as well as in laboratory animals. In fact, adult pairs of *S. mansoni* exposed to 1 $\mu$g/ml of niridazole for 100 hours ceased egg-laying, death of the worms occurring when exposed to 10 $\mu$g/ml for the same period of time. When rabbit sera from animals dosed with 500 mg/kg (single oral dose) were collected 6 hours after dosing and added to a synthetic medium containing schistosomes, female worms were found completely immobile after 72 hours of contact and male worms, after 96 hours. A high rate of schistosomicidal activity was observed in mice treated with daily oral doses of 100 mg/kg, for a period of 5 to 10 days. In desert rats, similar effects were obtained with 50 mg/kg for 15 consecutive days.

In rhesus monkeys, Bruce and Sadun (1966) and Sadun *et al.* (1966) found that niridazole was active against *S. mansoni* infections when treatment started on the day of exposure or a few days thereafter or when the worms reached maturity. Pellegrino *et al.* (1966) showed that, in mice dosed with 200 or 100 mg/kg/day, orally administered niridazole induced complete cessation of egg laying, with hepatic shift and death of the worms. In hamsters, the activity of the drug was less pronounced. In *Cebus* monkeys, however, niridazole proved very toxic. In fact, dose levels varying from 10 to 50 mg/kg/day, produced death of the animal within 1 to 3 days after the beginning of treatment (Pellegrino *et al.*, 1966). The pronounced toxicity observed in *Cebus* monkeys contrasts sharply with the good tolerance displayed by rhesus (Sadun *et al.*, 1966) and *Callithrix* monkeys (Pellegrino and Katz, 1968) when treated at dose levels 20 times higher.

The mode of action of niridazole on *S. mansoni* worms was investigated by Striebel and Kradolfer (1966) and Striebel (1969). The results obtained may be summarized as follows: (*1*) the vitellogenic gland of the female worm is the organ most sensitive to niridazole treatment, eggshell formation being inhibited by low doses; (*2*) masses of vitelline and ovary cells are excreted by the female worm; (*3*) the testes of male worms are affected only by high doses; (*4*) in mice, daily doses of one-tenth $ED_{90}$, for 10 consecutive days, lead to a reduction in the length of worms and in the size of the female worm ovary, these effects having a direct relationship to the dose applied; (*5*) the changes in the worms are not related to their hepatic shift; (*6*) the females are destroyed, in the liver, by leukocyte infiltration and autolysis, and the males are immobilized by a connective tissue reaction; (*7*) in the monkey liver, both male and female worms are destroyed by leukocytic infiltration (Striebel and Kradolfer, 1966; Striebel, 1969).

Niridazole is selectively taken up by the worms and their eggs (Hess *et al.,* 1966). This accumulation inside schistosome eggs produces an abnormal shape of the eggshell and/or ooblast, and a small amount of vitelline granules are scattered over the ooblast (Monteiro *et al.,* 1968).

Niridazole does not interfere with glycolysis; glycogen, however, is reduced in the worm musculature. In fact, there is a positive dose–effect relationship with respect to the degree of glycogen depletion (Bueding and Fisher, 1969). This effect is accounted for by decreased phosphorylase inactivation produced by niridazole (Bueding and Fisher, 1970).

In man, niridazole is slowly absorbed from the intestinal tract and is rapidly destroyed in the liver. The drug concentration in the portal blood is several times higher than in the peripheral blood. The process of absorption takes several hours, its maximum duration being 10–15 hours. The metabolites produced in the human body are eliminated from the blood more slowly than the unchanged active substance. These metabolites are excreted in the urine as well as in the bile (Faigle and Keberle, 1966, 1969; Martins da Rocha and Gill, 1966). Metabolic studies showed that, in mild forms of *S. haematobium* and *S. mansoni* infections in man, the drug metabolism is not subject to any marked individual fluctuations (Faigle *et al.,* 1970a). In patients with hepatosplenic forms of *S. mansoni,* metabolic analyses showed that the concentrations of the active substance in the peripheral blood were much higher and that probably there exists a causal connection between the elevated concentrations and the occurrence of side effects, especially in the psychoneurological field. The high concentrations, in such cases, are due to portal–systemic shunts. Through these shunts, part of the active substance bypasses the liver and is not so rapidly broken down as in patients with no shunt (Faigle *et al.,* 1970b).

Data about experimental and clinical studies with niridazole can be found in the reports presented at the Lisbon Meeting (1965), the Round Table on Ciba 32,644-Ba (Ambilhar) in Rio (1966), and the Conference on Niridazole (1967), which were published, respectively, in *Acta Trop.,* Suppl. **9** (1966), *Folha Med.* **53,** (1966), and *Ann. N. Y. Acad. Sci.* **160** (1969).

Clinical trials performed in Brazil, Africa, Philippines, Japan, and Britain, under different schedules of treatment with niridazole, showed that *S. haematobium* is more susceptible to treatment than *S. mansoni,* and that *S. japonicum* is the most resistant of the three.

The main side effects observed were nausea, vomiting, anorexia, headache, myalgia, and loss of body weight. The most dangerous were, however, those connected with neuropsychical disorders (convulsions, hallucinations, etc.).

The schedule recommended by most researchers for *S. mansoni* clinical treatment is 25 mg/kg/day, divided into 2 daily doses administered for 7 consecutive days, which allows approximately 60–90% rate of cure.

In Brazil, Prata (1966, 1969) showed that better results are obtained with a more prolonged period of administration than with increased daily doses, and Cunha (1966a) suggested a schedule of 15 mg/kg/day for 15 consecutive days.

In the Rio Meeting (1966), most papers presented showed that niridazole produces psychoneurological side effects, more frequently in the hepatosplenic form of the disease, but also in the intestinal and hepatointestinal forms. It was reported that children, and adult patients in the acute phase of *S. mansoni* infection, are more resistant to treatment (Baranski, 1966; Campos, 1966; Coutinho, 1966; Cunha, 1966a; Galvão, 1966; Katz, 1966; Kloetzel, 1966; Magaldi, 1966; Marques, 1966; Neves, 1966; Nohmi, 1966; Rodrigues da Silva, 1966b; Silva, 1966; Teixeira, 1966). That children are most resistant to treatment was also remarked by Jordan (1966) and Jarumilinta *et al.* (1968), Clarke and Blair (1969), and Prata (1969).

It is interesting to point out that, in Iran, 6488 *S. haematobium* patients were treated with 30 mg/kg/day for 4 days, and only 12 of them suffered convulsions (Arfaa *et al.*, 1970). Also, in Mozambique, about 1000 *S. haematobium* patients tolerated niridazole well, since it was not necessary to interrupt treatment for any of them (Ruas and Franco, 1966).

In Tanzania, 5 out of 92 *S. mansoni* patients treated with 25 mg/kg/day, for 7 consecutive days, suffered convulsions and hallucinations or mental confusion. Cure rates were higher among patients eliminating less than 10,000 eggs per day than among those with 100,000 to 500,00 eggs daily in their feces (McMahon and Kilala, 1966). In fact, a direct correlation could be seen to exist between the number of *S. mansoni* eggs in the feces and the number of patients considered cured (Jordan, 1966; Prata, 1969).

In Puerto Rico, Ramos-Morales *et al.* (1969) treated 15 *S. mansoni* patients with 25 mg/kg/day for 7 days, and, although they were able to detect a decrease in the number of eggs, no cure was achieved. In mice, a Tanzanian strain of *S. mansoni* proved more resistant to niridazole than a Puerto Rican strain (Taylor and Nelson, 1971).

Attempts have been made to minimize the neuropsychical disturbances by using, concomitantly with niridazole, various drugs such as antihistamines, diallylbarbiturate, benzodiazepine, and phenobarbitone, but results were not completely satisfactory (McMahon, 1967; Zacharias *et al.*, 1967a,b; Katz *et al.*, 1967a; Abdallah *et al.*, 1968; Julião *et al.*, 1969; Teixeira *et al.*, 1969).

Three pregnant women were treated with niridazole (30-40 mg/kg/day × 7–10 days). Two of them had normal delivery and 1 suffered a miscarriage after a fall from a bus (Neves and Costa, 1969).

It has been demonstrated that there is frequently an increase in the glycemia levels of patients treated with niridazole (Martins *et al.*, 1968; Carneiro Filho *et al.*, 1969) and that this drug can trigger hemolysis in patients whose red blood cells are deficient in glucose-6-phosphate dehydrogenase, of the Caucasian type (Sonnet and Doyen, 1969; McCaffrey *et al.*, 1972).

Alterations of electrocardiographic tracings are common and involve depression or inversion of the T wave and sometimes ischemia. Alterations of the electroencephalogram are more frequent in patients with the hepatosplenic form of the disease and mainly appear in the form of paroxysmal discharges, indicating that the drug has an epileptogenic effect (Coutinho, 1966; Marques, 1966; Arruda *et al.*, 1967; Basmy *et al.*, 1968).

A depression of spermatogenesis was noted in experimental and clinical trials. In fact, mice, rats, and dogs presented temporary but marked inhibition of spermatogenesis, the drug action directly affecting the germinative epithelium of the testes (Lambert *et al.*, 1965; Yokogawa *et al.*, 1966). Rodrigues da Silva (1966a) and Prates and Franco (1966), studying spermatograms or testes biopsies from humans, showed that inhibition of spermatogenesis in man is reversible and not as accentuated as in animals.

*In vitro* tests with *Salmonella typhimurium* histidine auxotrophes showed niridazole to act as a frameshift mutagen. In host-mediated assays, using a single oral dose of 10 mg/kg, niridazole also produced mutations (Conner *et al.*, 1974; Legator *et al.*, 1974).

An attempt to establish spaced-dosage treatment with niridazole (7 doses of 25 mg/kg twice weekly) failed, since psychoneurological side effects occurred and cure rates were markedly low (Abdallah *et al.*, 1968).

According to a report from Ciba Laboratories, in about 200,000 cases treated with niridazole, there occurred 6 drug-related deaths (WHO, 1972).

The conclusion of the Rio Meeting (1966) participants was that "the nature of the problems observed when niridazole is used for *S. mansoni* treatment precludes its use for mass chemotherapy."

## C. Lucanthone and Hycanthone

Lucanthone (Miracil D, Nilodin) (Fig. 6) is the hydrochloride of 1-(β-diethylaminoethylamino)-4-methylthiaxanthone and was the first metal-free compound used as an antischistosomal agent (Kikuth *et al.*, 1946; Mauss, 1948).

In clinical trials, it was shown that lucanthone is more active in *S. haematobium* than in *S. mansoni* and that it was necessary to administer it for several days. Side effects, such as anorexia, nausea, vomiting, abdominal distress, hallucination, dizziness, tremors of the hands, mental confusion, insomnia, yellow staining of the skin and mucosae, are very common and not infrequently severe (Alves, 1949, 1950, 1958; Koch and Kux, 1951; Rodrigues da Silva, 1953; Blair, 1958; Davis, 1963; Davis *et al.*, 1965; Janssens *et al.*, 1965; Lees, 1966).

Although attempts to minimize these side effects and increase therapeutic activity were made for more than 20 years, mainly by researchers at Bayer Laboratories, a real improvement was only obtained with the discovery of hycanthone by Sterling Winthrop Laboratories.

Hycanthone (Etrenol) (Fig. 6), a hydroxymethyl analog of Miracil D, was obtained by the microbiological oxidation of the parent compound by *Aspergillus sclerotiorum* (Rosi *et al.*, 1965). In mice and hamsters, complete cures were achieved, respectively, with oral doses of 150 mg/kg/day × 5 days and 12.5 mg/kg/day × 5 days. Intramuscular injection proved 5 times more effective than giving the drug by oral route (Berberian *et al.*, 1967a,b).

Oogram studies showed hycanthone to be 10 times more effective in hamsters than in mice (Pellegrino *et al.*, 1967a). Parasitological cures were obtained in *Cebus* monkeys treated with oral doses of 10 and 5 mg/kg/day, for 5 consecutive days (Pellegrino *et al.*, 1967a).

Comparing the activity of hycanthone with that of lucanthone, in mice, Foster *et al.* (1971a) found that, by oral administration, the $ED_{50}$

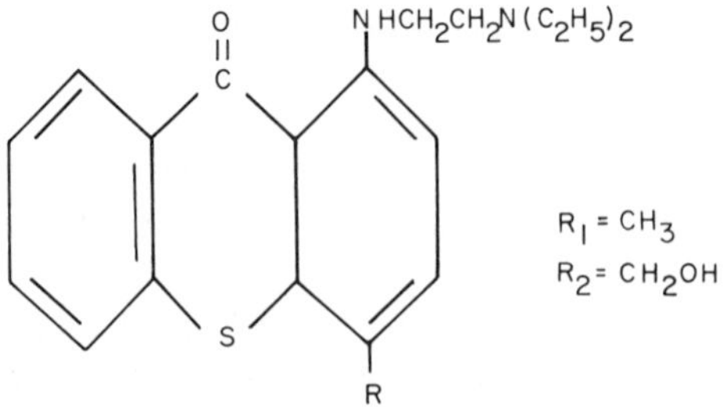

Fig. 6. Chemical structure of lucanthone ($R_1$) and hycanthone ($R_2$).

and $ED_{99}$ of lucanthone were 189 mg/kg and 524 mg/kg, respectively, whereas the $ED_{50}$ and $ED_{99}$ of hycanthone were 30 mg/kg and 208 mg/kg. Male *S. mansoni* worms are more susceptible to hycanthone than female worms (Foster *et al.*, 1971a; Lee, 1972), although drug concentration in the female is 5 times higher (Yarinsky *et al.*, 1970).

Hycanthone is not active against *S. mansoni in vitro* (Archer and Yarinsky, 1972), it is also inactive in mice infected with Japanese and Philippine strains of *S. japonicum* (Yarinsky *et al.*, 1972).

By administering tritium-labeled hycanthone to mice infected with *S. mansoni,* Yarinsky *et al.*, (1970) observed that peak concentrations of the drug in the blood plasma were reached within 30 minutes and that these concentrations were higher than those in the blood red cells. The drug detected in the worms was unchanged hycanthone. At the end of 24 hours the schistosomes contained more drug than was present in the blood. In further studies on mice with the same hycanthone doses, *S. mansoni* worms were seen to have 3 times more drug per microgram worm weight than *S. japonicum* and, also, a great amount of drug was found in *S. mansoni* testicular tissue.

Hycanthone produced an increase in the level of 5-hydroxytryptamine in *S. mansoni,* this increase coinciding with the worms' shift from the mesenteric veins to the liver (Chou *et al.*, 1973).

Differences in the response of four *S. mansoni* strains (Puerto Rico, Liberia, St. Lucia, and Belo Horizonte) were observed when four known active schistosomicidal drugs (lucanthone, niridazole, stibophen, and hycanthone) were used in experimentally infected mice. In fact, treatment with hycanthone at dosages of 20 to 30 mg/kg resulted in a marked decrease in the number of male worms of the Puerto Rico strain, which was not observed with the St. Lucia and Liberia strains. Response differences were also observed with the other drugs employed (Lee *et al.*, 1971).

Preliminary clinical trials with hycanthone were carried out in South Africa and in Brazil. Maritz (1969, 1970) treated Bantu school children, infected with *S. haematobium,* with enteric-coated tablets (2.5–3.0 mg/kg/day × 4 days) and a hycanthone salt for intramuscular injection (2.0–3.5 mg/kg, single dose). The chief side effects observed with both formulations were anorexia, nausea, vomiting, and abdominal pain. Transient increase in serum glutamic oxalacetic transaminase (SGOT) and serum glutamic pyruvic transaminase (SGPT) values was observed in a few patients. Cure rate was about 95%.

In Brazil, Katz *et al.* (1968a) administered hycanthone capsules to 52 *S. mansoni* patients (2 and 3 mg/kg/day × 5 days), the percentage of cure being about 80%. The side effects observed and the toxicity data obtained were similar to those reported from Maritz's trial. In further trials, Katz *et al.* (1969) treated 26 patients with a single, intramuscular hycanthone–methanesulfonate dose of 2.0 mg/kg, and 30 patients with a dose of 3.0 mg/kg. The cure rates were 91.8 and 96.4%, respectively. Transient electrocardiographic changes consisting of flattening of the ST segment and T wave were also observed (Katz *et al.*, 1969; Salgado *et al.*, 1968, 1972). Similar findings concerning cure rates and side effects were also described by other Brazilian researchers (Argento *et al.*, 1968; Figueiredo *et al.*, 1968; Figueiredo and Prata, 1969; Garcia and Aguirre, 1969; Oliveira *et al.*, 1969; Coutinho and Barreto, 1971). Jaundice was present in a few patients (Figueiredo *et al.*, 1968; Almeida *et al.*, 1970; Coutinho and Barreto, 1971; Cunha *et al.*, 1971b).

Cunha *et al.* (1971a) claim that the minimal effective dose of hycanthone is 1.5 mg/kg, the use of higher doses being of no advantage.

In Venezuela, Pedrique and Sanz (1970) administered hycanthone (2.5–3 mg/kg) to 134 patients with *S. mansoni* infection. The drug was well tolerated and the percentage of cure, as judged from rectal biopsy, was 97.5%.

In Santa Lucia, Cook and Jordan (1971) treated 94 *S. mansoni* patients with a single dose of hycanthone (3.0 mg/kg, i.m.). At the end of 6 months, 26 (28%) patients were no longer passing eggs, whereas the remainder showed over 90% decrease in the number of eggs in their feces. Hycanthone did not induce hemolysis in patients with G-6-P deficiency.

In Surinam, Oostburg (1972), cured all but 3 of 216 patients treated with a single dose of hycanthone (3.0 mg/kg, i.m.). Transient elevations of SGPT and SGOT were common, reaching high levels in 3 cases.

In Rhodesia, Clarke *et al.* (1969) obtained 88% cure (58 out of 66) of *S. haematobium* infection and 72% (42 out of 58) of *S. mansoni* infection in four groups treated with oral doses of 2.5 mg/kg/day, for 3 or 4 days, and with a single intramuscular injection of 3.0 or 3.5 mg/kg. MacDonald *et al.* (1973) achieved 49% cure of *S. mansoni* infection with the same intramuscular dose, and no apparent cure rate dependence on age was recorded. After repeated treatment with hycanthone, the cure rates for *S. haematobium* and/or *S. mansoni* were not found to be significantly different from those of the first course of treatment (MacDonald *et al.*, 1973).

In Uganda, Ongom (1971) treated 32 *S. mansoni* patients with a single intramuscular hycanthone dose of 3.0 mg/kg; jaundice was observed in 1 case. The cure rate was 70.5% and the egg output of most noncured patients was reduced nearly to zero.

In Kenya, Rees *et al.* (1970), in a comparative study on *S. mansoni* patients, found that with hycanthone, 3 months after a single intramuscular injection (3.0 mg/kg), 73% of the patients provided negative results; with niridazole (25 mg/kg/day × 5 days), 27% and, with placebos, 22%. High incidence of vomiting (about 60%) was observed in the patients treated with hycanthone.

In Sudan, Omer *et al.* (1972) treated 95 *S. mansoni* patients (3.0 mg/kg, i.m.), but followed up only 11, for 6 months, all of them having been considered as cured.

In Egypt, Mousa *et al.* (1970), in the Nile Delta area, treated 936 school children heavily infected with *S. haematobium,* with a single dose of 3.5 mg/kg. After 3 months, the cure rate was around 40%. The noncured children received a second injection. Considering both schedules of treatment, the joint percentage of cure was over 80%. Abdallah *et al.* (1971) observed 40 and 54% cure when hycanthone was administered in single doses of 3.0 mg/kg and 3.5 mg/kg, respectively, to a total of 209 schistosome patients. No age dependence was observed but the intensity of infection was important so far as cure rate was concerned (Abdallah *et al.,* 1971). Sherif *et al.* (1971) achieved 89% cure after treating 1095 bilharzial patients, infected with either *S. haematobium* or *S. mansoni,* or both, with doses of 2.7 mg/kg to 4 mg. In one group, hycanthone was administered with the multidose gun. Farid *et al.* (1973) treated 20 Egyptian male farmers, infected with both schistosome species, with a single intramuscular injection of 3.0 mg/kg. Three months after treatment, only 2 out of 10 *S. haematobium* patients and 1 out of 10 *S. mansoni* patients seemed to be cured. Serial liver biopsies confirmed the development of hepatic-cell injury in 1 out of 4 patients that presented increase bromsulphalein (BSP) retention and serum transaminase levels.

In newly infected patients, hycanthone displays poor activity. In fact, when 15 *S. mansoni* patients were treated with a single intramuscular injection of 2.5 mg/kg, only 6 (40%) of them were cured 2–8 months after infection, whereas, among 13 patients with 1-year infection (11–13 months) and treated with the same dosage, 11(84.7%) no longer presented eggs in their feces (Katz, 1971). After treating 13 patients with clinical and epidemiological evidence of recent (2–3 months) schistosomiasis infection, Oliveira *et al.* (1971) achieved only a low percentage of cure with a single-dose schedule. They then recommended that, in acute cases, patients should be treated with 2 doses of hycanthone, allowing 1 week between doses.

Pilot projects for schistosomiasis control in the endemic areas of different countries showed the possibility of treating the great majority of infected patients after clinical examiations. The drug toxic effects and counterindications, howerver, preclude its use for mass treatment.

In Brazilian endemic areas in three different states (Minas Gerais, Bahia, and Rio de Janeiro), it was demonstrated that a single intramuscular hycanthone injection of 2.5 to 3.0 mg/kg is a relatively well-tolerated schedule that produces more than 90% cure; its most common side effects are anorexia, nausea, vomiting, headache, muscle pain, dizziness, and local pain (Garcia and Aguirre, 1969; Bina and Prata, 1970, 1974; Katz *et al.,* 1970b).

Among more than 300,000 patients so far treated with hycanthone, 40 severe adverse reactions of various kinds have been reported, including 20 fatalities (2–5 days after treatment), 17 of them being associated with hepatic necrosis, which, in some cases, was also aggravated by other diseases (WHO, 1972).

Fatal cases after hycanthone administration were published by Cunha (1970), Mendonça *et al.* (1970), Medeiros *et al.* (1972), Gane (1971, 1973), Lapierre *et al.* (1973), Andrade *et al.* (1974), Godoy *et al.* (1974), Marinho *et al.* (1974a,b), Bina and Prata (1974). Other patients presented jaundice and liver involvement but recovered after a few weeks (Figueiredo *et al.,* 1968; Almeida *et al.,* 1970; Coutinho and Barreto, 1971; Cunha *et al.,* 1971b; Medeiros *et al.,* 1972; Farid *et al.,* 1972). From these reports, counterindications are well established in some cases, although in others they can only be presumed. These are previous liver pathology, respiratory-tract infections, use of other drugs (phenothiazine derivatives, male and female hormones), and consumptive diseases (lupus erythematosus disseminatus, chronic osteomyelites, etc.).

Summing up, hycanthone is a hepatotoxic drug sometimes producing only elevation of transaminase levels, sometimes inducing jaundice and, in some patients causing, severe hepatic injury, such as yellow atrophy, with consequent death. A real estimation of the frequency of those side effects is not available so far.

Mutagenic effects of hycanthone were initially detected by Hartman *et al.* (1971) on *Salmonella* and *Escherichia coli* T4 bacteriophage. Further studies showed that hycanthone produces chromosomal aberrations in lymphoma cell cultures (Clive *et al.,* 1972), in leukocyte cultures (Sieber *et al.,* 1973), interference in cellular differentiation during the embryonic stage of chicks and arachnidan eggs (Medina *et al.,* 1972), mitosis blockade, chromosomal breaks and anaphases with chromosomal bridges in *Allium cepa* root tips (Medina *et al.,* 1972; Rocha and Katz, 1973), malformation of snails (Souza and Katz, 1973), mutagenic effects on *Neurospora crassa* (Ong and de Serres, 1972) and on *Saccharomyces cerevisiae* (Igali and von Borstel, 1974).

No mutagenic effects were observed in *Habrobracon serinopae* females (Smith, 1972), nor were chromosomal aberrations seen in the whole spermatogenic cycle of mice treated with hycanthone (Generoso *et al.*, 1972). No mutations were observed in 16,196 offspring of male mice intraperitoneally injected with 150 mg/kg of hycanthone, thus indicating that the test for gene mutation induction using the specific locus method was negative (Russell and Kelly, 1972; Russell, 1973).

Frota-Pessoa *et al.* (1973) found no significant effect of hycanthone on the frequency of blood cells presenting chromosomal abnormalities in 13 patients treated with 2.5 mg/kg.

Results from two strains of female mice show that hycanthone has a marked effect on fertility, since it produces an increase in the frequency of dead implantation (Generoso *et al.,* 1972). The question whether this is caused by its toxic effect or by its chemical property for inducing dominant-lethal mutations in oocytes in large follicles has not been solved yet (Generoso *et al.,* 1972).

Moore (1972) found that total fetus mortality, at the dose level of 50 mg/kg, reached 44.6% and, furthermore, that 49.0% of the litter fetuses were abnormal in some way (exencephalia, hydrocephthalmia, rib fusion, and branching). Sieber's *et al.* (1973) experiments on pregnant female mice, did not reveal any teratogenic action when hycanthone was applied, but its embryotoxicity was manifested by increasing incidence of intrauterine death.

Haese *et al.* (1973) observed that, when hycanthone was administered to infected mice as a 60 mg/kg single dose, a higher frequency of hepatomas was found as compared with uninfected hycanthone-treated mice and/or uninfected, untreated control animals. This experiment was repeated by Yarinsky *et al.* (1974), and the frequency of liver tumor in the three groups of mice was the same. The difference between the two studies was the time of follow-up. In fact, in Haese's *et al.* (1973) experiments, tumors started to appear after 17 months, whereas, in the studies of Yarinsky *et al.* (1974), the seventeenth month was the last month of observation.

Rogers and Bueding (1971) administered high doses of hycanthone to *S. mansoni*-infected mice, collected the eggs shed by the surviving worms, and then infected snails and mice with this new generation of worms. The second generation was totally resistant to hycanthone action. Yarinsky repeated such experiments using *S. mansoni* from the same origin and also from another source than that already used by

Rogers and Bueding (1971). He confirmed the resistance of one strain, but he also reported that, with *S. mansoni* maintained in the Sterling-Winthrop Research Institute, resistance had not been induced (Archer and Yarinsky, 1972).

Further studies demonstrated that resistance to hycanthone was maternally transferred, and remained stable for several generations. Resistance was also observed when immature schistosomes (28 days infection) within mice were exposed to the drug. In this manner, four out of five strains of *S. mansoni* became resistant (Jansma *et al.*, 1974).

Recently, Katz *et al.* (1973a) reported, for the first time, resistance in mice of a *S. mansoni* strain isolated from 2 patients who had been treated twice with hycanthone and once with niridazole but who were not cured by this triple treatment.

In 1972, WHO promoted two meetings for the discussion of problems related to possible teratogenic, mutagenic, and carcinogenic effects as well as other undesirable toxic effects of hycanthone when administered to humans. All participants but one agreed that, on the basis of available data on hycanthone, no genetic effect of the drug in man if any, could be reliable estimated, there being no reason for precluding its use in clinical therapy of schistosomiasis (WHO, 1972). More recently, another meeting for the same purpose, sponsored by the U.S.–Japan Cooperative Medical Science Program and the Environmental Mutagen Society, was held at Bethesda, Maryland, U.S.A. (1974), and its papers and conclusions have been published in the *Journal of Toxicology and Environmental Health* **1** (1975).

It is interesting to remark that some analogs of hycanthone present a very marked reduction in mutagenic and toxic activities without decreasing antischistosomal potency (Bueding, 1975).

### D. Oxamniquine

A more recent schistosomicide, oxamniquine is also known as 6-hydroxymethyl-2-isopropylaminomethyl-7-nitro-1,2,3,4-tetrahydroquinoline, U.K. 4271, Mansil (Fig. 7). Richards and Foster (1969) and Baxter

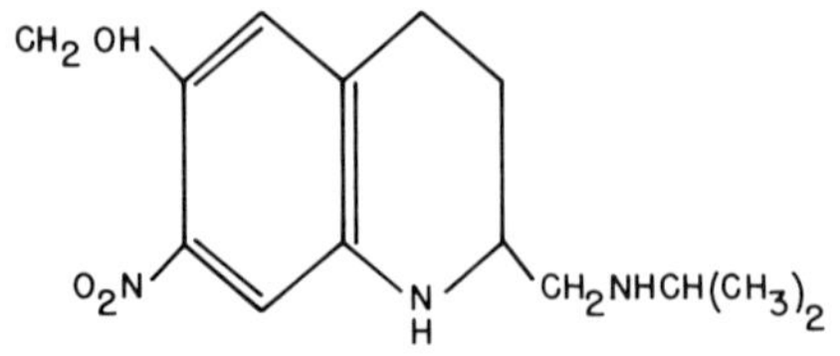

Fig. 7. Chemical structure of oxamniquine.

and Richards (1971) described a new series of 2-aminomethyltetrahydroquinoline derivatives displaying strong antischistosomal activity. From about fifty active members of this series, U.K. 3883 was selected as one of the most promising schistosomicidal compounds. This drug is curative in a single oral or intramuscular dose in rodents and monkeys, and also presents high chemoprophylactic activity (Foster *et al.,* 1971b,c; Pellegrino and Katz, 1972). Studying the metabolism of U.K. 3883 in mice, rats, rabbits, and rhesus monkeys, Kaye and Woolhouse (1972) observed that all these species converted this compound into its 6-hydroxymethyl analog, which showed greater schistosomicidal activity *in vivo* than the parent drug. This analog was named U.K. 4271 or oxamniquine.

Foster (1973) summarized as follows the experimental data on oxaminiquine: (*1*) in mice, the oral potency of the drug was 2–3 times higher than that of hycanthone, 5–11 times more than that of niridazole, and 8–11 times more than that of lucanthone; (*2*) in hamsters, its oral potency was similar to that in mice, but its intramuscular activity was much greater; (*3*) in rhesus monkeys and *Cercopithecus,* the oral curative dose was several times higher than the intramuscular one, whereas *Cebus* monkeys were more sensitive to oxamniquine than the former species; (*4*) female worms are more resistant to the treatment than male ones; (*5*) the drug was effective against all stages of immature worms in mice and monkeys; (*6*) the therapeutic index is much higher with the intramuscular formulation; (*7*) *in vitro*, oxamniquine is only moderately schistosomicidal, no difference being observed in the reaction of male and female worms; (*8*) in chronic toxicity tests, significant abnormalities were observed only after repeated treatment with dosages far in excess of curative levels; (*9*) there were no teratogenic properties; (*10*) methemoglobinemia was not induced; (*11*) activity against *S. haematobium* was less than against *S. mansoni,* and no effect was observed in *S. japonicum* (Foster, 1973).

Concordant therapeutic results were also obtained by Fripp (1973) and by Pellegrino *et al.* (1973) in rodents and monkeys, and on chemoprophylaxis in mice by Jewsbury (1973).

A preliminary clinical trial was performed, in Brazil, on 24 patients with active schistosomiasis mansoni (Katz *et al.,* 1973b). The compound was administered in capsules [50 mg twice a day (b.i.d.), for 2 days, and 100 mg, b.i.d., for 2 days] and intramuscular injections (5 and 7.5 mg/kg). Tenderness at the site of injection was the only side effect observed. In oral formulation, the drug brought about a decrease in white- and red-cell counts in 2 patients out of 10. Parasitological control of patients treated with the oral formulation revealed, 1 month later, a decrease in the number of eggs in the feces of 9 patients out of 10. Nevertheless, 4–6 months after the end of treatment the egg drop persisted in only 3 cases. The best schedule of treatment was a single intramuscular dose of 7.5 mg/kg, since all patients thus treated were considered cured, including 4 cases in the early phase of schistosomiasis (5–9 months after infection) (Katz *et al.,* 1973b).

Further clinical trials were performed on 104 patients with active schistosomiasis mansoni. The schedule applied was 7.5 mg/kg, i.m. Moderate to severe pain at the site of injection was recorded in all cases but 5, this pain lasting from 1 to 16 days. Other side effects were rare, slight, and of no clinical significance. Laboratory trials, performed 3–4 days after treatment, revealed an increase in the mean total number of leukocytes and neutrophiles, and in creatinophosphokinase (CPK). Transient and discrete elevation of the plasma transaminase levels was also observed in a few patients. Electrocardiographic tracings revealed slight alterations of QRS, T, and S waves. Among 71 patients followed up, 66 were considered as parasitologically cured, including 11 individuals in the early phase of the disease (4–6 months after infection) (Katz *et al.,* 1973c).

In 1973, Pfizer Laboratories sponsored a meeting about oxamniquine, in Brazil, whose scope was to evaluate clinical trials already performed in Brazil and Africa. The papers presented were published in a special issue of *Rev. Inst. Med. Trop. Sao Paulo* **15,** Suppl. 1 (1973). The data presented by the Brazilian researchers were similar to those previously mentioned, but other important observations were added.

Coutinho *et al.* (1973) treated 57 patients with the hepatointestinal, and 17 with the hepatosplenic form of schistosomiasis mansoni, with 7.5 mg of oxamniquine/kg, i.m. No important reaction was observed in the liver, kidney, bone marrow, heart, or nervous system which could indicate toxicity. All patients were cured.

Coura *et al.* (1973) used the same dose in 102 hepatointestinal and 12 hepatosplenic cases. The SGPT of 3 out of 97 patients were elevated and SGOT in 1 out of 56 patients, but no figure beyond 150 units was observed after treatment. Liver biopsy, performed in 6 patients before and after oxamniquine administration, did not reveal histological alterations. The main side effects were local pain and induration at the site of injection.

Prata *et al.* (1973) used single dose schedules of 5, 7.5, and 10.0 mg/kg, i.m. Three patients in the acute phase were cured with 7.5 mg/kg. In chronic cases, 5 mg/kg produced 85% cure and 7.5 and 10.0 mg/kg, 95%.

Silva *et al.* (1973) administered 7.5 mg/kg, i.m., to 53 schistosomiasis patients. In one-third of the cases, slight elevations of SGOT and CPK were observed on the third day, and, in 20% of the treated patients an elevation of SGOT, on the tenth day. In one patient, SGPT rose to 490 units and the liver biopsy revealed slight nonspecific alterations. Thirty-eight of the 41 patients followed up did not excrete eggs in their stools after 6 months of treatment.

Pedro *et al.* (1973) treated 33 patients with the schedule of 7.5 mg/kg, i.m., and observed in 94 and 67% of the patients pain and nodules, respectively, at the site of injection. One patient developed an abscess and another electrocardiographic alterations compatible with subepicardic ischemia. A few patients showed an increase of the transaminase levels (less than 100 units), and 1 patient developed bilirubinemia of 1.6 mg%.

In Tanzania, Eyakuse (1973) tried oxamniquine at the dose level of 30 mg/kg, i.m., in 26 *S. mansoni* patients. No toxic effects were observed. Cure ranged from 80 to 100%, according to the parasitological control method employed.

In Rhodesia, Clarke *et al.* (1973) treated 59 children, infected with *S. haematobium* and *S. mansoni,* with 7.5 mg/kg, i.m. Side effects were slight and uncommon, but only a few patients completely ceased to pass eggs.

In Kenya, Rees *et al.* (1973) obtained 77% cure (as judged by only two stool examinations performed after treatment) when 53 schoolchildren, most of them infected by *S. mansoni,* were treated with 7.5 mg/kg of oxamniquine.

After discussing the data mentioned above, the conclusion was reached that, although oxamniquine, intramuscularly, produced few toxic side effects and a high percentage of cure in Brazil, the severe local pain would hardly allow its use on a large scale for field treatment.

Silva *et al.* (1974) tried oxamniquine in capsules, orally administered in 109 *S. mansoni* patients, divided into three groups: (*a*) 29 patients treated with 10 mg/kg; (*b*) 47 patients with 12–12.5 mg/kg; and (*c*) 33 patients with 15 mg/kg. The most frequent side effects were dizziness, nausea, and drowsiness, whose intensity and frequency increased with the dosage employed. In 3 out of 81 patients, there was found an elevation of transaminase levels (more than 100 units). Leukopenia was also observed in 3 patients, and hematuria and proteinuria in 8 patients. The percentages of cure obtained were 70.0, 81.5, and 100.0%, respectively, in the groups treated with 10, 12–12.5, and 15 mg/kg.

Katz *et al.* (1976) performed clinical trials with two oral formulations of oxamniquine (syrup and capsules) on 335 patients with active schistosomiasis mansoni. They used a number of different schedules: 10, 12.5, 15, and 20 mg/kg as single oral doses, and also 10 mg/kg b.i.d., 7.5 mg/kg b.i.d., and 10 mg/kg/day for 2 consecutive days. Dizziness, drowsiness, headache, and nausea, as well as few cases of hallucination and psychic excitation, were observed. This symptomatology appeared 1 or 2 hours after the drug administration and persisted, in most cases, less than 6 hours. The frequency and intensity of these side effects were directly related to the dose applied. The drug was better tolerated when ingested after a meal. In laboratory tests, slight elevations of transaminases and 1 case of leukopenia were observed after treatment. The electrocardiographic and electroencephalographic tracings were within the normal limits. A great difference between the cure rate in adults and in children was recorded. In fact, with the schedules of single doses of 10 and 15 mg/kg, the percentage of cure was 81.2 and 93.7 for adults, and 0.0 and 30.5 for children. The best schedules for treating children seem to be 7.5–10 mg/kg, b.i.d., and 10 mg/kg/day × 2 days, which provide a cure rate of about 85% and are better tolerated than a single dose of 20 mg/kg.

To date, about 2000 patients have been treated with oxamniquine by the oral route. This limited number does not permit us to draw a final conclusion as to its rank as a schistosomicidal drug, but the initial trials have shown that oxamniquine is a promising drug and that pilot projects for mass treatment as well as comparative studies with hycanthone in the field of toxicity, mutagenicity, and carcinogenicity must be performed.

## VIII. Compounds with Antischistosomal Activity

### A. Nitrofuran Derivatives

Robinson *et al.* (1970) have demonstrated that a nitrofuran derivative, *trans*-5-amino-3-[2-(5-nitro-2-furyl)vinyl]-1,2,4-oxadiazole (SQ 18,506) which was synthesized by Breuer (1969), presents antischistosomal action in laboratory animals. Further studies showed that this compound exerted chemotherapeutic activity when orally administered to mice, hamsters, and monkeys infected with *S. mansoni* or *S. japonicum* (Bueding *et al.*, 1971; Erickson *et al.*, 1971). The SQ 18,506 activity increased when the compound particle size was reduced to 3.5 $\mu$m or when it was administered in glycerol. Intramuscular injection of a single high dose of SQ 18,506 (1gm/kg) produced parasitological cure in mice, the drug being slowly absorbed and excreted for about 60 to 80 days. The drug is very active when given in the diet instead of by gavage. In fact, after the administration for 24 hours of a diet containing 1.2% of

SQ 18,506 to mice or hamsters experimentally infected with *S. mansoni*, the presence of abnormalities in the reproductive system of the female worms became evident. The hepatic shift started 48 hours later and was completed after 3 to 4 days. When the animals were thus fed for 5 days, parasitological cure was observed in 100% of the cases. SQ 18,506 appears to have a direct effect on worm eggs in the tissues. The drug did not present high toxicity with curative antischistosomal doses; it inhibits the activity of the phosphorylase-phosphatase enzyme of the worms (Bueding *et al.*, 1971). This nitrovinylfuran derivative displayed pronounced activity when administered to mice orally at various stages during development of the *S. mansoni* infection, i.e., in the period from 1 to 44 days after cercariae penetration. The drug activity on immature worms was stronger than that observed in 56–125 day infections. A single intramuscular dose of SQ 18,506 at 1–8 days prior to infection has a marked prophylactic effect (Lennox and Bueding, 1972).

It is interesting to remark that the wide spectrum of antischistosomal activity (immature and mature worms, and eggs) appears to be characteristic of nitrovinylfurans, since similar results were obtained with other alkyl-substituted nitrovinylfurans (Lei *et al.*, 1964; Hill *et al.*, 1966; Lennox and Bueding, 1972).

A series of 24 analogs of SQ 18,506 were prepared and evaluated in mice infected with *S. mansoni*. Compounds containing 2-imidazolyl and 2-pyridyl groups provided cure rates of around 25% at 400- and 250-mg dose levels, respectively. Better still, the 2-thiazolyl and 2-pyrimidyl derivatives produced 100% cure at 250 and 200 mg/kg, respectively (Henry *et al.*, 1973). SQ 18,506 showed high antischistosomal activity when administered orally to *Mastomys natalensis* infected with *S. mansoni* at doses of 500 mg/kg for 5 consecutive days. Pathophysiological studies demonstrated increase in the level of sorbitol dehydrogenase in the serum and in the number of leukocytes and eosinophilic granulocytes in these animals (Lämmler and Schuster, 1974).

It has recently been demonstrated by Ong (1974) that SQ 18,506 is a potent mutagen in *Neurospora crassa*.

### B. Thiazolines and Nitrothiazolines

At the Parke-Davis Laboratories, a series of nitrothiazolines and some thiazolines devoid of nitro groups were shown to be active against *S. mansoni* in mice and monkeys. In fact, 2-[3-(diethylaminomethyl)-*p*-anisidino]-5-nitrothiazole killed 33% of *S. mansoni* worms when administered to mice at 0.25% in their diet for 14 days (Werbel *et al.*, 1969).

Many 5-nitro-4-thiazolines showed high schistosomicidal activity when used for 3 to 14 days (Islip *et al.*, 1972; Werbel *et al.*, 1972).

Slight modifications in the niridazole molecule completely hinder schistosome activity. Generally, the $NO_2$ group in the 5-position must be present for activity. However, a desnitro derivative S-2 [(2-thiazolylcarbamoyl ethylamino)ethyl hydrogen thiosulfate] presents high activity in mice and monkeys experimentally infected with *S. mansoni* (Westland *et al.*, 1971).

Other derivatives of nitrothiazolines and nonnitrated thiazolines have also proved active against *S. mansoni* infection in mice (Islip *et al.*, 1973a,b), but no clinical data are available so far.

### C. Arylazonaphthylamine Derivatives

More than 500 naphthylazo compounds were synthesized and tested in laboratory animals at Parke-Davis Laboratories by Elslager *et al.* (1963a). Some compounds showed activity when administered to mice in the diet, during extended schedules (1–2 weeks), and a few of them also showed to be effective in rhesus monkeys experimentally infected with *S. mansoni*.

Although a lot of information has been gained by Eslager and his group concerning structure–activity relationship and metabolism of this class of compounds together with hundreds of derivatives, not a single promising drug for clinical schistosomiasis treatment has come to light from these studies (Elslager *et al.*, 1963a,b, 1964a,b, 1966, 1970a,b; Werbel, *et al.*, 1968, 1970).

### D. Thiophene Derivatives

At the Hoffman-La Roche Laboratories, over 100 compounds belonging to the class of thiophene derivatives have been synthesized, more than half of them having shown activity against *S. mansoni* infection of mice, hamsters, and *Cebus* monkeys. The most interesting effects were found with some 3,5-dinitro-2-thienylamine derivative. Two members of this chemical group, Ro 10-7062 [2-(2-morpholinoethylamino)-3,5-dinitrothiophene] and Ro 10-0761 [3(3,5-dinitro-2-thienyl) thiazoline] were more closely investigated. These drugs were orally administered for 5 consecutive days since they proved less active when giving in a single dose (Stohler and Szente, 1974).

The RO 10-0761 showed higher activity, both in mice and hamsters, and is about twice as active as niridazole, where Ro 10-7062 displayed lower activity. In mice, schistosome eggs deposited in the tissues were killed and 90–100% of schistosomules, from the second week of infection onward, were destroyed. Both compounds show *in vitro* activity against adult *S. mansoni* worms. Toxicological studies performed on rats, dogs, and *Cebus* monkeys showed that both drugs are better tolerated than niridazole, which was used as the comparative compound. Also, a Malagasy strain of *S. haematobium* proved to be susceptible to the treatment (Stohler and Szente, 1974).

In view of the data available from chemical studies and antischistosomal and toxicology measurements, Stohler and Szente (1974) suggest that at least one of these two members of the thiophene series should be tested in clinical trials.

### E. Organophosphorus Compounds

To this class of compounds belong the following drugs: Dipterex, dichlorvos, trichlorphon, Neguvon, chlorophos, Dylox, metriphonate. Werbel and Thompson (1967) investigated a wide variety of organophosphorus compounds against *S. mansoni* infection in mice. The most active compounds are the phosphate and thiophosphate derivative of *N*-hydroxynaphthalimide. None of these compounds has shown high activity in monkeys (Werbel and Thompson, 1967).

Cerf *et al.* (1962) and Talaat *et al.* (1963) demonstrated that another organophosphorus compound, trichlorphon, was active in clinical treatment of ancylostomiasis, ascariasis, trichuriasis, creeping eruption, and intestinal schistosomiasis.

No antischistosomal activity was observed in mice, gerbils, and *Cercopithecus aetiops* experimentally infected with *S. mansoni* and treated, per os, with trichlorphon, at doses of 100 mg/kg/day for 3 to 6 consecutive days (mice and gerbils) and 5–10 mg/kg/day for 10 days (monkeys). In patients infected with *S. haematobium* and *S. mansoni* and treated with 5 mg/kg/day for 12 consecutive days, the percentages of cure were 65 and 18%, respectively (Abdallah *et al.*, 1965). When the schedules employed were 200 and 100 mg/kg/day × 7 days, 100% of mice and hamsters, respectively, exhibited oogram changes. No significant activity was found in *Cebus* monkeys with doses of up to 30 mg/kg/day × 5 days. Transient interruption of egg laying by worms, as judged by rectal biopsies, was observed in 6 out of 12 patients infected with *S. mansoni,* after treatment with 5 fortnightly trichlorphon doses of 7.5 mg/kg (Katz *et al.*, 1968b).

Although trichlorphon has its place in *S. haematobium* human treatment (Forsyth and Rashid, 1967; Davis and Bailey, 1969), it is of no value for the clinical treatment of *S. mansoni*.

As was well demonstrated by Bueding *et al.* (1972), trichlorphon has similar activity in the inhibition of acetylcholinesterase and cholinesterases against both schistosome species, *in vitro*. Nevertheless, in mice, the worms were shifted to the liver or to the lungs, according to the species tested, and, whereas *S. mansoni* recovered and returned to the mesenteric veins, *S. haematobium* was immobilized and killed in the lungs (Denham and Holdsworth, 1971).

### F. Tubercidin

According to the rational approach, Jaffe *et al.* (1971) tested *in vitro* several purine analogs against *S. mansoni* and found tubercidin (7-deazaadenosine) to be one of the most active. In fact, at a concentration of $10^{-7}$ *M*, tubercidin induces separation of paired worms, alteration of the muscular activity, and inhibition of egg laying. In mice, after being absorbed into the red cells, tubercidin induced hepatic shift of the worms, suppression of egg laying, and a large increase in the number of mature and dead eggs (Jaffe *et al.*, 1971). Tubercidin also prevented the utilization of adenosine for adenosine nucleotide formation *in vitro* (Ross and Jaffe, 1972). When added to the culture medium, tubercidin interfered with the maintenance of normal ATP levels in worms (Stegman *et al.*, 1973). The necessity for tubercidin to be absorbed into the red cells in order to effect tolerability of the drug precludes its use for the large-scale treatment of schistosomiasis.

### G. SN 10,275

(6,8-Dichloro-2-phenyl-4-quinolyl)-2-piperidylcarbinol hydrochloride (SN 10,275; Merck Laboratories) was very active against mature and, especially immature infection of *S. mansoni* in mice, hamsters, and rhesus monkeys (Campbell and Cuckler, 1963; Pellegrino and Katz, 1968). However, its known photosensitizing action precludes its use in clinical schistosomiasis.

### H. Amphotericin B

According to Gordon and St. John (1963), amphotericin B (Squibb Laboratories) significantly prolongs the life of mice experimentally infected with *S. mansoni* and induces a decrease in the number of worms of treated animals. This activity of amphotericin B has not been confirmed (Pellegrino, 1965; Prata *et al.*, 1965). In clinical trials, Prata *et al.* (1965) administered, intravenously, 1.5 mg/kg/day for 20 days and concluded that the drug was totally ineffective.

### I. S-201

This dicarbonic acid hydrazide [bis-(β-carbohydrazidoethyl)sulfone; Hoechst Laboratories] was highly active in mice (Lämmler, 1963; Pellegrino and Faria, 1965), but it was only partially effective in rhesus (Bruce and Sadun, 1966) and *Cebus* monkeys (Pellegrino and Katz, 1968).

Clinical trials performed by Carvalho (1965) showed that S-201 is effective in patients with *S. mansoni,* but also very toxic.

### J. A-16,612

The A-16,612 [*N*-(3-chloro-4-methylphenyl)-*N'*-(ω-4'-*t*-amylphenoxyhexyl)piperazine hydrochloride, teroxalene; Abbott Laboratories] given according to a schedule of 200 mg/kg/day 5 days per os, killed 86.8% of *S. mansoni* worms in the liver of mice, and all animals presented oogram changes. Nevertheless, no antischistosomal activity was observed in infected hamsters, even at the dose of 1000 mg/kg/day × 7 days. In *Cebus* monkeys, slight activity was detected with doses of 500 and 1000 mg/kg/day × 5 days (Katz *et al.,* 1967b).

In patients with active schistosomiasis mansoni, no therapeutic activity could be detected with schedules of 750 mg/kg, which corresponded to neurologically toxic levels (Katz *et al.,* 1967b). The inefficacy of this drug was confirmed in humans infected with *S. haematobium* or *S. mansoni* in Egypt (Abdallah and El-Mawla, 1968).

When the 4-methyl group was replaced by the 4-hydroxymethyl, the antischistosomal activity of A-16,612 greatly increased, as observed in mice and hamsters (Rosi *et al.,* 1967). No clinical studies have so far been performed with this new compound.

### K. RD-12,869

In mice and *Cebus* monkeys, RD-12,869 [6-chloro-5-(β-diethylaminoethylamino)-8-methylquinoline; Boots Pure Drugs Co., Ltd.] presented high antischistosomal activity when dosed with 120, 60, or 30 mg/kg/day × 5 days per os in mice but proved inactive in hamsters (Bristow *et al.,* 1967; Pellegrino *et al.,* 1967b). Although several compounds (for example, lucanthone and A-16,612) increase their schistosomicidal activity when a methyl group in the para position to a dialkylaminoalkyamino moiety on an aromatic ring is replaced by the respective hydroxymethyl analog, this does not happen with RD-12,869 (Bailey *et al.*, 1970).

The toxic effects of RD-12,869 did not allow its use in human schistosomiasis.

## L. Tris(*p*-aminophenyl)carbonium Salts

Tris(*p*-aminophenyl)carbonium chloride (TAC chloride, CI-403-A; Parke-Davis Laboratories) presents both curative and protective activity in mice infected with *S. mansoni* (Elslager *et al.*, 1961). Since this salt induces vomiting and gastritis, it was replaced by the pamoate salt, which is also effective against *S. mansoni* and *S. japonicum* when injected into mice, monkeys, and man. The TAC pamoate acts against immature and mature *S. mansoni* worms and causes cessation of egg laying (Thompson *et al.*, 1962; Pellegrino and Faria, 1964). The drug reduces the glycogen content in the cuticular tubercles of male worms and causes a localized paralysis of the worms' acetabulum, pharynx, and oral suckers. The paralysis is correlated with the decrease of cholinesterase in the central ganglia and can be reversed, *in vitro,* by mecamylamine, a cholinergic blocking agent (Saz and Bueding, 1966).

Conflicting results were obtained in clinical trials: Burnett and Wagner (1961) and Rodrigues da Silva *et al.* (1963) reported activity against human *S. mansoni* infection whereas Bruaux and Gillet (1961) claimed that there had occurred only a temporary interruption of egg laying but no cures. All these authors employed schedules of 1–2 weeks' duration. Pesigan *et al.* (1967) found TAC pamoate very useful as a suppressive agent in *S. japonicum* infection in humans, when orally administered, once a week, for 16 to 24 weeks.

True synergistic effect has been observed when TAC salts were coadministered with antimonials to rodents and primates experimentally infected with *S. mansoni* (Thompson *et al.*, 1965), but no clinical trial using this association has been performed.

Prolonged administration of TAC induces an increase in the incidence of skin tumors in female rats (Kaump *et al.*, 1965), but no evidence of such effects have been observed in other laboratory animals or in humans (Werbel, 1970).

## M. *p*-Aminophenoxyalkane Derivatives

To this class of compounds belong the following drugs: amphothalide, M & B 2948A, R. P. 6171, M & B 9884, Schistomide (Wellcome

Foundation and May & Baker Laboratories). More than 300 di-(*p*-aminophenoxy) alkane derivatives were investigated as antischistosomal agents, several of them having displayed high activity in laboratory animals (Raison and Standen, 1954a,b, 1955; Collins *et al.*, 1959). In clinical trials, when 1-*p*-aminophenoxy-5-phthalimidopentans were orally administered at doses of 250 to 400 mg, spread over 5–6 days, a small percentages of cure of *S. haematobium* infection was observed (11–45%), but in *S. mansoni*-infected patients no action could be observed (Schneider and Sansarricq, 1959; Larivière *et al.*, 1960; El Bitashi *et al.*, 1961; Alves *et al.*, 1961; Silva and Prata, 1962; Cunha, 1966b). This compound produces retinotoxicity or visual-field diminution, and its clinical use is thus excluded (Collins *et al.*, 1959; Hill, 1964).

## N. Dehydroemetine

This drug is an emetine derivative [BT 436 (E. Merck A. G.) and Ro 19,334 (Hoffman La Roche Laboratories)] that is well tolerated according to therapeutic results of clinical trials, in both *S. mansoni* and *S. haematobium* infections. When dehydroemetine was orally or parenterally (s.c. or i.m.) administered for 14 to 21 days, the percentage of cure for both schistosome infections ranged from 70 to more than 90%, with low incidence of side effects (Gouveia and Teixeira, 1963; Salem, 1965; Abd-Rabbo and Montasir, 1967; Gilles, 1967; Blanc and Nosny, 1968).

On the other hand, Abdallah *et al.* (1966) reported that dehydroemetine must be given at the maximum tolerated dose to obtain therapeutic effect against *S. haematobium*, no significant effect having been detected in *S. mansoni* patients. Since dehydroemetine requires a long course of treatment, and efficacy and tolerance do not show any advantage over those of other antischistosomal drugs now available, its use must be discouraged.

## O. Other Active Compounds

The following compounds, among others, show some kind of activity when tested in animals experimentally infected with *S. mansoni*: rhodanines and hydantoins (Luttermoser and Bond, 1954), cortisone (Coker, 1957; Weinmann and Hunter, 1960), dexamethasone, and C-norprednisone acetate (Lagrange, 1963; Newsome, 1963), hexachloro-*p*-xylene (Hetol) as well as some of its derivatives (Lämmler, 1964; Elslager *et al.*, 1970c), a thiamine antimetabolite (Nabith and Zoroob, 1971), quinine, quinidine, cinchonine (Pellegrino and Katz, 1974).

## P. Egg Suppressants and Chemosterilants

### 1. *Nicarbazin*

This drug is an equimolecular complex of 4,4′-dinitrocarbanilide and 2-hydroxy-4,6-dimethylpyrimidine (Merck Laboratories). It was demonstrated that nicarbazin administered in the diet suppressed *S. mansoni* egg laying in experimentally infected mice (Campbell and Cuckler, 1967). This transient inhibitory effect was confirmed on mice and *Cebus* monkeys by Pellegrino and Katz (1969).

Warren (1970) claimed that when nicarbazin was administered to mice from the tenth to the fifteenth week after *S. mansoni* infection, egg suppression was irreversible. This finding could not be confirmed in our laboratories (Antunes *et al.*, 1974).

### 2. *Thiosinamine*

Thiosinamine (*N*-allylthiourea) blocks the normal process of egg-shell formation in *S. mansoni* by inhibiting a copper-containing enzyme, polyphenoloxidase (Machado *et al.*, 1970). The drug was active in mice, when incorporated in their diet (1% of the drug) and in hamsters, per oral route (50 and 25 mg/kg/day × 5 days), inducing an almost immediate cessation of egg laying. As soon as treatment was interrupted, resumption of oviposition occurred (Pellegrino and Machado, 1972).

### 3. *Antifertility Agents*

Ethylene 1,2-dimethanesulfonate, methylene dimethanesulfonate, hexamethylphosphoramide, *N,N*-ethyleneurea and its *N′,N′*-dimethyl derivative, and mitoclomine, drugs with known sterilant activity in male rodents, induced temporary inhibition of oviposition in *S. mansoni*-infected mice. The gonads of male and female worms are directly affected (Jackson *et al.*, 1968; Davies and Jackson, 1970).

### 4. *Dapsone*

This drug (4,4′-diaminodiphenyl sulfone, DDS) interferes with the egg-laying of *Schistosoma mansoni* in mice, hamsters, and *Cebus* monkeys experimentally infected. In mice the activity was evident when DDS was administered in the diet at a concentration as low as 0.05%. The activity was transitory, disappearing soon after the drug was withdrawn. A parasitological survey among lepers under specific treatment revealed a low index of infection by helminths. However, the treatment by DDS of patients harboring *S. mansoni* infection as well as other intestinal helminths was ineffective (Pellegrino and Katz, 1975).

### Q. Biological Agents and Materials

Numerous species of bacteria have been shown to colonize and ultimately destroy adult schistosomes. The therapeutic effect is handicapped by the fact that only live bacteria exhibit this activity, bacterial material being completely inactive (Ottens and Dickerson, 1969, 1972; Basch, 1971).

Biological materials, such as rhesus hemolysate, intact rhesus erythrocytes (Oliver-Gonzalez, 1967), Forssman-positive extract of guinea pig kidney (Cox and Oliver-Gonzalez, 1969), snail hemolymph (Oliver-Gonzalez, 1968), and specially disrupted membranes of rhesus monkey erythrocytes (Cox and Oliver-Gonzalez, 1970), were claimed to have antischistosomal effect.

However, as was pointed out by Chiriboga *et al.* (1971) and Dean and Gadd (1973), the activity of snail hemolymph and erythrocyte products on schistosomes is probably due to bacterial contamination.

## References


Abdallah, A. (1964), In Friedheim, 1973.

Abdallah, A., and El-Mawla, N. G. (1968). *J. Egypt. Med. Assoc.* **51,** 580–586.

Abdallah, A., and Saif, M. (1964). *J. Egypt Med. Assoc.* **47,** 427–438.

Abdallah, A., Saif, M., and Taha, A. (1959). *J. Egypt. Med. Assoc.* **42,** 631–635.

Abdallah, A., Saif, M., Taha, A., Ashmawy, H., Tawfik, J., Abdel-Fattah, F., Sabet, S., and Abdel-Medgio, M. (1965). *J. Egypt. Med. Assoc.* **48,** 263–273.

Abdallah, A., Saif, M., and El-Mawla, M. G. (1968). *J. Egypt. Med. Assoc.* **51,** 823–830.

Abdallah, A., Saif, M., and Koura, M. (1971). *J. Egypt. Med. Assoc.* **54,** 155–170.

Abdallah, H., Kordy, M. I., Saif, M., Aly, I. M., and El-Mawly, G. (1966). *J. Egypt. Public Health Assoc.* **41,** 11–18.

Abdallah, R. E., Iskander, S., and Haseeb, M. A. (1968). *J. Trop. Med. Hyg.* **71,** 44–45.

Abd-Rabbo, H., and Montasir, M. (1967). *J. Trop. Med. Hyg.* **70,** 117–121.

Almeida, F. M., Mincis, M., Vilela, M. P., Guimarães, R. X., Pferferman, A., Cabeça, M., Soares, M. A., Prócoli, T. I., Rodrigues, L. D., and Rodrigues, F. S. (1970). *Rev. Assoc. Med. Bras.* **16,** 315–320.

Alves, W. (1945). *S. Afr. Med. J.* **19,** 171–172.

Alves, W. (1946). *S. Afr. Med. J.* **20,** 146–147.

Alves, W. (1949). *S. Afr. Med. J.* **23,** 428–431.

Alves, W. (1950). *Ann. Trop. Med. Parasitol.* **44,** 34–41.

Alves, W. (1958). *Bull. W. H. O.* **18,** 1109–1111.

Alves, W., and Blair, D. M. (1946). Lancet **250,** 9–12.

Alves, W., and Blair, D. M. (1947). *S. Afr. Med. J.* **21,** 352–357.

Alves, W., Harper, J., and Hill, J. (1961). *Trans. R. Soc. Trop. Med. Hyg.* **55,** 40–43.

Andrade, Z. A., Santos, H. A., Borojenic, R., and Grimaud, J. A. (1974). *Rev. Inst. Med. Trop. Sao Paulo* **16,** 160–170.
Anrep, G. V., Barsoum, G. S., and Kenawy, M. R. (1941). *J. Egypt. Med. Assoc.* **24,** 172.
Antunes, C. M. F., Katz, N., Dias, E. P., and Pellegrino, J. (1974). *Ann. Trop. Med. Parasitol.* **68,** 237–238.
Archer, S., and Yarinsky, A. (1972). *Prog. Drug Res.* **16,** 12–66.
Arfaa, F., Farahmandian, I., and Soleimani, M. (1970). *Trans. R. Soc. Trop. Med. Hyg.* **64,** 130–133.
Argento, C. A., Garcia, S., Delvaux, R. P., Silva, J. R., and Coura, J. R. (1968). *Int. Congr. Trop. Med. Malaria, 8th, 1968*, p. 31.
Arruda, P. V., Magaldi, C., and Amato Neto, V. (1967). *Rev. Inst. Med. Trop. Sao Paulo* **9,** 381–387.
Badran, A. M. (1966). In Badran and Abdallah, 1967.
Badran, A. M., and Abdallah, A. (1967). *J. Egypt. Med. Assoc.* **50,** 360–368.
Bailey, D. M., Archer, S., Wood, D., Rosi, D., and Yarinsky, A. (1970). *J. Med. Chem.* **13,** 598–601.
Bang, F. B., and Hairston, N. G. (1946). *Am. J. Hyg.* **44,** 348–366.
Baranski, M. (1966). *Folha Med.* **53,** 101–110.
Barbosa, F. A. S. (1969). *Rev. Inst. Med. Trop. Sao Paulo* **11,** 442–443.
Barker, L. R., Bueding, E., and Timms, A. R. (1966). *Br. J. Pharmacol. Chemother.* **26,** 656–665.
Basch, P. F. (1971). *Nature (London)* **233,** 492–493.
Basmy, K., Shoeb, S. M., Mostafa, M. M., and Hassan, A. H. (1968). *J. Egypt. Med. Assoc.* **51,** 290–300.
Baxter, C. A. R., and Richards, H. C. (1971). *J. Med. Chem.* **14,** 1033–1042.
Bell, D. R. (1963). *Bull. W. H. O.* **29,** 525–530.
Bell, D. R. (1964). *Lancet* **1,** 643–644.
Bénex, J. (1960). *Bull. Soc. Pathol. Exot.* **53,** 309–314.
Bennett, J., and Bueding, E. (1971). *Comp. Biochem. Phys. A* **39,** 857–867.
Bennett, J. L., and Bueding, E. (1973). *Mol. Pharmacol.* **9,** 311–319.
Berberian, D. A., and Freele, H. (1964). *J. Parasitol.* **50,** 435–440.
Berberian, D. A., Freele, H., and Rosi, D. (1967a). *J. Parasitol.* **53,** 306–311.
Berberian, D. A., Freele, H., and Rosi, D. (1967b). *Am. J. Trop. Med.* **16,** 487–491.
Bina, J. C., and Prata, A. (1970). *Gaz. Med. Bahia* **70,** 127–130.
Bina, J. C., and Prata, A. (1974). *Rev. Soc. Brasi. Med. Trop.* **8,** 217–222.
Bittencourt, H. T. (1937). In Dias, 1949.
Blagg, W., Schledegel, E. L., Mansour, E. S., and Khalaf, G. F. (1955). *Am. J. Trop. Med. Hyg.* **4,** 23–28.
Blair, D. M. (1958). *Bull. W. H. O.* **18,** 989–1010.
Blanc, F., and Nosny, Y. (1968). *Presse Med.* **76,** 1419–1420.
Booth, G. H., and Schulert, A. R. (1968). *Proc. Soc. Exp. Biol. Med.* **127,** 700–704.
Bourgeois, J. G., and Bueding, E. (1971). *J. Pharmacol. Exp. Ther.* **176,** 455–463.
Brady, F. J., Lawton, A. H., Cowie, D. B., Andrews, H. L., Ness, A. T., and Ogden, G. E. (1945). *Am. J. Trop. Med.* **25,** 103–107.
Brener, Z. (1957). *Revta. Bras. Malar. Doenc. Trop.* **9,** 489–496.
Brener, Z. (1960). *Hospital (Rio de Janeiro)* **57,** 1069–1073.
Brener, Z. (1962). Thesis, Federal University of Minas Gerais, Belo Horizonte, Brazil.
Brener, Z. (1965). *Rev. Inst. Med. Trop. Sao Paulo* **6,** 167–170.
Brener, Z., and Alvarenga, R. J. (1962). *Rev. Inst. Med. Trop. Sao Paulo* **4,** 180–186.

Brener, Z., and Chiari, E. (1957). *Rev. Brasil. Malariol. Doencas Trop.* **9,** 485–488.
Brener, Z., and Pellegrino, J. (1958). *J. Parasitol.* **44,** 659–664.
Brener, Z., Pellegrino, J., and Oliveira, C. A. (1956). *Rev. Brasil. Malariol. Doencas Trop.* **8,** 583–587.
Breuer, H. (1969). *J. Med. Chem.* **12,** 708–709.
Bristow, N. W., Lessel, B., Richards, H. C., and Williams, G. A. H. (1967). *Nature (London)* **216,** 282–283.
Brown, M. C., Koura, M., Bell, D. R., and Gilles, H. M. (1973). *Ann. Trop. Med. Parasitol.* **67,** 369–370.
Browne, H. G., and Schulert, A. R. (1963). *Fed. Proc., Fed. Am. Soc. Exp. Biol.* **22,** 666.
Browne, H. G., and Schulert, A. R. (1964). *Am. J. Trop. Med. Hyg.* **13,** 558–571.
Browne, H. G., and Thomas, J. I. (1963). *J. Parasitol.* **49,** 371–374.
Bruaux, P., and Gillet, J. (1961). *Ann. Soc. Belge Med. Trop.* **41,** 397.
Bruce, J. I., and Sadun, E. H. (1963). *Am. J. Trop. Med. Hyg.* **12,** 184–187.
Bruce, J. I., and Sadun, E. H. (1966). *Am. J. Trop. Med. Hyg.* **15,** 324–332.
Bruce, J. I., Sadun, E. H., and Schoenbechler, M. J. (1962). *Am. J. Trop. Med. Hyg.* **11,** 25–30.
Bruce, J. I., Weiss, E., Stirewalt, M. A., and Lincicome, D. R. (1969). *Expl. Parasitol.* **26,** 29–40.
Brumpt, L. C., Degremont, A., Barbier, M., Coumbaras, A., and Lavarde, V. (1968). *Presse Med.* **76,** 797–800.
Bueding, E. (1949). *Physiol. Rev.* **29,** 195–218.
Bueding, E. (1950). *J. Gen. Physiol.* **33,** 475–495.
Bueding, E. (1952). *Br. J. Pharmacol. Chemother.* **7,** 563–566.
Bueding, E. (1959). *J. Pharm. Pharmacol.* **11,** 385–392.
Bueding, E. (1962). *In* "Biological Council Symposium on Drugs Parasites and Hosts," pp. 15–28. Churchill, London.
Bueding, E. (1967). *In* "Chemical Zoology," Vol. 2, p. 551. Academic Press, New York.
Bueding, E. (1969). *Biochem. Pharmacol.* **18,** 1541–1547.
Bueding, E. (1975). *J. Toxicol. Environ. Health* **1,** 329–334.
Bueding, E., and Charms, B. (1951). *Nature (London)* **167,** 149.
Bueding, E., and Fisher, J. (1969). *Ann. N.Y. Acad. Sci.* **160,** 536–543.
Bueding, E., and Fisher, J. (1970). *Mol. Pharmacol.* **6,** 532–539.
Bueding, E., and Koletsky, S. (1950). *Proc. Soc. Exp. Biol. Med.* **73,** 594–596.
Bueding, E., and MacKinnon, J. A. (1955a). *J. Biol. Chem.* **215,** 495–506.
Bueding, E., and MacKinnon, J. A. (1955b). *J. Biol. Chem.* **215,** 507–513.
Bueding, E., and Mansour, J. M. (1957). *Br. J. Pharmacol. Chemother.* **12,** 159–165.
Bueding, E., and Penedo, N. (1957). *Fed. Proc. Fed. Am. Soc. Exp. Biol.* **16,** 286.
Bueding, E., and Peters, L. (1951). *J. Pharmacol. Exp. Ther.* **101,** 210–229.
Bueding, E., Peters, L., and Waite, J. F. (1947). *Proc. Soc. Exp. Biol. Med.* **64,** 111–113.
Bueding, E., Peters, L., Koletsky, S., and Moore, D. V. (1953). *Br. J. Pharmacol. Chemother.* **8,** 15–18.
Bueding, E., Ruppender, H., and Mackinnon, J. (1954). *Proc. Natl. Acad. Sci. U.S.A.* **40,** 773–777.
Bueding, E., Schiller, E. L., and Bourgeois, J. G. (1967). *Am. J. Trop. Med. Hyg.* **16,** 500–515.
Bueding, E., Naquira, C., and Bouwman, S. (1971). *J. Pharmacol. Exp. Ther.* **178,** 402–410.
Bueding, E., Liu, C. L., and Rogers, S. H. (1972). *Br. J. Pharmacol.* **46,** 480–487.
Burnett, H. S., and Wagner, E. D. (1961). *Am. J. Trop. Med. Hyg.* **10,** 547–550.
Campbell, W. C., and Cuckler, A. C. (1963). *J. Parasitol.* **49,** 528.

Campbell, W. C., and Cuckler, A. C. (1967). *J. Parasitol.* **53,** 977–980.
Campos, R. (1966). *Folha Med.* **53,** 112–115.
Cançado, J. R., Cunha, A. S., Carvalho, D. G., and Cambraia, J. M. S. (1965). *Bull. W. H. O.* **33,** 557–566.
Carneiro Filho, D. A., Brandão, E. D., and Noleto, P. A. (1969). *Hospital (Rio de Janeiro)* **76,** 1593–1596.
Carvalho, D. G. (1965). Thesis, Federal University of Minas Gerais, Belo Horizonte, Brazil.
Cerf, J., Lebrun, A., and Bierich, L. (1962). *Am. J. Trop. Med. Hyg.* **11,** 514–517.
Chaia, G. (1956). *Rev. Brasil. Malariol. Doencas Trop.* **8,** 355–357.
Chaia, G., Chaia, A. B. Q., McAullife, J., Katz, N., and Gasper, D. (1968). *Rev. Inst. Med. Trop. Sao Paulo* **10,** 349–353.
Cheever, A. W., and Weller, T. H. (1958). *Am. J. Hyg.* **68,** 322–339.
Chernin, E., and Michelson, E. H. (1957a). *Am. J. Hyg.* **65,** 57–70.
Chernin, E., and Michelson, E. H. (1957b). *Am. J. Hyg.* **65,** 71–80.
Chiriboga, J., Ritchie, L. S., Oliver-Gonzalez, J., Brown, R., and Lopez, V. A. (1971). *Am. J. Trop. Med. Hyg.* **20,** 672–678.
Chou, T. T., Bennett, J. L., Pert, C., and Bueding, E. (1973). *J. Pharmacol. Exp. Ther.* **186,** 408–415.
Christopherson, J. B. (1918). *Lancet* **2,** 325–327.
Chu, C. C., Tseh, Y. L., Liang, Y. I., and Ting, K. S. (1957a). *Sheng Li Hsueh Pao* **21,** 12–18.
Chu, C. C., Liang, Y. I., and Ting, K. S. (1957b). *Sheng Li Hsueh Pao* **21,** 394–402.
Clarke, V. de V., and Blair, D. H. (1969). *Ann. N.Y. Acad. Sci.* **160,** 645–649.
Clarke, V. de V., and Blair, D. M., and Weber, M. C. (1969). *Cent. Afr. J. Med.* **15,** 1–6.
Clarke, V. de V., Blair, D. M., and Weber, M. (1973). *Rev. Inst. Med. Trop. Sao Paulo* **15,** (Suppl. 1), 73–77.
Clegg, J. A. (1959). *Bull. Res. Counc. Isr.,Sect. G* **8,** 1–6.
Clive, D., Flamm, W. G., and Machesco, M. R. (1972). *Mutat. Res.* **14,** 262–264.
Coelho, B., and Magalhães Filho, A. (1953). *Publ. Avulsas Inst. Aggeu Magalhães, Recife, Braz.* **2,** 61–97.
Coker, C. M. (1957). *Proc. Soc. Exp. Biol. Med.* **96,** 1–3.
Collins, R. F., Davis, M., Edge, N. D., Hill, J., and Turnbull, E. R. (1959). *Brit. J. Pharmacol.* **14,** 467–476.
Connor, T., Stoeckel, M., and Legator, S. M. (1974), *Annu. Meet. Environ. Mutagen Soc. 5th, 1974,* p.31.
Cook, J. A., and Jordan, P. (1971). *Am. J. Trop. Med. Hyg.* **20,** 84–88.
Coura, J. R., and Conceição, M. J. (1974). *Rev. Soc. Brasil. Med. Trop.* **8,** 153–158.
Coura, J. R., Argento, C. A., Figueiredo, N., Wanke, B., and Queiroz, G. C. (1973). *Rev. Inst. Med. Trop. Sao Paulo* **15,** (Suppl. 1), 41–46.
Coutinho, A. (1966). *Folha Med.* **53,** 89–95.
Coutinho, A. D., and Barreto, Y. S. (1971). *Rev. Inst. Med. Trop. Sao Paulo* **13,** 57–70.
Coutinho, A., Lima, C. A., and Alves, C. (1966). *Rev. Inst. Med. Trop. Sao Paulo* **8,** 89–98.
Coutinho, A., Dominques, A. L. C., and Bonfim, J. R. A. (1973). *Rev. Inst. Med. Trop. Sao Paulo* **15,** (Suppl. 1), 15–34.
Cowper, S. G. (1946). *Ann. Trop. Med. Parasitol.* **40,** 163–170.
Cox, K. B., and Oliver-Gonzalez, J. (1969). *Am. J. Trop. Med. Hyg.* **18,** 683–687.
Cox, K. B., and Oliver-Gonzalez, J. (1970). *Am. J. Trop. Med. Hyg.* **19,** 284–299.
Cram, E. B. (1947). *Nat. Inst. Health Bull.* **189,** 49–54.

Cram, E. B., and Figgat, W. B. (1947). *Nat. Inst. Health Bull.* **189,** 106–108.
Cram, E. B., Files, V. S., and Jones, M. F. (1947). *Nat. Inst. Health Bull.* **189,** 81–97.
Cunha, A. S. (1966a). *Folha Med.* **53,** 49–72.
Cunha, A. S. (1966b). *Rev. Inst. Med. Trop. Sao Paulo* **8,** 99–102.
Cunha, A. S. (1970). *In* "Esquistossomose mansoni," pp. 362–363. Editora da Universidade de São Paulo, São Paulo.
Cunha, A. S., and Carvalho, D. G. (1966). *Rev. Inst. Med. Trop. Sao Paulo* **8,** 113–121.
Cunha, A. S., Cançado, J. R., Pellegrino, J., and Oliveira, C. A. (1963). *Rev. Inst. Med. Trop. Sao Paulo* **5,** 75–84.
Cunha, A. S., Carvalho, D. G., and Cambraia, J. N. S. (1971a). *Rev. Inst. Med. Trop. Sao Paulo* **13,** 131–136.
Cunha, A. S., Carvalho, D. G., Cambraia, J. N. S., and Cançado, J. R. (1971b). *Rev. Inst. Med. Trop. Sao Paulo* **13,** 213–222.
Davies, P., and Jackson, H. (1970). *Parasitology* **61,**167–176.
Davis, A. (1961). *Ann. Trop. Med. Parasitol.* **55,** 256–261.
Davis, A. (1963). *East Afr. Med. J.* **40,** 628–634.
Davis, A., and Bailey, D. R. (1969). *Bull. W. H. O.* **41,** 209–224.
Davis, A., Newsome, J., Henderson, J. R., Kettle, J., and Wiggins, L. F. (1965). *East Afr. Med. J.* **42,** 10–30.
Dean, D. A., and Gadd, P. (1973). *Int. J. Parasitol.* **3,** 661–663.
De Carneri, I. (1958). *Arch. Ital. Sci. Med. Trop. Parassitol.* **39,** 400–424.
Denham, D. A., and Holdsworth, R. J. (1971). *Trans. R. Soc. Trop. Med. Hyg.* **65,** 696–697.
Dias, C. B. (1949). Thesis, Federal University of Minas Gerais, Belo Horizonte, Brazil.
Dias, C. B., Borrotchim, M., and Rodrigues da Silva, J. (1952). *Rev. Bras. Med.* **9,** 723–726.
Dickerson, G. (1965). *Nature (London)* **206,** 953–954.
Dodin, A., Ratovondrahety, J., Morreau, J. P., and Richaud, J. (1966). *Acta Trop.* Suppl. 9, 35 44.
El-Abdin, A. Z., Samy, G., Mousa, A. H., El-Raziky, E. H., Roshoy, M. Z., Abd-El-Rahman, H., Hafez, S., and Adham, I. A. (1974). *Egypt. J. Bilharziasis* **1,** 117–133.
El Ayadi, M. S. (1947). *J. Egypt. Med. Assoc.* **30,** 562–566.
El Bitashi, M. D., Abdallah, A., Saif, M., and Taha, A. (1961). *J. Egypt. Med. Assoc.* **42,** 705–718.
Elslager, E. F., Short, F. W., Worth, D. F., Meisenhelder, J. E., Najarian, H., and Thompson, P. E. (1961). *Nature, (London)* **190,** 628–629.
Elslager, E. F., Capps, D. B., Werbel, L. M., Worth, D. F., Meisenhelder, J. E., Najarian, H., and Thompson, P. E. (1963a). *J. Med. Chem.* **6,** 217–219.
Elslager, E. F., Capps, D. B., Kurtz, D. H., Werbel, L. M., and Worth, D. F. (1963b). *J. Med. Chem.* **6,** 646–653.
Elslager, E. F., Capps, D. B., Werbel, L. M., Worth, D. F., Meisenhelder, J. E., and Thompson, P. E. (1964a). *J. Med. Chem.* **7,** 487–493.
Elslager, E. F., Capps, D. B., and Werbel, L. M. (1964b). *J. Med. Chem.* **7,** 658–662.
Elslager, E. F., Capps, D. B., Kurtz, D. H., Short, F. W., Werbel, L. W., and Worth, D. F. (1966). *J. Med. Chem.* **9,** 378–391.
Elslager, E. F., Werbel, L. M., and Worth, D. F. (1970a). *J. Med. Chem.* **13,** 104–109.
Elslager, E. F., Battaglia, J., Phillips, A. A., and Werbel, L. M. (1970b). *J. Med. Chem.* **13,** 587–592.
Elslager, E. F., Hutt, M. P., and Werbel, L. M. (1970c). *J. Med. Chem.* **13,** 542–544.
Ercoli, N. (1967). *Nature (London)* **216,** 398–399.

Ercoli, N. (1968). *Proc. Soc. Exp. Biol. Med.* **129,** 284–290.
Ercoli, N., and Payares, G. (1974). *Exp. Parasitol.* **35,** 171–178.
Erfan, M., and Talaat, S. (1950). *Trans. R. Soc. Trop. Med. Hyg.* **44,** 123–126.
Erickson, D. G., Bourgeois, J. G., and Sadun, E. H. (1971). *J. Pharmacol. Exp. Ther.* **178,** 411–416.
Etges, F. J., and Ritchie, L. S. (1966). *Bull. W. H. O.* **34,** 963–966.
Eyakuse, V. M. (1973). *Rev. Inst. Med. Trop. Sao Paulo* **15** (Suppl. 1), 67–72.
Faigle, J. W., and Keberle, H. (1966). *Acta Trop.* Suppl. 9, 8–22.
Faigle, J. W., and Keberle, H. (1969). *Ann. N.Y. Acad. Sci.* **160,** 544–557.
Faigle, J. W., Blair, D. M., Clarke, V. de V., Davidson, L. A. G., Dukes, D. C., and Keberle, H. (1970a). *Ann. Trop. Med. Parasitol.* **64,** 373–382.
Faigle, J. W., Coutinho, A. D., Keberle, H., and Barreto, F. T. (1970b). *Ann. Trop. Med. Parasitol.* **64,** 383–393.
Fairley, N. H. (1951). *Trans. R. Soc. Trop. Med. Hyg.* **45,** 279–303.
Faria, J., and Pellegrino, J. (1963). *Rev. Inst. Med. Trop. Sao Paulo* **5,** 281–286.
Farid, Z., Schulert, A., Bassily, S., and McConnell, E. (1965). *Ann. Trop. Med. Parasitol.* **59,** 301–303.
Farid, Z., Bassily, S., McConnell, E., and Davis, J. (1967). *Ann. Trop. Med. Parasitol.* **61,** 310–314.
Farid, Z., Smith, J. H., Bassily, S., and Sparks, H. A. (1972). *Br. Med. J.* **2,** 88–89.
Farid, Z., Bassily, S., Young, S., and El Masry, N. A. (1973). *Ann. Trop. Med. Parasitol.* **67,** 233–236.
Figueiredo, J. M. F., and Prata, A. (1969). *Gaz. Med. Bahia* **69,** 16–19.
Figueiredo, J. M. F., Carvalho, E. A., Carvalho, J. S., Macedo, V., Goncalves, H. J. D., and Montenegro, M. A. (1968). *Gaz. Med. Bahia* **68,** 124–131.
Files, V. S. (1951). *Parasitology* **41,** 264–269.
Files, V. S., and Cram, E. B. (1949). *J. Parasitol.* **35,** 555–560.
Forsyth, D. M., and Rashid, C. (1967). *Lancet* **2,** 909–912.
Forsyth, D. M., and Simpson, W. T. (1961). *Ann. Trop. Med. Parasitol.* **55,** 410–412.
Foster, R. (1973). *Rev. Inst. Med. Trop. Sao Paulo* **15,** (Suppl. 1), 1–9.
Foster, R., and Broomfield, K. E. (1971). *Ann. Trop. Med. Parasitol.* **65,** 367–384.
Foster, R., and Cheetham, B. L. (1973). *Trans. R. Soc. Trop. Med. Hyg.* **67,** 674–684.
Foster, R., Cheetham, B. L., Mesmer, E. T., and King, D. F. (1971a). *Ann. Trop. Med. Parasitol.* **65,** 45–58.
Foster, R., Cheetham, B. L., King, D. F., and Mesmer, E. T. (1971b). *Ann. Trop. Med. Parasitol.* **65,** 59–70.
Foster, R., Mesmer, E. T., Cheetham, B. L., and King, D. F. (1971c). *Ann. Trop. Med. Parasitol.* **65,** 221–232.
Foster, R., Cheetham, B. L., and King, D. F. (1973). *Trans. R. Soc. Trop. Med. Hyg.* **67,** 685–693.
Fraga de Azevedo, J., Gil, F. B., Barreira, F., Rocha, R. M., and Monteiro, O. S. (1966). *Ann. Inst. Med. Trop., Lisbon* **23,** 3–10.
Frank, G. H. (1963). *Bull. W. H. O.* **29,** 531–537.
Friedheim, E. A. H. (1967). *Trans. R. Soc. Trop. Med. Hyg.* **61,** 575–579.
Friedheim, E. A. H. (1973). *In* "Chemotherapy of Helminthiasis" (R. Cavier and F. Hawking, eds.), Vol. I, pp. 29–144. Pergamon, Oxford.
Friedheim, E. A. H., and De Jongh, R. T. (1959). *Ann. Trop. Parasitol.* **53,** 316–324.
Friedheim, E. A. H., Rodrigues da Silva, J., and Martins, A. V. (1954). *Am. J. Trop. Med. Hyg.* **3,** 714–727.

Friedheim, E. A. H., Salem, H. H., and El Sherif, A. F. (1959). *Lancet* **2,** 410.
Fripp, P. J. (1967a). *Exp. Parasitol.* **21,** 380–390.
Fripp, P. J. (1967b). *Comp. Biochem. Physiol.* **23,** 897–898.
Fripp, P. J. (1973). *J. Trop. Med. Hyg.* **76,** 316–320.
Frota-Pessoa, O., Ferreira, N. R., Silva, L. C., Chamone, D. A. F., Robles, M. B. P., Moro, A. M., and Otto, P. A. (1973). *Encontro Nacional sobre Esquistossomose, 1st, 1973*, pp. 113–115.
Galvão, F. (1966). *Folha Med.* **53,** 116–125.
Gane, N. F. C. (1971). *Cent. Afr. J. Med.* **17,** 108–109.
Gane, N. F. C. (1973). *Proc. Int. Congr. Trop. Med. Malaria, 9th, 1973*, p. 152.
Garcia, O. S., and Aguirre, G. H. (1969). *Rev. Brasil. Malariol. Doencas Trop.* **21,** 571–582.
Gellhorn, A., Tupikova, N. A., and Van Dyke, H. B. (1946). *J. Pharmacol. Exp. Ther.* **87,** 169–180.
Gellhorn, A., Rose, H. M., and Culbertson, J. T. (1947). *J. Trop. Med. Hyg.* **50,** 27–31.
Generoso, W. M., De Serres, F. J., Huff, S. W., and Cain, K. T. (1972). *Oak Ridge Nat. Lab. Biol. Div., Annu. Progr. Rep.*, pp. 125–126.
Gentilini, M., Capron, A., Le Parco, J. C., Vernes, A., Biguet, J., and Domart, A. (1967). *Bull. Soc. Pathol. Exot.* **60,** 241–263.
Gilles, H. M. (1967). *Trans. R. Soc. Trop. Med. Hyg.* **61,** 571–573.
Godoy, P., Oliveira, M. C., Raso, P., Marinho, R. P., and Neves, J. (1974). *Rev. Inst. Med. Trop. Sao Paulo* **16,** 114–120.
Goldsmith, E. I., Luz, F. F. C., Prata, A., and Kean, B. H. (1967). *J. Am. Med. Assoc.* **199,** 235–240.
Gönnert, R. (1955a). *Z. Tropenmed. Parasitol.* **6,** 33–52.
Gönnert, R. (1955b). *Z. Tropenmed. Parasitol.* **6,** 257–279.
Gordon, B. L., and St. John, P. A. (1963). *Nature (London)* **200,** 790–791.
Gouveia, O. F., and Teixeira, D. (1963). *Hospital (Rio de Janeiro)* **63,** 639–653.
Haese, W. H., Smith, D. L., and Bueding, E. (1973). *J. Pharmacol. Exp. Ther.* **186,** 430–440.
Halawani, A. E. (1946). *J. Egypt. Public Health Assoc.* **21,**219–226.
Halawani, A. E. (1964). In Friedheim, 1973.
Halawani, A. E., Abdallah, A., Shakir, M. H., and Saif, M. (1955). *J. Egypt. Med. Assoc.* **38,** 711-717.
Hartman, P. E., Levine, K., Hartman, Z., and Berger, H. (1971). *Science* **172,** 1058–1060.
Henry, D. W., Brown, V. H., Cory, M., Johansson, J. G., and Bueding, E. (1973). *J. Med. Chem.* **16,** 1287–1291.
Hess, R., Faigle, J. W., and Lambert, C. (1966). *Nature (London)* **210,** 964–965.
Hill, J. (1956). *Ann. Trop. Med. Parasitol.* **50,** 39–48.
Hill, J. (1964). In Friedheim, 1973.
Hill, J., Rust, M. A., Pellegrino, J., and Faria, J. (1966). *J. Parasitol.* **52,** 822.
Hillman, G. R., and Senft, A. W. (1973). *J. Pharmacol. Exp. Ther.* **185,** 177–184.
Hillman, G. R., Olsen, N. J., and Senft, A. W. (1974). *J. Pharmacol. Exp. Ther.* **188,** 529–535.
Hoffman, V. A., Pons, J. A., and Janer, J. L. (1934). *P. R. J. Public Health Trop. Med.* **9,** 283–291.
Hsiao, S. H., and Lo, W. C. (1962). *Recent Exp. Res. Ther. Schistosomiasis, Recent Important Special Topic Rep. Sci. Res. Parasitic Diseases* (L. C. Fong and S. P. Mao, eds.) Shangai Sci. Tech. Intelligence Res. Cent.

Huang, L. S., and Chen, C. (1963). *Yao Hsueh Hsueh Pao* **10,** 622.
Igali, S., and von Borstel, R. C. (1974). *Ann. Meet. Environ. Mutagen Soc. 5th, 1974,* pp. 26–27.
Islip, P. J., Closier, M. D., Neville, M. C., Werbel, L. M., and Capps, D. B. (1972). *J. Med. Chem.* **15,** 951–954.
Islip, P. J., Closier, M. D., and Weale, J. E. (1973a). *J. Med. Chem.* **16,** 1027–1030.
Islip, P. J., Closier, M. D., and Neville, M. C. (1973b). *J. Med. Chem.* **16,** 1030–1034.
Jackson, H., Davies, P., and Block, M. (1968). *Nature (London)* **218,** 977.
Jaffe, J. J., Meymarian, E., and Doremus, H. M. (1971). *Nature (London)* **230,** 408–409.
Jansma, W. B., Hulbert, P. B., and Bueding, E. (1974). *Fed. Proc. Fed. Am. Soc. Exp. Biol.* **33,** No. 3, Part 1.
Janssens, P. G., Muynck, A., and Sieniawski, J. (1965). *Trop. Geogr. Med.* **17,** 112–120.
Jarumilinta, R., Ruas, A., and Lambert, C. R. (1968). *Ann. Trop. Med. Parasitol.* **62,** 154–157.
Jesus, J. A., and Hernandez-Morales, F. (1959). *G. E. N.* **13,** 119–120.
Jewsbury, J. M. (1972). *Ann. Trop. Med. Parasitol.* **66,** 409–419.
Jewsbury, J. M. (1973). *Ann. Trop. Med. Parasitol.* **67,** 431–438.
Jordan, P. (1966). *Br. Med. J.* **1,** 276–278.
Jordan, P., and Randall, K. (1962). *Trans. R. Soc. Trop. Med. Hyg.* **56,** 523–528.
Julião, A. F., Vallaba, L. P. Crossmann, A. P., and Bassoi, O. N. (1969). *Hospital (Rio de Janeiro)* **76,** 2229–2234.
Kagan, I. G., and Geiger, S. J. (1965). *J. Parasitol.* **51,** 622–627.
Kagan, I. G., and Pellegrino, J. (1961). *Bull. W. H. O.* **25,** 611–674.
Kato, K. (1960). In Martin and Beaver, 1968.
Katz, N. (1965). Unpublished data.
Katz, N. (1966). *Folha Med.* **53,** 34–37.
Katz, N. (1971). *Rev. Soc. Bras. Med. Trop.* **5,** 55–60.
Katz, N. (1972). *Rev. Assoc. Med. Minas Gerais* **23,** 27–34.
Katz, N., and Pellegrino, J. (1974a). *Adv. Parasitol.* **12,** 369–390.
Katz, N., and Pellegrino, J. (1974b). *Rev. Inst. Med. Trop. Sao Paulo* **16,** 245–252.
Katz, N., and Pellegrino, J. (1974c). *Rev. Inst. Med. Trop. Sao Paulo* **16,** 346–353.
Katz, N., Bittencourt, D., Oliveira, C. A., Dias, R. P., Ferreira, H., Grimbaum, E., Dias, C. B., and Pellegrino, J. (1966a). *Folha Med.* **53,** 561–567.
Katz, N., Pellegrino, J., and Memória, J. M. P. (1966b). *J. Parasitol.* **52,** 917–919.
Katz, N., Cançado, F. A. X., and Pellegrino, J. (1967a). *Folha Med.* **54,** 795–805.
Katz, N., Pellegrino, J., Oliveira, C. A., and Cunha, A. S. (1967b). *J. Parasitol.* **53,** 1229–1232.
Katz, N., Pellegrino, J., Ferreira, M. T., Oliveira, C. A., and Dias, C. B. (1968a). *Am. J. Trop. Med. Hyg.* **17,** 743–746.
Katz, N., Pellegrino, J., and Pereira, J. P. (1968b). *Rev. Soc. Bras. Med. Trop.* **2,** 237–245.
Katz, N., Pellegrino, J., and Oliveira, C. A. (1969). *Am. J. Trop. Med. Hyg.* **18,** 924–929.
Katz, N., Coelho, P. M. Z., and Pellegrino, J. (1970a). *J. Parasitol.* **56,** 1032–1033.
Katz, N., Antunes, C. M. F., Andrade, R. M., Pellegrino, J., and Coelho, P. M. Z. (1970b). *J. Parasitol.* **56,** 434.
Katz, N., Chaves, A., and Pellegrino, J. (1972). *Rev. Inst. Med. Trop. Sao Paulo* **14,** 397–400.
Katz, N., Dias, E. P., Araújo, N., and Souza, C. P. (1973a). *Rev. Soc. Bras. Med. Trop.* **7,** 382–387.

Katz, N., Pellegrino, J., Grimbaum, E., Chaves, A., and Zicker, F. (1973b). *Rev. Inst. Med. Trop. Sao Paulo* **15,** 25–29.

Katz, N., Pellegrino, J., Grimbaum, E., Chaves, A., and Zicker, F. (1973c). *Rev. Inst. Med. Trop. Sao Paulo* **15,** (Suppl. 1), 35–40.

Katz, N., Grimbaum, E., Chaves, A., Zicker, F., and Pellegrino, J. (1976). *Rev. Inst. Med. Trop. Sao Paulo,* in press.

Kaump, D. H., Schardein, J. L., Woosley, E. T., and Fisken, R. A. (1965). *Cancer Res.* **25,** 1919–1924.

Kaye, B., and Woolhouse, N. M. (1972). *Xenobiotica* **2,** 169–178.

Khalil, M. B. (1931). In Dias, 1949.

Khalil, M. B., and Betache, M. H. (1930). *Lancet* **218,** 234–235.

Khayyal, M. T. (1964), *Br. J. Pharmacol.* **22,** 342–348.

Khayyal, M. T. (1965a). *Nature (London)* **205,** 1331–1332.

Khayyal, M. T. (1965b). *Bull. W. H. O.* **33,** 589–591.

Khayyal, M. T. (1969). *Bull. W. H. O.* **40,** 959–963.

Khayyal, M. T., Girgis, N. I., and McConnell, E. (1967). *Bull. W. H. O.* **37,** 387–392.

Khayyal, M. T., Saleh, S., and El-Masri, A. M. (1973). *Bull. W. H. O.* **48,** 415–420.

Kikuth, W., and Gönnert, R. (1948). *Ann. Trop. Med. Parasitol.* **42,** 256–267.

Kikuth, W., Gönnert, R., and Mauss, H. (1946). *Naturwissenschaften* **33,** 253–254.

Kloetzel, K. (1966). *Folha Med.* **53,** 125–127.

Koch, K. R., and Kux, P. (1951). *Z. Tropenmed. Parasitol.* **3,** 94–100.

Lagrange, E. (1963). *C. R. Seances Soc. Biol. Paris* **157,** 425–427.

Lambert, C. R. (1964). *Ann. Trop. Med. Parasitol.* **58,** 292–303.

Lambert, C. R. (1967). *Trans. R. Soc. Trop. Med. Hyg.* **61,** 559–562.

Lambert, C. R., and Stauffer, P. (1964). *Ann. Trop. Med. Parasitol.* **58,** 292–303.

Lambert, C. R., Wilhelm, M., and Striebel, H. (1964). *Experientia* **20,** 452–453.

Lambert, C. R., and Stauffer, P. (1964). *Ann. Trop Med. Parasitol.* **58,** 292–303.

Lambert, C. R., Sinari, U. S. P., and Tripod, J. (1965). *Acta Trop.* **22,** 155–161.

Lämmler, G. (1958). *Z. Tropenmed. Parasitol.* **9,** 294–310.

Lämmler, G. (1963). *Proc. Int. Congr. Trop. Med. Malaria, 7th, 1963* p. 36.

Lämmler, G. (1964). *Z. Tropenmed. Parasitol.* **15,** 337–368.

Lämmler, G. (1968). *Adv. Chemother.* **3,** 153–251.

Lämmler, G., and Petranyi, G. (1971). *Bull. W. H. O.* **44,** 739–750.

Lämmler, G., and Schuster, J. (1974). *Z. Tropenmed. Parasitol.* **25,** 66–74.

Lampe, P. H. J. (1926). *J. Trop. Med. Hyg.* **29,** 4–10.

Lapierre, J., Holler, C., Saison, E., and Hien, T. V. (1973). *Nouv. Presse Med.* **2,** 901–905.

Lariviére, M., Hocquet, P., and Michel, R. (1960). *Bull. Soc. Pathol. Exot.* **53,** 996–1010.

Lasbrey, F. O., and Colleman, R. B. (1921). *Br. Med. J.* **1,** 299–301.

Lee, H. G. (1972). *Bull. W. H. O.* **46,** 397–402.

Lee, H. G., Cheever, A. W., and Fairweather, W. R. (1971). *Bull. W. H. O.* **45,** 147–155.

Lees, R. E. M. (1966). *Trans. R. Soc. Trop. Med. Hyg.* **60,** 233–236.

Legator, M. S., Stoeckel, M., and Connor, T. (1974). *Annu. Meet. Environ. Mutagen Soc. 5th, 1974*, pp. 30–31.

Lei, H. H., Chang, L. C., Hsu, M. L., Chang, S. P., Tzin, K. C., and Yen, M. (1964). *Sci Sinica* **13,** 523–524.

Lemos, V., Dorico, D. M., Losada, H. V., Martins, R., Miranda, S. L., Costa, V. P., and Alvariz, F. G. (1969). Presented at the XXI Brasilian Congress of Gastroenterology, Recife.

Lennox, R. W., and Bueding, E. (1972). *Am. J. Trop. Med. Hyg.* **21,** 302–306.
Liang, Y. I., Chu, H. C., Tsen, G. Y. I., and Ting, K. S. (1957a). *Sheng Li Hsueh Pao* **21,** 24–32.
Liang, Y. I., Shen, M. L., Chen, E. H., and Ting, K. S. (1957b). *Sheng Li Hsueh Pao* **21,** 235.
Lichtenberg, F., and Ritchie, L. S. (1961). *Am. J. Trop. Med. Hyg.* **10,** 859–869.
Lippincott, S. W., Ellerbrook, L. D., Rhees, M., and Mason, P. (1947). *J. Clin. Invest.* **26,** 370–378.
Lu, C. Y., Lin, C. J., Shu, H. C., and Lao, J. H. (1965). *Yao Hsueh Hsueh Pao* **12,** 416.
Luttermoser, G. W. (1954). *J. Parasitol.* **40,** 130–137.
Luttermoser, G. W. (1959). *J. Parasitol.* **45,** 301–309.
Luttermoser, G. W., and Bond, H. W. (1954). *J. Parasitol.* **40,** 33–34.
Luttermoser, G. W., and De Witt, W. B. (1961). *Am. J. Trop. Med. Hyg.* **10,** 541–546.
Luttermoser, G. W., Bruce, J. I., and McMullen, D. B. (1960). *Am. J. Trop. Med. Hyg.* **9,** 39–45.
McCaffrey, R. P., Farid, Z., and Kent, D. C. (1972). *Trans. R. Soc. Trop. Med. Hyg.* **66,** 795–797.
MacDonald, F., Clarke, V. de V., Gaddie, P., and Atkinson, G. (1973). *Cent. Afr. J. Med.* (Suppl.), **19,** 22–32.
Machado, A. B., Silva, M. L., and Pellegrino, J. (1970). *J. Parasitol.* **56,** 392–393.
McMahon, J. E. (1967). *Trans. R. Soc. Trop. Med. Hyg.* **61,** 648–652.
McMahon, J. E., and Kilala, C. P. (1966). *Br. Med. J.* **2,** 1047–1049.
Magaldi, C. (1966). *Folha Med.* **53,** 115–116.
Mainzer, F., and Krause, M. (1940). *Trans. R. Soc. Trop. Med.* **33,** 405–418.
Maldonado, J. F., and Acosta Matienzo, J. (1948). *Am. J. Trop. Med.* **28,** 645–657.
Maldonado, J. F., Acosta Matienzo, J., and Vélez Herrera, F. (1950a). *P. R. J. Public Health Trop. Med.* **25,** 359–366.
Maldonado, J. F., Acosta Matienzo, J., and Vélez Herrera, F. (1950b). *P. R. J. Public Health Trop. Med.* **26,** 85–91.
Mansour, T. E., and Bueding, E. (1953). *Br. J. Pharmacol. Chemother.* **8,** 431–434.
Mansour, T. E., and Bueding, E. (1954). *Br. J. Pharmacol.* **9,** 459–462.
Mansour, T. E., Bueding, E., and Stavitsky, A. B. (1954). *Br. J. Pharmacol. Chemother.* **9,** 182–186.
Mao, Y. C., Sheng, S. C., Tu, C. K., Fang, J. C., Fang, K. Y., Shen, J. S., Chou, S. N., and Huang, C. Y. (1959). *Chin. Med. J.* **78,** 532–541.
Marinho, R. P., Godoy, P., Raso, P., and Neves, J. (1974a). *Rev. Inst. Med. Trop. Sao Paulo* **16,** 54–59.
Marinho, R. P., Godoy, P., Raso, P., and Neves, J. (1974b). *Rev. Inst. Med. Trop. Sao Paulo* **16,** 354–361.
Maritz, J. C. (1969). *S. Afr. Med. J.* **43,** 1320.
Maritz, J. C. (1970). *S. Afr. Med. J.* **44,** 126–128.
Marques, R. J. (1966). *Folha Med.* **53,** 81–89.
Martin, L. K., and Beaver, C. P. (1968). *Am. J. Trop. Med. Hyg.* **17,** 382–391
Martins, H. J. C., Freitas, O. N., and Alvariz, F. G. (1968). Presented at the XX Brasilian Congress of Gastroenterology, São Paulo.
Martins da Rocha, R., and Gill, F. B. (1966). *Acta Trop.* Suppl. 9, 23–27.
Mauss, H. (1948). *Chem. Ber.* **81,** 91–31.
Medeiros, J. L., Laurentys, L. L., Nunes, A., Alves Filho, N., and Boucinhas, J. (1972). Presented at the VIII Congress of the Brasilian Society of Tropical Medicine, Belo Horizonte.

Medina, H. S. G., Vianna, M. J. B., Tse, H. C., Cerósimo, F., Brumer, A., Jr., and Bacila, M. (1972). *Cienc. Cult. (Sao Paulo)* **24,** 350.
Meira, J. A. (1951). Thesis, University of São Paulo, São Paulo, Brazil.
Meisenhelder, J. E., and Thompson, P. E. (1963). *J. Parasitol.* **49,** 567–570.
Mendonça, J. S. S., Amato Neto, V., Levy, A., and Martins Filho, J. (1970). *Rev. Medica IAMSPE* **1,** 131–133.
Michaels, R. M. (1969). *Exp. Parasitol.* **25,** 58–71.
Michaels, R. M., and Prata, A. (1968). *J. Parasitol.* **54,** 921–930.
Michelson, E. H. (1961). *Am. J. Hyg.* **73,** 66–74.
Molokhia, M. M., and Smith, H. (1969). *Bull. W. H. O.* **40,** 123–128.
Monteiro, W., Pellegrino, J., and Silva, M. L. (1968). *J. Parasitol.* **54,** 175–176.
Moore, D. V., and Meleney, H. E. (1955). *J. Parasitol.* **41,** 235–245.
Moore, D. V., Yolles, T. K., and Meleney, H. E. (1949). *J. Parasitol.* **35,** 156–170.
Moore, D. V., Thillet, C. J., Carney, D. M., and Meleney, H. E. (1953). *J. Parasitol.* **39,** 215–221.
Moore, J. A. (1972). *Nature (London)* **239,** 107–109.
Morales, F. H., and Oliver-Gonzalez, J. (1972). *Bol. Asoc. Med. P. R.* **64,** 5–7.
Mousa, A. H., El-Abdin, A. Z., El-Garem, A. A., El-Raziky, E. A., and Fadl, A. A. (1970). *O.A.U. Symp. Schistosomiasis*, Addis Ababa, Ethiopia.
Nibih, I., and Zoroob, H. (1971). *Experientia* **27,** 143–144.
Nagaty, H. F., and Rifaat, M. A. (1960). *J. Egypt. Med. Assoc.* **43,** 678–695.
National Schistosomiasis Research Committee (1959a). *Chin. Med. J.* **78,** 368–379.
National Schistosomiasis Research Committee (1959b). *Chin. Med. J.* **78,** 461–489.
Neves, J. (1966). *Folha Med.* **53,** 37–48.
Neves, P. F., and Costa, P. D. (1969). *Hospital (Rio de Janeiro)* **75,** 857–861.
Newsome, J. (1953). *Trans. R. Soc. Trop. Med. Hyg.* **47,** 428–430.
Newsome, J. (1962a). *Nature (London)* **195,** 722–723.
Newsome, J. (1962b). *In* "Bilharziasis" (G. E. W. Wolstenholme and M. O'Connor, eds), pp. 310–317. Little, Brown, Boston, Massachusetts.
Newsome, J. (1962c). *Nature (London)* **195,** 1175–1179.
Newsome, J. (1963). *Trans. R. Soc. Trop. Med. Hyg.* **57,** 425–432.
Newton, W. L. (1953). *Exp. Parasitol.* **2,** 242–257.
Nimmo-Smith, R. H., and Raison, C. G. (1968). *Comp. Biochem. Physiol.* **24,** 403–416.
Nohmi, N. (1966). *Folha Med.* **53,** 72–79.
Oesterlin, M. (1934). *Arch. Schiffs-Trop.-Hyg.* **38,** 433–441.
Okpala, I. (1959). *West Afr. Med. J.* **8,** 94–101.
Oliveira, C. A., Chamone, D. A. F., Lemos, M. Z., Melo, J. R. C., Zeitune, J. M. R., Costa, W. O. P., and Cangussú, W. A. (1969). *Rev. Inst. Med. Trop. Sao Paulo* **11,** 130–139.
Oliveira, C. A., Zeitune, J. M. R., Chamone, D. A. F., Melo, J. R. C., and Salgado, J. A. (1971). *Rev. Inst. Med. Trop. Sao Paulo* **13,** 202–212.
Oliver-Gonzalez, J. (1967). *Am. J. Trop. Med. Hyg.* **16,** 565–567.
Oliver-Gonzalez, J. (1968). *Proc. Soc. Exp. Biol. Med.* **128,** 1029–1033.
Oliver-Gonzalez, J., Ramos, F. L., and Coker, C. M. (1955). *Am. J. Trop. Med. Hyg.* **4,** 908–912.
Olivier, L., and Stirewalt, M. A. (1952). *J. Parasitol.* **38,** 19–23.
Olivier, L., Haskins, W. T., and Gurian, J. (1962). *Bull. W. H. O.* **27,** 87–94.
Omer, A. H., Abdullah, E. A., Elhassan, A. M., and Wasfi, A. M. (1972). *J. Trop. Med. Hyg.* **75,** 165–168.
Ong, T. M. (1974). *Annu. Meet. Environ. Mutagen Soc. 5th, 1974,* pp. 23–24.

Ong, T. M., and de Serres, F. J. (1972). *Oak Ridge Nat. Lab. Biol. Div. Annu. Progr. Rep.*, p. 80

Ongom, V. L. (1971). *East Afr. Med. J.* **48,** 247–250.

Oostburg, B. F. (1972). *Trop. Geogr. Med.* **24,** 148–151.

Ottens, H., and Dickerson, G. (1969). *Nature (London)* **223,** 506–507.

Ottens, H., and Dickerson, G. (1972). *Trans. R. Soc. Trop. Med. Hyg.* **66,** 85–107.

Otto, G. F., and Maren, T. H. (1950). *Am. J. Hyg.* **51,** 353–395.

Otto, G. F., Maren, T. H., and Brown, H. W. (1947). *Am. J. Hyg.* **46,** 193–211.

Ottolina, C., and Atencio, H. M. (1943). *Rev. Policl. Caracas.* **12,** 1–35.

Paraense, W. L., and Corrêa, L. R. (1963). *Rev. Inst. Med. Trop. Sao Paulo* **5,** 15–22.

Pedrique, M. R., and Sanz, M. (1970). G. E. N. **24,** 379–386.

Pedrique, M. R., Barbera, S., and Ercoli, N. (1970). *Ann. Trop. Med. Parasitol* **64,** 255–261.

Pedro, R. J., Amato Neto, V., Freddi, N. A., Bertazzoli, S. B., and Dias, L. C. S. (1973). *Rev. Inst. Med. Trop. Sao Paulo* **15,** (Suppl. 1), 63–66.

Pellegrino, J. (1956). *J. Parasitol.* **51,** 683–684.

Pellegrino, J., and Brener, Z. (1956). *J. Parasitol.* **42,** 564.

Pellegrino, J., and Faria, J. (1964). *J. Parasitol.* **50,** 587.

Pellegrino, J., and Faria, J. (1965). *Am. J. Trop. Med. Hyg.* **14,** 363–369.

Pellegrino, J., and Gonçalves, M. G. R. (1965). *J. Parasitol.* **51,** 1014.

Pellegrino, J., and Katz, N. (1968). *Adv. Parasitol.* **6,** 233–290.

Pellegrino, J., and Katz, N. (1969). *Rev. Inst. Med. Trop. Sao Paulo* **11,** 215–221.

Pellegrino, J., and Katz, N. (1972). *Rev. Inst. Med. Trop. Sao Paulo* **14,** 59–66.

Pellegrino, J., and Katz, N. (1974). *Rev. Inst. Med. Trop. Sao Paulo* **16,** 301–304.

Pellegrino. J., and Katz, N. (1975). *Rev. Inst. Med. Trop. Sao Paulo* **17,** 199–205.

Pellegrino, J., and Machado, A. (1972). *Rev. Bras. Pesqui. Med. Biol.* **5,** 43–45.

Pellegrino, J., Oliveira, C. A., Faria, J., and Cunha, A. S. (1962). *Am. J. Trop. Med. Hyg.* **11,** 201–215.

Pellegrino, J., Oliveira, C. A., and Faria, J. (1963). *J. Parasitol.* **49,** 365–370.

Pellegrino, J., De Maria, M., and Faria, J. (1965a). *J. Parasitol.* **51,** 1015.

Pellegrino, J., Katz, N., Oliveira, C. A., and Okabe, K. (1965b). *J. Parasitol.* **51,** 617–621.

Pellegrino, J., Katz, N., and Raick, A. (1966). *Folha Med.* **52,** 333–342.

Pellegrino, J., Katz, N., and Scherrer, J. F. (1967a). *J. Parasitol.* **53,** 55–59.

Pellegrino, J., Katz, N., and Scherrer, J. F. (1967b). *J. Parasitol.* **53,** 1225–1228.

Pellegrino, J., Katz, N., and Dias, E. P. (1973). *Rev. Inst. Med. Trop. Sao Paulo* **15,** (Suppl. 1), 10–14.

Pereira, L. H., Pellegrino, J., Valadares, T. E., Mello, R. T., and Coelho, P. M. Z. (1974). *Rev. Inst. Med. Trop. Sao Paulo* **16,** 123–126.

Pesigan, T. P., Banzon, A. T., Santos, J., Noseñas, J., and Zataba, R. G. (1967). *Bull. W. H. O.* **36,** 263–274.

Petranyi, G. (1969). Thesis, Justus Liebig University, Giessen, Germany.

Powers, K. G. (1965). *J. Parasitol.* **51,** 53.

Prata, A. (1956). *Hospital (Rio de Janeiro)* **6,** 259–266.

Prata, A. (1957). Thesis, Serviço Nacional de Educação Sanitaria, Rio de Janeiro, Brazil.

Prata, A. (1966). *Hospital (Rio de Janeiro)* **69,** 175–177.

Prata, A., Oliveira, C. A., Rodrigues da Silva, J., Campos, R., and Amato Neto, V. (1965). *Hospital (Rio de Janeiro)* **68,** 1097–1106.

Prata, A., Machado, R., and Macedo, V. (1966). *Acta Trop. Suppl.* **9,** 180–186.

Prata, A., Figueiredo, J. F. M., Brandt, P. C., and Lauria, L. (1973). *Rev. Inst. Med. Trop. Sao Paulo* **15,** (Suppl. 1), 47–57.

Prates, M. D., and Franco. L. T. (1966). *Acta Trop. Suppl.* **9,** 287–288.
Radke, M. G., Broome, P. B., and Belanger, G. S. (1971). *Exp. Parasitol.* **30,** 1–10.
Raison, C. G., and Standen, O. D. (1954a). *Br. J. Pharmacol.* **10,** 191–199.
Raison, C. G., and Staden, O. D. (1954b). *Trans. R. Soc. Trop. Med. Hyg.* **48,** 446–447.
Raison, C. G., and Staden, O. D. (1955). *Br. J. Pharmacol. Chemother.* **10,** 191–199.
Ramos-Morales, F., Correa-Coronas, R., and Jesus, L. G. (1969). *Ann. N.Y. Acad. Sci.* **160,** 670–685.
Rees, P. H., Roberts, J. M. D., Oomen, L. F. A., and Mutinga, M. J. (1970). *East Afr. Med. J.* **47,** 634–638.
Rees, P. H., Roberts, J. M. D., Woodger, B. A., and Pamba, H. O. (1973). *Rev. Inst. Med. Trop. Sao Paulo* **15,** (Suppl.1), 78–82.
Richards, H. C., and Foster, R. (1969). *Nature (London)* **222,** 581–582.
Ritchie, L. S., and Berrios-Duran, L. A. (1961). *J. Parasitol.* **47,** 363–365.
Ritchie, L. S., Berrios-Duran, L. A., and Deweese, R. (1963). *Am. J. Trop. Med. Hyg.* **12,** 264–268.
Ritchie, L. S., Hernandez, A., and Rosa Amador, R. (1966a). *Am. J. Trop. Med. Hyg.* **15,** 614–617.
Ritchie, L. S., Knight, W. B., McMullen, D. B., and Lichtenberg, F. (1966b). *Am. J. Trop. Med. Hyg.* **15,** 43–49.
Robinson, C. H., Bueding, E., and Fisher, J. (1970). *Mol. Pharmacol.* **6,** 604–616.
Robinson, D. L. H. (1960). *Ann. Trop. Med. Parasit.* **54,** 112–117.
Rocha, L. R. S. C., and Katz, N. (1973). *Ciênc. Cult. (Sao Paulo)* **25,** 348–350.
Rodrigues da Silva, J. (1948). *Vida Med.* **15,** 6–20.
Rodrigues da Silva, J. (1953). *Rev. Bras. Med.* **9,** 577–581.
Rodrigues da Silva, J. (1958). *Proc. Int. Congr. Trop. Med. Malaria, 6th, 1958*, pp. 89–100.
Rodrigues da Silva, J. (1966a). *Acta Trop.* Suppl. 9, 283–286.
Rodrigues da Silva, J. (1966b). *Folha Med.* **53,** 128–130.
Rodrigues da Silva, J., and Dias, C. B. (1957). *Rev. Assoc. Med. Bras.* **3,** 33–36.
Rodrigues da Silva, J., Prata, A., Argento, C. A., Brasil, H. A., and Ferreira, L. F. (1963). *Proc. Int. Congr. Trop. Med. Malaria, 7th, 1963*, p. 119.
Rodrigues da Silva, J., Argento, C. A., and Brasil, H. A. (1964). *Rev. Bras. Malariol. Doencas Trop.* **16,** 295–300.
Rodriguez Molina, R. Acevedo, C. E., Torres, J. M., Lopez-Sanabria, V., and Ramirez-Rodriguez, E. (1950). *Am. J. Trop. Med.* **30,** 881–886.
Rodriguez Molina, R., Lichtemberg, F., Gonzalez, J, and Rivera de Sala, A. (1959). *Am. J. Trop. Med. Hyg.* **8,** 565–569.
Rodriguez Molina, R., Oliver-Gonzalez, J., and Rivera de Sala, A. (1962). *J. Am. Med. Assoc.* **182,** 1001–1004.
Rogers, S. H., and Bueding, E. (1971). *Science* **172,** 1057–1058.
Rosanelli, J. D., and Price, D. L. (1963). *Am. J. Trop. Med.* **12,** 758–760.
Rosi, D., Peruzzotti, G., Dennis, E. W., Berberian, D. A., Freele, H., and Archer, S. (1965). *Nature (London)* **208,** 1005–1006.
Rosi, D., Lewis, T. R., Lorenz, R., Freele, H., Berberian, D. A., and Archer, S. (1967). *J. Med. Chem.* **10,** 877–880.
Ross, A. F., and Jaffe, J. J. (1972). *Biochem. Pharmacol.* **21,** 3059–3069.
Rowan, W. B. (1958). *J. Parasitol.* **44,** 247.
Ruas, A., and Franco, L. T. A. (1966). *Ann. Trop. Med. Parasitol.* **60,** 288–292.
Russell, W. L. (1973). *Proc. Int. Congr. Trop. Med. Malaria, 9th, 1973*, p. 175.
Russell, W. L., and Kelly, E. M. (1972). *Oak Ridge Nat. Lab., Biol. Div., Annu. Progr. Rep.,* pp. 113–114.

Sadun, E. H., Bruce, J. I. Moose, J. W., and McMullen, W. B. (1966). *Acta Trop. Suppl.* **9,** 69–77.
Salem, H. H. (1965). *Trans. R. Soc. Trop. Med. Hyg.* **59,** 307–317.
Salem, H. H., and El Sherif, A. F. (1961). *J. Egypt. Public Health Assoc.* **36,** 129–146.
Salem, H. H., El Sherif, A. F., Abd-Rabbo, H., Morcoss, W., and El-Ninny, H. M. (1961). *J. Egypt. Public Health Assoc.* **36,** 39–62.
Salgado, J. A., Velloso, C., Oliveira, C. A., Chamone, S. A. F., Lemos, M. S., Katz, N., and Pellegrino, J. (1968). *Rev. Inst. Med. Trop. Sao Paulo* **10,** 312–315.
Salgado, J. A., Velloso, C., Galizzi, J., Jr., Oliveira, J. P. M., and Tavares, E. C. P. (1972). *Rev. Soc. Bras. Med. Trop.* **6,** 129–133.
Sandt, D. G., Bruce, J. I., and Radke, M. G. (1965). *J. Parasitol.* **51,** 1012–1013.
Saoud, M. F. A. (1965). *J. Helminthol.* **39,** 363–376.
Saz, H. J., and Bueding, E. (1966). *Pharmacol. Rev.* **18,** 871–894.
Schneider, J., and Sansarricq, H. (1959). *Med. Trop.* **19,** 412–424.
Schubert, M. (1948a). *Am. J. Trop. Med.* **28,** 121–136.
Schubert, M. (1948b). *Am J. Trop. Med.* **28,** 137–156.
Schubert, M. (1948c). *Am. J. Trop. Med.* **28,** 157–162.
Schubert, M., Golberg, E., and Schreiber, F. G. (1949). *Am. J. Trop. Med.* **29,** 115–127.
Schwink, T. M. (1955). *J. Parasitol.* **41,** 26.
Scott, J. A. (1942a). *Am. J. Hyg.* **35,** 337–366.
Scott, J. A. (1942b). *Am. J. Trop. Med.* **22,** 647–655.
Senft, A. W. (1963). *Ann. N.Y. Acad. Sci.* **113,** 272–288.
Senft, A. W. (1965). *Ann. Trop. Med. Parasitol.* **59,** 164–168.
Senft, A. W. (1966). *Comp. Biochem. Physiol.* **18,** 209–216.
Senft, A. W., and Hillman, G. R. (1973). *Am. J. Trop. Med. Hyg.* **22,** 734–742.
Senft, A. W., Miech, R. P., Brown, P. R., and Senft, D. G. (1972). *Int. J. Parasitol.* **2,** 249–260.
Senft, A. W., Senft, D. G., and Miech, R. P. (1973a). *Biochem. Pharmacol.* **22,** 437–447.
Senft, A. W., Crabtree, G. W., Agarwal, K. C., Scholar, E. M., Agarwal, R. P., and Parks, R. E., Jr. (1973b). *Biochem. Pharmacol.* **22,** 449–458.
Sherif, A. F., El-Sawy, M. F., Barakat, P. H., and Barakat, R. (1971). *Bull. High Inst. Public Health Alexandria* **1,** 9–21.
Shoeb, H. A., Keira, M. A., Gingis, N. I., Henry, W., and Mousa, A. H. (1970). *J. Egypt. Med. Assos.* **53,** 108–112.
Sieber, S. M., Whang-Peng, J., Johns, D. G., and Adamson, R. H. (1972). *Biochem. Pharmacol.* **22,** 1253–1262.
Silva, L. C. (1966). *Folha Med.* **53,** 111–112.
Silva, L. C., Camargo, M. E., Hoshino, S., Gunji, J., Lopes, J. D., Chamone, D. F., Martinez, J. O., Ferri, R. G., Rothstein, W., Silva, G. R., Genevia, A. C., and Cardoso, E. J. (1971). *Rev. Inst. Med. Trop. Sao Paulo* **13,** 121–130.
Silva, L. C., Sette, H., Jr., Chamone, D. A. F., Alquezar, A. S., and Monteiro, A. A. (1972). *Rev. Inst. Med. Trop. Sao Paulo* **15,** (Suppl. 1), 58–62.
Silva, L. C., Sette, H., Jr., Chamone, D. A. F., Alquezar, A. S., Punskas, J. A., and Raia, S. (1974). *Rev. Inst. Med. Trop. Sao Paulo* **16,** 103–109.
Silva, P., and Prata, A. (1962). *Rev. Med. Bahia* **18,** 40–44.
Smith, R. H. (1972). *Oak Ridge Nat. Lab. Biol. Div. Annu. Progr. Rep.* pp. 105–107.
Smith, T. M., and Brooks, T. G., Jr. (1969). *Parasitology* **59,** 293–298.
Smithers, S. R. (1960). *Trans. R. Soc. Trop. Med. Hyg.* **54,** 68–70.
Smithers, S. R., and Terry, R. J. (1965). *Parasitology* **55,** 701–710.
Sonnet, J., and Doyen, A. (1969). *Ann. N.Y. Acad. Sci.* **160,** 786–798.

Souza, C. P., and Katz, N. (1973). *Cienc. Cult.* **25,** 345–348.
Standen, O. D. (1949). *Ann. Trop. Med. Parasitol.* **43,** 268–283.
Standen, O. D. (1951a). *Ann. Trop. Med. Parasitol.* **45,** 80–83.
Standen, O. D. (1951b). *Trans. R. Soc. Trop. Med. Hyg.* **45,** 225–241.
Standen, O. D. (1952). *Ann. Trop. Med. Parasitol.* **46,** 48–53.
Standen, O. D. (1953). *Ann. Trop. Med. Parasitol.* **47,** 26–43.
Standen, O. D. (1955). *Ann. Trop. Med. Parasitol.* **49,** 183–192.
Standen, O. D. (1962). *In* "Bilharziasis" G. E. W. (Wolstenholme and M. O'Conner, eds.), pp. 266–286. Little, Brown, Boston, Massachusetts.
Standen, O. D. (1963). *Exp. Chemother.* **1,** 701–892.
Standen, O. D. (1967). *Trans. R. Soc. Trop. Med. Hyg.* **61,** 563–569.
Stegman, R. J., Senft, A. W., Brown, P. R., and Parks, R. E., Jr. (1973). *Biochem. Pharmacol.* **22,** 459–468.
Stirewalt, M. A., and Bronson, J. F. (1955). *J. Parasitol.* **41,** 328.
Stohler, H. R., and Frey, J. R. (1963). *Ann. Trop. Med. Parasitol.* **57,** 466–480.
Stohler, H. R., and Frey, J. R. (1964a). *Ann. Trop. Med. Parasitol.* **58,** 280–291.
Stohler, H. R., and Frey, J. R. (1964b). *Ann. Trop. Med. Parasitol.* **58,** 431–438.
Stohler, H. R., and Szente, A. (1974). *Proc. Int. Congr. Parasitol. 3rd, 1974*, p. 1303.
Stoll, N. R., and Hausheer, W. C. (1926). *Am. J. Hyg.* (Suppl.), **11,** 134–145.
Striebel, H. P. (1969). *Ann. N.Y. Acad. Sci.* **160,** 491–518.
Striebel, H. P., and Kradolfer, F. (1966). *Acta Trop. Suppl.* **9,** 54–58.
Stunkard, H. W. (1946). *J. Parasitol.* **32,** 539–552.
Talaat, S. M., Amin, N., and El Masry, B. (1963). *J. Egypt. Med. Assoc.* **46,** 827–832.
Tarrant, M. E., Wedley, S., and Woodage, T. F. (1971). *Ann. Trop. Med. Parasitol.* **65,** 233–244.
Taylor, M. G., and Nelson, G. S. (1971). *Trans. R. Soc. Trop. Med. Hyg.* **65,** 169–174.
Teixeira, D., Gouveia, O. F., Cunha, M. A. R., Galper, E., and Miyahira, A. R. (1969). *Hospital (Rio de Janeiro)* **76,** 29–38.
Teixeira, R. (1966). *Folha Med.* **53,** 95–98.
Thommen, H., Stohler, H. R., Würsch, J., and Frey, J. R. (1964). *Ann. Trop. Med. Parasitol.* **58,** 439–452.
Thompson, P. E., Meisenhelder, J. E., and Najarian, H. (1962). *Am. J. Trop. Med. Hyg.* **11,** 31–45.
Thompson, P. E., Meisenhelder, J. E., Moore, A. K., and Waitz, J. A. (1965). *Bull. W. H. O.* **33,** 517–535.
Timms, A. R., and Bueding, E. (1959). *Br. J. Pharmacol. Chemother.* **14,** 68–73.
Tonelli, E., and Neves, J. (1966). *Rev. Assoc. Med. Minas Gerais* **17,** 1–9.
Vogel, H. (1942). *Zentralbl. Bakteriol., Parasitenk. Infektionskr., Abt. I* **148,** 29–35.
Vogel, H. (1949). *Zentralbl. Bakteriol., Parasitenk. Infektionskr., Abt. I* **154,** 118–126.
Vogel, H. (1958). *Bull. W. H. O.* **18,** 1097–1103.
Waitz, J. A., Ober, R. E., Meisenhelder, J. E., and Thompson, P. E. (1965). *Bull. W. H. O.* **33,** 537–546.
Walker, J. (1928). *Ann. Soc. Belge Med. Trop.* **8,** 273–289.
Warren, K. S. (1970). *J. Infect. Dis.* **121,** 514–521.
Warren, K. S., and Newill, V. A. (1967). "A Bibliography of the World's Literature from 1852 to 1962," Vols. 1 & 2. Case Western Reserve Univ. Press, Cleveland, Ohio.
Watson, J. M., and Pringle, A. (1950). *J. Trop. Med.* **53,** 233–238.
Watson, J. M., Abdel Azim, M., and Halawani, A. (1948). *Trans. R. Soc. Trop. Med. Hyg.* **42,** 37–54.
Weinmann, C. J., and Hunter, G. W. (1960). *Exp. Parasitol.* **9,** 239–242.

Werbel, L. M. (1970). *In* "Topics in Medicinal Chemistry" (J. L. Rabinowitz and R. M. Myerson, eds.), Vol. 3, pp. 125–168. Wiley (Interscience), New York.
Werbel, L. M., and Thompson, P. E. (1967). *J. Med. Chem.* **10,** 32–36.
Werbel, L. M., Elslager, E. F., and Worth, D. F. (1968). *J. Med. Chem.* **11,** 950–955.
Werbel, L. M., Elslager, E. F., Phillips, A. A., Worth, D. F., Islip, P. J., and Neville, M. C. (1969). *J. Med. Chem.* **12,** 521–524.
Werbel, L. M., Battaglia, J., Elslager, E. F., and Youngstrom, C. (1970). *J. Med. Chem.* **13,** 592–598.
Werbel. L. M., Degnan, M. B., Harger, G. F., Capps, D. B., Islip, P. J., and Closier, M. D. (1972). *J. Med. Chem.* **15,** 955–963.
Westland, R. D., Werbel, L. M., and Dice, J. R. (1971). *J. Med. Chem.* **14,** 916–920.
WHO (1966). Tech. Rep. Ser. 317, pp. 1–71, Geneva.
WHO (1972). *Bull. PAHO* **6,** 82–89.
Yarinsky, A., Hernandez, P., and Dennis, E. W. (1970). *Bull. W. H. O.* **42,** 445–449.
Yarinsky, A., Hernandez, P., Ferrari, R. A., and Freele, H. W. (1972). *Jpn. J. Parasitol.* **21,** 101–108.
Yarinsky, A., Drobeck, H. P., Freele, H., Wiland, J., and Gumaer, K. I. (1974). *Toxicol. Appl. Pharmacol.* **27,** 169–182.
Yokogawa, M., Yoshimura, H., and Sano, M. (1966). *Acta Trop. Suppl.* **9,** 78–88.
Zacharias, N., Carvalho, P. R., and Penteado, J. F. (1967a). *Hospital (Rio de Janeiro)* **71,** 657–662.
Zacharias, N., Carvalho, P. R., Penteado, J. F., and Machado, W. A. (1967b). *Hospital (Rio de Janeiro)* **72,** 1465–1468.
Zeng, Y. L., and Lu, Z. X. (1965). *Yao Hsueh Hsueh Pao* **12,** 727–733.
Zicker, F., Katz, N., and Wolf, J. (1974). *Congr. Bras. Soc. Trop. Med. 10th, 1974,* Abst. No. 138.
Zussman, R. A., Bauman, P. M., and Petruska, J. C. (1970). *J. Parasit.* **56,** 75–79.

# The Behavioral Toxicity of Monoamine Oxidase-Inhibiting Antidepressants

DENNIS L. MURPHY

*Section on Clinical Neuropharmacology*
*Laboratory of Clinical Science*
*National Institute of Mental Health*
*National Institutes of Health Clinical Center*
*Bethesda, Maryland*

I. Introduction . . . . . 72
A. Classes and Uses of Clinically Effective Monoamine Oxidase-Inhibiting Drugs . . . . . 74
B. Methodologic Limitations in the Study of Adverse Behavioral Effects of Antidepressant Drugs . . . . . 74
II. Methods . . . . . 75
III. Iproniazid-Related Adverse Behavioral Changes . . . . . 76
A. Incidence of Adverse Behavioral Changes . . . . . 76
B. Incidence of Adverse Behavioral Changes as a Function of Iproniazid Dosage and Treatment Duration . . . . . 77
C. Patient Subgroup Differences in Adverse Behavioral Changes . . . . . 77
D. Specific Behavioral Changes with Iproniazid . . . . . 80
IV. Phenelzine-Related Adverse Behavioral Changes . . . . . 83
A. Incidence of Adverse Behavioral Changes . . . . . 83
B. Incidence of Adverse Behavioral Changes as a Function of Phenelzine Dosage and Treatment Duration . . . . . 86
C. Patient Subgroup Differences in Adverse Behavioral Changes . . . . . 87
D. Specific Behavioral Changes with Phenelzine . . . . . 88
V. Tranylcypromine-Related Adverse Behavioral Changes . . . . . 90
VI. Adverse Behavioral Changes Associated with Other Monoamine Oxidase-Inhibiting Antidepressants . . . . . 90
A. Pargyline . . . . . 92
B. Isocarboxazid . . . . . 92
C. Procarbazine . . . . . 93
D. Nialamide . . . . . 94
E. Pheniprazine . . . . . 94
VII. Comparison of Adverse Behavioral Effects during Monoamine Oxidase-Inhibitor Treatment with Those during Treatment with Other Antidepressant Drugs . . . . . 95
A. Tricyclic Antidepressants . . . . . 95
B. L-Dopa and L-Tryptophan . . . . . 95
C. *d*-Amphetamine and Lithium Carbonate . . . . . 96
VIII. Behavioral Effects of Monoamine Oxidase-Inhibiting Drugs in Animals of Possible Relevance to Their Behavioral Toxicity in Man . . . . . 97

IX. Biochemical Effects of Monoamine Oxidase-Inhibiting Drugs in Animals and Man of Possible Relevance to Their Behavioral Effects . . . . . . 97
X. Discussion and Conclusions . . . . . . . . . . . . . . . . . 98
References . . . . . . . . . . . . . . . . . . . . 101

## I. Introduction

The concept of behavioral toxicity is used to designate undesirable drug side effects that take the form of psychological and behavioral alterations. Some examples of behavioral toxicity that have been widely reported include the apparent precipitation of paranoid psychoses and excessive hyperactivity by amphetamine (Snyder, 1972), of depressive reactions by reserpine (Goodwin and Bunney, 1971), and of a variety of behavioral changes by L-dopa (Murphy, 1973). A related term, neurotoxicity, has been used to describe drug side effects that alter brain structure or produce evident neurological impairment, which may or may not be accompanied by behavioral or psychological changes.

There has been some debate over the term behavioral toxicity because of its possible overapplication to behavioral changes that may be only distantly associated with drug treatment (e.g., lethargy as an indirect effect of anemia produced by an antitumor drug). In addition, what may be considered behavioral toxicity at one time (e.g., excessive sedation during chronic chlorpromazine administration) may be a component of the therapeutic effect of the drug at another time, as in an agitated, psychotic individual (Cole, 1960; Fingl and Woodbury, 1965). Shader and Dimascio (1970) have provided the following definition of the term:

> Behavioral toxicity is a phrase used to denote those pharmacological actions of a drug that, when administered within the dosage range of which it has been found to possess clinical utility, produce through mechanisms not immediately specifiable alterations in perceptual and cognitive functions, psychomotor performance, motivation, mood, interpersonal relationships, or intrapsychic processes of an individual to the degree that they interfere with or limit the capacity of the individual to function within his setting or constitute a hazard to his physical well being in the process.

There are some difficulties in identifying behavioral side effects resulting from drugs administered for psychological or behavioral disorders. Although the neurotoxicity of antineoplastic agents (Weiss *et al.*, 1974) and the behavioral and psychological consequences of drugs such as L-dopa (Murphy, 1973), whose major effects are directed against medical or neurological disorders, can often be identified as behavioral changes occurring apparently *de novo,* there is greater difficulty in untangling the undesirable from the beneficial behavioral effects of psychoactive agents used in treating patients with psychiatric disorders. Preexisting symptoms or symptoms that develop during different phases of depression, for instance, overlap with symptoms reported as side effects with some antidepressant agents (Raskin, 1972). In addition, behavioral and psychological changes are characteristically difficult to view objectively and quantitatively.

This review will consider the nature and incidence of the adverse effects reported with a major class of drugs used primarily as antidepressant and antihypertensive agents, the so-called monoamine oxidase (MAO)-inhibiting drugs. For comparative purposes, several other drugs with some antidepressant properties including the tricyclic antidepressants, lithium carbonate, amphetamine, L-tryptophan, and L-dopa, will also be considered briefly. This review does not include data on the therapeutic efficacy of MAO-inhibiting drugs nor on other side effects of these drugs such as cardiovascular changes. Hence, it makes no attempt to present a balanced view of the usefulness of these drugs in the treatment of depression and other disorders—the subject of many reviews (e.g., Klein and Davis, 1969).

The question of the behavioral effects of MAO-inhibiting drugs in man is of current interest because of a number of recent developments leading to a resurgence of clinical trials with these drugs. Specific factors in drug metabolism (e.g., genetically based differences in the rate of acetylation) have been identified as contributing factors to individual differences in the side effects and clinical efficacy of these drugs (Johnstone and Marsh, 1973; Price-Evans *et al.,* 1964). Greater understanding of synaptic physiology and of the biochemistry of MAO has led to new hypotheses concerning the mode of action of these drugs (Costa and Sandler, 1972; Hendley and Synder, 1968; Murphy and Weiss, 1972). In particular, the discovery of two apparent forms of the enzyme, MAO-A and MAO-B, and the identification of drugs that selectively affect MAO-A to increase brain serotonin and norepinephrine concentrations or MAO-B to increase $\beta$-phenylethylamine and dopamine concentrations (Yang and Neff, 1974), have stimulated clinical studies of these drugs as well as attempts to develop even more specific MAO-inhibiting drugs. In addition, the ability to assess directly the magnitude of MAO inhibition produced during treatment with these drugs (Murphy and Weiss, 1972; Robinson *et al.,* 1968, 1973) and observations suggesting that genetically controlled variations in endogenous MAO activity might be associated with behavioral alterations (Murphy, 1973; Murphy *et al.,* 1974a; Nies *et al.,* 1973, 1974) have also served to foster increased interest in the specific nature of the behavioral changes associated with drugs that reduce MAO activity.

### A. Classes and Uses of Clinically Effective Monoamine Oxidase-Inhibiting Drugs

Iproniazid, isocarboxazid, nialamide, phenelzine, and pheniprazine are some of the hydrazine MAO-inhibiting agents that have been studied in man. Tranylcypromine and $\alpha$-ethyl tryptamine are simple amines, and pargyline, clorgyline, and deprenyl are substituted amines that inhibit MAO. Clorgyline and Lilly 51641 are relatively selective MAO type A inhibitors, whereas deprenyl and pargyline have greater specificity as inhibitors of MAO type B.

All of these drugs have been identified as having some antidepressant and psychoactive potency. In addition, several have been used as antihypertensive and antianginal agents (Biel, 1967). Current clinical appraisal (Klein and Davis, 1969) holds the MAO-inhibiting agents as generally less effective antidepressants than the tricyclics or electroconvulsive therapy. In England they are used more extensively in the treatment of individuals with "atypical depressions" and phobias. However, the clinical opinion that there are individual patients or subgroups of patients who respond best or exclusively to MAO-inhibiting drugs and not to other antidepressants has been frequently expressed (Dally and Rohde, 1961; Sargeant, 1961) and a familial association of such responses has also been described (Pare and Mack, 1971). There is current interest in identifying more precisely clinical subgroups of psychiatric patients who might be especially responsive to MAO-inhibiting drugs (Raskin, 1972; Robinson *et al.*, 1973).

### B. Methodologic Limitations in the Study of Adverse Behavioral Effects of Antidepressant Drugs

As side effects are, by definition, not the main focus of a clinical drug trial, the mode of behavioral data collection, its evaluation, and its reporting is extremely variable from study to study. Behavioral side effects of psychoactive drugs such as the antidepressants are often only irregularly reported, and may be summed up in a clinical trial report in a column labeled "no response or worse" in an otherwise carefully executed study. One survey of 473 articles bearing on the effectiveness of antidepressant agents noted that only 19% of these articles made specific mention of the presence or absence of undesirable reactions of any type (Smith, 1969). Peculiarly, the advent of more sophisticated rating scales may have been contributed to this problem. Some widely used depression rating scales contain no items regarding behavioral phenomena other than those pertaining to depression. Thus, mild forms of manic or psychotic phenomena occurring during a trial with an antidepressant drug could conceivably not appear in the data from a controlled, double-blind study using only such rating instruments.

Incidence figures for the behavioral side effects in the studies reviewed below range from 0 to 83% of the patients treated. Factors possibly resulting in this wide incidence variation include differences in patient groups studied, differences in subclasses of these drugs (including dose and duration of administration differences), as well as, of course, differences in data collection and reporting. It has been suggested that adverse effects of all types may be generally underreported (Klein and Davis, 1969). This may well be especially true of the more ephemeral and extremely varied behavioral side effects of drugs.

Different problems exist in evaluating another source of information on the adverse behavioral effects of drugs—the case report. The coincidental occurrence of a striking behavioral change, such as an acute psychosis during a period of drug administration, is occasionally reported. Greater certainty is suggested by the disappearance of symptoms when the drug is stopped or the reappearance of symptoms upon rechallenge with the drug, but in most instances causality in single cases is difficult to ascertain. Double-blind studies, comparing antidepressant and antianxiety drugs with placebo in psychiatric patients, have revealed that apparent side effects of all types range in incidence from 0 to 30% of placebo-treated patients. Although behavioral side effects are less frequently reported, and certainly acute psychosis as an apparent side effect of placebo is very uncommon, a coincidental occurrence or a psychologically induced occurrence of a marked behavioral change in a nonblind, nonplacebo-controlled case report can seldom be completely excluded.

## II. Methods

For the present review, two basic approaches were followed. To gain an estimate of the frequency of occurrence of behavioral side effects during treatment with MAO-inhibiting antidepressants, clinical reports of the three most clinically effective of these drugs (Klein and Davis, 1969), iproniazid, phenelzine, and tranylcypromine, were systematically surveyed. All of the placebo-controlled, double-blind studies with these drugs listed in several reviews (Cole, 1964; Davis *et al.*, 1968; Klein and Davis, 1969; Ross, 1965) were examined. The incidence and type of behavioral side effects, their time course, and their relation to drug dose, duration of treatment, and type of clinical population studied were tabulated.

In addition, reviews of side effects of psychoactive drugs (Kettner, 1969–1974; Meyler, 1964, 1966; Meyler and Herxheimer, 1968, 1971; Shader and Dimascio, 1970) and the Index Medicus volumes for 1960–1974 were surveyed for all journal article titles listed under "MAO-Inhibiting Drugs" that suggested the occurrence of a behavioral side effect of these three drugs. Reports concerning other MAO-inhibiting drugs studied for antidepressant effects, including isocarboxazid, nialamide, pheniprazine, α-ethyl tryptamine, pargyline, clorgyline, and deprenyl as noted in the sources listed above were also reviewed and excerpted, but a systematic survey of all clinical studies of these less commonly studied drugs was not attempted.

## III. Iproniazid-Related Adverse Behavioral Changes

Iproniazid (1-isonicotinyl-2-isopropylhydrazine) was the first MAO-inhibiting agent studied extensively in man. Behavioral side effects in patients receiving iproniazid as an antituberculosis drug in 1952–53 (O'Conner *et al.,* 1953; Selikoff and Robitzek, 1952) provided much of the initial impetus for studies of its possible antidepressant effects in psychiatric patients (Loomer *et al.,* 1957). A high incidence of behavioral toxicity, together with its severe liver toxicity, contributed to its replacement in the treatment of tuberculosis by its less toxic congener, isoniazid, and its replacement in the treatment of depression by other MAO-inhibiting drugs (Crane, 1956a).

### A. Incidence of Adverse Behavioral Changes

The frequency of behavioral side effects observed during iproniazid treatment in studies of its clinical efficacy in patients with tuberculosis and patients with psychiatric disorders is summarized in Table I. In the 11 studies that mentioned the presence or absence of behavioral side effects, the average incidence of behavioral side effects was 27%, ranging from 2 to 83%. Many of the placebo-controlled, double-blind studies as reviewed elsewhere (Davis *et al.,* 1968) did not mention behavioral side effects. In the one study that compared behavioral changes observed during iproniazid administration with those occurring in a placebo-treated group, all 28 behavioral changes were found in the iproniazid group, including instances of physical aggression ($N = 12$), increased psychomotor activity ($N = 6$), irritability ($N = 5$), tension ($N = 1$), continuous sexual aggression ($N = 1$), and hallucinations with reactivation of psychosis ($N = 3$) (Freymuth *et al.,* 1959).

### B. Incidence of Adverse Behavioral Changes as a Function of Iproniazid Dosage and Treatment Duration

The two studies reporting very high behavioral side-effect incidence figures were those using the highest iproniazid dosage (4–6 mg/kg or an estimated 280–420 mg/day) compared to doses of 50–150 mg/day in eight studies and 200–280 mg/day in the remaining two studies (Table I). Feldman (1959) observed a sixfold higher incidence of side effects of all types (30 vs 5) in 50 patients receiving 150 mg vs 75 mg/day of iproniazid; 4 of the 5 behavioral side effects occurred in the patient group receiving 150 mg/day. The two studies with the lowest incidence of behavioral side effects (Cheifetz *et al.*, 1954; Kiloh *et al.*, 1960) were those with the shortest iproniazid treatment duration, averaging less than 4 weeks in both studies. Although few studies provided explicit data on the time of onset of behavioral changes, none of the changes observed were noted to have occurred before 3 weeks of treatment.

### C. Patient Subgroup Differences in Adverse Behavioral Changes

Several reports noted the occurrence of hypomanic or manic episodes in patients with histories of similar episodes occurring spontaneously. For example, Bates and Douglas (1961) observed that 3 of 6 individuals developing hypomania had manic–depressive histories. In only 2 of the 6 did the hypomanic state remit within a week of drug withdrawal. In 1 patient with no previous history of hypomania, the symptoms persisted and this patient eventually discharged himself "in a state of elation."

Rees and Benaim (1960) observed that endogenous depressed patients had a higher overall incidence (17%, 5 of 30 patients) of hypomania (3 patients) or mania (2 patients) than did patients with reactive, atypical or neurotic depressions (2%, 1 of 50 patients). These authors also noted that the occurrence of paranoid ideation during iproniazid treatment was highly prevalent in their subgroup of "atypical" depressed patients. Six of 9 such patients became paranoid and, in 3 of the 6, "marked schizophrenic thought disorder" also developed. Rees and Benaim (1960) also commented on a subgroup of patients who showed consistent improvement with the drug, relapse with its discontinuation, and subsequent improvement when the drug was reinstituted. However, they could not define any distinctive diagnostic or clinical features prior to treatment that differentiated this subgroup from other patients.

It should be specifically noted that there are many similarities in the behavioral responses to iproniazid in patients with such medical disorders as tuberculosis and rheumatoid arthritis compared to patients with

TABLE I

INCIDENCE OF ADVERSE BEHAVIORAL EFFECTS REPORTED DURING IPRONIAZID TREATMENT

| Population | Iproniazid dose (mg/day) | Treatment duration (weeks) | Incidence of behavioral side effects (%) | Behavioral changes[a] | Reference |
|---|---|---|---|---|---|
| 27 Tuberculosis patients | 4[b] | — | 11 | Manic psychosis (1); paranoid psychosis (2) | O'Connor *et al.* (1953) |
| 49 Tuberculosis patients | 200 (maximum) | 2–22 | 2 | Psychosis (1) | Cheifetz *et al.* (1954) |
| 34 Tuberculosis patients | 4–6[b] | 4–26 | 62 | Manic psychosis (5); paranoid psychosis (2); other (14) | Bloch *et al.* (1954) |
| 18 Tuberculosis patients with psychopathology | 4–6[b] | 3–52 | 83 | Mania (1); hypomania (1); excited or overactive (11); other (2) | Crane (1956b) |
| 50 Mixed psychiatric patients | 75–150 | 12 | 10 | Hypomania (2); other (3) | Feldman (1959) |
| 100 Mixed psychiatric patients | 50–150 | — | 50 | "Acute psychotic reactions manifested by hyperactivity, combativeness, noisiness and insomnia" (50) | Belisle *et al.* (1958) |

| | | | | | |
|---|---|---|---|---|---|
| 30 Mixed psychiatric patients | 150 | — | 30 | Manic episode (1); increased hallucinations (7); other (1) | Tavener (1959) |
| 28 Chronic and regressed schizophrenic patients | 150 | 8 | —[c] | Physical aggression, increased psychomotor activity, irritability, hallucinations, other | Freymuth *et al.* (1959) |
| 26 Depressed patients | 100–150 | 3–4 | 4[d] | Hypomania (1) | Kiloh *et al.* (1960) |
| 60 Depressed patients | 75–150 | 6 | 15[d] | Mania (2); hypomania (3); paranoid ideas (6) | Rees and Benaim (1960) |
| 31 Depressed patients | 75–150 | 10 | 19[d] | Mania (1); restlessness (4); other (1) | Wittenborn *et al.* (1961) |
| 54 Depressed patients | 150 | 20 | 11 | Hypomania (2); elation (2); other (2) | Bates and Douglas (1961) |
| | | Mean | 27% | | |

[a] Number of cases in parentheses. See also Table II.

[b] Expressed as milligrams per kilogram per day.

[c] Behavioral symptoms not listed per patient (results omitted from mean).

[d] Placebo-controlled study.

different psychiatric disorders (Tables I and II). In addition, one study of normal volunteers treated briefly with iproniazid (10 mg/kg) noted euphoric responses in 8 of the 10 individuals (Friend *et al.,* 1958).

### D. Specific Behavioral Changes with Iproniazid

In patients treated with iproniazid, the predominant severe behavioral side effects consisted of manic or paranoid episodes (Table II). The most frequently described cluster of side effects consisted of overactive, excited, euphoric, and hypomanic behavior which was noted in ten of the twelve studies. Irritability, restlessness, insomnia, and tension was the second most common cluster of symptoms. A smaller number of patients developed depression, drowsiness, and lethargy or inability to concentrate and increased anxiety. Several individuals were noted to develop cyclical periods of increased activity alternating with depression (Crane, 1956a). Confusion and hallucinations were noted in only one instance, and, in general, Crane's reviews (1956a, 1956b) suggested that the behavioral and psychological side effects of iproniazid occurred in the context of a clear sensorium.

By contrast, the occasional psychosis reported with the related antituberculosis drug, isoniazid, which is not a mitochondrial MAO inhibitor, is commonly characterized by confusion, disorientation, and neurological symptoms such as tremors (Hunter, 1952; Pleasure, 1954). Some case reports describing "schizophrenia" precipitated by isoniazid predominantly documented confusional symptoms and neurological changes (Wiedorn and Ervin, 1954). In addition to the qualitative differences in the CNS side effects of these two drugs, a much lower overall incidence of behavioral toxicity of all types has been observed during isoniazid treatment (Bloch *et al.,* 1954; Coates *et al.,* 1954; MRC Report, 1952).

Withdrawal of iproniazid treatment was noted to be accompanied by psychological and behavioral changes that were somewhat different from those occurring during drug treatment. Both insomnia and excessive dreaming, headaches, irritability, depression, and other symptoms were noted most frequently in the period immediately after drug discontinuation (Crane, 1956b; Fisher *et al.,* 1952).

Crane (1956b) has provided the most detailed case histories of the behavioral and psychological responses of tubercular patients to iproniazid. In his review of 14 patients with behavioral changes, he notes:

> the manifestations ranged from overt psychotic behavior (in 3 patients) to subtle changes in the dream life. . . . Eleven patients presented a picture of overactivity or excitement whereas 3 became depressed and fatigued. The typical reaction of the overactive group

TABLE II

SPECIFIC TYPES OF BEHAVIORAL SIDE EFFECTS REPORTED DURING IPRONIAZID TREATMENT

| | No. of individuals with each specific behavioral change[a] | | | | | | | | | | | |
|---|---|---|---|---|---|---|---|---|---|---|---|---|
| Specific behavior | (a) | (b) | (c) | (d) | (e) | (f) | (g) | (h) | (i) | (j) | (k) | (l) |
| Paranoid episodes | 2 | — | 2 | — | — | — | — | — | — | 6 | — | — |
| Psychosis | — | 1 | — | — | — | 50 | — | — | — | — | — | — |
| Mania or manic psychosis | 1 | — | 5 | 1 | — | — | 1 | — | — | 2 | 1 | — |
| Hypomania | — | — | — | 1 | 2 | — | — | — | 1 | 3 | — | 2 |
| Euphoria or elation | — | — | 3 | 4 | — | — | — | — | — | — | — | 2 |
| Overactivity | — | — | — | 11 | — | — | — | — | — | — | — | — |
| Irritability | — | — | 3 | — | — | — | 1 | 5 | — | — | — | — |
| Restlessness | — | — | — | — | — | — | — | — | — | — | 4 | — |
| Increased psychomotor activity with aggression | — | — | — | — | — | — | — | 6 | — | — | — | — |
| Physical aggression | — | — | — | — | — | — | — | 12 | — | — | — | — |
| Inability to concentrate | — | — | 1 | — | — | — | — | — | — | — | — | — |
| Apprehension and sense of impending disaster | — | — | — | — | 3 | — | — | — | — | — | — | — |
| Tension | — | — | 1 | — | — | — | — | 1 | — | — | — | 1 |
| Increased depression | — | — | — | 3 | — | — | — | — | — | — | — | — |
| Mild confusional episode | — | — | — | — | — | — | — | — | — | — | — | 1 |
| Continuous sexual aggression | — | — | — | — | — | — | — | 1 | — | — | — | — |
| Hallucinations | — | — | 1 | — | — | — | 7 | 3 | — | — | — | — |
| Suicide | — | — | — | — | — | — | — | — | — | 1 | — | — |
| Other | — | — | — | — | — | — | — | — | — | — | 1 | — |

[a] Key to references:
(a) O'Connor *et al.* (1953)
(b) Cheifetz *et al.* (1954)
(c) Bloch *et al.* (1954)
(d) Crane (1956b)
(e) Feldman (1959)
(f) Belisle *et al.* (1958)
(g) Tavener (1959)
(h) Freymuth *et al.* (1959)
(i) Kiloh *et al.* (1960)
(j) Rees and Benaim (1960)
(k) Wittenborn *et al.* (1961)
(l) Bates and Douglas (1961)

was: increased response to external stimuli, excessive but superficial involvement in the environment, feeling of well-being, increased resistance to fatigue, tremendous appetite and poor sleep.

Case reports on additional patients indicated marked sexual stimulation, euphoria, and increased energy. For example, 1 patient described a tremendous increase in appetite and energy associated with euphoria and a sense of extreme productivity, with no time to carry out all of his projects. Cyclical depressions alternating with periods of elation occurred in 2 patients, and typical hypomanic symptoms with meddlesome, demanding, and difficult-to-manage behavior, paranoid trends, and hostile behavior were also as noted in different individuals as responses to iproniazid treatment (Crane, 1956b).

Ferreira and Freeman (1958) summarized their overall impression of the psychological effects of iproniazid in a group of psychotic depressed patients as follows:

> Analysis of the changes in individual items of behavior showed an improvement in motor activity, mimetic expression, responsivity, socialization, attention, speech, mood, feeling and perception. Hostility, on the other hand, was slightly increased. In the items of thought processes, the trend showed a shift from obsessive ideas, somatic delusions and despairing self-blame to illogical thinking, ideas of reference and shifting of blame. From this point of view, the drug altered the type of thinking, but not necessarily in a beneficial manner, toward a "schizoid" type of ideational content.

Feldman (1959) reported that iproniazid in a mixed psychiatric population had apparently selective effects on accessibility, affect, sociability, and amicability; lesser effects on negativism, hostility, delusions, and realistic planning; produced only occasional improvement in judgment, tension, and hallucinations; and led to no change in insight or compulsivity.

The study by Wittenborn *et al.* (1961) provides the most comprehensive report of quantitatively rated behavioral and psychological data on the effects of iproniazid observed in a population of depressed women. In comparison to patients receiving placebo, the drug produced significant Minnesota Multiphasic Personality Inventory psychasthenia (but not depression) scale score reductions, and Clyde mood scale elevations in "friendly," "energetic," and "clear-thinking" scores and a reduction in "jittery" but no change in "depression" scores. Physicians' global ratings did reveal significant reductions in depression, whereas anxiety ratings on the Wittenborn scale were unchanged. Externally directed motivation, an ego-defense measure derived from the Rosenzweig picture test, was increased in the iproniazid treatment group. Psychomotor speed, as measured by a reduction in verbal response latency test scores, was increased. Some cognitive and perceptual test performances, including the numerical ability subtest of the Differential Ability Test and the number of Necker cube reversals thought relevant to the slowing of such functions in depression were also improved more by iproniazid treatment than by placebo. These changes were interpreted by Cole (1964) as representing a psychomotor stimulant effect of iproniazid, an effect not apparent in a similar study of imipramine conducted by the same investigators (Wittenborn *et al.*, 1962).

## IV. Phenelzine-Related Adverse Behavioral Changes

Phenelzine ($\beta$-phenylethylhydrazine) is an irreversible, hydrazine-type inhibitor of MAO. It has been available for almost 20 years, and currently may be the most used MAO-inhibiting antidepressant possibly because its use has been only occasionally associated with acute hypertensive episodes.

As a "second-generation" MAO-inhibiting antidepressant, it has been subject to more controlled studies than iproniazid. Reviews in 1968 and 1974 and an Index Medicus search revealed fourteen studies carried out under placebo-controlled, double-blind conditions (Davis *et al.*, 1968; Raskin *et al.*, 1974). Of these, seven mentioned adverse behavioral effects during the trials. In general, unlike the earlier reports of iproniazid trials, these papers rarely described details of the response of individual patients to phenelzine treatment, and most reported only statistical summaries of responses based on various rating scale changes.

### A. Incidence of Adverse Behavioral Changes

The overall incidence of behavioral toxicity as derived from those studies reporting behavioral side effects was 11%, with a range of 4 to 40%. A generally similar incidence of behavioral side effects was observed in placebo-controlled studies (15%, $N = 7$) compared to other studies (9%, $N = 9$; Table III).

Although the overall incidence of all behavioral side effects was lower than with iproniazid, the changes most frequently observed were similar to those described for iproniazid, namely hypomanic and manic episodes. Increased restlessness, hyperactivity, agitation, and irritability also occurred frequently. A smaller number of patients developed confusional states (Table III).

A possibly important qualification to the adverse behavioral change incidence figures is provided by several studies that included comparisons with placebo or other antidepressant drugs. For example, Raskin (1972) reported a 21–23% incidence of "agitation or excitement" in 110 depressed patients prior to a double-blind study treatment, and a 9% incidence of the same behaviors during treatment with either phenelzine or placebo. Unfortunately, no other details and no subdivision of these symptoms are provided, and, hence, it is not possible from these data to differentiate possible hyperactivity representing, for example, a hypo-

TABLE III

INCIDENCE OF ADVERSE BEHAVIORAL EFFECTS REPORTED DURING PHENELZINE TREATMENT

| Population | Phenelzine dose (mg/day) | Treatment duration (weeks) | Incidence of behavioral side effects (%) | Behavioral changes[a] | Reference |
|---|---|---|---|---|---|
| 60 Depressed patients | 75 | 76 | 18 | Hypomania (4); mania (1); increased anxiety (5); increased "inner tension and drive" (1) | Sarwer-Foner *et al.* (1959) |
| 29 Schizophrenic patients with depressive symptoms | 60 | 24–36 | 17 | Increased aggressiveness, hostility, agitation, and occasional assaultiveness (4); euphoria (1) | Bailey *et al.* (1959) |
| 46 Depressed patients | 75 | — | 6 | Toxic, nocturnal delirium with choreiform movements (1); toxic delirium with "mescaline-like psychosis" with vivid hallucinations and perceptual distortions (1); "wooly" thinking and forgetfulness (1) | Clarke (1960) |

| | | | | | |
|---|---|---|---|---|---|
| 31 Depressed patients | 45 | 4–24 | 13 | Severe agitation (2); marked euphoria (2) | Cole and Weiner (1960) |
| 46 Depressed patients | — | 5 | 6 | Hypomania/mania (3) | Imlah (1960) |
| 40 Depressed patients | 30–90 | 5–26 | 8 | Increased tension and agitation (3) | Levy and Lohrenz (1960) |
| 132 Depressed patients | 45 | 4 | 4[b] | Hypomania (5) | Middlefell *et al.* (1960) |
| 68 Depressed patients | 30–90 | — | 10 | Hypomania (5); irritable outbursts (2) | Woods and Lewis (1961) |
| 54 Depressed patients | 45 | 20 | 13 | Hypomania (3); increased tension (1); elation (1) | Bates and Douglas (1961) |
| 20 Depressed patients | 90 | 6 | 5[b] | Increased anxiety, guilt feelings and insomnia (1) | Rees and Davies (1961) |
| 30 Mixed psychiatric patients | 60 | 8 | 40[b] | Confusion (5); tension or anxiety (4); hyperactivity (3) | Greenblatt *et al.* (1962) |
| 20 Depressed patients | 45 | — | 10 | Mania (1); increased anxiety (1) | Ducoudray *et al.* (1963) |
| 47 Depressed patients | 45–60 | 4 | 4[b] | Elation (2) | Martin (1963) |
| 38 Depressed patients | 60–75 | 8 | 21[b] | Hyperactivity (8) | Greenblatt *et al.* (1964) |
| 110 Depressed patients | 45 | 5 | 8 | Agitation or excitement (9) | Raskin (1972) |
| 28 Depressed patients | 60 | 4 | 25[b] | Mania (3); hypomania (1); increased anxiety, agitation, and delusions (3) | Murphy *et al.* (1975) |
| | Mean | | 13% | | |

[a] Number of cases in parentheses.
[b] Placebo-controlled double-blind study.

manic episode during drug treatment from the expected occurrence of agitation as part of depressive symptomatology. In a comparison of phenelzine with imipramine, isocarboxazid, placebo, and electroconvulsive therapy, hyperactivity occurred in 21% of the patients receiving phenelzine but was not mentioned as a side effect of the other treatments (Greenblatt *et al.,* 1962). In one comparison of phenelzine with imipramine, 3 of 22 phenelzine-treated patients were reported as "worse," vs none of 25 imipramine-treated patients (Leitch and Seager, 1963), whereas, in another such comparison, 2 of 47 patients treated with phenelzine developed elation vs 5 of 49 patients receiving imipramine (Martin, 1963).

In some instances, data on patients dropped from a study can provide some indication of the occurrence of behavioral toxicity. For instance, in a study comparing phenelzine, diazepam, and placebo (Raskin *et al.,* 1974), which did not report any specific behavioral side effects during treatment, approximately twice as many patients dropped out during the first 4 weeks of either phenelzine or placebo treatment compared to diazepam treatment; this difference was reversed in the second 4 weeks of treatment, with more diazepam-treated patients being discontinued from the study. In another study that reported no behavioral side effects (Kay *et al.,* 1973), 3 times as many depressed outpatients were early dropouts because of "side effects, worse or overdoses" in the amitriptyline compared to phenelzine groups, but the only patient developing mania was a phenelzine-treated patient.

### B. Incidence of Adverse Behavioral Changes as a Function of Phenelzine Dosage and Treatment Duration

No explicit comparisons of behavioral change incidence differences in relation to drug dosage were noted in these studies. One report mentioned that hyperactivity regularly occurred at a phenelzine dosage of 60 mg/day or higher (Bailey *et al.,* 1959).

Of interest in regard to the question of what dosage of phenelzine constitutes adequate treatment, which was raised in several discussions of the varying effectiveness of phenelzine in different studies (Raskin *et al.,* 1974; Rees and Davies, 1961; Robinson *et al.,* 1973), is the observation that the rapid eye movement, sleep-suppressing effects of phenelzine only occurred at higher dosage levels of 60 to 90 mg/day (Akindele *et al.,* 1970; Wyatt *et al.,* 1971).

Although little detailed information was supplied, the few instances that the time of onset of adverse behavior changes was noted indicated that the changes occurred after a minimum of 1 to 4 weeks of treatment.

In one study in which daily behavioral ratings were available, the greatest number of adverse behavioral effects occurred in the second and third weeks, although the three episodes of mania (all of which occurred in bipolar patients) developed after 3 to 4 weeks of treatment, which was also the time of onset of antidepressant effects (Table IV) (Murphy *et al.*, 1974b).

### C. Patient Subgroup Differences in Adverse Behavioral Changes

In a number of instances, hypomanic and manic forms of behavioral change occurred during phenelzine treatment in individuals who had a history of such episodes prior to drug treatment (Imlah, 1960; Middlefell

TABLE IV

Times of Specific Behavioral Changes during One Study of Phenelzine Administration (60 mg/day) to Depressed Patients[a]

| | Placebo for (weeks) | | Phenelzine for (weeks) | | | | Placebo for (weeks) | |
|---|---|---|---|---|---|---|---|---|
| Ratings | −2 | −1 | 1 | 2 | 3 | 4 | +1 | +2 |
| Significantly lower ratings (improvement): | | | | | | | | |
| Depression scale | — | 1 | 1 | 0 | 3 | 7 | 1 | 1 |
| Anxiety scale | — | 0 | 1 | 1 | 2 | 6 | 1 | 0 |
| Psychosis scale | — | 1 | 0 | 0 | 2 | 0 | 1 | 1 |
| | | 2 | 2 | 1 | 7 | 13 | 3 | 2 |
| Significantly higher ratings (worse): | | | | | | | | |
| Depression scale | — | 0 | 1 | 3 | 4 | 2 | 3 | 1 |
| Anxiety scale | — | 1 | 1 | 3 | 3 | 1 | 3 | 1 |
| Psychosis scale | — | 0 | 0 | 4 | 2 | 2 | 0 | 1 |
| Mania scale | — | 0 | 0 | 0 | 1 | 2 | 0 | 0 |
| | | 1 | 2 | 10 | 10 | 7 | 6 | 3 |
| Grand totals: | | 3 | 4 | 11 | 17 | 20 | 9 | 5 |

[a] Figures indicate the number of patients in each week who manifested a statistically significant mean rating change from the preceding week on the individual scales. Ratings were done twice daily, and 28 depressed patients (22 unipolar and 6 bipolar) were included in the trial. Data from Murphy *et al.* (1974b).

*et al.,* 1960; Murphy *et al.,* 1974b; Woods and Lewis, 1961). Very few of the studies included individuals other than depressed patients. However, in a study focused on the effects of phenelzine on sleep in normals, 2 of 5 individuals were described as being overelated during the phenelzine treatment period (Akindele *et al.,* 1970).

### D. Specific Behavioral Changes with Phenelzine

Detailed descriptions of adverse behavioral changes occurring during phenelzine treatment are provided in only three reports (Ayd, 1961; Bailey *et al.,* 1959; Johnson and Eilenberg, 1960).

Bailey *et al.* (1959) treated 30 "schizophrenics characterized by depression, withdrawal, disinterest, apathy or very similar dominant symptoms" using 60-mg/day doses for 6 to 9 months, except that nonresponders received 100 mg/day for the last month. Activity was increased in all patients, and approximately 70% of the patients developed exacerbations of psychopathology. Nonetheless, most of the patients were seen as improved to some degree in their symptoms of depression, withdrawal, and apathy. Four patients became so aggressive, hostile, agitated, and occasionally assaultive that the dosage had to be reduced or discontinued, as was the case also in 1 patient who became euphoric. Hyperactivity was particularly associated with doses above 60 mg/day. The 1 patient discussed in greatest detail benefited from several MAO-inhibiting antidepressants, including iproniazid and pheniprazine as well as phenelzine. A self-initiated trial of 40 mg phenelzine to which 50 mg iproniazid was added precipitated a hypomanic episode with excess activity, sexual stimulation, and a requirement of "only 2 to 3 hours sleep without any fatigue, not wishing to spend her time in bed since there were so many interesting things to do." Phenelzine alone was not associated with hypomanic symptoms, but produced a " 'festive type of energy,' wanting to get out and be with other people, enjoying her social contacts greatly, and able to concentrate much better on her reading."

Johnson and Eilenberg (1960) described 3 outpatients receiving phenelzine for depression who developed acute psychoses during treatment. All of the episodes developed after more than 8 weeks of treatment and remitted rapidly after discontinuation of the drug. Two of the episodes were primarily hypomanic in character, whereas the other episode consisted of a confusional state with misidentification of people, increased nighttime activity with no sleep, together with disorientation and clouding of consciousness observed upon admission to the hospital. The individuals developing hypomania had no past history of hypomania.

One became overactive, talkative, and threatening shortly after the phenelzine dose was raised from 45 to 75 mg/day. She developed flight of ideas, guilt feelings, paranoid concerns, labile mood with rapid fluctuations between depression, elation, and irritability together with distractability and no capacity for sustained concentration. The other patient began to feel less depressed after 6 weeks of treatment with 45 mg/day and gradually developed euphoria, expansive ideas, and some paranoid suspicions over the next 4 weeks. She then had an abrupt onset of feeling "exhilaratingly happy" and became overactive, overtalkative, and aggressive, requiring admission to the hospital, discontinuation of phenelzine, and treatment with chlorpromazine.

Ayd (1961) described 6 patients taking phenelzine and 1 taking isocarboxazid who developed excited, elated episodes. None had a prior history of elation or excitement, and 5 had recovered uneventfully from prior depressions either spontaneously or during treatment with shock therapy and other antidepressant drugs. Ayd observed that the symptoms superficially resembled those of hypomanic or manic episodes but felt that they represented "a toxic psychokinetic reaction similar to the excitatory effects of stimulants like amphetamines." The case histories detail symptoms such as feeling like "I can do anything," talking fast, paranoid delusions, threatening to kill, not sleeping, irritability, "spending money like a fool," feeling "like a millionaire, even though I don't have the money," "never . . . more confident, more energetic, and more alert," and hypersensitive. Most of the excited episodes required several weeks of hospital treatment with tranquilizers, and they were generally followed by a return of depressive symptoms. In Ayd's experience, these toxic psychopathological episodes occurred infrequently but constituted a definite hazard of treatment with antidepressant drugs such as phenelzine.

One quantitatively assessed study of the psychological effects of phenelzine examined 25 moderately depressed patients who were treated under randomized double-blind conditions with either phenelzine, imipramine, or placebo for 3 to 5 weeks and evaluated before and at the end of the treatment using a number of standardized psychological tests and a clinical interview (Bellak and Rosenberg, 1966). Although overall clinical improvement was not significantly different with any of the treatments, some specific differences in drug effects were observed. A quantitative scoring assessment of the Rorschach test revealed a statistically significant increase in total responses, drive-related responses, and aggressive responses in the phenelzine-treated patients compared to both other treatment groups, which was interpreted as indicating that phenelzine facilitated emotional arousal. In addition, phenelzine treatment was associated with increases in some global ego strength subscales hypothesized to reflect the capacity to regulate and integrate conflicts. Imipramine treatment was also associated with improvement in these psychic defensive characteristics.

## V. Tranylcypromine-Related Adverse Behavioral Changes

Tranylcypromine is a nonhydrazine, phenylalkylamine inhibitor of MAO, which was first studied as an antidepressant in 1958 and was approved for clinical use in 1961. One early review (Atkinson and Ditman, 1965) summarized clinical trials data indicating behavioral side effect frequencies of insomnia (12%), agitation (5%), drowsiness (3%), and anxiety (2%). Several of the controlled studies surveyed made no mention of behavioral side effects whatsoever.

In the studies reporting behavioral side effects, an overall incidence of 13% was found (Table V). Increased restlessness and overstimulation were most frequently reported, with a smaller number of patients developing irritability and paranoid ideation. Only 1 patient was reported as developing hypomania (Bartholomew, 1962), although 4 other patients in one study were described as exhibiting the beginning of manic episodes with paranoid features at the time the drug was discontinued (Himmelhoch *et al.*, 1972).

Drug dosages used were in the 30–60 mg range, but there was no evidence of a clear dose relationship or of patient population differences in susceptibility to adverse behavioral effects. In one study, the incidences of restlessness and insomnia were essentially the same for tranylcypromine (30–40 mg/day) as for the comparison drug, *d*-amphetamine (15 mg/day) (Overall *et al.*, 1966). Similarly, tranylcypromine and pargyline (another nonhydrazine MAO-inhibiting drug) were associated with overstimulation in equal numbers of patients in another study (Janecek *et al.*, 1963a).

## VI. Adverse Behavioral Changes Associated with Other Monoamine Oxidase-Inhibiting Antidepressants

Other drugs inhibiting MAO that have been studied in man include isocarboxazid, nialamide, pargyline, α-ethyl tryptamine, and procarbazine. These MAO inhibitors have been less widely used and reported upon as antidepressants (with the possible exception of isocarboxazid and nialamide) than those drugs already reviewed. No systematic attempt was made to evaluate the incidence of behavioral toxicity with

TABLE V

INCIDENCE OF ADVERSE BEHAVIORAL EFFECTS REPORTED DURING TRANYLCYPROMINE TREATMENT

| Population | Drug dose (mg/day) | Treatment duration (weeks) | Incidence of behavioral side effects (%) | Behavioral changes[a] | Reference |
|---|---|---|---|---|---|
| 32 Depressed patients | 30–60 | 6 | 3 | Hypomania (1) | Bartholomew (1962) |
| 51 Mixed psychiatric patients | 30 | 2–4 | 16 | Overstimulation characterized by increased talkativeness and restlessness (8) | Chu and Fogel (1963) |
| 25 Depressed patients | 15–30 | 2 | 4 | Increased anxiety (1) | Gottfries (1963) |
| 40 Depressed patients | 20–60 | 3 | 13 | Overstimulation (5) | Janecek *et al.* (1963a) |
| 30 Mixed psychiatric patients | 10–40 | 4 | 17 | Overstimulation (3); restlessness (2) | Janecek *et al.* (1963b) |
| 50 Schizophrenic patients with depression | 10–60 | 10 | 2 | Assaultive and difficult to manage (1) | Schiele (1963) |
| 22 Depressed patients | 30–40 | 4 | 27 | Restlessness (6) | Overall *et al.* (1966) |
| 21 Depressed patients | 20–60 | — | 24 | Irritability and paranoid ideation (5) (with 4 patients progressing to the "beginning of a manic episode with paranoid features") | Himmelhoch *et al.* (1972) |
| | | Mean | 13% | | |

[a] Number of cases in parentheses.

these other drugs, but several reports specifically dealing with adverse behavioral effects are of note.

### A. Pargyline

Sutnick *et al.* (1964) reported 3 cases of acute psychotic reactions that were thought to be related to the treatment of 33 medical patients with pargyline. This drug is a nonhydrazine, propargylamine MAO-inhibiting agent primarily used in antihypertensive therapy. One individual gradually developed nervousness and agitation as pargyline dosage was increased from 25 to 200 mg/day. After 4 weeks of treatment at 200 mg/day, drug discontinuation was followed on the third day by the abrupt onset of visual and auditory hallucinations and paranoid delusions, which gradually improved during hospitalization and treatment with chlorpromazine and psychotherapy. A second individual receiving 75 mg of the drug per day for 7 months developed auditory hallucinations and paranoid delusions that diminished within 7 days of discontinuing treatment. A third woman receiving multiple drugs for hypertension developed an acute exacerbation of paranoid thinking, confusion, and disorientation 3 weeks after treatment with 25 mg/day pargyline was begun. It should be noted that the second and third patients described in the preceding had prior psychiatric symptomatology that may have been exacerbated by the drug, whereas the first individual, who had no prior psychiatric history, developed psychotic symptoms only after abrupt discontinuation of the drug.

Bryant *et al.* (1963) described nervousness (24%) and insomnia (42%) as frequent side effects of pargyline treatment and also mentioned the occurrence of typical manic episodes in 2 of 33 hypertensive patients receiving pargyline. Dunlop (1963) and Dunlop *et al.* (1965) also reported that pargyline given to 70 depressed inpatients and outpatients was accompanied by side effects including agitation (9 patients), increase in schizoid behavior (1 patient), and insomnia (10 patients) or sedation (8 patients). Kline (1963) noted that 3 patients out of 50 treated with pargyline developed psychotic symptoms, including 1 case of mania and 2 of paranoid psychosis. The patient developing mania had previously experienced a manic episode during treatment with another MAO-inhibiting antidepressant.

### B. Isocarboxazid

In a review of forty-six clinical trials of isocarboxazid, Kurland *et al.* (1967) reported that only three were randomized, double-blind studies using quantitative assessment measures and acceptable statistical analysis. A review of these three studies (Greenblatt *et al.*, 1962, 1964; Overall *et al.*, 1962; Rothman, 1962; Rothman *et al.*, 1961), however, did not reveal any mention of the presence or absence of behavioral side effects during isocarboxazid treatment. Kurland *et al.* (1967) gave isocarboxazid, 30 mg/day for 3 weeks to depressed patients and observed a somewhat higher incidence of agitation during treatment with isocarboxazid (16 of 59 patients, 27%) compared to placebo (7 of 50, 14%). Among dropouts, 7 of 10 patients left isocarboxazid treatment because they were "worse," but only 2 of 11 dropouts receiving placebo were so rated. Specific symptoms in the worse groups were not reported.

### C. Procarbazine

Procarbazine is a methyl hydrazine [*N*-isopropyl-$\alpha$-(2-methylhydrezino)-*p*-toluanide hydrochloride] MAO-inhibiting drug that is used as an antitumor agent. Mann and Hutchison (1967) reported an acute manic episode in a patient with Hodgkin's disease who had no previous psychiatric difficulties. He developed an increased sense of well-being (despite early nausea) during the first 10 days of treatment. After 3 weeks, he felt his energy increase was abnormal, and he felt he was on "pep pills." His activity level increased further, and he became overtalkative, uninhibited, grandiose, aggressive, demanding, restless, and insomniac. He saw his physician after 5 weeks of treatment and expressed concern about his excessive talking and the appropriateness of his behavior, describing himself as "full of pep" and "driving all the time" with some feelings of grandeur. The next day, immediately following the extraction of 3 teeth (for which he received 4 ml of 2% Xylocaine with 1:100,000 adrenaline), he was observed to be acting bizarrely and on admittance to a hospital was psychotic, with overactivity, pressure of speech, emotional lability, and aggressive demanding behavior but no disorientation or hallucinations. His symptoms did not change during 4 days of treatment with paraldehyde, chloral hydrate, and pyridoxine but responded after several days' treatment with chlorpromazine. Because the patient had a remission of Hodgkin's disease during procarbazine treatment and was nonresponsive to other agents, he was treated several months later with procarbazine, 100 mg/day, together with thioridazine, 150 mg/day, but again developed overstimulation. In other reports of procarbazine use in cancer treatment, mood lability has also been described (Weiss *et al.*, 1974).

## D. Nialamide

Gradwell (1960) reported a manic–depressive patient who had been chronically depressed for 5 years and who was started on the hydrazine MAO-inhibiting drug, nialamide, 300 mg/day. Two days later she received 1.5 mg reserpine and on the following day became hypomanic and shortly thereafter manic. Discontinuation of the drugs did not lead to any change, and she remained manic for several weeks. In this same report, the occurrence of psychosis was also noted in another patient receiving nialamide, 1 patient receiving phenelzine, and 2 receiving imipramine.

Olson (1962) compared antidepressant responses and side effects in depressed patients receiving either 100 or 300 mg/day nialamide. The high dosage group showed not only greater improvement but also a higher frequency of side effects, including hyperactivity, and a greater number of dropouts from the study because of complications.

## E. Pheniprazine

In an examination of the possibility that hallucinations observed during MAO-inhibitor treatment might be a direct pharmacological result of the drug (Ayd, 1961; Brune and Himwich, 1962; Janzarik, 1959), Marjerrison (1966) studied visual imagery production in 18 psychiatric patients receiving 12 mg pheniprazine for 7 days. Compared to placebo, pheniprazine treatment was associated with an increase in the intensity and the structural detail of visual imagery. Urinary tryptamine excretion during drug treatment was significantly correlated with both the intensity ($r = +0.56$, $p < 0.05$) and amount ($r = +0.52$, $p < 0.05$) of visual imagery reported. Those individuals reporting the greatest increase in visual imagery were discriminated from the others on the basis of greater urinary tryptamine increases (an indirect measure of MAO inhibition) and greater changes in some EEG measures (less alpha and greater beta activity) as well as greater decreases in Bender Gestalt scores, higher field dependency on the Witkin rod and frame test, and lower-ranking Symptom Rating Scale scores. These results were interpreted as indicating an association between drug-induced imagery production, increased cortical activation, increased attentiveness or vigilance reflected in the EEG, and possibly psychological improvement. That these changes might be a direct result of degree of MAO inhibition is suggested by the association of these psychophysiological changes with the amount of urinary tryptamine excreted during drug treatment.

## VII. Comparison of Adverse Behavioral Effects during Monoamine Oxidase Inhibitor Treatment with Those during Treatment with Other Antidepressant Drugs

### A. Tricyclic Antidepressants

The Boston Collaborative Drug Surveillance Program (1972) reported a total incidence of 5% (13 out of 260 patients) of behavioral side effects such as disorientation and agitation (8), psychoses and hallucinations (4), and exacerbation of depression (1) during treatment with tricyclic antidepressants. Klein and Fink (1962) studied 180 patients (102 with schizophrenia, 67 with depression, and 11 others) who received large doses of imipramine (80% received a modal maximum of 300 mg/day). Six percent (10 of 180) developed manic episodes and 11% developed agitated disorganization. Four of the 19 patients (20%) with diagnoses of a manic–depressive disorder developed mania during treatment. Bunney *et al.* (1970, 1972) reviewed reports of hypomania and mania occurring during tricyclic drug administration and reported an overall approximate incidence of 5% (160 episodes in 3450 patients). Among the patients for whom past histories were provided, approximately two-thirds of those developing mania had a prior history of mania, whereas among those developing hypomania, less than one-third had prior episodes of either mania or hypomania.

### B. L-Dopa and L-Tryptophan

Behavioral activation of all types, including restlessness, insomnia, irritability, and hypomania as well as some instances of confusional behavior, delusions, paranoid states, and other psychotic phenomena have been reported during the treatment of neurological and psychiatric patients with L-dopa, the catecholamine precursor (Murphy, 1973). Approximately 15% of patients treated with L-dopa exhibit some form of behavioral toxicity (Murphy, 1973). A particularly high incidence of brief hypomanic episodes was observed in bipolar depressed patients (those with a past history of hospitalization for mania) during treatment with high doses of L-dopa compared to a negligible incidence in unipolar depressed patients (those with no histories of mania) (Murphy *et al.*, 1971).

L-Tryptophan has been reported to have both antidepressant and antimanic effects in some but not all studies (Chase and Murphy, 1973). Although one of the first clinical studies with this indoleamine precursor noted some instances of euphoric and "drunken" behavior (Smith and

Prockop, 1962), most subsequent studies have observed no appreciable behavioral toxicity of any type with this drug (Murphy *et al.,* 1974c). In contrast to L-dopa, L-tryptophan appears to have some sleep-enhancing properties (Wyatt *et al.,* 1970) and no hypomania or mania-eliciting effects (Murphy *et al.,* 1974c).

### C. *d*-Amphetamine and Lithium Carbonate

*d*-Amphetamine has been used in the past for acute antidepressant and stimulant effects, and, although there are still a few advocates of its use in depressed patients under certain limited conditions (Hollister, 1973), tolerance to its effects as well as behavioral toxicity severely limit its clinical antidepressant efficacy (General Research Group Report, 1964). Sustained, high-dosage administration is capable of provoking hallucinations and paranoid psychoses in amphetamine addicts and also in normals (Connell, 1958; Griffith *et al.* 1970). Acute administration leads to a variety of behavioral and subjective responses, ranging from mood elevation and activation (to the point of hypomanic behavior in a few individuals) to dysphoric agitation or even a sedative effect in others (Lasagna *et al.,* 1955; van Kammen and Murphy, 1975). In one study of depressed patients in which 15 mg/day *d*-amphetamine was compared to 30 mg/day tranylcypromine, an approximately equal incidence of behavioral toxicity was observed with both drugs (Overall *et al.,* 1966).

Lithium carbonate has antidepressant as well as antimanic effects and is most used in the long-term, prophylactic treatment of individuals with recurrent affective disorders (Gershon and Shopsin, 1973). Although high doses produce a characteristic toxic state consisting of confusion, tremor, and ataxia that may progress to convulsions and coma, in the moderate dose range used therapeutically significant behavioral toxicity in the absence of neurological symptoms has been generally only observed in some schizophrenic patients who develop increased psychotic and confusional symptoms with a general reduction in effective functioning (Shopsin *et al.,* 1971). Lithium is definitely unlike the MAO-inhibiting and tricyclic antidepressants as well as *d*-amphetamine in that it is rarely if ever associated with the development of hypomanic or manic episodes, increased agitation or anxiety, or psychotic phenomena (except, as noted above, in some schizophrenic patients). Lithium carbonate administration, in fact, has been described to antagonize the euphoriant, activating, and hypomania-producing effects of L-dopa and of *d*- and *l*-amphetamine (van Kammen and Murphy, 1975).

## VIII. Behavioral Effects of Monoamine Oxidase-Inhibiting Drugs in Animals of Possible Relevance to Their Behavioral Toxicity in Man

The general effects of MAO inhibitors on animal behavior observed in over thirty-five studies have been summarized by Pletscher *et al.* (1966) as consisting of increased spontaneous motor activity and enhanced irritability and aggressivity—changes most marked after repeated administration of the drugs. However, discrepant changes, for example, decreased motor activity, have also been observed and, as with the biochemical changes reviewed in the following, there are definite species, drug, treatment duration, and dosage determinants of the behavioral effects of these drugs.

Monoamine oxidase inhibitors markedly potentiate the locomotor and other behavioral effects of monoamine precursors such as L-dopa. The MAO inhibitors also prevent or reverse reserpine and benzoquinolazine sedation, hypotension, hypothermia, and miosis. In fact, motor excitation rather than sedation results from reserpine administration to a MAO-inhibitor pretreated rodent—an interesting model to consider as an explanation for manic behavior occurring during MAO inhibitor treatment, presuming that some amine-releasing event capable of producing effects similar to reserpine might occur in man.

Many specific behaviors, such as conditioned avoidance responses, sexual activity, eating, stress-related defecation, and brain self-stimulation are also affected by MAO-inhibiting drugs (Pletscher *et al.*, 1966). In addition, more complex behaviors such as social interactions in nonhuman primates are also influenced by MAO-inhibiting drugs (Redmond *et al.*, 1971).

## IX. Biochemical Effects of Monoamine Oxidase-Inhibiting Drugs in Animals and Man of Possible Relevance to Their Behavioral Effects

The MAO-inhibiting antidepressants are a group of drugs with different chemical structures that share MAO-inhibiting potency. Some of these drugs have other properties that may contribute to their behavioral effects, such as direct amphetamine-like sympathetic stimulation effects (e.g., tranylcypromine, phenelzine), amine uptake-inhibiting effects (Hendley and Snyder, 1968), effects on the transport of amines and related substances across the blood–brain barrier (Cotzias *et al.*, 1974) and the gut (Huebers *et al.*, 1974), as well as some nonamine-related effects (Pletscher *et al.,* 1966). However, much evidence suggests that their major behavioral actions following chronic administration result from the consequences of MAO inhibition (Pletscher *et al.,* 1966).

Reductions in MAO activity not only interfere with the normal deamination and degradation of biogenic amines but can initiate a secondary chain of events that may modify synaptic function, including alterations in amine synthesis and the intracellular storage of increased amounts of natural amines or exogenous and uncommon amines ("false transmitters"). Different MAO inhibitors have different effects on the different biogenic amine systems in brain as well as on related systems such as those utilizing $\gamma$-aminobutyric acid as a neuromodulator. Marked species differences also exist. For example, motor activity changes following MAO inhibitor treatment have been attributed to catecholamine-related changes rather than to serotonin or tryptamine changes (Spector *et al.,* 1963), although in some species and some tissues different MAO-inhibiting drugs may have negligible effects or may act through other neurotransmitter mechanisms (Kopin, 1966; Pletscher *et al.,* 1966). The heterogeneity of MAO, the availability of different routes of metabolism (especially for the catecholamines), differences in drug treatment time and in drug metabolism, and the existence of different neurotransmitter systems subserving different behavioral functions or interacting with other neurotransmitter systems are a few of the variables that have been identified as contributing to species and tissue differences in response to these drugs.

In man, MAO-inhibiting drugs have been demonstrated to reduce brain and platelet MAO activity (Ganrot *et al.,* 1962; Robinson *et al.,* 1968), to increase brain or platelet levels of dopamine, serotonin, and octopamine (Ganrot *et al.,* 1962; Gjessing, 1964; Jones *et al.,* 1972; MacLean *et al.,* 1965; Murphy *et al.,* 1975; Sjoerdsma *et al.,* 1959), and to lead to reductions in the levels of deaminated metabolites of the biogenic amines in the cerebrospinal fluid (Kupfer and Bowers, 1972). Psychophysiological concomitants of MAO inhibition, particularly a marked and sustained reduction in rapid eye movement sleep (REM) (an effect not duplicated by any other drug), have been reported (Kupfer and Bowers, 1972; Wyatt *et al.,* 1971). The MAO-inhibiting drugs potentiate the effects of many drugs ranging from insulin to narcotics and including most biogenic amine-related agents (Stockley, 1973).

## X. Discussion and Conclusions

It is difficult to generalize and to draw firm conclusions from the information reviewed here because of the marked methodologic limitations in working from nonsystematically obtained data. Some tentative judgments, nonetheless, may be helpful for future comparative studies of the behavioral toxicity of psychoactive drugs.

Monoamine oxidase-inhibiting antidepressants are associated with significant, dose-related behavioral toxicity that exceeds that found in placebo-treated individuals and which may be similar in incidence, although not necessarily similar in form, to that reported with tricyclic antidepressants. Much of the behavioral toxicity of these drugs has been studied in psychiatric patients, and the overall incidence estimates may represent an interaction with a preexisting disorder. This point is certainly well illustrated in the case of bipolar, manic–depressive individuals who are especially prone to develop manic episodes during MAO inhibitor treatment, as well as during treatment with other antidepressant or stimulant drugs, such as the tricyclics, amphetamines, and L-dopa. The same point is also apparent in studies of schizophrenic patients, who appear to be activated by the drugs and respond with both some beneficial effects as well as some adverse exacerbations of psychopathology. It should be noted that all forms of psychiatric treatment may be associated with behavioral toxicity, and although there are no comprehensive comparative studies, not only drug treatment but also electroconvulsive therapy and the various psychotherapies [especially some of the more provocative therapies, e.g., the encounter approach (Lambert *et al.,* 1976; Lieberman, 1973)] have been reported to precipitate adverse behavioral changes.

The MAO inhibitors also very clearly induce some behavioral changes in nonpsychiatric patients, including normal volunteers and patients with tuberculosis, hypertension, and cancer. It is quite striking, in fact, that the predominant behavioral changes observed in these individuals are similar to those observed in the psychiatric patient groups, including hypomania or mania, euphoria, irritability, hallucinations, and paranoid episodes (see Table II). The euphoriant effects on normal volunteers observed in several studies primarily oriented toward the biochemical or sleep effects of these drugs are particularly of note (Akindele *et al.,* 1970; Friend *et al.,* 1958).

Direct relationships between adverse behavioral effects and drug dosage were observed with several of these MAO-inhibiting antidepressants. Duration of treatment was less clearly related to the occurrence of behavioral changes, although most commonly several weeks of treatment preceded such changes. However, the acute ingestion of high doses of MAO inhibitors has commonly been described as leading to agitation, delirium, and hallucinations associated with other signs of CNS stimulation including hyperreflexia, dilated pupils, and markedly increased temperature, blood pressure, heart rate, and respiratory rate. Convulsions and coma may also occur (Hollister, 1966; Shader and Dimascio, 1970).

It is not readily possible to compare the incidence and nature of the adverse behavioral effects associated with the different MAO-inhibiting drugs. The three drugs reviewed in greatest detail were studied at different times, with different assessment procedures, and different organization of reports. Although the somewhat lower incidence of behavioral side effects with phenelzine and tranylcypromine compared to iproniazid might represent real drug effects, the many non-drug-related issues contributing to the methodologic difficulties in assessing incidence data may also contribute to this apparent difference.

Not only MAO-inhibitor drug treatment but also its withdrawal may be associated with frequent behavioral changes. The co-occurrence of markedly increased REM sleep at the time of drug cessation (which seems to be rebound phenomenon following the nearly total suppression of REM sleep during drug treatment) provides some insight into the symptoms noted during this period (Akindele *et al.*, 1970; Crane, 1956b; Fisher *et al.*, 1952; Kupfer and Bowers, 1972). There are fewer hints concerning the specific neurochemical mechanisms involved in the adverse effects encountered during MAO-inhibitor treatment, or, for that matter, in the therapeutic effects of these drugs. Whether the adverse effects reflect an individual supersensitivity to or an excess of whichever effects of these drugs contribute to their therapeutic actions is not known.

Some plausible models for the excitant effects of these drugs can be suggested from data indicating that MAO-inhibitor treatment in man and animals can turn the depressant effects of reserpine into stimulant effects (Gradwell, 1960; Voelkel, 1959) and can markedly enhance the effects of biogenic amine precursors such as L-dopa (Stockley, 1973). As L-dopa by itself has some hypomania-inducing properties (Murphy, 1973; Murphy *et al.*, 1971) and as endogenous factors such as stress can also induce catecholamine synthesis, the potential for the adverse behavioral effects of the MAO inhibitors to result from an interaction with such endogenous or even dietary factors seems plausible. An organizing principle for effects of this type is the interpretation that MAO, unlike many catabolic enzymes, has indirect regulatory functions on biogenic amine storage and synthesis that are impaired by MAO-inhibiting drugs. Thus, these MAO inhibitors render the organism more vulnerable to other events which can alter amine functions and which may have behavioral consequences, both beneficial and adverse (Clarke and Sampath, 1973; Grahame-Smith, 1971; Murphy and Weiss, 1972; Murphy *et al.,* 1974a).

ACKNOWLEDGMENTS

This review was completed with generous assistance from Ms. Janice Grice, Wendy Hillerman, Robin Ulanow, and Irene Bellesky.

REFERENCES

Akindele, M. O., Evans, J. I., and Oswald, I. (1970). *Electroencephalogr. Clin. Neurophysiol.* **29,** 47.

Atkinson, R. M., and Ditman, K. S. (1965). *Clin. Pharmacol. Ther.* **6,** 631.

Ayd, F. J., Jr. (1961). *J. Neuropsychiatry* **2,** 119.

Bailey, S. d'A., Bucci, L., Gosline, E., and Kline, N. S. (1959). *Ann. N. Y. Acad. Sci.* **80,** 652.

Bartholomew, A. A. (1962). *Med. J. Aust.* **49,** 655.

Bates, T. J. N., and Douglas, A. D. McL. (1961). *J. Ment. Sci.* **107,** 538.

Belisle, J., Townley, M., Kozlowski, V., and Markel, P. (1958). *Am. J. Psychiatry* **115,** 544.

Bellak, L., and Rosenberg, S. (1966). *Psychosomatics* **7,** 106.

Biel, J. H. (1967). *In* "Psychopharmacological Agents" (M. Gordon, ed.), Vol. 2, pp. 519–522. Academic Press, New York.

Bloch, R. G., Dooneief, A. S., Buchberg, A. S., and Spellman, S. (1954). *Ann. Intern. Med.* **40,** 881.

Boston Collaborative Drug Surveillance Program (1972). *Lancet* **1,** 529.

Brune, G. G., and Himwich, H. E. (1962). *J. Nerv. Ment. Dis.* **134,** 447.

Bryant, J. M., Schvartz, N., Torosdag, S., Fertig, H., Fletcher, L., Jr., Schwartz, M. S., and Quan, R. B. F. (1963). *Ann. N. Y. Acad. Sci.* **107,** 1023.

Bunney, W. E., Jr., Murphy, D. L., Goodwin, F. K., and Borge, G. F. (1970). *Lancet* **1,** 1022.

Bunney, W. E., Jr., Goodwin, F. K., Murphy, D. L., House, K. M., and Gordon, E. K. (1972). *Arch. Gen. Psychiatry* **27,** 304.

Chase, T. N., and Murphy, D. L. (1973). *Annu. Rev. Pharmacol.* **13,** 181.

Cheifetz, I., Paulin, C., Tuatay, H., and Rubin, E. H. (1954). *Dis. Chest* **23,** 390.

Chu, J., and Fogel, E. J. (1963). *J. Indiana State Med. Assoc.* **56,** 40.

Clarke, D. E., and Sampath, S. S. (1973). *J. Pharmacol. Exp. Ther.* **187,** 539.

Clarke, J. (1960). *Br. Med. J.* **1,** 1204.

Coates, E. O., Jr., Brickman, G. L., and Meade, G. M. (1954). *Arch. Intern. Med.* **93,** 541.

Cole, J. O. (1960). *In* "Drugs and Behavior" (L. Uhr and J. G. Miller, eds.), p. 375. Wiley, New York.

Cole, J. O. (1964). *J. Am. Med. Assoc.* **190,** 124.

Cole, R. A., and Weiner, M. F. (1960). *Am. J. Psychiatry* **117,** 361.

Connell, P. H. (1958). "Amphetamine Psychosis." Chapman & Hall, London.

Costa, E., and Sandler, M. (1972). "Monoamine Oxidases—New Vistas." Raven, New York.

Cotzias, G. C., Tang, L. C., and Ginos, J. Z. (1974). *Proc. Natl. Acad. Sci. U.S.A.* **71,** 2715.

Crane, G. E. (1956a). *Am. J. Psychiatry* **112,** 494.
Crane, G. E. (1956b). *J. Nerv. Ment. Dis.* **124,** 322.
Dally, P. G., and Rohde, P. (1961). *Lancet* **1,** 18.
Davis, J. M., Klerman, G. L., and Schildkraut, J. J. (1968). "Psychopharmacology" (D. H. Efron, ed.). US Govt. Printing Office, Washington, D.C.
Ducoudray, J., Noyer, J., and Mimart, J. (1963). *Presse Med.* **71,** 12.
Dunlop, E. (1963). *Ann. N. Y. Acad. Sci.* **107,** 1107.
Dunlop, E., DeFelice, E. A., Berge, J. R., and Resnick, O. (1965). *Psychosomatics* **6,** 1.
Feldman, P. E. (1959). *Ann. N. Y. Acad. Sci.* **80,** 712.
Ferreira, A. J. DeL., and Freeman, H. (1958). *Am. J. Psychiatry* **114,** 933.
Fingl, E., and Woodbury, D. M. (1965). "Pharmacological Basis of Therapeutics" (L. S. Goodman and A. Gilman, eds.). Macmillan, New York.
Fisher, M. M., Mamlock, E. R., Tendlau, A., Tebrok, E. H., Drumm, A. E., and Spiegelman, A. (1952). *N. Y. Med. J.* **52,** 1517.
Freymuth, H. W., Walker, H., Baumecker, P., and Stein, H. (1959). *Dis. Nerv. Syst.* **20,** 123.
Friend, D. G., Zileli, M. S., Hamlin, J. T., and Reutter, F. W. (1958). *J. Clin. Exp. Psychopathol.* **19,** 61.
Ganrot, P. O., Rosengren, E., and Gottfries, C. G. (1962). *Experientia* **18,** 260.
General Research Group Report (1964). *Practitioner* **192,** 151.
Gershon, S., and Shopsin, B. (1973). "Lithium." Plenum, New York.
Gjessing, L. R. (1964). *J. Psychiatr. Res.* **2,** 149.
Goodwin, F. K., and Bunney, W. E., Jr. (1971). *Semin. Psychiatry* **3,** 435.
Gottfries, C. G. (1963). *Acta Psychiatr. Scand.* **39,** 463.
Gradwell, B. G. (1960). *Br. Med. J.* **2,** 1018.
Grahame-Smith, D. G. (1971). *J. Neurochem.* **18,** 1053.
Greenblatt, M., Grosser, G. H., and Wechsler, H. (1962). *Am. J. Psychiatry* **119,** 144.
Greenblatt, M., Grosser, G. H., and Wechsler, H. (1964). *Am. J. Psychiatry* **120,** 935.
Griffith, J. D., Cavanaugh, J. H., Held, J., Oates, J. A. (1970). *In* "Amphetamines and Related Compounds," p. 897. Raven, New York.
Hendley, E. D., and Snyder, S. H. (1968). *Nature (London)* **220,** 1330.
Himmelhoch, J. M., Detre, T., Kupfer, D. J., Swartzburg, M., and Byck, R. (1972). *J. Nerv. Ment. Dis.* **155,** 216.
Hollister, L. E. (1966). *Clin. Pharmacol. Ther.* **7,** 142.
Hollister, L. E. (1973). "Clinical Use of Psychotherapeutic Drugs." Thomas, Springfield, Illinois.
Huebers, H., Huebers, E., Huebers, U., and Rummel, W. (1974). *Naunyn–Schmiedeberg's Arch. Pharmacol.* **282,** 36.
Hunter, R. A. (1952). *Lancet* **2,** 960.
Imlah, N. W. (1960). *Lancet* **1,** 826.
Janecek, J., Schiele, B. C., and Vestre, N. D. (1963a). *J. New Drugs* **3,** 309.
Janecek, J., Schiele, B. C., Bellville, T., and Anderson, R. (1963b). *Curr. Ther. Res., Clin. Exp.* **5,** 608.
Janzarik, W. (1959). *Can. Psychiatr. Assoc. J.* **4,** 195.
Johnson, J., and Eilenberg, M. D. (1960). *Br. Med. J.* **2,** 857.
Johnstone, C. C., and Marsh, W. (1973). *Lancet* **1,** 567.
Jones, A. B., Pare, C. M. B., Nicholson, W. J., Price, K., and Stacey, R. S. (1972). *Br. Med. J.* **1,** 17.
Kay, D. W. K., Garside, R. F., and Fahy, T. J. (1973). *Br. J. Psychiatry* **123,** 63.

Kettner, H., ed. (1969–1974). *Adverse Reaction Titles,* Vols. 4–9.
Kiloh, L. G., Child, J. P., and Latner, G. (1960). *J. Ment. Sci.* **106,** 1139.
Klein, D. F., and Davis, J. M. (1969). "Diagnosis and Drug Treatment of Psychiatric Disorders." Williams & Wilkins, Baltimore, Maryland.
Klein, D. F., and Fink, M. (1962). *Am. J. Psychiatry* **119,** 432.
Kline, N. S. (1963). *Ann. N. Y. Acad. Sci.* **107,** 1090.
Kopin, I. (1966). *Pharmacol. Rev.* **16,** 179.
Kupfer, D. J., and Bowers, M. B., Jr. (1972). *Psychopharmacologia* **27,** 183.
Kurland, A. A., Destounis, N., Shaffer, J. W., and Pinto, A. (1967). *J. Nerv. Ment. Dis.* **145,** 292.
Lambert, M. J., Bergin, A. E., Collin, J. L. (1976). "The Therapist's Contribution to Effective Psychotherapy" (A. S. Gurman and A. M. Razin, eds.). Pergamon, Oxford. (In press).
Lasagna, L., von Felsinger, J. M., and Beecher, H. K. (1955). *J. Am. Med. Assoc.* **157,** 1006.
Leitch, A., and Seager, C. P. (1963). *Psychopharmacologia* **4,** 72.
Levy, L., and Lohrenz, J. (1960). *Can. Med. Assoc. J.* **82,** 1031.
Lieberman, M. A. (1973). "Encounter Groups: First Facts." Basic Books, New York.
Loomer, H. P., Saunders, J. C., and Kline, N. S. (1957). *Am. Psychiatr. Assoc. Res. Rep.* **8,** 129.
MacLean, R., Nicholson, W. J., Pare, C. M., Stacey, R. S. (1965). *Lancet* **2,** 205.
Mann, A. M., and Hutchison, J. L. (1967). *Can. Med. Assoc. J.* **97,** 1350.
Marjerrison, G. (1966). *J. Nerv. Ment. Dis.* **142,** 254.
Martin, M. E. (1963). *Br. J. Psychiatry* **109,** 279.
Meyler, L. (1964). "Side Effects of Drugs," Vol. 4. Excerpta Medica, Amsterdam.
Meyler, L. (1966). "Side Effects of Drugs, " Vol. 5. Excerpta Medica, Amsterdam.
Meyler, L., and Herxheimer, A. (1968). "Side Effects of Drugs," Vol. 6. Excerpta Medica, Amsterdam.
Meyler, L., and Herxheimer, A. (1971). "Side Effects of Drugs," Vol. 7. Excepta Medica, Amsterdam.
Middlefell, R., Frost, I., Egan, G. P., and Eaton, H. (1960). *J. Ment. Sci.* **106,** 1533.
MRC Report (1952). *Br. Med. J.* **2,** 281, 735.
Murphy, D. L. (1973). *Annu. Rev. Med.* **24,** 209.
Murphy, D. L., and Weiss, R. (1972). *Am. J. Psychiatry* **128,** 1351.
Murphy, D. L., Brodie, H. K. H., Goodwin, F. K., Bunney, W. E., Jr. (1971). *Nature (London)* **229,** 135.
Murphy, D. L., Belmaker, R., and Wyatt, R. J. (1974a). *J. Psychiatr. Res.* **11,** 221.
Murphy, D. L., Brand, E., Baker, M., van Kammen, D., and Gordon, E. (1974b). *J. Pharmacol.* **5,** Suppl. 1, 102 (abstr.); "Neuropsychopharmacology" (J. R. Boissier, H. Hippius, P. Pichot, eds.), pp. 788–799. Am. Elsevier, New York.
Murphy, D. L., Baker, M., Goodwin, F. K., Miller, H., Kotin, J., and Bunney, W. E., Jr. (1974c). *Psychopharmacologia* **34,** 11.
Murphy, D. L., Cahan, D. H., and Molinoff, P. B. (1975). *Clin. Pharmacol. Ther.* **18,** 587.
Nies, A., Robinson, D. S., Lamborn, K. R., and Lampert, R. P. (1973). *Arch. Gen. Psychiatry* **28,** 834.
Nies, A., Robinson, D. S., Harris, L. S., and Lamborn, K. R. (1974). *Adv. Biochem. Psychopharmacol.* **12,** 59.
O'Connor, J. B., Howlett, K. S., Jr., and Wagner, R. R. (1953). *Annu. Rev. Tuberculosis* **68,** 270.

Olson, G. W. (1962). *Am. J. Psychiatry* **118,** 1044.

Overall, J. E., Hollister, L. E., Pokorny, C. K. (1962). *Clin. Pharmacol. Ther.* **3,** 16.

Overall, J. E., Hollister, L. E., Shelton, J., Johnson, M., and Kimbell, I., Jr. (1966). *Dis. Nerv. Syst.* **27,** 653.

Pare, C. M. B., and Mack, J. W. (1971). *J. Med. Genet.* **8,** 306.

Pleasure, H. (1954). *Arch. Neurol. Psychiatry* **72,** 313.

Pletscher, A., Gey, F. K., and Burkand, W. P. (1966). *Handb. Exp. Pharmacol.* **19,** 38.

Price-Evans, D. A., Davison, K., and Pratt, R. T. C. (1964). *Clin. Pharmacol. Ther.* **6,** 430.

Raskin, A. (1972). *J. Clin. Psychopharmacol.* **12,** 22.

Raskin, A., Schulterbrandt, Reatig, N., Crook, T. H., and Odle, D. (1974). *Arch. Gen. Psychiatry* **30,** 66.

Redmond, D. E., Jr., Maas, J. W., Kling, A., and Dekirmenjian, H. (1971). *Psychosom. Med.* **33,** 97.

Rees, L., and Benaim, S. (1960). *J. Ment. Sci.* **106,** 193.

Rees, L., and Davies, B. (1961). *J. Ment. Sci.* **107,** 560.

Robinson, D. S., Lovenberg, W., Keiser, H., and Sjoerdsma, J. (1968). *Biochem. Pharmacol.* **17,** 109.

Robinson, D. S., Nies, A., Ravaris, C. L., and Lamborn, K. (1973). *Arch. Gen. Psychiatry* **29,** 407.

Ross, I. S. (1965). *Am. J. Psychiatry* **119,** 251.

Rothman, T. (1962). *J. Neuropsychiatry* **3,** 234.

Rothman, T., Grayson, H., Ferguson, J. (1961). *Compr. Psychiatry* **2,** 27.

Sargeant, W. (1961). *Br. Med. J.* **1,** 225.

Sarwer-Foner, G. J., Korantyi, E. K., Mezzaros, A., and Grauer, I. I. (1959). *Can. Med. Assoc. J.* **81,** 991.

Schiele, B. C. (1963). *Ann. N. Y. Acad. Sci.* **107,** 1131.

Selikoff, I. J., and Robitzek, E. H. (1952). *Dis. Chest* **21,** 385.

Shader, R., and Dimascio, A. (1970). "Psychotropic Drug Side Effects (Clinical and Theoretical Perspectives)." Williams & Wilkins, Baltimore, Maryland.

Shopsin, B., Kim, S., and Gershon, S. (1971). *Br. J. Psychiatry* **119,** 435.

Sjoerdsma, A., Lovenberg, W., Oates, J. A., Crout, J. R., and Udenfriend, S. (1959). *Science* **130,** 225.

Smith, A. (1969). *Psychopharmacol. Bull.* **4,** 1–53.

Smith, B., and Prockop, D. J. (1962). *New Engl. J. Med.* **267,** 1338.

Snyder, S. H. (1972). *Arch. Gen. Psychiatry* **27,** 169.

Spector, S., Hirsch, C. W., and Brodie, B. B. (1963). *Int. J. Neuropharmacol.* **2,** 81.

Stockley, I. H. (1973). *Pharm. J.* **210,** 590; **211,** 95.

Sutnick, A. I., Weiss, L. B., Schindler, P. D., and Soloff, L. A. (1964). *J. Am. Med. Assoc.* **188,** 610.

Tavener, R. H. (1959). *Can. Psychiatr. Assoc. J.* **4,** 8.

van Kammen, D., and Murphy, D. L. (1975). *Psychopharmacologia* **44,** 215.

Voelkel, A. (1959). *Ann. N. Y. Acad. Sci.* **80,** 680.

Weiss, H. D., Walker, M. D., and Wierhik, P. H. (1974). *New Engl. J. Med.* **291,** 75.

Wiedorn, W. S., and Ervin, F. (1954). *Arch. Neurol. Psychiatry* **72,** 321.

Wittenborn, J. R., Plante, M., Burgess, F., and Livermore, N. (1961). *J. Nerv. Ment. Dis.* **133,** 316.

Wittenborn, J. R., Plante, M., Burgess, F., and Maurer, H. A. (1962). *J. Nerv. Ment. Dis.* **135,** 131.

Woods, L. W., and Lewis, D. J. (1961). *Can. Med. Assoc. J.* **84,** 212.
Wyatt, R. J., Engleman, K., Kupfer, D. J., Fram, D. H., Sjoerdsma, A., and Snyder, F. (1970). *Lancet* **2,** 842.
Wyatt, R. J., Fram, D. H., Kupfer, D. J., and Snyder, F. (1971). *Arch. Gen. Psychiatry* **24,** 145.
Yang, H.-Y. T., and Neff, N. H. (1974). *J. Pharmacol. Exp. Ther.* **189,** 733.

# Biology, Diagnosis, and Chemotherapeutic Management of Pancreatic Malignancy

John S. Macdonald,* Lawrence Widerlite,*† and Philip S. Schein*

I. Introduction . . . . . . . . . . 107
II. Adenocarcinoma of the Pancreas . . . . . . . . . . 108
A. Diagnosis . . . . . . . . . . 109
B. Chemotherapy . . . . . . . . . . 114
III. Islet Cell Tumors . . . . . . . . . . 127
Chemotherapy . . . . . . . . . . 129
IV. Conclusion . . . . . . . . . . 136
References . . . . . . . . . . 137

## I. Introduction

Adenocarcinoma of the pancreas has demonstrated an increasing incidence in the United States during the past three decades, particularly in Black males. It presently ranks as the fourth (*109*) most common cause of cancer death, exceeded only by lung, large bowel, and breast cancer. Over 19,000 cases are diagnosed each year, and essentially all patients can be expected to die of their disease. In recognition of the importance of the disease as a health problem in this country, the National Pancreatic Cancer Project has been established by the National Cancer Advisory Board.

Several epidemiologic studies have been carried out in an attempt to identify specific etiological factors that may be responsible for the increasing incidence of this disease. There is evidence (*165*) that chemical carcinogens are causative agents. Studies (*79*) conducted on members of the American Chemical Society suggest that exposure to certain chemicals increases the risk of pancreatic cancer. Furthermore, cigarette smoking and a diet high in cholesterol have demonstrated a positive correlation with the occurrence of pancreatic cancer. Animal studies have clearly demonstrated that the pancreas is a target organ for

* Division of Medical Oncology, Vincent T. Lombardi Cancer Research Center, Georgetown University, Washington, D.C.

† Gastroenterology Section, Veterans Hospital, Washington, D.C.

chemical carcinogenesis. Agents such as 1-methyl-1-nitrosourea (*119*) and di-*N*-propylnitrosamine (*116*) are capable of producing adenocarcinoma of the pancreas in specific rodent species.

Although the true incidence of pancreatic islet cell tumors is unknown, islet cell adenomas may be found in as many as 1.5% of carefully performed autopsies. Most, however, do not become clinically manifest (*144*). The incidence of islet cell carcinomas is estimated to be less than 1/100,000 population (*101*). Despite the infrequency with which these tumors are encountered in individual centers, islet cell neoplasms have been the subject of extensive investigations and discussion in the medical literature. This has resulted, in part, from recognition of the devastating and difficult-to-manage distinctive clinical syndromes which these tumors may present. In addition, the investigation of these diseases has significantly increased our understanding of the physiology of the different cell types that constitute the islets of Langerhans and the function of the hormones they produce. A proportion of these tumors appear to be inherited in association with adenomas that concurrently affect other endocrine organs: Wermer's syndrome or multiple endocrine adenomatosis Type I (*7*). In addition there is evidence from animal studies that functioning islet cell tumors can be produced by chemical carcinogens (*118*). The purpose of this review is to bring together much of the rapidly accumulating information on the chemotherapeutic management of the exocrine and endocrine neoplasms of the pancreas.

## II. Adenocarcinoma of the Pancreas

It is estimated that three-quarters of the nonendocrine malignancies of the pancreas are classified as duct cell adenocarcinomas (*31*). The remaining 25% are diagnosed as giant cell, microadeno, adenosquamous, mucinous, and anaplastic carcinomas. Only 1% of the tumors have been classified as acinar cell malignancies. There is considerable speculation as to the cell of origin of adenocarcinomas. Many pathologists regard the duct cell as precursor cell for the tumor. However, there is some evidence that acinar cells, under the stimulus of a carcinogen, can dedifferentiate to the ductal form of histology (*119*) from which they arose embryologically.

The clinical manifestations of adenocarcinoma of the pancreas (*12, 15, 18, 87, 93*) have been extensively reviewed, and it is clear that pancreatic cancer is rarely diagnosed at an early stage. The initial symptoms may be nonspecific and are frequently disregarded until anorexia, weight loss, pain, or jaundice become overtly manifest. An early diagnosis requires a high index of suspicion on the part of the physician and the willingness of the patient to undergo a series of diagnostic procedures for what might otherwise appear to be relatively mild complaints.

Pain is an important feature of pancreatic carcinoma. It typically presents in the epigastrium, with radiation to the back in approximately 25% of cases. It increases in severity, frequently requiring the use of narcotics, and neurosurgical palliative procedures may be required in carefully selected patients.

Anorexia and weight loss are common accompaniments of pancreatic cancer and may become the most debilitating features of the disease. Occasionally the weight loss may be associated with signs of pancreatic exocrine insufficiency and malabsorption. There are no data yet available to estimate accurately how frequently malabsorption is an important clinical problem and to what magnitude the various forms of therapy for pancreatic carcinoma may compromise pancreatic exocrine function. Diabetes secondary to pancreatic endocrine insufficiency may occur but is found in less than 20% of patients.

Obstructive jaundice can be expected to occur in greater than 75% of patients in whom the tumor arises in the head of the pancreas and may be associated with a palpable gall bladder (Courvoisier's sign). Jaundice may be "painless," but more frequently is preceded or coexists with abdominal discomfort.

Physical examination is generally unrewarding in the diagnosis of pancreatic cancer. By the time physical signs can be demonstrated, the disease is usually inoperable because of local spread or distant metastasis. Because of the retroperitoneal location of the pancreas, a palpable abdominal mass is unusual and is present in only 20% of patients. Hepatomegaly may be present resulting from biliary tract obstruction or liver metastasis, and the presence of an abnormal supraclavicular lymph node may be an initial sign of distant metastasis.

### A. Diagnosis

A great deal of clinical investigative effort has been directed toward defining the usefulness of available or newly developing diagnostic procedures for detection of pancreatic cancer. Routine hematological and clinical chemistry tests are too insensitive and nonspecific to be of diagnostic value. As a result, radiographic procedures have been the mainstay for diagnosis.

Conventional upper gastrointestinal (UGI) series has low diagnostic accuracy (*125*) and most often detects only a large carcinoma that has caused gross pancreatic enlargement and secondary infiltration of the surrounding structures. Abnormalities commonly found on UGI series involve the posterior gastric wall, (*122, 125, 139*) retrogastric space, antrum, and duodenal loop. Hypotonic duodenography, a modification of the UGI, has a diagnostic accuracy of 75% in cancer of the pancreatic head and about 90% in ampullary carcinoma. Unfortunately, most patients are already symptomatic at the time of this procedure. Hypotonic duodenography is not sensitive enough and cannot be used to evaluate lesions of the body and tail.

Ultrasonography, a new noninvasive procedure, has been useful in detecting pancreatic disease. Typical echo patterns have now been defined for acute pancreatitis, fibrosis, and tumors of the head, body, and tail of the pancreas (*22, 45*).

Selenomethionine-$^{75}$Se (*83*) scanning allows assessment of size, shape, and position of the pancreas and defines the extent of morphological damage. It can detect neoplasms over 2 cm in size and is particularly helpful for lesions in the body and tail of the pancreas.

An unequivocal normal scan is a reliable finding to exclude pancreatic disease. However, abnormal scans pose difficulties in defining pathological entities (*71*). Differentiation between pancreatitis and diffuse involvement of the pancreas with carcinoma is, at best, difficult; furthermore, 30% false positive findings have been reported. Concentration of the isotope in the liver with overlap interference has been a problem that is being resolved with new photosubtractive techniques. Continued investigation into this field to improve the specificity of isotopes and resolution may make this a valuable screening procedure.

The use of computerized axial tomography in the detection of pancreatic masses is currently undergoing evaluation at Georgetown University Hospital. The ACTA scanner (*77*) has provided good definition of pancreatic masses in several patients with pathologically proven pancreatic cancer. This research tool is currently undergoing a prospective evaluation to determine its usefulness in both detection and following of patients with unresectable pancreatic cancer as compared to other noninvasive techniques such as ultrasound.

Endoscopic cholangiopancreatography (ERCP) performed with a fiberoptic duodenoscope, with cannulation of the ampulla of Vater and retrograde injection of contrast material into the pancreatic ducts, is a new and developing technique (*167*). Most procedures have been performed in patients with advanced disease, and as a result its value in the early detection of pancreatic carcinoma is unknown. The overall accuracy of this procedure in the diagnosis of pancreatic carcinoma is still being determined, but some authors (*125, 167*) claim a 90% yield. The major findings of pancreatic cancer demonstrated by ERCP include pancreatic duct stenosis (solitary or multiple), delayed contrast outflow, ductal occlusion or displacement, necrotic cavity formation, and deformity of the common bile duct by a tumor in the pancreatic head (*3, 10, 110, 145*). Combined with ERCP, investigators have used carcinoembryonic antigen (CEA) (*72*) determinations on pancreatic juice, cytology (*42*) of duodenal juice, pancreatic juice, and bile, plus secretin testing with collection of ductular fluids and measurement of bicarbonate (*108*). One report claims a 79% (*42*) accuracy with the combination of ERCP and cytology; however, limitations arise in cases with early stage lesions, neoplasms located in the body and tail of the pancreas, and in those in which exocrine activity is significantly impaired. Combined ERCP–CEA–secretin testing is a new diagnostic approach undergoing evaluation. Duodenal drainage techniques utilizing the secretin test have been found to be positive (*37*) in 85–95% of patients with pancreatic carcinoma involving the head of the organ but have not been shown to be helpful at an early stage of disease when cure is possible.

Transhepatic cholangiography is a technique that may be of value in demonstrating compression, distortion, or obstruction of the common bile duct by tumor in an enlarged head of the pancreas.

Selective and superselective angiography (*53, 112*) are highly accurate procedures allowing differentiation of carcinoma of the pancreas from pancreatitis in approximately 85% of cases, and 1–2 cm size cancers may be detected. Magnification techniques and the pharmacoangiographic (*53, 84*) use of vasoconstrictors and vasodilators significantly improve diagnostic confidence and accuracy, allowing differentiation of the normal and abnormal pancreas in 95% of cases, and a diagnostic accuracy of up to 95% in pancreatic adenocarcinoma (*16, 53*). Many angiographic features of carcinoma have been described (*53, 125, 153*). These include: arterial narrowing and encasement, suggesting compression or invasion of the vessels by the neoplasm (*16, 84*); neovascularity, an uncommon finding consisting of small tortuous vessels in a fine network; and arterial obstructions of the celiac, superior mesenteric, hepatic, splenic, gastroduodenal, or small intrapancreatic branches. Rarely tumor opacification (i.e., tumor blush) is noted. In addition, involvement of the splenic, portal, and superior mesenteric veins is often found, especially in tumors of the body and tail, which may grow to large sizes before diagnosis because of a paucity of early symptoms. Vascular displacement is uncommon, since the carcinoma infiltrates rather than displaces surrounding tissue (*153*). Hepatic metastases and gallbladder enlargement can be evaluated by hepatic arterial configuration and configuration of the cystic artery. In addition to its diagnostic value, pancreatic angiography is a useful tool for predicting tumor resectability (*53, 148, 154*). Patients with encasement limited to intrapancreatic arteries, tumor vessels, and involvement of the gastroduodenal artery, but not extrapancreatic arteries, are amenable to surgical exploration and possible resection.

The possibility of using circulating marker substances for diagnosis and follow-up of patients with pancreatic carcinoma is being examined. Ona *et al.* (*111*) demonstrated elevated CEA (>2.5 ng/ml) in the majority of a series of patients with pancreatic cancer. The elevation of CEA was shown to correlate with extent of disease: 71% of patients with metastatic disease had CEA > 10 ng/ml, whereas all patients without apparent metastasis had CEA < 9 ng/ml. Unfortunately, CEA lacks specificity and has also been demonstrated to be elevated in patients with nonmalignant disease of the pancreas, and 18 of 42 (43%) patients with pancreatitis were demonstrated to have elevated CEA by Delwicke *et al.* (*34*). The usefulness of monitoring CEA to follow therapy of pancreatic cancer has not been clearly defined.

$\alpha$-Fetoglobulin is a fetal protein that has been demonstrated to be elevated in hepatocellular carcinoma and embryonal cell carcinomas. Recently, McIntire *et al.* (*85*) demonstrated elevated $\alpha$-fetoglobulin (>40 ng/ml) in 25% of patients with pancreatic carcinoma. This relationship between $\alpha$-fetoglobulin and pancreatic carcinoma deserves further investigation to establish the efficacy of this serum marker in following the course of patients with cancer of the pancreas.

Both CEA and $\alpha$-fetoglobulin are nonspecific markers, and it is clear that the ideal tumor marker would be a specific tumor antigen circulating in patients with pancreatic malignancies. In 1974, Banwo *et al.* (*8*) demonstrated evidence for an oncofetal antigen circulating in the serum of patients with pancreatic cancer. Homogenates of fetal pancreas were used to immunize rabbits, and the resultant antisera was absorbed with human albumin and adult pancreas. The absorbed antisera were shown, using Ouchterlony gel diffusion techniques, to form precipitant lines with the serum of 36 of 37 patients with pancreatic carcinoma. No precipitant lines were seen in 38 controls, including patients with pancreatitis, obstructive jaundice, cirrhosis, carcinoma of the colon, gastric carcinoma, and hepatoma. This work needs to be confirmed with more sensitive techniques including radioimmunoassay. However, a sensitive and specific test for circulating specific oncofetal antigen or tumor-specific antigen offers the hope of increased detection of cases in whom resection with curative intent is possible.

Although these indirect means of detecting pancreatic cancer are becoming more useful, definitive diagnosis requires tissue confirmation of malignancy. In the past, surgical dogma has always held that biopsy of the pancreas was a hazardous procedure with an unacceptable rate of morbidity and mortality (*17, 138*). Complications cited in the literature include pancreatic cutaneous fistulas, pancreatitis, and postoperative wound infection in as many as 25% of cases. Surgeons have been tempted to make the "clinical diagnosis" of pancreatic carcinoma solely from inspection and palpation of the organ at the time of laparotomy. However, the forms of postoperative therapy currently being employed mandate for a definitive diagnosis and exclusion of chronic pancreatitis as the etiology of a pancreatic mass. Recently, a large series (*68*) of patients have been reported from the Mayo Clinic who experienced little morbidity after undergoing pancreatic biopsy. Of 527 patients in the total series, 112 underwent exploratory laparotomy with pancreatic biopsy as the only surgical procedure, 64 had Vim-Silverman needle biopsies, and 48 had wedge biopsies performed. There were 7 complications including postoperative pancreatitis (2 patients), subphrenic abscess (1 patient), and wound infection (4 patients) for a total complication rate of 6.2% with no deaths. This rate of complication compared favorably to a complication rate of 4.1% secondary to pancreatic biopsy in 415 patients who had biopsy followed by definitive surgical procedures. The frozen section interpretation of pancreatic biopsy specimens was highly satisfactory with only 1 false negative in 201 patients interpreted as having benign specimens on frozen section. Thus, it is clear that a tissue diagnosis by pancreatic biopsy can be accomplished at the time of laparotomy with very acceptable morbidity. The morbidity (*68*) of biopsy may be further reduced in head lesions if transduodenal needle biopsy is the only biopsy procedure performed.

Less invasive means of making a pathological diagnosis of pancreatic carcinoma are undergoing initial trials with promising results. Twenty (*91*) cases of pancreatic carcinoma diagnosed at peritoneoscopy have recently been reported from investigators in Germany. Both Menghini needle biopsies and thin-needle aspirates for cytology were performed under direct peritoneoscopic visualization with no evidence of bleeding, fistula formation, or elevation of serum amylase.

Thin-needle cytological aspirate of pancreatic tissue has also been performed under ultrasonic guidance (*62, 142*). Smith *et al.* (*142*) reported aspirating pancreatic tissue for cytology on 6 patients who had pancreatic tumors. Five of 6 patients had positive cytology for carcinoma, and the procedure resulted in no morbidity. It is very encouraging that rapid progress is being made in relatively noninvasive techniques in making a definitive pathological diagnosis of pancreatic carcinoma as these techniques may in the future aid greatly in developing intelligent plans of patient diagnosis and management.

## B. Chemotherapy

### 1. *Single-Agent Chemotherapy*

5-Fluorouracil (5-FU) has been the single agent most frequently used in the treatment of adenocarcinoma of the pancreas. Using variations of a standard intravenous loading course (15 mg/kg day × 5, followed by 7.5 mg/kg every other day × 4) as originally described by Curreri *et al.* (*33*), response rates ranging between 0 and 67% have been reported (Table I). Moertel and Reitemeier (*97*) found a similar wide variation in response rate, in their review of results reported in the case of 5-FU therapy in colorectal carcinoma. Although the 5-FU response rates in the treatment of advanced pancreatic cancer have been variable, a 20–30% response rate is generally accepted as valid (Table I). It must be remembered that response rate in pancreatic cancer may be difficult to define since patients frequently do not have many parameters of followable disease, and disease progression is often manifested only by progressive wasting and cachexia, whereas tumor regression may be heralded merely by increased well being, weight gain, and decreased

TABLE I

5-Fluorouracil Therapy in Pancreatic Carcinoma

| No. responses | Response rate (%) | Reference (year) |
|---|---|---|
| 5/9 | 67 | *67* (1960) |
| 9/17 | 52 | *123* (1962) |
| 3/6 | 50 | *28* (1960) |
| 23/50 | 46 | *66* (1964) |
| 5/17 | 29 | *124* (1965) |
| 1/4 | 25 | *30* (1966) |
| 5/23 | 22 | *96* (1967) |
| 1/5 | 20 | *161* (1961) |
| 2/11 | 18 | *103* (1968) |
| 3/19 | 16 | *98* (1964) |
| 1/7 | 14 | *120* (1967) |
| 1/20 | 5 | *107* (1968) |
| 0/6 | 0 | *73* (1961) |
| 0/5 | 0 | *44* (1963) |

constitutional symptoms. 5-Fluorouracil must be considered the standard single agent in the treatment of pancreatic cancer, and the response rate of approximately 20–30% induced by 5-FU is the standard to which the results of other forms of chemotherapy must be compared.

In addition to 5-FU, there have been relatively few single agents that have been adequately tested in pancreatic carcinoma. However, the antitumor antibiotic mitomycin C is an agent that has been found to be efficacious, with clinical activity comparable to 5-FU (Table II). As noted in the table, the drug has usually been given in a loading course. This method of administration has caused serious toxicity. Myelosuppression is the common severe and dose-limiting toxic effect seen with this drug. The myelosuppression is represented by both leukopenia and thrombocytopenia and, similar to the nitrosoureas, is delayed in onset. The nadir of white blood cell and platelet counts is not seen until 3 to 4 weeks after the drug is given, and recovery from myelosuppression may be prolonged. It can be easily understood that loading dose therapy with mitomycin C may lead to a profound myelosuppression that may result in significant morbidity. Repeated courses of loading therapy may result in cumulative bone marrow injury. Mitomycin C can produce a significant mucositis with the development of oral ulceration and hemorrhage, which may predispose the patient to superinfection. The drug has caused particular concern among some workers (*100*) because of its vesicant activity if injected subcutaneously rather than intravenously. This toxicity can be profound and has resulted in local ulceration and necrosis requiring grafting. It is very important for the physician or paramedical person administering mitomycin C to determine with certainty that the drug is being injected intravenously and that there is no inadvertent infiltration of subcutaneous tissues.

TABLE II

MITOMYCIN C THERAPY IN PANCREATIC CARCINOMA

| Drug regimen | No. responses / No. patients | Response rate (%) | Reference (year) |
|---|---|---|---|
| 0.05–0.1 mg/kg/d × 10–25 | 3/8 | 38 | *162* (1970) |
| 0.01–0.50 mg/kg/d × 2–40 | 6/18 | 33 | *23* (1968) |
| (a) 0.05 mg/kg/d × 6, then every other day to 50 mg total; or (b) 0.15 mg/kg/d × 5 every 8–12 weeks | 2/8 | 16 | *100* (1968) |
| 0.05 mg/kg/d × 6, then every other day to 50 mg total | 1/10 | 10 | *104* (1969) |

Many of the problems with severe myelosuppression with mitomycin C may be eliminated if the drug is given in an intermittent rather than loading schedule. Mitomycin C in doses of 10–20 mg/m$^2$ administered every 6–8 weeks can be given with minimal toxicity. The myelosuppression encountered is mild, and recovery is generally complete in 4 to 5 weeks. This treatment schedule is quite adaptable for use in combination chemotherapy with other myelosuppressive agents, and we are currently carrying out studies in gastrointestinal cancer using mitomycin C in combination with 5-FU, Adriamycin, and streptozotocin.

The nitrosoureas have been shown to have activity in a number of gastrointestinal cancers (*24*), but have been found to be relatively inactive in pancreatic cancer. 1,3-Bis(2-chloroethyl)-1-nitrosourea (BCNU) as a single agent has been reported to have no activity in pancreatic carcinoma in studies reported from the Mayo Clinic (*75, 94*). Most other nitrosoureas have not been adequately tested to determine their single agent activity. However, the naturally occurring nitrosourea, streptozotocin, has produced objective response in both adenocarcinoma and islet cell carcinoma of the pancreas (*19, 137*). Broder and Carter (*19*) reported objective responses in 4 of 13 (31%) patients, Stolkinsky *et al.* (*147*) reported 2 out of 5 (40%) responses, and Dupriest *et al.* (*38*) reported 2 out of 4 (50%) responses in patients with adenocarcinoma of the pancreas (Table III).

Alkylating agents have not been adequately studied in pancreatic carcinoma, and less than 20 patients treated with these drugs have been reported in the literature (Table IV). The response rate has generally been less than 20% in this small number of patients with the notable exception of the 67% response reported by Moore *et al.* (*102*) in patients treated with chlorambucil. The Eastern Cooperative Oncology Group (*39*) currently has an active protocol in advanced pancreatic cancer with L-phenylalanine mustard as one of the arms of treatment. This drug was arbitrarily chosen as a representative alkylating agent that is easily

TABLE III

STREPTOZOTOCIN THERAPY IN PANCREATIC CARCINOMA

| Drug regimen | No. responses / No. patients | Response rate (%) | Reference (year) |
|---|---|---|---|
| 1–1.5 gm/m$^2$ weekly | 2/4 | 50 | *38* (1975) |
| 1–2.0 gm/m$^2$ weekly | 2/5 | 40 | *147* (1972) |
| 1–2.0 gm/m$^2$ weekly | 4/13 | 31 | *19* (1971) |

TABLE IV

ALKYLATING AGENT THERAPY IN PANCREATIC CARCINOMA

| Drug regimen | No. responses / No. patients | Response rate (%) | Reference (year) |
|---|---|---|---|
| Chlorambucil | | | |
| 0.2mg/kg/d × 42 as tolerated | 4/6 | 67 | *102* (1968) |
| Mechlorethamine | | | |
| 0.1 mg/kg/d × 4–6 every 2–3 months | 1/1 | — | *164* (1948) |
| 0.1 mg/kg/d × 4 | 0/2 | 0 | *6* (1949) |
| Cyclophosphamide | | | |
| 0.8–9.3 mg/kg/d × 5–35 i.v. loading dose, p.o. maintenance | 0/1 | 0 | *11* (1960) |
| 200 mg/d i.v. to WBC 2000, then 100–200 mg/d p.o. | 0/2 | 0 | *4* (1961) |
| (a) 100–200 mg/d p.o. and/or (b) 30 mg/kg × 1 i.v., then 10–12 mg/kg every 1–2 weeks | 1/2 | — | *143* (1963) |

administered and well tolerated. This protocol compares L-phenylalanine mustard 9 mg/m$^2$ orally × 4 days every 5 weeks against combination chemotherapy with streptozotocin + 5-FU + 1-(2-chloroethyl)-3-(4-methylcyclohexyl)-1-nitrosourea (methyl-CCNU) or streptozotocin + 5-FU. This study should help to define the role of phenylalanine mustard in pancreatic cancer, but studies should be initiated to attempt to confirm the role of chlorambucil and other alkylating agents in this disease.

Recently, data published by Djerassi *et al.* (*36*) suggested that high-dose methotrexate may have activity against pancreatic cancer. Five patients with metastatic pancreatic carcinoma were treated with methotrexate at 50 mg/kg followed by leucovorin "rescue." It is difficult to assess objective parameters of response in this study, but of the 5 patients treated, 3 are reported alive at 1 year after initiation of therapy and 2 are "improved and functional" at 8 and 10 months. Since the median survival (*92*) of untreated patients with inoperable pancreatic cancer is 3–4 months, Djerassi's report is of some interest and deserves attempts at confirmation. No data are given relating to drug toxicity observed in these patients, but other workers have reported significant toxicity when high-dose methotrexate with leucovorin is used in adults. Pittman *et al.* (*115*) reported 20% significant nephrotoxicity as measured by a rise in serum creatinine of greater than 25% above the pretreatment value. The dose of 50 mg/kg methotrexate used by Djerassi is relatively low and, therefore, his toxicity may not be as significant as that seen by Pittman.

Neocarzinostatin is an antitumor polypeptide antibiotic known to inhibit DNA synthesis. This drug has been studied in Japan in patients with acute leukemia, gastric cancer, and pancreatic cancer. The experience in advanced pancreatic cancer is somewhat promising and deserves further study. Of 88 patients (*69*) treated, 11 (12.5%) obtained remissions. There were 3 complete responses of 1 year duration and 8 partial responses. Further evaluations of Neocarzinostatin in pancreatic cancer are being carried out.

It can be appreciated that evaluable experience with single-agent chemotherapy of pancreatic adenocarcinoma is extremely limited. There is a relative paucity of single agents that have received adequate Phase II evaluation in this disease. This deficiency should be altered by the systematic testing of single agents for activity in pancreatic cancer through the auspices of national cooperative group studies.

### 2. *Combination Chemotherapy*

Physicians dealing with patients with advanced pancreatic cancer are working under significant handicaps. As previously noted, there are only a limited number of single chemotherapeutic agents that have been demonstrated to have activity in this disease. Also the data on combination chemotherapy in pancreatic cancer are sparse, and the data that have been developed are frequently difficult to evaluate because of design faults and the small number of patients in the studies that have been performed. Controlled randomized trials are certainly important in the Phase III evaluation of any therapy, but it must be remembered that patients with unresectable pancreatic cancer have a median survival of 3 to 4 months (*92*), and it is reasonable to perform pilot studies of new chemotherapeutic regimens without concurrent controls since an effective regimen will be readily apparent because of improved survival.

Table V presents a compilation of thirteen series of patients treated with combination chemotherapy for advanced pancreatic carcinoma over the last 10 years. Only the Mayo Clinic investigators, Moertel, Reitemeier, Hahn *et al.* (*75, 120, 121*) have reported prospective randomized controlled studies. The initial experiences (*121*) with the combination of 5-FU and BCNU or of 5-FU, BCNU, and mitomycin C showed no benefit over 5-FU alone. Although Lokich and Skarin (*81*) reported 3 of 4 responses with 5-FU and BCNU in patients with pancreatic cancer, other workers (*75, 120, 121*), performing randomized

TABLE V

Combination Chemotherapy in Adenocarcinoma of the Pancreas

| Drug regimen[a] | No. responses / No. patients | Response rate (%) | Reference (year) |
|---|---|---|---|
| 5-FU 10 mg/kg/wk; Testolactone 150–200 mg/d or testolactone 100 mg/d and spironolactone 100–150 mg/d | 10/13 | 77 | *154* (1973) |
| 5-FU (9–10 mg/kg/d × 5); BCNU (37.5–40 mg/m²/d × 5) | 5/7 | 70 | *121* (1970)<br>*81* (1972) |
| Cyclophosphamide (300 mg d 1 and 5); Vincristine (0.025 mg/kg d 2 and 5); Methotrexate (0.5 mg/kg d 1 and 5); 5-FU (10 mg/kg d 1 and 5) | 2/3 | 67 | *29* (1969) |
| 5-FU (10 mg/kg/d × 5); BCNU (40 mg/m²/d × 5) | 10/30 | 33 | *78* (1974) |
| 5-FU (9 mg/kg/d × 5); Mitomycin C (60 μg/kg/d × 5); BCNU (20 mg/m²/d × 5) | 1/3 | 33 | *121* (1970) |
| 5-FU (300 mg × 3–5 d); Vincristine (0.5–1 mg/m² d 2 and 5); Cyclophosphamide (150–300 mg d 1 and 5) | 1/3 | 33 | *152* (1968) |
| 5-FU (10 mg/kg/d × 5); BCNU (40 mg/m²/d × 5) | 4/15 | 27 | *80* (1974) |
| 5-FU (10–15 mg/kg/wk); Vinblastine (0.15–0.3 mg/kg) | 3/11 | 27 | *2* (1972) |
| 5-FU (9 mg/kg/d × 5); Mitomycin C (110 μg/kg/d × 5) | 0/2 | 0 | *121* (1970) |
| Mitomycin C (25 μg/kg/d × 5); BCNU (25 mg/m²/d × 5) | 0/1 | 0 | *121* (1970) |
| 5-FU (loading dose); Fluorometholone (25 mg every 12 hr p.o. × 2 months) | 0/4 | 0 | *120* (1967) |
| Methotrexate (1.25 mg/d p.o.); Cyclophosphamide (50 mg/d p.o.) | 0/2 | 0 | *48* (1970) |
| 5-FU (15–20 mg/kg/wk); Cytosine arabinoside (30–60 mg/m²/wk s.c.) | 1/1 | — | *51* (1972) |

[a] 5-FU, 5-fluorouracil; BCNU, 1-bis(2-chloroethyl)-1-nitrosourea.

concurrently controlled trials, have not demonstrated similar response rates. It is important to note that some of the combination regimens reported (Table V) employ drugs that have not been shown to have any significant single-agent activity and, therefore, would be unlikely to be active in a combination.

The most encouraging data on combination chemotherapy in pancreatic cancer have been reported by Kovach *et al.* (*75*). They performed a prospectively controlled study comparing 5-FU, BCNU, and the combination 5-FU + BCNU in patients with advanced pancreatic carcinoma. The 5-FU and BCNU were given in loading courses whether used singly or in combination. Objective responses were seen in 5 of 31 (16.1%) patients receiving 5-FU, in 0 of 21 patients receiving BCNU alone, and in 10 of 30 (33.3%) patients receiving 5-FU + BCNU. Although there were no statistically significant differences in response rate between the combination and 5-FU alone and no significant differences in patient survival among patients on the three arms of the study, the suggestion of improved response rate with combination chemotherapy is encouraging and should stimulate the development of more combination chemotherapy protocols with the known active agents. An uncontrolled confirmation of Kovach's *et al.* work was provided by Lokich (*80*) again using 5-FU and BCNU. Nine of 15 (60%) evaluable patients were reported to have shown either objective response (4/15) or stabilization of disease (5/15) following therapy with 5-FU and BCNU combination chemotherapy. The responders had a longer median survival (11 months) than the nonresponders (4 months), although the overall numbers in each group are too small to make this difference significant.

An intriguing study utilizing combination chemotherapy in advanced pancreatic carcinoma was reported by Waddell (*157*). This retrospectively controlled study employed a control group of 26 patients treated with weekly 5-FU and Coumadin. These patients were compared to a treatment group of 13 patients treated with weekly 5-FU plus daily oral testolactone or testolactone and spironolactone. The patients appeared to be well matched for extent of disease and operative procedures. The median survival in the 5-FU and Coumadin patients was 5 months, whereas the median survival in the 5-FU and lactone group had not been reached by 21 months. This difference is statistically significant ($p < 0.001$). It is not clear why the combination of 5-FU and testolactone appears to have this striking effect, although there is some *in vitro* (*155*) evidence that testolactone may inhibit purine synthesis. Rat liver aspartate transcarbamylase, the enzyme responsible for *de novo* synthesis of purines, has been shown to be inhibited by testolactone, and the drug may have a significant role in inhibiting nucleic acid synthesis. The combination of 5-FU and testolactone is currently being tested in a controlled prospective trial by the Eastern Cooperative Oncology Group (ECOG) and the results of this study will be very valuable in assessing possible activity of 5-FU and testolactone in advanced pancreatic cancer.

A number of National Cooperative Groups have active protocols in pancreatic cancer, and a review of their studies will provide information on the current status and new directions in the treatment of this disease. The Gastrointestinal Tumor Study Group (GITSG) has developed three protocols for pancreatic adenocarcinoma. Two of the protocols evaluated combined radiation therapy and 5-FU chemotherapy and the third study, which has already been completed, was a Phase II evaluation of single-agent chemotherapy in advanced pancreatic cancer.

Several groups (*43, 99*) have shown a synergistic effect of 5-FU and supervoltage radiation on increasing the survival of patients with pancreatic cancer. The GITSG's two radiation + 5-FU protocols attempted to test this observation in two clinical situations. The first protocol (Fig. 1) is a randomized evaluation of the efficacy of 5-FU + 4000 rads of supervoltage radiation therapy as a adjuvant in patients who have undergone a radical pancreatectomy. It is known that approximately 80% of patients who undergo "curative" resection will die of recurrent disease if no further therapy is given. Currently there are not enough patients entered into this study, and the follow-up has been too short to

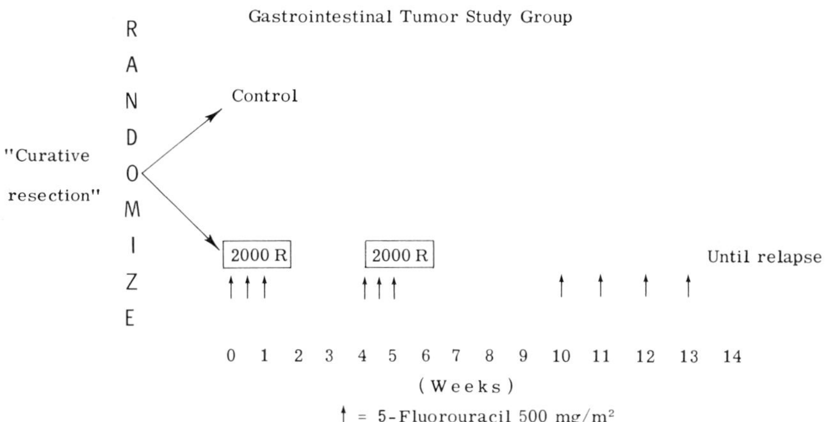


FIG. 1. Drug regimen of 5-FU plus supervoltage radiation therapy in patients with radical pancreatectomy.

draw any conclusions. However, this protocol should be very useful in defining the role of adjuvant therapy in pancreatic carcinoma.

The second GITSG protocol (Fig. 2) compares therapy with two doses of radiation therapy with or without 5-FU in patients with locally unresectable pancreatic cancer. Haslam *et al.* (*63*) reported in 1973 that 6000 rads radiation to the pancreas bed in patients with locally unresectable disease resulted in a 25% 2-year survival. This GITSG protocol (Fig. 2) tests a similar 6000-rad course of irradiation in a randomized study versus a standard 5-FU and 4000-rad regimen and 6000 rads + 5-FU. Complete evaluation of the patients entered in this protocol is not available at this time, but early results indicate that 4000 rads + 5-FU is superior to either of the 6000-rad regimen.

The third GITSG protocol was a prospective randomized Phase II trial of three single agents in advanced pancreatic cancer. Actinomycin D, methotrexate, and Adriamycin were evaluated in this study, and sufficient data accrual has occurred to show that none of these agents has very significant activity in the doses and schedules used in the study. However, there was a suggestion that Adriamycin may be a potentially useful agent since 15% of patients showed evidence of response. This protocol has now been terminated and the GITSG is now in the process of designing a new advanced disease protocol using combination chemotherapy.

The ECOG has developed protocols to examine combination chemotherapy in patients with pancreatic carcinoma. A protocol study compar-

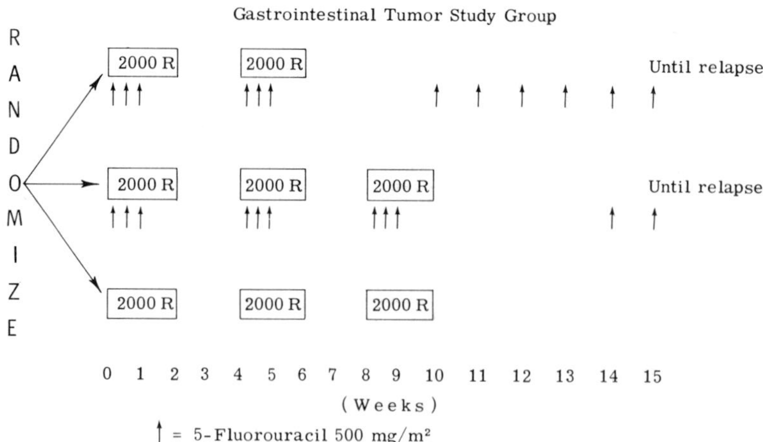


FIG. 2. Radiation therapy with and without 5-FU chemotherapy in patients with locally unresectable pancreatic cancer.

ing 5-FU + streptozotocin vs cyclophosphamide + streptozotocin vs methyl-CCNU in patients with advanced pancreatic cancer with measurable disease has recently been completed (Fig. 3). The overall response rate of all patients entered on the protocol was only 17%, and the median survival times varied between 9 and 15 weeks (*40*). Although the overall results of this study are discouraging, the streptozotocin plus 5-FU arm was found to have a slightly better response rate than the other two arms and was associated with tolerable toxicity.

The current active ECOG protocol for patients with measurable disease (Fig. 4) compares melphalan to 5-FU + streptozotocin and 5-FU + streptozotocin + methyl-CCNU. This study has only recently been activated and there are currently no data available concerning results. The second active ECOG protocol is designed for patients who have no objectively followable parameters of disease. This protocol (Fig. 5) is a comparative evaluation of 5-FU alone versus 5-FU and streptozotocin combined with an evaluation of spironolactone as an adjuvant to the chemotherapy of pancreatic cancer. Melphalan with and without spironolactone will be evaluated in patients who progress on primary therapy. The protocol is designed to evaluate under controlled circumstances the previously described observations of Waddell (*157*)

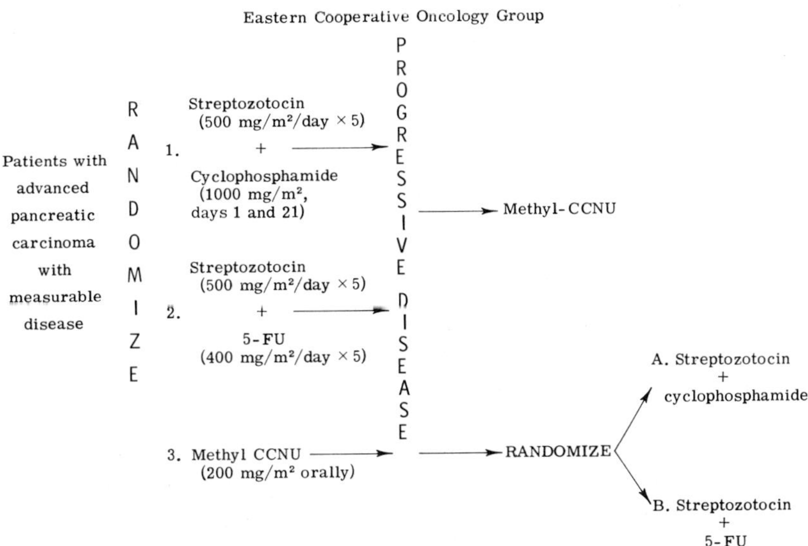


FIG. 3. Comparison of 5-FU + streptozotocin versus cyclophosphamide + streptozotocin versus methyl-CCNU in patients with advanced pancreatic cancer.

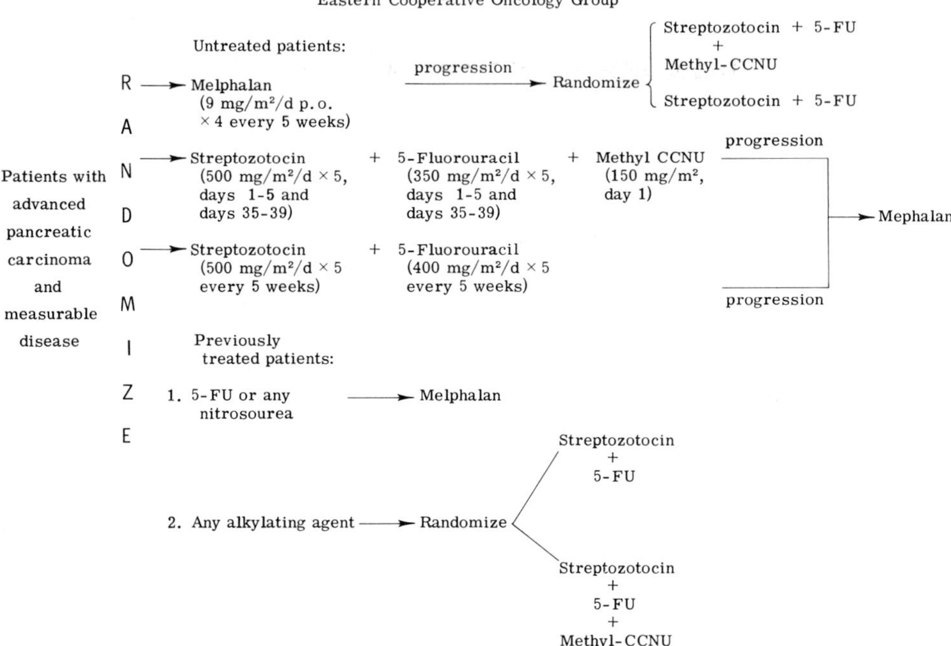


FIG. 4. Comparison of drug regimens of melphalan versus 5-FU + streptozotocin versus 5-FU + streptozotocin + methyl-CCNU in patients with advanced pancreatic cancer.

that lactones (spironolactone and/or testolactone) combined with 5-FU markedly increase survival in patients with advanced pancreatic cancer. This study was activated in October, 1974, and there is currently not adequate data accrual to evaluate response rates or survival.

The Central Oncology Group (COG) has an active protocol in advanced pancreatic cancer (Fig. 6). This study randomizes patients with adenocarcinoma and islet cell carcinoma, with stratification for measurable and nonmeasurable disease. 5-Fluorouracil alone is compared to 5-FU, streptozotocin, and tubercidin. Tubercidin is known to be an active agent in islet cell tumors (*95*) but its activity in adenocarcinoma of the pancreas has not yet been defined. Eighty patients with adenocarcinoma and 3 with islet cell carcinoma have been entered into the study. Only 1 of the 23 (4.3%) patients (*26*) evaluable on the 5-FU alone arm achieved a remission. Six of 22 (26%) patients on the combination program responded. This response rate is statistically significant ($p = 0.03$). The median survival in the 5-FU group was 15 weeks, and the median survival in the combination group was 35 weeks. However, this was not a statistically significant difference because of the small number in each group.

The Veteran's Administration Adjuvant Cancer Chemotherapy Study Group has had a clinical trial in the chemotherapy of pancreatic cancer underway since January, 1973. This trial randomizes patients between no therapy and combination chemotherapy with 5-FU and 1-(2-chloroethyl)-3-cyclohexyl-1-nitrosourea (CCNU) (Fig. 7). Patients with histologically proven, unresectable carcinoma of the pancreas are eligible for this protocol. As of April, 1975 (*156*), 60 patients had been entered into the treatment arms of this protocol. Twenty-five patients received 5-FU and CCNU, and 35 patients were left as untreated controls. No response rates are reported and survival was the parameter followed. After 3 months on study, 62.5% of the treated group and 49.9% of the control group were alive. The median survival was 4.2 months for the treated group and 3.0 months for the control group. None of these differences are statistically significant.

It is hoped that two major points will be apparent from this review of the chemotherapy of pancreatic adenocarcinoma. First, it is clear that there are only a limited number of drugs that have been adequately tested for activity in this disease. Second, only small numbers of

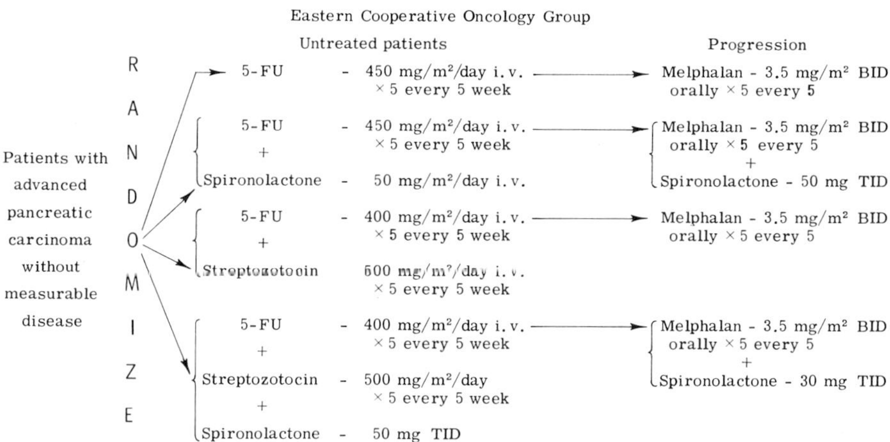


FIG. 5. Comparison of drug regimens of 5-FU with and without spironolactone versus 5-FU + streptozotocin with and without spironolactone in patients with advanced pancreatic cancer. Melphalan with and without a lactone is evaluated in patients who progress on primary therapy. (TID, 3 times a day; BID, twice a day.)

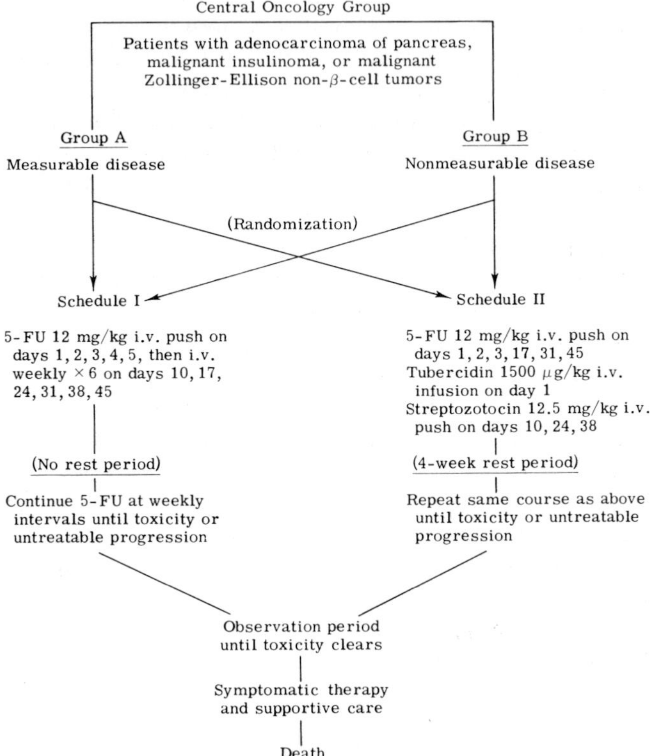


FIG. 6. Comparison of drug regimens of 5-FU alone with 5-FU + streptozotocin + tubercidin in patients with various forms of advanced pancreatic cancer.

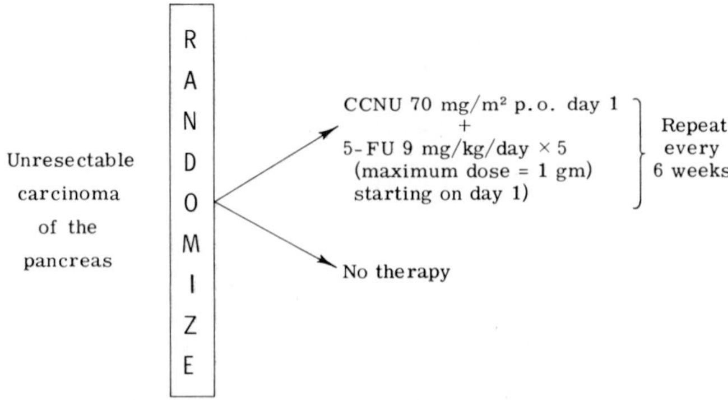


FIG. 7. Drug regimen of 5-FU + CCNU compared with untreated controls in patients with unresectable carcinoma of the pancreas.

patients have been treated in combination chemotherapy protocols and only recently has there been a major thrust by individual institutions and cooperative oncology groups to design and test well-conceived combination chemotherapy protocols in pancreatic cancer.

## III. Islet Cell Tumors

The pancreatic islets of Langerhans are composed of a variety of cells that may be distinguished by their distinctive histochemical staining and by the appearance of their secretory granules with electron microscopy. The islet cells are thought to arise from the neural crest, and they share in common with pituitary corticotrophes, thyroid parafollicular cells, gastrointestinal argyrophile and argentaffin cells, and adrenal medullary cells (*113, 114*) the ability to concentrate and decarboxylate precursors of biogenic amines (*113*). This function is designated APUD, indicating the capacity for amine precursor uptake and decarboxylation.

Any of the constituent cells of the islet may undergo neoplastic transformation in a functioning or nonfunctioning tumor. Virtually all benign islet cell tumors and approximately 75% of malignant islet cell tumors are recognized during life by a syndrome related to hypersecretion of one or more hormones. These hormones may be divided into two groups—those native to the pancreatic islet and those ectopically secreted (*134*).

The most common clinical syndrome is the excessive secretion of insulin, an endogenous hormone. Approximately 10% of insulinomas or beta-cell tumors are interpreted as malignant (*76*). The fundamental feature of the insulinoma is fasting hypoglycemia. Many patients will experience their initial symptoms during the morning hours prior to breakfast, or after exercise. The clinical features of this disease, representative of the recurrent episodes of lowered blood glucose, have been well described, and in many cases will be misinterpreted as psychiatric or neurological in origin for long periods of time (*89*). The diagnosis of insulinomas benign or malignant, as the cause of hypoglycemia is dependent on the concurrent measurement of plasma immunoreactive insulin (IRI). The hallmark of the insulinoma is a state where the IRI is inappropriately high at a time when the blood glucose is low, thus distinguishing this condition from other cases of fasting hypoglycemia, including extrapancreatic neoplasms, liver disease, adrenal and pituitary insufficiency, and glycogen storage diseases (*60*). In investigations of patterns of insulin secretion in insulinoma, the proinsulin-like component (PLC), a presumed precursor protein of insulin (*146*), has been demonstrated to comprise a disproportionately high percentage of the total circulating basal IRI (*55, 56*). Although not specific for insulinoma, having also been found associated with hypokalemia (*57*), assay of PLC may improve the future success in diagnosis of this disease and has already served as an important measure for assessing a patient's response to therapy (*15*). Successful treatment should bring the percent PLC down to normal levels.

Based on the responsiveness of the neoplastic beta cell to specific stimuli, a number of dynamic tests have been developed for diagnosis, which are also useful in following response to treatment in patients with insulinoma (*32, 47*). The tolbutamide test, with measurement of glucose and insulin, has proved the most efficient and will correctly identify approximately 80% of insulin-secreting tumors. False negatives with this test can be reduced by the simultaneous determination of percent PLC (*61*), and the use of additional provocative procedures such as L-leucine, glucose, or glucagon stimulation.

The second most common clinical syndrome associated with excessive endogenous hormone secretion of a hormone is the Zollinger-Ellison syndrome. The clinical manifestations of intractable peptic ulceration, diarrhea, and marked gastric hypersecretion, in association with a non-beta-cell neoplasm results from the hypersecretion of gastrin (*41, 88, 169*). Diagnostic measures include gastric acid analysis with Histalog stimulation, which is reported to demonstrate a basal acid output (BAO) value greater than 15 mEq/hour with basal acid concentration/stimulated acid concentration ratio greater than 60% in many patients (*86, 126, 163*). However, overlap of values in normal patients and those with a duodenal ulcer occurs occasionally. An elevated level of serum or plasma gastrin by the radioimmunoassay technique is the most sensitive and accurate diagnostic measure, most patients with the Z-E syndrome demonstrating gastrin levels greater than 300 pg/ml. Also useful as diagnostic tools are secretin or glucagon infusion tests that produce increased gastrin levels in patients with Z-E as opposed to decreased levels in other hypergastrin states. The calcium infusion test (*159, 162*) is useful in instances in which the fasting serum gastrin value is elevated to an equivocal level. At least twofold, elevation of borderline serum gastrin levels, with the absolute gastrin value exceeding 500 pg/ml, is strong evidence for the presence of gastrinoma (*159*).

"Pancreatic cholera" is the third most common syndrome associated with ectopic hormone secretion. This clinical entity is characterized by diffuse watery diarrhea, hypokalemia, and metabolic acidosis in patients with non-beta islet cell tumors (*134*). It has been distinguished from the Zollinger-Ellison syndrome in which diarrhea may be associated with gastric hypersecretion, by the absence of increased gastric acid, ulcer disease, and hypergastrinemia (*168*). The hormone or hormones responsible for the clinical manifestations in the pancreatic cholera syndrome have not been clearly defined (*70*). Secretin, glucagon, cholecystokinin, calcitonin, prostaglandins, gastric inhibitory peptide (GIP), and, most recently, vasoactive intestinal peptide (VIP) have all been proposed as the responsible agent (*129*).

The other major clinical syndromes associated with islet cell tumors include Cushing's syndrome due to ACTH secretion, and carcinoid syndrome resulting from serotonin production (*134*).

## Chemotherapy

Other than as a measure to maintain a patient for definitive surgery, chemotherapy of islet cell neoplasms is reserved for those cases in whom the tumor has metastasized or cannot be found at operation. Excessive hormone production may generally produce as much morbidity as the actual physical tumor, necessitating the use of two distinct forms of drug treatment: anticancer and antihormonal. The former is directed against the primary tumor and its metastases; the latter may offer palliation through the inhibition of synthesis, release, or direct cellular action of the specific hormone produced in excess (*130*).

### 1. *Antihormonal Management*

*a. Insulin-Secreting Islet Cell Tumors.* The recurrent attacks of hypoglycemia that characterize this disease can often be managed during the early stages with diet and supportive agents such as corticosteroids, growth hormone, and glucagon. Diazoxide represents a major advance in palliation. The principal hyperglycemic action of this antidiuretic benzothiadiazine is a direct inhibition of insulin release; there is no influence on insulin synthesis, and the hormone accumulates within the beta cell (*9, 58*). A second, extrapancreatic mechanism that has been observed in animals involves the beta-adrenergic stimulation of hepatic gluconeogenesis and a decrease in peripheral glucose utilization (*158*). Although the plasma insulin levels in many cases of malignant insulinoma can be lowered to asymptomatic concentrations, the tumors will continue to grow and metastasize because diazoxide has no antitumor activity. The anticonvulsant, diphenylhydantoin, a known hyperglycemic agent in man, has been identified as an inhibitor of insulin release from both the labile and storage beta-cell pools (*78*). Studies in patients with benign insulinomas have shown that the drug can blunt the response to tolbutamide and other provocative stimuli of insulin secretion (*27, 74*). The usefulness of diphenylhydantoin as a palliative agent in insulinoma has not yet been demonstrated. In patients with undiagnosed seizure disorders, however, this drug may partially mask both the clinical and diagnostic chemical features of insulinoma.

During its initial clinical trials as an antileukemic agent, L-asparaginase was shown to depress protein synthesis, through reduction in levels of serum albumin, clotting factors, and plasma insulin (*50*). We have recently used the enzyme to treat a patient with malignant insulinoma whose hypoglycemia was refractory to other measures (*134*). A reduction in the plasma insulin level, with a resultant rise in blood glucose, was noted by the fourth treatment day, without a decrease in albumin, prolongation of the prothrombin time, or evidence of pancreatitis. However, apparent hepatotoxicity developed, requiring discontinuation of therapy; this was followed by a rapid return to the previous hyperinsulinemic state. The principal mechanism for the reduction of plasma insulin appeared to be a decrease in synthesis; there was no apparent objective reduction in tumor mass during the period of treatment. A similar response to L-asparaginase has been reported by Sadoff (*128*). This experience suggests that L-asparaginase may be helpful as a short-term palliative agent.

*b. Gastrin-Secreting Islet Cell Tumors.* Until recently, there has been no antihormonal therapy to inhibit gastrin activity. However, within the last 2 years, a promising pharmacological inhibitor of gastrin activity has been developed. Metiamide, a thiourea analog of histamine, was synthesized by Black (*14*) and was shown to be an inhibitor of the $H_2$ histamine receptor. It has previously been shown (*52*) that there are two pharmacologically different histamine receptors. The $H_1$ receptor is inhibited by common antihistamines and is responsible for the contraction of gut and bronchial smooth muscle. The $H_2$ receptor is not inhibited by the ordinary antihistamines but is inhibited by metiamide. The $H_2$ receptor is responsible for the inhibition of contraction of the rat uterus, gastric acid secretion, and increased auricular rate. Several workers (*86, 149*) have shown in man that metiamide is capable of significantly (> 80%) inhibiting gastric acid secretion in normals and in patients with peptic ulcer disease. Mainardi *et al.* (*86, 87*) reported an acute reduction in gastric acid secretion for 2.5 hours after a single dose of 200 mg orally. Thompson *et al.* (*151*) reported on the chronic use of metiamide in a patient who clinically was felt to have Zollinger-Ellison syndrome with recurrent gastric and jejunal ulceration and with elevated gastrin and gastric acid levels with 90% of the serum gastrin being "big gastrin." Basal and pentagastrin-stimulated gastric acid secretion was shown to be reduced by 90% with the infusion of 100 mg metiamide per hour. The patient was then placed on metiamide 200 mg by mouth 4 times per day, and endoscopically documented healing of gastric and jejunal ulcers was demonstrated after 1 month's therapy. The patient had been receiving metiamide chronically for 4 months at the time of publication of this report without any toxicity being described. Although this patient did not have histological confirmation of an islet cell tumor, the serum gastrin levels, gastric acid hypersecretion, and the clinical course are certainly suggestive of the Zollinger-Ellison syndrome and the patient's clinical response to, and toleration of metiamide therapy is impressive. It is hoped that metiamide, or a similar agent, may eventually obviate the present policy of end organ removal (total gastrectomy) for palliation. There is some concern that chronic therapy with metiamide may lead to tachyphylaxis in some patients. At the present time metiamide has been given without toxicity in most reports. However, Mainardi *et al.* (*81*) have documented transient agranulocytosis in 2 patients receiving the drug on a chronic basis.

*c. Adrenocorticotropic Hormone-Secreting Islet Cell Tumors.* Aminoglutethimide (Elipten) had been used for several years as an anticonvulsant; however, with continued use, adrenal insufficiency and goitrous hypothyroidism have been observed. Further studies have demonstrated that the drug produces distinctive histological changes in the adrenal gland and inhibition of the enzymic conversion of cholesterol to $\Delta^5$-pregnenolone (*25*). Aminoglutethimide has been shown to be an effective palliative treatment in Cushing's syndrome secondary to adrenocortical carcinoma, adenoma, and ectopic ACTH production by extraadrenal carcinomas, with the potential for a rapid and sustained suppression of corticosteroid synthesis (*54*). Because the drug has the capacity to alter the extraadrenal metabolism of cortisol, measurement of urinary 17-OHCS excretion alone may overestimate the effectiveness of therapy; plasma cortisol concentrations are a more reliable index of drug effect for this hormone (*46*). The usual clinical dose is in the range of 1 to 2 gm/day, and the important toxicities include anorexia, dermatitis, somnolence, ataxia, and decreased thyroid function.

*d. Serotonin-Secreting Islet Cell Tumors.* The serotonin-related symptoms of the carcinoid syndrome include a watery diarrhea, abdominal colic, and malabsorption. When mild, these gastronintestinal manifestations may be successfully managed with simple measures, such as opiates and diphenoxylate hydrochloride with atropine (Lomotil) for long periods of time. With more severe symptoms, the use of peripheral antagonists of serotonin, methysergide and cycloheptadine, has been effective in controlling diarrhea and, in some cases, malabsorption (*21, 90*).

Another avenue of clinical investigation has been the use of agents that are known inhibitors of serotonin synthesis. *p*-Chlorophenylalanine (PCAC) is an inhibitor of the enzyme tryptophan 5-hydroxylase involved in the conversion of the amino acid to 5-hydroxytryptophan (5-HTP), the immediate precursor of serotonin. Engleman has demonstrated that PCAC at doses 2–4 gm/24 hours can reduce the urinary excretion of 5-hydroxyindoleacetic acid (as an indirect measurement of 5-hydroxyindole synthesis) by 51 to 81% in patients with carcinoid tumors (*140*). This was accompanied by good to excellent control of diarrhea and other gastrointestinal symptoms. Several toxicities of PCAC have been defined. In addition to lethargy and lightheadedness, chronic administration may be accompanied by such mental aberrations as depression, anxiety, and confusional states. The development of an allergic eosinophilia appearing 2–9 weeks after initiation of treatment with PCAC has been observed in 50% of patients. This abnormality is rapidly reversible with withdrawal of the drug, reappears promptly with rechallenge, and is a definite sign for cessation of PCAC therapy. Continued treatment in the face of eosinophilia has lead to the development of urticaria, asthma, and pulmonary infiltrates (Löffler's syndrome) (*140*).

### 2. *Antitumor Therapy*

Because of the relative rarity of islet cell tumors, the conventional cancer chemotherapy agents have not been extensively evaluated. The literature does contain individual case reports describing the effectiveness of 5-FU and alkylating agents in the management of individual patients (*49, 82, 95, 150*). The more systematic clinical trials in this disease have involved the use of compounds for which there has been some expectation for selective toxicity against the malignant islet cell tissue, based on toxicologic observations in normal animals. Historically, alloxan was the first agent with proven diabetogenic activity to be tested clinically (*166*). Although only rarely effective, it, nevertheless, demonstrated the potential efficacy of this approach to drug selection.

Tubercidin (7-deazaadenosine) is an antibiotic isolated from the fermentation broth of *Streptomyces tubericidus*. Biochemically the drug has been shown to substitute effectively for the corresponding adenosine compound in a number of enzymic reactions and it may be incorporated into DNA and RNA as a fraudulent purine with resultant inhibition of protein synthesis (*1*). Tubercidin inhibited the growth of KB cells *in vitro* and demonstrated antitumor activity against Sarcoma 180, Ehrlich ascites tumor, and Jensen sarcoma *in vivo*. Toxicologic studies carried out in dogs in preparation for clinical use of the compound demonstrated histological lesions in the pancreatic islets of Langerhans with resulting glucose intolerance. At the present time, tubercidin has received only a limited clinical trial, but several cases of islet cell carcinoma, including 1 patient with the Zollinger-Ellison syndrome, have been reported to demonstrate objective regression in tumor mass, lasting 6 months to over 1 year (*13, 59*). Recently, the Mayo Clinic has demonstrated remissions in 2 of 5 cases (*95*). Tubercidin's overall usefulness is limited by its severe toxicity to veins and local tissues and, therefore, has necessitated the development of elaborate measures for its administration (*59*). A unit of whole blood is removed from the patient and is incubated with the prescribed dose of drug for 1 hour at 37°C. Tubercidin is transported into the red blood cells and phosphorylated to the corresponding nucleotide. The blood is then retransfused, and the drug is slowly released from the red blood cells where it had been incorporated (*59*). Clinical toxicities have included renal damage, manifested by proteinuria and azotemia, nausea and vomiting, mild leukopenia and thrombocytopenia, and mild liver function abnormalities. The currently used dose schedule is 1500 μg/kg delivered days 1 and 8 in red blood cells, followed by 750 μg/kg at monthly intervals as tolerated.

The chemotherapeutic agent in most active clinical trials for the treatment of malignant insulinoma is streptozotocin, an antibiotic isolated from the fermentation cultures of *Streptomyces achromogenes*. Chemically, the compound is composed of the union of a known anticancer agent, 1-methyl-1-nitrosourea, and glucose (*64*). The diabetogenic properties of streptozotocin were discovered during its initial preclinical toxicologic evaluation (*117*). It was demonstrated that a single intravenous dose could produce a permanent diabetic state in rodents, dogs, and monkeys—an action mediated through the selective destruction of the pancreatic beta cell.

Biochemically, this acute diabetogenic activity of streptozotocin has been related to an acute reduction of pyridine nucleotides in the pancreatic islets. Both the depletion of NAD and the diabetes can be prevented in animals with the use of pharmacological doses of nicotinamide (*131, 132, 133, 136*). Studies using methyl ($^{14}$C) streptozotocin and (methyl-$^{14}$C) 1-methyl-1-nitrosourea have been conducted (*5*). The *in vivo* uptake of radiolabeled streptozotocin by pancreatic islets was found to be 3.8 times that of 1-methyl-1-nitrosourea, whereas uptake into the exocrine pancreas favored 1-methyl-1-nitrosourea over streptozotocin 2.4:1. The decreased islet uptake of 1-methyl-1-nitrosourea correlated with a 3.5 times increased molar dosage required to produce islet NAD comparable to that of a moderately diabetogenic dose of streptozotocin. In addition, it was possible to demonstrate for the first time that 1-

methyl-1-nitrosourea was capable of producing diabetes if a superlethal dose was administered and the animals were studied chemically and histologically before they expired from profound bone marrow toxicity. These studies indicated that the glucose carrier of streptozotocin facilitates uptake of the cytotoxic group, 1-methyl-1-nitrosourea, into islets.

An unexpected product of the investigations using nicotinamide–streptozotocin combinations was the development of a new rat model for islet cell tumors. It was found that rats held for long-term study after receiving the combined therapy demonstrated significant and persistent hypoglycemia after 1 year. They were subsequently found to have developed islet cell tumors that were actively producing insulin (*118*). It has been proposed that the nicotinamide pretreatment prevents the beta cell from being acutely destroyed by a lowering of pyridine nucleotides to critical levels, but methylation of DNA by the 1-methyl-1-nitrosourea end group was allowed to take place. This latter event is subsequently expressed by the transformation of the beta cell and the development of the islet tumor after 1 year of latency.

Because of the inherent diabetogenic properties of streptozotocin, an attempt has been made to exploit this "toxicity" in the treatment of malignant insulinomas (*135*). In a series of 29 cases of malignant insulinoma in whom measureable disease was present, 48% of patients had an objective reduction in tumor mass, and 17% were considered to have obtained complete remission status with streptozotocin therapy (*20*). The average duration of these remissions has been approximately 1 year. In regard to hormonal response, 62% of patients were reported to have a lessening in severity of hypoglycemia or a lowering of an initially elevated insulin. In 26% of cases, there was a return of these hormonal parameters to normal levels. The length of a functional response can be directly related to its magnitude, and for patients achieving a complete hormonal remission the median duration has exceeded 1 year. The available data relating to the influence of streptozotocin treatment on survival in malignant insulinoma are preliminary. However, the median of 744 days of responders vs 289 for nonresponders suggests that the drug will prove beneficial in prolonging life. As previously mentioned, one of the noteworthy characteristics of islet cell carcinomas are their biological capacity to synthesize a wide range of hormones, including insulin, gastrin, glucagon, ACTH, and serotonin. It is of interest that remissions with streptozotocin have not been limited to patients with excessive production of insulin or to beta-cell tumors. In the original case report demonstrating the successful use of streptozotocin, Murray-Lyon *et al.* (*105*) documented a concomitant reduction of initially elevated plasma insulin, gastrin, and glucagon values. In this connection, of the 29 patients with insulinoma, all 3 cases who were treated with streptozotocin and who had documented secretion of both insulin and gastrin responded. Remissions have been documented in patients with non-beta-cell neoplasms with associated pancreatic cholera (*70*), hypercalcemia (*35*), or ectopic production of ACTH (*160*) and serotonin (*137*). This therapeutic activity is not confined solely to the hormone-secreting tumors, since 5 of 8 patients with nonfunctioning islet cell carcinoma have also achieved some reduction in tumor size with treatment (*20*).

The clinical toxicity of streptozotocin has been carefully defined (*137*). Gastrointestinal toxicity was confined to nausea and vomiting, which was experienced by 87% of patients. Symptoms usually appeared 1–4 hours after drug administration, and in large part could not be prevented or controlled by the use of phenothiazine antiemetics. In 11% of patients, nausea and vomiting was severe, whereas in the remaining 76% of patients this toxicity was equally divided between mild and moderate degrees of severity. There was great variability between patients as to the susceptibility to this drug effect at the same dose and schedule. With the 5-day schedule, patient tolerance improves with each succeeding dose.

Heptatotoxicity, evidenced by elevations in serum glutamic oxalacetic transaminase and pyruvic transaminase was demonstrable in 13 of 88 patients (15%), in whom these determinations were serially performed. These liver function abnormalities appeared 1–2 days after completion of a course of treatment and rapidly returned to normal levels without attendant symptoms or corroborative evidence of acute or chronic hepatotoxicity. Liver histology of patients who died soon after treatment failed to demonstrate signs of hepatocellular necrosis.

In general, streptozotocin is not a bone marrow toxin. Mild reduction in white blood cell and platelet counts occurs in 9% of cases, with the nadir appearing 1–2 weeks after treatment.

Renal tubular damage is the most common serious drug toxicity, and its occurrence severely limits the potential for further treatment (*127, 137*). The earliest manifestation in our experience has been the development of proteinuria in the range of 400 to 1500 mg/24 hours, decreased creatinine clearance, and hypophosphatemia. With more significant nephrotoxicity, excretion of up to 10 gm of protein/24 hours has been documented. Mild renal toxicity is usually reversible in 2 to 4 weeks. However, with continued treatment, pronounced signs of proximal tubular damage are produced including aminoaciduria, phosphaturia, uricosuria, glycosuria, and renal tubular acidosis, all of which are potentially reversible. Two investigators have reported the development of nephrogenic diabetes insipidus after large doses of the drug, and varying degrees of azotemia have been observed (*106, 141*). Serious renal toxicity can be avoided by closely monitoring the urine for protein excretion and stopping treatment until full reversal to normal renal function has been documented.

Several cooperative groups have been conducting studies of combination chemotherapy for metastatic islet cell tumors. The ECOG has been comparing streptozotocin, 500 mg/m$^2$, i.v., days 1–5 every 6 weeks, vs the same dose of streptozotocin combined with 5-FU 400 mg/m$^2$, i.v., days 1–5. This study is still in progress, but approximately one-third of patients in each treatment group have demonstrated objective responses. The COG is comparing 5-FU as a single agent with a combination of 5-FU, tubercidin, and streptozotocin.

Studies of the clinical pharmacology of streptozotocin have been carried out. The serum half-life of intact drug was found to be 15 minutes with essentially no drug detectable by 2 hours after administration. Ten to 20% of each total dose was recovered in the urine, the majority excreted within 60 minutes after the start of the infusion (*137*). In the treatment of the pancreatic cholera syndrome, the intraarterial route of administration was employed and compared pharmacologically with intravenous therapy in 2 patients. It was found that with intraarterial treatment the peripheral blood levels of intact drug were reduced to less than 50% of those observed with the intravenous route (*70*). This was also reflected in a one-third reduction in urinary excretion of streptozotocin. This has been interpreted as a significant first-pass uptake of drug by the regional tissues, liver and tumor. The result is the delivery of higher drug concentrations to the target tissue and the organ responsible for drug inactivation, while sparing the peripheral tissues and, in particular, the kidney, the potential organ of treatment toxicity.

## IV. Conclusion

It is hoped that this review of the biology and treatment of pancreatic malignancies will succeed in stressing two major points: the first is that active treatment protocols are under way in these diseases that, until recently, were felt to be totally resistant to therapy; and, second, we wish to stress the need for continuing active investigation in the biology, diagnosis, and therapy of pancreatic cancer.

## References


*1.* Acs, G., Reich, E., and Mori, M. (1964). *Proc. Natl. Acad. Sci., U.S.A.* **52,** 493.
*2.* Al-Saraff, M., Vaughn, C. B., Reed, M. L., and Vaitkevicius, V. K. (1972). *Oncology* **26,** 99.
*3.* Anacker, H., Weiss, H. K., Kramann, B., and Rupp, N. (1974). *Am. J. Roentgenol. Radium Ther. Nucl. Med.* **122,** 375.
*4.* Anders, C., and Kemp, N. (1961), *Br. Med. J.* **2,** 1516.
*5.* Anderson, T., Schein, P. S., McMenamin, M. G., and Cooney, D. A. (1974). *J. Clin. Invest.* **54,** 672.
*6.* Ariel, I., and Kanter, L. (1949). *Am. J. Surg.* **77,** 509.
*7.* Ballard, H. S., Frame, B., and Hartsock, R. J. (1964). *Medicine (Baltimore)* **43,** 481.
*8.* Banwo, O., Versey, J., and Hobbs, J. R. (1974). *Lancet* **1,** 643.
*9.* Basabe, J., Lopey, N., Viktora, J., and Wolff, F. (1970). *Diabetes* **19,** 271.
*10.* Belsito, A. A., Cramer, G. G., and Dickinson, P. B. (1973). *Am. J. Roentgenol. Radium Ther. Nucl. Med.* **119,** 109.
*11.* Bergsagel, D., and Levin, W. (1960). *Cancer Chemother. Rep.* **8,** 120.
*12.* Berk, E. J., and Haubrich, W. S. (1965). *In* "Gastroenterology" (H. L. Bockus, ed.), Vol. 3, pp. 1021–1055. Saunders, Philadelphia, Pennsylvania.
*13.* Bisel, H. F., Ansfield, F. J., Mason, J. H., and Wilson, W. L. (1970). *Cancer Res.* **30,** 76.
*14.* Black, J. W. (1973). *Int. Symp. Histamine $H_2$ Receptor Antagonists* (C. J. Wood and M. A. Simpkins, eds.), pp. 23–27. Smith, Kline & French, London.
*15.* Blackard, W. G., Garcia, A. R., and Brown, C. L., Jr. (1970). *J. Clin. Endocrinol. Metab.* **31,** 215.
*16.* Bookstein, J. H., Reuter, S. B., and Martel, W. (1969). *Radiology* **93,** 757.
*17.* Bowden, L. (1954). *Ann. Surg.* **139,** 403.
*18.* Bowden, L. (1972). *Ca.* **22**(5), 275.
*19.* Broder, L. E., and Carter, S. K. (1971). "Streptozotocin: Clinical Brochure." Therapy Evaluation Program, Natl. Cancer Inst., Bethesda, Maryland.
*20.* Broder, L. E., and Carter, S. K. (1973). *Ann. Intern. Med.* **79,** 108.
*21.* Brown, R. E., Hill, S. R., Jr., Berry, K. W., and Bing, R. J. (1960). *Clin. Res.* **8,** 61.
*22.* Burger, J., and Blauenstein, U. W. (1974). *Am. J. Roentgenol. Radium Ther. Nucl. Med.* **122,** 406.
*23.* Carter, S. K. (1968). *Cancer Chemother. Rep., Part 3* **1,** 99.
*24.* Carter, S. K., Schabel, F. M., Broder, L. E., and Johnston, T. P. (1972). *Adv. Cancer Res.* **16,** 273.
*25.* Cash, R., Brough, A. J., Cohen, M. N. P., and Satoh, P. S. (1967). *J. Clin. Endocrinol. Metab.* **27,** 1239.
*26.* Central Oncology Group (1975). *Minutes of 1975 Meeting, Miami Beach, Florida,* p. 105.
*27.* Cohen, M. S., Bower, R. H., Fidler, S. M., Johnsonbaugh, R. E., and Sode, J. (1973). *Lancet* **1,** 40.
*28.* Cornell, G. N., Cahow, C. E., Frey, C., McSherry, C., and Beal, J. M. (1960). *Cancer Chemother. Rep.* **9,** 23.
*29.* Costanzi, J. J., and Coltman, C. A., Jr. (1969). *Cancer* **23,** 589.
*30.* Cressy, N. L., and Schell, H. W. (1966). *Cancer Chemother. Rep.* **50,** 683.
*31.* Cubilla, A. L., and Fitzgerald, P. J. (1975). *Cancer Res.* **35,** 2234.

*32*. Cunningham, G. R., Quickel, K. E., Jr., and Labovitz, H. E. (1971). *J. Clin. Endocrinol. Metab.* **33,** 530.

*33*. Curreri, A. R., Ansfield, F. J., McIver, F., Weisman, H. A., and Heidlberger, C. (1958). *Cancer Res.* **18,** 478.

*34*. Delwiche, R., Zamcheck, N., and Marcon, N. (1973). *Cancer* **31,** 328.

*35*. De Wys, W. D., Stoll, R., Au, W. Y., and Salisnjak, M. M. (1973). *Am. J. Med.* **55,** 671.

*36*. Djerassi, I., Kim, S. J., and Suvansii, V. (1974). *Proc. AACR and ASCO* **15,** 78.

*37*. Dreiling, D. A. (1970). *Scand. J. Gastroenterol. (Suppl.)* **6,** 115.

*38*. DuPriest, R. W., Huntington, M., Massey, W. H., Weiss, A. J., Wilson, W. L., and Fletcher, W. S. (1974). *Cancer* **35,** 358.

*39*. Eastern Cooperative Oncology Group (1974). *Minutes of Meeting, Columbia, Maryland, November 11–12*, p. M-34.

*40*. Eastern Cooperative Oncology Group (1974). *Minutes of Meeting, Columbia, Maryland, November 11–12,* p. 62.

*41*. Ellison, E. H., and Wilson, S. D. (1967). *Surg. Clin. North Am.* **47,** 1115.

*42*. Endo, Y., Morii, T., Tamura, H., and Shigeru, O. (1974). *Gastroenterology* **67,** 944.

*43*. Falkson, G., Falkson, H. C., and Fichardt, T. (1970). *S. Afr. Med. J.* **2,** 444.

*44*. Field, J. B. (1963). *Cancer Chemother. Rep.* **33,** 45.

*45*. Filly, R. A., and Freimanis, A. K. (1970). *Radiology* **96,** 575.

*46*. Fishman, L. M., Liddle, G. W., Island, D. P., Fleischer, N., and Kuchel, O. (1967). *J. Clin. Endocrinol. Metab.* **27,** 1967.

*47*. Floyd, J. C., Jr., Fajans, S. S., Knopf, R. F., and Conn, J. W. (1964). *J. Clin. Endocrinol. Metab.* **24,** 747.

*48*. Foley, J. F., Lemon, H. M., and Miller, D. (1970). *Cancer Chemother. Rep., Part I* **54,** 41.

*49*. Fonkalsrud, E. W., Dilley, R. B., and Longmire, W. P., Jr. (1964). *Ann. Surg.* **159,** 730.

*50*. Gailani, S., Nussbaum, A., Ohnuma, T., and Freeman, A. (1971). *Clin. Pharmacol Ther.* **12,** 487.

*51*. Gailani, S., Holland, J. F., Falkson, G., Leone, L., Burningham, R., and Larsen, V. (1972). *Cancer* **29,** 1308.

*52*. Gibson, R., Hirschowitz, B. I., and Hutchison, G. (1974). *Gastroenterology* **67,** 93.

*53*. Goldstein, H. M., Neiman, H. L., and Bookstein, J. J. (1974). *Radiology* **112,** 275.

*54*. Gorden, P., Becker, C. E., Levey, G. S., and Roth, J. (1968). *J. Clin. Endocrinol. Metab.* **28,** 921.

*55*. Gorden, P., Freychet, P., and Nankin, H. (1971). *J. Clin. Endocrinol. Metab.* **33,** 983.

*56*. Gorden, P., Sherman, B., and Roth, J. (1971). *J. Clin. Invest.* **50,** 2113.

*57*. Gorden, P., Sherman, B. M., and Simopoulos, A. (1972). *Clin. Endocrinol. Metab.* **34,** 235.

*58*. Graber, A. L., Porte, E., Jr., and Williams, R. H. (1966). *Diabetes* **15,** 143.

*59*. Grage, T. B., Rochlin, D. B., Weiss, A. J., and Wilson, W. L. (1970). *Cancer Res.* **30,** 79.

*60*. Grunt, J. A., Pallotta, J. A., and Soeldner, J. S. (1970). *Diabetes* **19,** 122.

*61*. Gutman, R. A., Lazarus, N. R., Penhas, J. C., Fajans, S., and Recant, L. (1971). *N. Engl. J. Med.* **284,** 1003.

*62*. Hancke, S., Holm, H., and Koch, F. (1975). *Surg, Gynecol. Obstet.* **140,** 361.

*63*. Haslam, J. B., Cavanaugh, P. J., and Stroup, S. L. (1973). *Cancer* **32,** 1341.

*64.* Herr, R. R., Jahnke, H. K., and Argondelis, A. S. (1967). *J. Am. Chem. Soc.* **89,** 4808.
*65.* Howard, J. M., and Jordan, G. L. (1960). *In* "Surgical Diseases of the Pancreas," pp. 449–498. Lippincott, Philadelphia, Pennsylvania.
*66.* Hurley, J. D. (1964). *Acta Unio Int. Contra Cancrum* **20,** 363.
*67.* Hurley, J. D., and Ellison, E. H. (1960). *Ann. Surg.* **152,** 568.
*68.* Isaacson, R., Weiland, L., and McIlraty, D. (1974). *Arch. Surg. (Chicago)* **109,** 227.
*69.* Ishii, K., and Nakamura, N. (1974). *Cancer Chemother. (Tokyo)* p. 433.
*70.* Kahn, C. R., Levy, A. G., Gardner, J. D., Gorden, P., and Schein, P. S. (1975). *N. Engl. J. Med.* **292,** 941.
*71.* Kaplan, E. (1972). *Gastroenterology* **63,** 911.
*72.* Kawanishi, H., Sell, J. E., and Pollard, H. M. (1975). *Gastroenterology* **68,** A20.
*73.* Knoepp, L. F., Kastl, W. H., Rayburn, A. L., Sayegh, S. F., and Letson, W. M. (1961). *Cancer Chemother. Rep.* **12,** 89.
*74.* Knopp, R. H., Sheinin, J. C., and Freinkel, N. (1972). *Arch. Intern. Med.* **130,** 904.
*75.* Kovach, J. S., Moertel, C. G., Schutt, A. J., Hahn, R. G., and Reitemeier, R. J. (1974). *Cancer* **33,** 563.
*76.* Laurent, J., Debry, G., and Floquent, J. (1971). "Hypoglycemic Tumours." Excerpta Medica, Amsterdam.
*77.* Ledley, R. S., Dichiro, G., Luessenhop, A. J., and Twigg, H. L. (1974). *Science* **186,** 207.
*78.* Levin, S. R., Grodsky, G. M., Hagura, R., and Smith, D. (1972). *Diabetes* **21,** 856.
*79.* Li, F. P., Fraumeni, J. F., Mantel, N., and Miller, R. W. (1969). *J. Natl. Cancer Inst.* **43,** 1159.
*80.* Lokich, J., Chawke, P. L., Brooks, J., and Frei, E. (1974). *Ann. Surg.* **179**(4), 450.
*81.* Lokich, J. J., and Skarin, A. T. (1972). *Cancer Chemother. Rep., Part 1* **56,** 653.
*82.* Longmire, W. P., (1968). *Ann. Intern. Med.* **68,** 203.
*83.* McCarthy, M., Brown, P., Melmed, R. N., Agnew, J. E., and Bouchier, I. A. D. (1972). *Gut* **13,** 75.
*84.* MacGregor, A. M. C., and Hawkins, I. F. (1973). *Surg. Gynecol. Obstet.* **137,** 917.
*85.* McIntire, K. R., Waldmann, T. A., Moertel, C. G., and Go, V. L. W. (1975). *Cancer Res.* **35,** 991.
*86.* Mainardi, M., Maxwell, V., Sturdevant, R. A. L., and Isenberg, J. I. (1974).*N. Engl. J. Med.* **291,** 373.
*87.* Mainardi, M., Maxwell, V., Sturdevant, R. A. L., and Isenberg, J. I. (1975). *Am. J. Dig. Dis.* **20,** 280.
*88.* Marks, I. N., Louw, J. H., Selzer, G., and Banks, S. (1961). *Gastroenterology* **41,** 77.
*89.* Marks, V., and Rose, F. C. (1965). "Hypoglycemia." Blackwell, Oxford.
*90.* Melmon, K. L., Sjoerdsma, A., Oates, J. A., and Laster, L. (1965). *Gastroenterology* **48,** 18.
*91.* Meyerburg, J., Ziegler, V., Kirstaedter, H., and Palme, G. (1973). *Endoscopy* **5,** 86.
*92.* Moertel, C. G. (1969). *In* "Advanced Gastrointestinal Cancer/Clinical Management and Chemotherapy" (C. G. Moertel and R. J. Reitemeier, eds.), pp. 3–14, Harper & Row, New York.
*93.* Moertel, C. G. (1973). *In* "Cancer Medicine" (J. F. Holland and E. Frei, eds.), pp. 1559–1590. Lea & Febiger, Philadelphia, Pennsylvania.
*94.* Moertel, C. G. (1973). *Cancer Chemother. Rep., Part 3* **4,** 27.
*95.* Moertel, C. G. (1975). *Cancer* **36,** 675.

*96.* Moertel, C. G., and Reitemeier, R. J. (1967). *Surg. Clin. North Am.* **47,** 929.
*97.* Moertel, C. G., and Reitemeier, R. J. (1969). *In* "Advanced Gastrointestinal Cancer/Clinical Management and Chemotherapy." (C. G. Moertel and R. J. Reitemeier, eds.), pp. 73–76. Harper & Row, New York.
*98.* Moertel, C. G., Reitemeier, R. J., and Hahn, R. G. (1964). *Gastroenterology,* **46,** 371.
*99.* Moertel, C. G., Childs, D. S., Reitemeier, R. J., Colby, M., and Holbrook, M. (1969). *Lancet* **2,** 865.
*100.* Moertel, C. G., Reitemeier, R. J., and Hahn, R. G. (1969). *In* "Advanced Gastrointestinal Cancer/Clinical Management and Chemotherapy" (C. G. Moertel and R. J. Reitemeier, eds.), pp. 168–175. Harper & Row, New York.
*101.* Moldow, R. E., and Connelly, R. R. (1968). *Gastroenterology* **55,** 677.
*102.* Moore, G., Bross, I. D. J., Ausman, R., Nadler, S., Jones, R., Jr., Slack, N., and Rimm, A. A. (1968). *Cancer Chemother. Rep., Part 1* **52,** 661.
*103.* Moore, G. E., Bross, I. D. J., Ausman, R., Nadler, S., Jones, R., Jr., Slack, N., and Rimm, A. A. (1968). *Cancer Chemother. Rep., Part 1* **52,** 641.
*104.* Moore, G. E., Bross, I. D. J., Ausman, R., Nadler, S., Jones, R., Jr., Slack, N., and Rimm, A. A. (1968). *Cancer Chemother. Rep., Part 1* **52,** 675.
*105.* Murray-Lyon, I. M., Eddleston, A. L., Williams, R., Brown, M., Hogbin, B. M., Bennett, A., Edwards, J. C., and Taylor, K. W. (1968). *Lancet* **2,** 895.
*106.* Murray-Lyon, I. M., Cassar, J., Coulson, R., Williams, R., Ganguli, P. C., Edwards, J. C., and Taylor, K. W. (1971). *Gut* **12,** 717.
*107.* Nadler, S. H., and Moore, G. E. (1968). *Surg. Gynecol. Obstet.* **127,** 1210.
*108.* Nakano, S., Horiguchi, Y., Takeda, T., Suzuki, T., and Nakajima, S. (1974). *Scand. J. Gastroenterol.* **9,** 383.
*109.* National Cancer Institute, Biometry Branch (1974). *Natl. Cancer Survey Adv. Three-Year Rep. (Excluding Carcinoma in Situ), Bethesda, Maryland, 1969–1971.* DHEW Publication No. (NIH) 74-637.
*110.* Ogoshi, K., Masajuki, N., Hara, Y., and Nebel, O. T. (1973). *Gastroenterology* **64,** 210.
*111.* Ona, F., Dhar, P., Moore, T. L., Kupchik, H. A., and Zamchek, N. (1973). *Cancer* **31,** 324.
*112.* Paul, R. E., Miller, H. H., Kahn, P. C., and Callow, A. D. (1965). *N. Engl. J. Med.* **272,** 283.
*113.* Pearse, A. G. E. (1969). *J. Histochem. Cytochem.* **17,** 303.
*114.* Pearse, A. G. E. (1969). *Nature (London)* **221,** 1210.
*115.* Pitman, S. W., Parker, L. M., Tattersall, J., Jaffee, N., and Frei, E., III (1975). *Cancer Chemother. Rep., Part 1* **6,** 43.
*116.* Pour, P., Kruger, W., Althoff, J., Cardesa, A., and Mohr, U. (1975). *Cancer Res.* **35,** 2259.
*117.* Rakieten, N., Rakieten, M. L., and Nadkarni, M. V. (1963). *Cancer Chemother. Rep.* **29,** 91.
*118.* Rakieten, N., Gordon, B. S., Beaty, A., Cooney, D. A., Davis, R. D., and Schein, P. S. (1971). *Proc. Soc. Exp. Biol. Med.* **137,** 280.
*119.* Reddy, V. K., and Rao, M. S. (1975). *Cancer Res.* **35,** 2269.
*120.* Reitemeier, R. J., Moertel, C. G., and Hahn, R. G. (1967). *Cancer Chemother. Rep.* **51,** 77.
*121.* Reitemeier, R. J., Moertel, C. G., and Hahn, R. G. (1970). *Cancer Res.* **30,** 1425.
*122.* Rennell, C. L. (1974). *Am. J. Roentgenol. Radium Ther. Nucl. Med.* **121,** 256.

*123.* Rochlin, D. B., Shiner, J., Langdon, E., and Ottoman, R. (1962). *Ann. Surg.* **156,** 105.
*124.* Rochlin, D. B., Smart, C. R., and Silva, A. (1965). *Am. J. Surg.* **109,** 43.
*125.* Rosch, J. (1975). *J. Surg. Oncol.* **7,** 121.
*126.* Ruppert, R. D., Greenberger, N. J., Beman, F. M., and McCullough, F. M. (1967). *Ann. Intern. Med.* **67,** 808.
*127.* Sadoff, L. (1970). *Cancer Chemother. Rep., Part 1* **54,** 457.
*128.* Sadoff, L. (1973). *J. Clin. Endocrinol. Metab.* **36,** 334.
*129.* Said, S. I., and Faloona, G. (1975). *N. Engl. J. Med.* **293,** 155.
*130.* Schein, P. S. (1972). *Cancer* **30,** 1616.
*131.* Schein, P. S., Cooney, D. A., and Vernon, M. L. (1967). *Cancer Res.* **27,** 2324.
*132.* Schein, P. S., Alberti, K. G. M. M., and Williamson, D. H. (1971). *Endocrinology* **89,** 8.
*133.* Schein, P. S., Cooney, D. A., McMenamin, M. G., and Anderson, T. (1973). *Biochem. Pharmacol.* **22,** 2625.
*134.* Schein, P. S., DeLellia, R. A., Kahn, C. R., Gorden, P., and Kraft, A. R. (1973). *Ann. Intern. Med.* **79,** 239.
*135.* Schein, P., Kahn, R., Jordan, P., Wells, S., and DeVita, V. T. (1973). *Arch. Intern. Med.* **132,** 555.
*136.* Schein, P. S., Rakieten, N., Cooney, D. A., Davis, R., and Vernon, M. L. (1973). *Proc. Soc. Exp. Biol. Med.* **143,** 514.
*137.* Schein, P. S., O'Connell, M. J., Blom, J., Hubbard, S., MaGrath, I. T., Bergevin, P., Wiernik, P. H., Ziegler, J. L., and DeVita, V. T. (1974). *Cancer* **34,** 993.
*138.* Schultz, N., and Sanders, R. (1963). *Ann. Surg.* **158,** 1053.
*139.* Shirley, D. V. (1974). *Br. J. Radiol.* **47,** 437.
*140.* Sjoerdsma, A., Lovenberg, W., Engelman, K., Carpenter, W. T., Wyatt, R. J., and Gessa, G. L. (1970). *Ann. Intern. Med.* **73,** 607.
*141.* Smith, C. K., Stoll, R. W., Vance, J., and Williams, R. H. (1971). *Diabetologia* **7,** 118.
*142.* Smith, E., Bantrum, R., Chang, Y., D'Orsi, C. J., Lokich, J., Abruezese, A., and Dantono, J. (1975). *N. Engl. J. Med.* **292,** 825.
*143.* Solom, J., Alexander, M., and Steinfeld, J. (1963). *J. Am. Med. Assoc.* **183,** 165.
*144.* Spencer, H. (1955). *J. Pathol. Bacteriol.* **69,** 259.
*145.* Stadelnamm, P., Safrany, A., and Loffler, A. (1974). *Endoscopy* **6,** 84.
*146.* Steiner, D. F., and Oyer, P. E. (1967). *Proc. Natl. Acad. Sci., U.S.A.* **57,** 473.
*147.* Stolkinsky, D. C., Sadoff, L., Braunwald, J., and Bateman, J. R. (1972). *Cancer* **30,** 61.
*148.* Suzuki, T., Kawabe, K., Imamura, M., and Honjo, I. (1972). *Ann. Surg.* **176,** 37.
*149.* Thjodleifsson, B., and Wormsley, K. G. (1974). *Br. Med. J.* **2,** 304
*150.* Thomas, R. L., Robinson, A. E., Johnsrude, I. S., Goodrich, J. K., and Lester, R. G. (1968). *Am. J. Roentgenol. Radium Ther. Nucl. Med.* **104,** 646.
*151.* Thompson, M. H., Venables, C. W., Miller, I. T., and Reed, J. D. (1975). *Lancet (Letter to the Editor)* **1**(1), 35.
*152.* Tucker, W. G., Talley, R. W., Brownlee, R. W., Burrows, J. H., Stott, P. B., Moorhead, E. L., and San Diego, E. L. (1968). *Cancer Chemother. Rep., Part 1* **52,** 593.
*153.* Tylen, U. (1973). *Acta Radiol., Diagn.* **14,** 449.
*154.* Tylen, U., and Arnesjo, B. (1973). *Scand. J. Gastroenterol.* **8,** 691.
*155.* Van Rymenant, M., Keymolen, P., Procheret, J., DeSchutter, A., and Kram, R.

(1971). *Acta Endocrinol. (Copenhagen)* **66,** 498.
*156.* V. A. Surgical Adjuvant Cancer Chemotherapy Study Group (1975). *Minutes of 38th Meeting, Atlanta, Georgia, April 20 and 21.*
*157.* Waddell, W. R. (1973). *Surgery* **74**(3), 420.
*158.* Walfish, P. G., Natale, R., and Chang, C. (1970). *Diabetes* **19,** 228.
*159.* Walsh, J., and Grossman, M. (1975). *N. Engl. J. Med.* **292,** 1377.
*160.* Walter, R. M., Ensinck, J. W., Ricketts, H., Kendall, J. W., and Williams, R. H. (1973). *Am. J. Med.* **55,** 667.
*161.* Weiss, A. J., Jackson, L. G., and Carabasi, R. (1961). *Ann. Intern. Med.* **55,** 731.
*162.* Whittington, R. M., and Close, H. P. (1970). *Cancer Chemother. Rep., Part 1* **54,** 195.
*163.* Winship, D. H., and Ellison, E. H. (1967). *Lancet* **1,** 1128.
*164.* Wintrobe, M., and Huguley, C. (1948). *Cancer* **1,** 634.
*165.* Wynder, E. L. (1975). *Cancer Res.* **35,** 2228.
*166.* Zimmer, F. E. (1964). *Ann. Intern. Med.* **61,** 543.
*167.* Zimmon, D. S., Breslaw, J., and Kessler, R. E. (1975). *J. Am. Med. Assoc.* **233,** 447.
*168.* Zollinger, R. M. (1975). *Am. J. Surg.* **129,** 102.
*169.* Zollinger, R. M., and Ellison, E. H. (1955). *Ann. Surg.* **142,** 709.

# Mechanisms of Action of Immunopotentiating Agents in Cancer Therapy

WILNA A. WOODS*

*Virus and Disease Modification Section, Viral Biology Branch*
*National Cancer Institute, National Institutes of Health*
*Bethesda, Maryland*

I. Introduction . . . . . . . . . . . . . . . . . . . . . . 143
II. Biological Stimulators . . . . . . . . . . . . . . . . . . 144
A. Bacteria or Bacterial Products . . . . . . . . . . . . . 144
B. Fungal Products . . . . . . . . . . . . . . . . . . . 148
C. Animal Products—Immune RNA . . . . . . . . . . . . 149
D. Plant Products—Lentinan . . . . . . . . . . . . . . 150
III. Chemical Stimulators . . . . . . . . . . . . . . . . . . 151
A. Polymers . . . . . . . . . . . . . . . . . . . . . 151
B. Miscellaneous . . . . . . . . . . . . . . . . . . . 153
IV. Conclusions . . . . . . . . . . . . . . . . . . . . . . 154
References . . . . . . . . . . . . . . . . . . . . . . 155

## I. Introduction

For the past decade, more and more emphasis has been placed on defining the response of the tumor-bearing host to his own malignant cells. Coincidentally, an impressive literature has developed on stimulating the immune response(s) to effect "last cell kill," thereby preventing relapses due to outgrowth of residual and drug-resistant cancerous cells that have escaped primary cytoreductive therapy. Further, since many cancer patients are immunosuppressed either by the disease process itself or by cytoreductive therapy (Eilber and Morton, 1970; Cheema and Hersh, 1971), secondary infectious disease presents a real threat to successful therapeutic management; therefore, return of immune function as soon as possible after suppressive therapy is necessary.

Delicate balance of immune responses to tumor-cell antigens appears to exist. On the one hand, "killer" thymus-derived (T) lymphocytes specifically primed to destroy tumor cells are present in most cancer patients who are not severely anergic (Hellström and Hellström, 1971).

* Present address: RNA Virus Studies Section, Collaborative Research Branch, National Cancer Institute, National Institutes of Health, Bethesda, Maryland.

Furthermore, macrophages are also capable of both nonspecific and specific tumoricidal activity (Evans, 1971). Antibodies, on the other hand, may be either beneficial [complement-dependent cytotoxic antibody (Kassel *et al.*, 1973), macrophage-cytophilic antibody (Mitchell *et al.*, 1975a, b), cell-mediated cytotoxic antibody (MacLennan and Harding, 1973), or unblicking antibody (Bansal and Sjögren, 1971)] or detrimental ["blocking" antibody (Hellström and Hellström, 1970)]. Careful monitoring of each of these factors during immunostimulation must be maintained to ensure that a favorable balance exists at all times. A further consideration in designing combined modality therapeutic regimens is that cytoreductive therapy targeted for rapidly dividing cells should not be administered immediately after immunostimulatory therapy aimed at increasing the number of specifically reactive immunocytes, lest the essential clone reacting to the tumor antigens be destroyed (Amiel and Berardet, 1972).

This survey will be primarily aimed toward those reports defining (*1*) the immune compartment primarily affected by each immunostimulant and (*2*) the biochemical mechanism in those few cases for which data are available. The reader is directed to several excellent reviews of experimental and clinical reports describing immunostimulatory regimens (Borsos and Rapp, 1973; Immunopotentiators, 1973; Hersh, *et al.* 1973; Moore *et al.*, 1973; Yarbro *et al.*, 1974; Chirigos, 1975).

## II. Biological Stimulators

### A. Bacteria or Bacterial Products

#### 1. *Mycobacterium bovis*

Although bacillus Calmette-Guérin (BCG) was one of the first immunostimulants to be tested for therapeutic value in animals (Old *et al.*, 1959, 1961) and in humans (for review, see Borsos and Rapp, 1973), basic studies on the mechanism of action and identity of the active substance(s) have only recently been reported. By careful pathological and electron microscopic examination of tumors and draining lymph nodes of strain-2 guinea pigs bearing carcinogen-induced hepatomas, Hanna and associates (Hanna *et al.*, 1972; Snodgrass and Hanna, 1973) demonstrated that the macrophage is probably the primary activated immune cell. Keller and Hess (1972) described similar macrophage infiltration of Walker carcinosarcomas in rats treated with BCG. Mastrangelo *et al.* (1974) showed a correlation between macrophage infiltration and tumor regression in melanoma patients treated with intralesional BCG.

The primary tumoricidal effect by BCG-activated macrophages is nonspecifically directed toward malignant cells as opposed to normal cells. Several groups have demonstrated nonspecific *in vitro* cytotoxicity by macrophages from mice infected with BCG (Hibbs *et al.*, 1972; Alexander, 1973; Cleveland *et al.*, 1974; Hibbs, 1974; Germain *et al.*, 1975). Fisher *et al.* (1974) note increased macrophage production in bone marrow from tumor-bearing mice. Although the nonspecific activity appears to be mediated by macrophages alone (Germain *et al.*, 1975; Pimm and Baldwin, 1975), many of the specific reactions of tumor rejection may be the result of stimulation of secondary effector cells (T or B lymphocytes) by the activated macrophages (Ariyan and Gershon, 1973) attracted to the tumor by the presence of the mycobacteria (Stjernsward, 1966; Bansal and Sjögren, 1973; Chess *et al.*, 1973, Mitchell *et al.*, 1973; Mackaness *et al.*, 1974).

One of the secondary effects, enhanced tumor growth (Ter-Grigorov and Drlin 1968; Piessens *et al.*, 1970), has been attributed to the production of "blocking antibody" (Chee and Bodurtha, 1974). Stimulation of the humoral immune system by treatment with BCG before tumor inoculation may predispose toward an unfavorable balance between antibody and tumor, resulting in formation of blocking antigen–antibody complexes.

Timing of BCG treatment in relation to tumor inoculation (Lemonde and Clode-Hyde, 1966; Mathé, 1969; Piessens *et al.*, 1970; Larson *et al.*, 1972; Bansal and Sjögren, 1973; Chaparas *et al.*, 1973) or cytoreductive therapy (Pearson *et al.*, 1972, 1973, 1974, 1975) seems to be important to effect the ameliorative effect of immune stimulation rather than tumor enhancement. Suppression of palpable tumors by BCG treatment alone depends on intralesional inoculation (Zbar and Tanaka, 1971; Zbar *et al.*, 1971, 1972; Bartlett *et al.*, 1972). Strains of BCG and modes of preparation also affect immunostimulatory activity (Mackaness, 1973; Mathé *et al.*, 1973). Use of defined components rather than whole living bacilli may allow standardization of effects. Several groups have produced adjuvant effects with subcellular fractions of mycobacteria. Bartlett and Zbar (1973) were able to use mycobacterial cell walls as adjuvant for tumor-specific vaccines in a transplantable guinea pig hepatoma model system. The studies of Weiss and associates (Weiss *et al.*, 1961, 1966; Steinkuller *et al.*, 1969; Yashphe, 1971; Weiss, 1972; Yron *et al.*, 1973, 1975; Minden *et al.*, 1974) and others (Lavrin *et al.*, 1973; Hopper *et al.*, 1975) on methanol-extracted residues of mycobacterial cell walls have shown that subcellular fractions can be active stimulators of tumor immunity, without some of the adverse reactions encountered in treatment with living organisms (Sparks *et al.,* 1973). However, the enhancement phenomenon can also occur (Jacobs and Kripke, 1972). This fraction appears to be similar, if not identical, to the "purified" wax of Suter and White (1954), which was shown to be the substance responsible for elicitation of delayed-type hypersensitivity. A water-soluble fraction (Hiu, 1972; Adam *et al.,* 1973; Juy *et al.,* 1974; Modolell *et al.,* 1974; Werner *et al.,* 1974; Sharma *et al.,* 1975) and a methanol-soluble fraction (Esber *et al.,* 1974; Bogden *et al.,* 1974), which also appear to elicit increased rejection of tumor grafts, are other promising approaches to stimulation of the immune system without complications due to infection of living mycobacteria.

In addition, several groups have isolated active, chemically defined substances. Bekierkunst *et al.* (1971) used trehalose -6,6-dimycolic acid (cord factor) to produce suppression of lung adenomas in mice. Vilkas *et al.* (1973) found immunoadjuvanticity in a galactofuranose disaccharide purified from wax D. Finally, Adam *et al.* (1974) have chemically defined the active material in the water-soluble fractions as peptidoglycans. As more active fractions are identified, it may become possible to elicit specific immune responses to repress tumor growth without adverse effects.

### 2. *Corynebacterium parvum*

Adjuvant activity by killed *Corynebacterium parvum* was first described by Halpern *et al.* (1964). Antitumor activity ascribed to immunological control has been described by many groups in animals (for review see Scott, 1974) and humans (Mathé, 1971; Israel and Halpern, 1972; Israel, 1973, 1974). As with BCG, the target cell of *C. parvum* stimulation is the macrophage (Smith and Woodruff, 1968; Basic *et al.,* 1974; Likhite, 1974; Olivotto and Bomford, 1974; Ghaffar *et al.,* 1974, 1975; Wolmark and Fisher, 1974). This may be mediated by a chemotactic factor released by the bacteria (Wilkinson *et al.,* 1973; Migliore-Samour *et al.,* 1974). However, in contrast to BCG, *C. parvum* does not have a stimulatory effect on lymphocytes (O'Neill *et al.,* 1973; Howard *et al.,* 1973a, b), and, therefore, stimulation of enhancing antibodies would not be expected.

Another advantage of *C. parvum* over mycobacteria is that repeated doses can be used to augment stimulatory activity (Wolmark and Fisher, 1974). This property increases the usefulness, since the stimulatory activity is transient and weak (Halpern *et al.*, 1966; Milas *et al.*, 1974; Currie and Bagshawe, 1970; Pearson *et al.*, 1975).

### 3. *Endotoxin*

The mechanism of action of bacterial endotoxins on tumor growth appears to be complex, and the outcome of endotoxin treatment of tumor-bearing hosts depends on dose and time of application in relation to stage of tumor development. Thus, treatment with *Bordetella pertussis* prior to spontaneous tumor development (Sinkovics *et al.*, 1970) decreased the incidence of neoplasm in the AKR mouse. Strausser and Bober (1972), Watanabe (1969), and Donner *et al.* (1972) also described inhibition of tumors in animals treated with bacterial lipopolysaccharides (LPS). On the other hand, augmentation of tumor growth followed treatment with LPS (Donner *et al.*, 1972) or pertussis vaccine (Floersheim, 1967; Hirano *et al.*, 1967). However, immunological specificity of these reactions was not attempted, although the presence of humoral blocking factors was implicated.

In view of the report of Mota *et al.* (1974) that pertussis adjuvanticity may be ascribed to its LPS content, one may assume that the enhancement phenomenon is mediated through production of humoral blocking factor. Indeed, LPS has a strong direct stimulatory activity on B-cell mitosis (Chiller *et al.*, 1973). However, the adjuvant activity on antibody production and antibody-forming cells may also be partially attributed to stimulation of both macrophages and helper T lymphocytes. Dresser *et al.* (1970) implicated localization of antigen-sensitive cells in the paracortical regions of lymph nodes of mice injected with *B. pertussis*. Newburger *et al.* (1974), Armerding and Katz (1974), and Skidmore *et al.* (1975) also noted potentiation of helper T cells by LPS. In addition, Alexander and Evans (1971), Allison *et al.* (1973), as well as Skidmore *et al.* (1975), noted macrophage activity of LPS. The activity of LPS (and probably pertussis vaccine) on all of these cell types is not surprising in view of many reports that the biochemical activity of LPS is mediated through the cyclic adenosine 3′,5′-monophosphate (cAMP) system of all elements of the reticuloendothelial system (Braun, 1973b; Zenser and Metzger, 1974; Chisari *et al.*, 1974; Cook *et al.*, 1975).

Timing of treatment in relation to tumor development determines whether the balance of immunological responses favors the cytotoxic elements or the enhancing factors. Thus, cytotoxic antibody activity may predominate with early treatment and result in decreased incidence of spontaneous leukemia in AKR mice (Sinkovics *et al.*, 1970). Inhibition of tumor growth at later stages of tumor development (Watanabe, 1969; Strausser and Bober, 1972; Donner *et al.*, 1972) may be due to increased macrophage activity, cytotoxic antibody activity, or to direct cytotoxicity of LPS on the tumor cells (Ralph *et al.*, 1974).

These complex interactions may serve as a reminder that little is known of the effects on tumor growth during interaction of the various compartments of the immune system. More definitive work is needed in this area before complex stimulants, with equally complex effects, may be administered with confidence for a favorable therapeutic outcome.

## B. Fungal Products

### 1. *Statolon*

A product of *Penicilium stoloniferum*, statolon, was originally described as a nonviral stimulator of interferon. However, Banks *et al.* (1968) and Kleinschmidt (1968) reported that the active factor was, indeed, a double-stranded RNA from viruslike particles found in the fungi. Wheelock (1967) originally ascribed the inhibitory effect of statolon treatment on Friend virus leukemia in DBA mice to induction of an interferon-induced antiviral effect. However, lack of correlation of interferon titers with induction of long-term remissions characterized by persistent latent infections (Wheelock *et al.*, 1969) led to investigation of immune mechanisms of disease control (Wheelock *et al.*, 1972, 1973; Toy *et al.*, 1973). The enhancement of humoral cytotoxic and virus-neutralizing antibodies reported in these later studies was shown to be coupled with reversal by statolon treatment of early immunodepression resulting from Friend virus infection (Weislow *et al.*, 1973; Weislow and Wheelock, 1975a). Another effect of statolon on immune cells is enhancement of macrophage function (Levy and Wheelock, 1975; Wheelock *et al.*, 1975). Stimulation of a cell-mediated immunity was shown to be augmented by addition of chlorite-oxidized oxyamylose (Weislow and Wheelock, 1975b), a polyacetal acid with interferon-inducing and macrophage-activating properties (Billiau *et al.*, 1970, 1971). This represents one of the rare studies of treatment with a combination of immunostimulatory drugs and opens the door for other similar regimens, utilizing agents active on either different target cells or biochemical reactions. It is possible that the augmentation is due to activation of macrophages, eliciting an early nonspecific "mopping up" of tumor cells, followed by increased antibody production (Wheelock, 1975).

2. *Protozoa*

Tumor resistance in mice bearing chronic infection by intracellular parasites, *Toxoplasma gondii* and *Besnoitia jellisoni*, was first described by Hibbs and co-workers (1971a,b). Resistance to spontaneous tumor development in C3H/He and AKR mice, as well as to challenge with Friend leukemia virus and Sarcoma 180 transplantation, was ascribed to the enhancement of cell-mediated immunity. No studies on specificity of tumor resistance were included, although Hibbs (1973) reported that nonspecifically activated macrophages were responsible for the resistance. The *in vitro* cytotoxic effect of the activated macrophages was directed nonspecifically toward all transformed, but not toward normal cells. Krahenbuhl and Remington (1974) were able to demonstrate an early *in vitro* cytostasis within 6 hours of addition of activated macrophages to cultures of several different tumor target cells; the effect lasted at least 19 weeks. Peritoneal lymphocytes were not involved in the reaction and were not capable of inhibiting tumor cell DNA synthesis. Similar results were reported by Droller and Remington (1975) using a mouse bladder tumor cell line; an *in vivo* effect was also noted. The nonspecific activation is similar to that noted by Morahan *et al.* (1974), using pyran copolymer treatment (see Section III, A, 2).

### C. Animal Products—Immune RNA

The use of RNA extracted from immune lymphocytes to "sensitize" lymphocytes from normal individuals or to increase the degree of immune responsiveness of individuals with prior exposure to an antigen offers another approach to augmentation of the immune responsiveness of tumor-bearing hosts. Two different species of RNA have been described to be effective transmitters of immune information between allogeneic or xenogeneic lymphoid cells: first, the low molecular weight dialyzable transfer factor (TF) in humans (Lawrence *et al.*, 1963) and, second, a somewhat higher (8–12 S) molecular weight, nondialyzable molecule that also has activity in several animal model systems (Alexander *et al.*, 1967; Pilch and Ramming, 1970; Bell and Dray, 1969). Both have been shown to sensitize lymphocytes from the "normal" individuals and tumor-bearing hosts to respond to antigens on the surface of tumor cells. The advantage of such preparations for tumor immunotherapy lies in transferring specific immune reactivity across histocompatibility barriers. The major disadvantage, however, as with any immune stimulatory agent, is the possibility of "transferring" unwanted information (Pilch and Ramming, 1971).

Transfer factor therapy in cancer patients has been reviewed by Krementz *et al.* (1974). However, the mechanism of activation, the donor cell type(s), and the target reactor cell(s) have not as yet been defined (Spitler *et al.,* 1975; Fudenberg, 1975). Ascher *et al.* (1974) also noted that precise characterization of the exact chemical nature and mode of action of the active moiety has been hampered by lack of both an animal model system and of a good *in vitro* assay for activity. Their antigen-triggered lymphocyte proliferation test appears to show good correlation with the immune status of the donor. They conclude that either new antigen receptor sites appear, resulting in the creation of new reactive clones, or a preexisting lymphoid clone is selectively activated and enhanced. Bloom (1973) had suggested that, in some instances, TF acts with an adjuvant effect. By using an *in vitro* mixed-lymphocyte assay, Dupont *et al.* (1974) have also reported that TF has a nonspecific stimulatory effect resulting in maturation of lymphocytes in patients with immune deficiency disease. Apparently, with new *in vitro* assay tools in hand, studies defining the chemical nature and mode of action of TF may be expected in the near future.

The specific transfer of immunological responsiveness using RNA from allogeneic or xenogeneic immune lymphocytes (Alexander *et al.,* 1967) has been reviewed by Pilch *et al.* (1974), Ohno *et al.* (1973), and Schlager *et al.* (1975). The active RNA species was determined by Thor and Dray (1973) to be 8–12 S. The target cell may be a T cell since RNA-transferrred *in vitro* cytotoxicity has been reported by Schlager *et al.* (1975), although the presence of antibody in the system was not conclusively ruled out. The B cells may also be sensitized, since transfer of specific antibody production has been demonstrated (Bell and Dray, 1969, 1970). Because clinical trials are now in progress (Pilch *et al.,* 1975), the need for critical studies of mechanism of action and donor cell identity as well as confirmation of the target cell(s) under specific conditions is critical.

### D. Plant Products—Lentinan

Japanese workers have clinically defined lentinan, a polysaccharide extracted and purified from the mushroom *Lentinus edodes* (Beck.) Sing. (Chihara *et al.,* 1970; Hamuro *et al.,* 1971), and demonstrated that the substance conferred resistance to Sarcoma 180 in Swiss and SWM/Ms mice. This resistance was reported by Maeda and Chihara (1971) to be mediated by T lymphocytes. Thymectomy or antilymphocyte serum treatment abrogated the protective effect of lentinan. However, specificity for the challenge tumor was not reported. The effect on antibody production or on macrophage activity was not investigated. If this polysaccharide is, indeed, a specific T-cell stimulator, its usefulness in therapy may prove to be important, since blocking factors might not be encountered.

## III. Chemical Stimulators

### A. Polymers

1. *Polynucleotides*

The mechanism of the antitumor activity of the double-stranded polynucleotides, polyinosinic–polycytidylic (poly I:poly C) and poly-adenylic–polyuridylic (poly A:poly U) acids, is not clear, but is probably the result of both an antitumor cell metabolic effect and an augmentation of the host's immune response to the tumor. The growth of spontaneous (Gelboin and Levy, 1970; La Cour *et al.,* 1975; Levy and Riley, 1970; Mathé *et al.,* 1971; Sandberg and Goldin, 1971), transplantable (Levy *et al.,* 1969; Potmesil and Goldfeder, 1972), and virus-induced tumors (Pearson *et al.,* 1969; Gazdar *et al.,* 1972a; DeClercq and Stewart, 1974) is inhibited by polynucleotide treatment. Poly A:poly U has fewer toxic side effects than poly I:poly C and has recently been studied more extensively. Rhim and Huebner (1971) found that the interferon-inducing activity of poly I:poly C did not correlate with the antitumor activity; macromolecular synthesis of malignant cells is markedly inhibited *in vitro* (Teng *et al.,* 1973) by poly I:poly C. This metabolic effect may contribute to the tumor inhibition. In addition, the immune stimulatory effect of polynucleotides (Braun *et al.,* 1968; Braun, 1973a) may contribute to the growth inhibitory and stimulatory effects (Gazdar *et al.,* 1972b). Stimulation of antibody production (Turner *et al.,* 1970) and enhancement of antibody-forming cells (Braun *et al.,* 1968; Johnson *et al.,* 1968; Braun *et al.,* 1971; Schmidtke and Johnson, 1971; Collavo *et al.,* 1972, 1973) indicate that the polynucleotides are capable of B-cell stimulation. *In vitro* DNA synthesis (Dean *et al.,* 1972; Woods *et al.,* 1974) has also been used extensively as a measure of polynucleotide stimulation of various compartments of the immune system. Scher *et al.* (1973) and Ruhl *et al.* (1974) used the technique with partitioned lymphocyte populations to demonstrate that B cells may be the primary responding cell. Antibody stimulation may, thus, be a direct effect and/or an indirect effect via macrophage activation (Johnson and Johnson, 1971; Chess *et al.,* 1972; Marchalonis *et al.,* 1973). The same remarks may pertain to activation of T cells as reported by Turner *et al.* (1970),

Cone and Johnson (1971, 1972), Cone and Wilson (1972), Hamaoka and Katz (1973), Han *et al.* (1973), Wagner and Cone (1974). Such widespread effects may reflect the end results of the effect of the polynucleotides on cAMP (Ishizuka *et al.,* 1971). The specific effects on immune responses to tumor cells themselves have not often been investigated, however, and the appearance of tumor-specific immunity should be demonstrated before the immune response can be implicated in antitumor effects.

Tennant *et al.* (1974) noted that another polynucleotide, poly(2′-*O*-methyladenylic acid), stimulated the immune response of BALB/c mice to Moloney sarcoma virus-induced tumors as well as to virus envelope antigens. Thus, this relatively nontoxic polynucleotide may be a new addition to the armamentarium of antitumor drugs, with a dual mechanism of inhibition of oncornaviral replication and transformation as well as immunological enhancement.

### 2. *Pyran Copolymer*

The effect pyran (maleic divinyl ether copolymer) has on the reticuloendothelial system mimics that of *C. parvum* in that the macrophage is the primary cell affected, although both antibody production and T cells have been reported to be enhanced; the biochemical target reaction, however, has not been identified. Pyran was first used as a chemotherapeutic antiviral agent against Friend virus-induced leukemia (Regelson, 1967; Chirigos *et al.,* 1969; Hirsch *et al.,* 1972). The protection was attributed to interferon induction. By contrast, Gazdar *et al.* (1972a) and Schuller *et al.* (1975) described tumor enhancement. The latter authors attributed the effect to an increase in target cells for virus transformation, although an immunological effect was not excluded. Nonviral tumors have also been inhibited by pyran (Kapila *et al.,* 1974; Sandberg and Goldin, 1971; Morahan *et al.*, 1974; Kaplan *et al.,* 1974). Regelson *et al.* (1970) first described the stimulatory effect of pyran on the reticuloendothelial system. Antibody stimulation was described by Braun *et al.* (1970), and Kapusta and Mendelson (1969) showed inhibition of T-cell function by demonstrating diminution of adjuvant disease in rats treated with pyran. Kapila *et al.* (1971) and Morahan *et al.* (1974) demonstrated that the basis of the pyran stimulation of the immune system rests in the capacity to stimulate macrophages to destroy tumor cells selectively; this activation of macrophages may also be contributory to antibody enhancement. Schultz, Woods, and Chirigos (unpublished results) have demonstrated that the macrophage cytotoxicity elicited in tumor-bearing mice can be specific for the tumor, and that the specificity can be blocked by antimouse globulin, suggesting an influence of cytophilic antibody in the specific reaction.

3. *Dextrans*

High molecular weight dextrans have been implicated in stimulation of B cells (Diamantstein *et al.,* 1971; Gall *et al.,* 1972; Battisto and Pappas, 1973; Diamantstein and Wagner, 1973; Vogt *et al.,* 1973; Dorries *et al.,* 1974; Bradfield *et al.,* 1974; Diamantstein *et al.,* 1974; Ralph *et al.,* 1974; Wittman *et al.,* 1975) resulting in increased antibody synthesis and DNA synthesis. Two members of the group have been shown to be active in tumor inhibition: levan (Leibovici *et al.,* 1975) and DEAE-dextran (Ebbesen, 1974). However, immunological specificity studies were not included, and, therefore, use of these substances in immunotherapy must await further clarification. Immunological enhancement must also be considered as a possible complication.

## B. Miscellaneous

1. *Tilorones*

Like the dextrans and polynucleotides, the tilorones have been implicated in immune inhibition of neoplasms, without clear evidence for immunological involvement (Morahan *et al.,* 1974; Chirigos *et al.,* 1973; Gazdar *et al.*, 1972b; Munson *et al.*, 1974). Gazdar *et al.* (1972a) also reported tumor enhancement under some conditions, suggesting an enhancement of antibody production or a suppression of cell-mediated immunity. Indeed, Hoffman *et al.* (1965) and Diamantstein (1973) reported enhancement of antibody-forming cells as measured by the Jerne technique and hemolysin titration. Megel *et al.* (1974) confirmed these observations and further reported that cell-mediated immunity was depressed. Munson *et al.* (1974) reported stimulation of macrophages as well as enhancement of antibody plaque-forming cells. Levine (1975) and Mitchell *et al.* (1975b) also reported T-cell depletion following tilorone treatment.

The tumor inhibitory activity could be due to direct cytotoxicity (Adamson, 1971; Chandra *et al.,* 1972). Schaffer *et al.* (1974) also reported that tilorone inhibits DNA polymerases; the drug preferentially interacted with adenine:thymine base pair sequences. Thus, the antitumor activity may mainly reflect the direct effect on tumor cells and on the immune response through macrophage activation. Until specific antitumor antibody and/or cell-mediated immunity have been reported to be increased, however, the tilorones must be considered to have little or no beneficial effect on host immune defenses to tumors.

### 2. *Levamisole*

Since the publication of the report by Renoux and Renoux (1971) that the anthelmintic L-2,3,5,6-tetrahydro-6-phenylimidazole [2,1-*b*] thiazole hydrochloride (levamisole, LMS) possessed immunostimulatory activity, many laboratories have reported augmented immune responses in cancer patients (Lichtenfeld, 1973, 1975; Brugmans *et al.,* 1973; Brugmans and Symoens, 1975; Hirshaut *et al.,* 1973; Tripodi *et al.,* 1973; Spitler *et al.,* 1975). Other investigators have reported that LMS stimulates *in vitro* DNA synthesis of lymphocytes (Woods *et al.,* 1975a,b; Sunshine *et al.,* 1975; Lieberman and Mae-Hsu, 1975; Haden, 1975). The effect is most pronounced under suppressive conditions (Woods *et al.,* 1975c; Sunshine *et al.,* 1975; Lichtenfeld *et al.,* 1973, 1975). Although the DNA synthetic stimulation appears to be restricted to lymphocytes (Woods *et al.,* 1975c), Schultz, Chirigos, and Mohr (personal communication) have found that macrophages from tumor-bearing levamisole-treated animals are specifically activated.

The effect seems mediated through the cAMP regulatory system (Woods *et al.,* 1975c; Sunshine *et al.,* 1975; Hadden, 1975). Woods *et al.* (1975c) determined that the cAMP and cGMP phosphodiesterase regulatory enzyme(s) are affected. In view of the mild stimulatory activity only under suppressive conditions with early restoration of immune competence, LMS appears to show great promise for combined chemoimmunotherapy of cancer.

## IV. Conclusions

Many immunostimulatory materials, both biological and chemical, have been shown to have activity in enhancing tumor immunity. Many of these agents influence the immune response through the cAMP–cGMP regulatory system (Ishizuka *et al.,* 1971; Seyberth *et al.,* 1973; Strom *et al.,* 1973; Watson *et al.,* 1973; Bourne *et al.,* 1974; Diamantstein and Ulmer, 1975; Gillette *et al.,* 1974; Henney *et al.,* 1974; Oliveira-Lima *et al.,* 1974; Remold-O'Donnell and Remold, 1974). One of the most exciting and promising approaches to cancer chemotherapy would thus appear to be explorations into the mechanisms and limitations of agents modifying the cAMP–cGMP system in tumor-specific immune systems.

ACKNOWLEDGMENTS

The author gratefully acknowledges many helpful discussions and suggestions of Dr. M. A. Chirigos of the National Cancer Institute. The skillful and speedy preparation of the manuscript by Mrs. P. Yasem and Miss M. A. Young is also acknowledged with appreciation.

REFERENCES

Adam, A., Ciorbaru, R., Petit, J. F., Lederer, E., Chedid, L., *et al.* (1973). *Infect. Immun.* **7,** 855–861.

Adam, A., Amar, C., Ciorbaru, R., Lederer, E., Petit, J. F., and Vilkas, E. (1974). *C. R. Acad. Sci. Ser. D* **278,** 799–801.

Adamson, R. H. (1971). *J. Natl. Cancer Inst.* **46,** 431–434.

Alexander, P. (1973). *Natl. Cancer Inst. Monogr.* **39,** 127–133.

Alexander, P., and Evans, R. (1971). *Nature (London), New Biol.* **232,** 76–78.

Alexander, P., Delorme, E. J., Hamilton, L. D. G., and Hall, J. G. (1967). *Nature (London)* **213,** 569–572.

Allison, A. C., Davies, P., and Page, R. C. (1973). *J. Infect. Dis.* **128,** 212–219.

Amiel, J. L., and Berardet, M. (1972). *Ann. Inst. Pasteur, Paris* **122,** 701–714.

Ariyan, S., and Gershon, R. K. (1973). *J. Natl. Cancer Inst.* **51,** 1145–1148.

Armerding, D., and Katz, D. H. (1974). *J. Exp. Med.* **139,** 24–43.

Ascher, M. S., Schneider, W. J., Valentine, F. T., and Lawrence, H. S. (1974). *Proc. Natl. Acad. Sci., U. S. A.* **71,** 1178–1182.

Banks, G. T., Buck, K. W., Chain, E. B., Himmelweit, F., *et al.* (1968). *Nature (London)* **218,** 542–543.

Bansal, S. C., and Sjögren, H. O. (1971). *Nature (London)* **233,** 76–77.

Bansal, S. C., and Sjögren, H. O. (1973). *Int. J. Cancer* **11,** 162–171.

Bartlett, G. L., and Zbar, B. (1973). *J. Natl. Cancer Inst.* **50,** 1385–1390.

Bartlett, G. L., Zbar, B., and Rapp, H. J. (1972). *J. Natl. Cancer Inst.* **48,** 245–257.

Basic, I., Milas, L., Grdina, D. J., *et al.* (1974). *J. Natl. Cancer Inst.* **52,** 1839–1842.

Battisto, J. R., and Pappas, F. (1973). *J. Exp. Med.* **138,** 176–193.

Bekierkunst, A., Levij, I. S., Yarkoni, E., Vilkas, E., and Lederer, E. (1971). *Science* **174,** 1240–1242.

Bell, C., and Dray, S. (1969). *J. Immunol.* **103,** 1196–1211.

Bell, C., and Dray, S. (1970). *J. Immunol.* **105,** 541–556.

Billiau, A., Desmyter, J., and DeSomer, P. (1970). *J. Virol.* **5,** 321–328.

Billiau, A., Eyssen, H., David, G., and DeSomer, P. (1971). *Proc. Soc. Exp. Biol. Med.* **137,** 626–630.

Bloom, B. R. (1973). *N. Engl. J. Med.* **288,** 908–909.

Bogden, A. E., Esber, H. J., Taylor, H. J., and Gray, J. H. (1974). *Cancer Res.* **34,** 1627–1631.

Borsos, T., and Rapp, H. J., eds. (1973). Conference on the Use of BCG in Therapy of Cancer. *Natl. Cancer Inst. Monogr.* **39.** US Govt. Printing Office, Washington, D. C.

Bourne, H. R., Lichtenstein, L. M., Melmon, K. L., Henney, C. S., *et al.* (1974). *Science* **184,** 19–28.

Bradfield, J. W., Souhami, R. L., and Addison, I. E. (1974). *Immunology* **26,** 383–392.

Braun, W. (1973a). *Ann. N. Y. Acad. Sci.* **207,** 17–28.

Braun, W. (1973b). *J. Infect. Dis.* **218,** S188–197.

Braun, W., Nakano, M., Jaraskova, L., Yajima, Y., and Jiminez, L. (1968). *In* "Nucleic Acids in Immunology" (O. J. Plescia and W. Braun, eds.), pp. 347–363. Springer-Verlag, Berlin and New York.

Braun, W., Regelson, W., Yajima, Y., *et al.* (1970). *Proc. Soc. Exp. Biol. Med.* **133,** 171–175.

Braun, W., Ishizuka, M., Yajima, Y., Webb, D., and Winchurch, R. (1971). *In* "Biological Effects of Polynucleotides" (R. F. Beers and W. Braun, eds.), pp. 139–156. Springer-Verlag, Berlin and New York.

Brugmans, J., and Symoens, J. (1975). *In* "Modulation of Host Immune Resistance in the Prevention or Treatment of Induced Neoplasia" (M. A. Chirigos, ed.). Fogarty Int. Center Proc. No. 28. U.S. Govt. Printing Office, Washington, D.C.

Brugmans, J., Schuermans, V., DeCock, W., Thienpoint, D., Janssen, P., Verhagen, H., Van Nimmer, H., Larewagie, A. C., and Stevens, E. (1973). *Life Sci.* **13,** 1499–1504.

Chandra, P., Zinino, F., Gaur, V. P., Zaccara, A., *et al.* (1972). *FEBS Lett.* **28,** 5–9.

Chaparas, S. D., Chirigos, M., Pearson, J., and Sher, N. (1973). *Natl. Cancer Inst. Monogr.* **39,** 87–88.

Chee, D. O., and Bodurtha, A. J. (1974). *Int. J. Cancer* **14,** 137–143.

Cheema, A. R., and Hersh, E. M. (1971). *Cancer* **28,** 851–855.

Chess, L., Lovy, C., Schmukler, M., Smith, K., and Mardiney, M. R., Jr. (1972). *Transplantation* **14,** 748–755.

Chess, L., Back, G. N., Ungaro, P. C., Buckholz, D. H., and Mardiney, M. R., Jr. (1973). *J. Natl. Cancer Inst.* **51,** 57–65.

Chihara, G., Hamuro, J., Maeda, Y. Y., Arai, Y., and Fukuorka, F. (1970). *Cancer Res.* **30,** 2776–2781.

Chiller, J. M., Skidmore, B. J., Morrison, D. C., and Weigle, W. O. (1973). *Proc. Natl. Acad. Sci., U.S.A.* **70,** 2129–2133.

Chirigos, M. A., ed. (1975). "Modulation of Host Immune Resistance in the Prevention or Treatment of Induced Neoplasia." Fogarty Int. Center Proc., No. 28. US Govt. Printing Office, Washington, D.C.

Chirigos, M. A., Turner, W., Pearson, J., and Griffin, W. (1969). *Int. J. Cancer* **4,** 267–278.

Chirigos, M. A., Pearson, J. W., and Pryor, J. (1973). *Cancer Res.* **33,** 2615–2618.

Chisari, F. V., Northrup, R. S., and Chen, L. C. (1974). *J. Immunol.* **113,** 729–739.

Cleveland, R. P., Meltzer, M. S., and Žbar, B. (1974). *J. Natl. Cancer Inst.* **52,** 1887–1895.

Collavo, D., Finco, B., and Chiecco-Bianchi, L. (1972). *Nature (London) New Biol.* **237,** 154–155.

Collavo, D., Biasi, G., Pennelli, N., and Chiecco-Bianci, L. (1973). *Tumori* **59,** 77–96.

Cone, R. E., and Johnson, A. G. (1971). *J. Exp. Med.* **133,** 665–676.

Cone, R. E., and Johnson, A. G. (1972). *Cell. Immunol.* **3,** 283–293.

Cone, R. E., and Wilson, J. D. (1972). *Int. Arch. Allergy Appl. Immunol.* **43,** 123–130.

Cook, R. G., Stavitsky, A. B., and Schoenberg, M. D. (1975). *J. Immunol.* **114,** 426–434.

Currie, G. A., and Bagshawe, K. D. (1970). *Br. Med. J.* **1,** 541–544.

Dean, J. H., Wallen, W. C., and Lucas, D. O. (1972). *Nature (London) New Biol.* **237,** 218–219.

DeClercq, E., and Stewart, W. E. (1974). *J. Nat. Cancer Inst.* **52,** 591–594

Diamantstein, T. (1973). *Immunology* **24,** 771–775.

Diamantstein, T., and Ulmer, A. (1975). *Immunology* **28,** 113–119.

Diamantstein, T., and Wagner, B. (1973). *Nature (London) New Biol.* **241,** 117–118.
Diamantstein, T., Meinhold, H., and Wagner, B. (1971). *Eur. J. Immunol.* **1,** 429–432.
Diamantstein, T., Blitstein-Willinger, E., and Schultz, G. (1974). *Nature (London)* **250,** 596–597.
Donner, M., Hottier, D., and Burg, C. (1972). *Eur. J. Cancer* **2,** 141–147.
Dorries, R., Schimpl, A., and Wecker, E. (1974). *Eur. J. Cancer* **4,** 230–233.
Dresser, D. W., Taub, R. N., and Krantz, A. R. (1970). *Immunology* **18,** 663–670.
Droller, M. J., and Remington, J. S. (1975). *Cancer Res.* **35,** 49–53.
Dupont, B., Ballow, M., Hansen, J. A., *et al.* (1974). *Proc. Natl. Acad. Sci., U. S. A.* **71,** 867–871.
Ebbesen, P. (1974). *Br. J. Cancer* **30,** 68–72.
Eilber, F. R., and Morton, D. L. (1970). *Cancer* **25,** 362–367.
Esber, H. J., Hagopian, M., and Bogden, A. E. (1974). *J. Natl. Cancer Inst.* **53,** 209–212.
Evans, R. (1971). *Immunology* **20,** 75–83.
Fisher, B., Taylor, S., Levine, M., Saffer, E., and Fischer, E. R. (1974). *Cancer Res.* **34,** 1668–1670.
Floersheim, G. L. (1967). *Nature (London)* **216,** 1235–1236.
Fudenberg, H. (1975). *In* "Modulation of Host Immune Resistance in the Prevention or Treatment of Induced Neoplasia" (M. A. Chirigos, ed.). Fogarty Int. Center Proc., No. 28. US Govt. Printing Office, Washington, D.C.
Gall, D., Knight, P. A., and Hampson, F. (1972). *Immunology* **23,** 569–575.
Gazdar, A. F., Steinberg, A. P., Spahn, G. S., and Baron, S. (1972a). *Proc. Soc. Exp. Biol. Med.* **139,** 1132–1137.
Gazdar, A. F., Weinstein, A. J., Sims, H. L., and Steinberg, D. (1972b). *Proc. Soc. Exp. Biol. Med.* **139,** 279–285.
Gelboin, H. V., and Levy, H. B. (1970). *Science* **167,** 205–207.
Germain, R. N., Williams, R. M., and Benacerraf, B. (1975). *J. Natl. Cancer Inst.* **54,** 709–720.
Ghaffar, A., Cullen, R. T., Dunbar, N., and Woodruff, M. F. A. (1974). *Br. J. Cancer* **29,** 199–205.
Ghaffar, A., Cullen, R. T., and Woodruff, M. F. A. (1975). *Br. J. Cancer* **31,** 15–24.
Gillette, R. W., McKenzie, G. O., and Swanson, M. H. (1974). *J. Reticuloendothel. Soc.* **16,** 289–299.
Hadden, J. (1975). *In* "Modulation of Host Immune Resistance in the Prevention or Treatment of Induced Neoplasia" (M. A. Chirigos, ed.). Fogarty Int. Center Proc., No. 28. US Govt. Printing Office, Washington, D.C.
Halpern, B. N., Prevot, A. R., Biozzi, G., Stiffel, C., *et al.* (1964). *J. Reticuloendothel. Soc.* **1,** 77–96.
Halpern, B. N., Biozzi, G., Stiffel, C., and Mouton, D. (1966). *Nature (London)* **212,** 853–854.
Hamaoka, T., and Katz, D. H. (1973). *Cell. Immunol.* **7,** 246.
Hamuro, J., Maeda, Y. Y., Arai, Y., Fukuka, F., and Chihara, G. (1971). *Chem.-Biol. Interact.* **3,** 69–71.
Han, I. H., Johnson, A. G., Cook, J., and Han, S. S. (1973). *J. Infect. Dis.* **128,** 232–237.
Hanna, M. G., Zbar, B., and Rapp, H. J. (1972). *J. Natl. Cancer Inst.* **48,** 1441–1455.
Hellström, I., and Hellström, K. E. (1971). *In* "*In Vitro* Methods in Cell-Mediated Immunity" (B. R. Bloom and P. R. Olade, eds.), pp. 409–414. Academic Press, New York.
Hellström, K. E., and Hellström, I. (1970). *Annu. Rev. Microbiol.* **24,** 378–398.

Henney, C. S., Gaffney, J., and Bloom, B. R. (1974). *J. Exp. Med.* **140,** 837–852.
Hersh, E. M., Gutterman, J. U., and Mavligit, G., eds. (1973). "Immunotherapy of Cancer in Man—Scientific Basis and Current Status." Thomas, Springfield, Illinois.
Hibbs, J. B., (1973). *Science* **180,** 868–870.
Hibbs, J. B. (1974). *Science* **184,** 468–471.
Hibbs, J. B., Lambert, L. H., and Remington, J. S. (1971a). *J. Clin. Invest.* **50,** 45a.
Hibbs, J. B., Lambert, L. H., and Remington, J. S. (1971b). *J. Infect. Dis.* **124,** 587–592.
Hibbs, J. B., Lambert, L. H., and Remington, J. S. (1972). *Proc. Soc. Exp. Biol. Med.* **139,** 1049–1052.
Hirano, M., Sinkovics, J. G., Shullenberger, C. C., and Howe, C. D. (1967). *Science* **158,** 1061–1064.
Hirsch, M. S., Black, P. H., Wood, M. L., and Monaco, A. P. (1972). *J. Immunol.* **108,** 1312–1318.
Hirshaut, Y., Pinsky, C., Marquardt, H., *et al.* (1973). *Proc. Am. Assoc. Cancer Res.* **14,** 109.
Hiu, I. J. (1972). *Nature (London) New Biol.* **238,** 241–242.
Hoffman, P. F., Pitter, H. W., and Krueger, R. F. (1965). *In* "Advances in Antimicrobial and Antineoplastic Chemotherapy" (M. Hejzlar, M. Semonsky, and S. Masek, eds.), p. 217. Urban & Schwarzenberg, Munich.
Hopper, D. G., Pimm, M. V., and Baldwin, R. W. (1975). *Br. J. Cancer* **31,** 176–181.
Howard, J. G., Christy, G. H., and Scott, M. T. (1973a). *Cell. Immunol.* **7,** 290–301.
Howard, J. G., Scott, M. T., and Christy, G. H. (1973b). *In* "CIBA Foundation Symposium on Immunopotentiation," pp. 100–120. Associated Scientific, Amsterdam.
Immunopotentiators (1973). "CIBA Foundation Symposium." Associated Scientific, Amsterdam.
Ishizuka, M., Braun, W., and Matsumoto, T. (1971). *J. Immunol.* **107,** 1027–1035.
Israel, L. (1973). *Cancer Chemother. Rep., Part 2* **4,** 283–285.
Israel, L. (1974). *Sem. Hop. Ther.* **50,** 159–161.
Israel, L., and Halpern, B. (1972). *Nouv. Presse Med.* **1,** 19–23.
Jacobs, D. J., and Kripke, M. L. (1972). *Fed. Proc., Fed. Am. Soc. Exp. Biol.* **31,** 640.
Johnson, A. G., Schmidtke, J., Merritt, K., and Han, I. (1968). *In* "Nucleic Acids in Immunology" (O. J. Plescia and W. Braun, eds.), pp. 379–385. Springer-Verlag, Berlin and New York.
Johnson, H. G., and Johnson, A. G. (1971). *J. Exp. Med.* **133,** 649–664.
Juy, D., Bona, C., and Chedid, L. (1974). *C. R. Acad. Sci., Ser. D* **278,** 2859–2862.
Kapila, K., Smith, C., and Rubin, A. A. (1971). *J. Reticuloendothel. Soc.* **9,** 447–450.
Kaplan, A. S., Morahan, P. S., and Regelson, W. (1974). *J. Natl. Cancer Inst.* **52,** 1919–1923.
Kapusta, M. A., and Mendelson, J. (1969). *Arthritis Rheum.* **12,** 463–471.
Kassel, R. L., Old, L. J., Carswell, E. A., *et al.* (1973). *J. Exp. Med.* **138,** 925–938.
Keller, R., and Hess, M. W. (1972). *Br. J. Exp. Pathol.* **53,** 570–571.
Kleinschmidt, W. J., Ellis, L. F., Van Frank, R. M., and Murphy, E. B. (1968). *Nature (London)* **220,** 167–168.
Krahenbuhl, J. L., and Remington, J. S. (1974). *J. Immunol.* **113,** 507–516.
Krementz, E. T., Mansell, P. W. A., Hornung, M. O., Samuels, M. S., *et al.* (1974). *Cancer* **33,** 394–401.
LaCour, F., DeLage, G., and Chianle, C. (1975). *Science* **187,** 256–257.
Larson, C. L., Baker, R. E., Ushijima, M., Baker, M. D., and Gillespie, C. (1972). *Proc. Soc. Exp. Biol. Med.* **140,** 700–702.

Lavrin, D. H., Rosenberg, S. A., Connor, R. J., and Terry, W. D. (1973). *Cancer Res.* **33,** 472–477.

Lawrence, H. S., Al-Askari, S., David, S., *et al.* (1963). *Trans. Assoc. Am. Physicians* **76,** 84–91.

Leibovici, J., Sinai, Y., Wolman, M., and Davidai, G. (1975). *Cancer Res.* **35,** 1921–1925.

Lemonde, P., and Clode-Hyde, M. (1966). *Cancer Res.* **26,** 585–589.

Levine, S. (1975). *In* "Modulation of Host Immune Resistance in the Prevention or Treatment of Induced Neoplasia" (M. A. Chirigos, ed.). Fogarty Int. Center Proc., No. 28. US Govt. Printing Office, Washington, D.C.

Levy, H. B., and Riley, F. (1970). *Proc. Soc. Exp. Biol. Med.* **135,** 141-145.

Levy, H. B., Law, L. W., and Rabson, A. S. (1969). *Proc. Natl. Acad. Sci., U. S. A.* **62,** 357-360.

Levy, M. H., and Wheelock, E. F. (1975). *J. Immunol.* **114,** 962–965.

Lichtenfeld, J. L., Desner, M., Mardiney, M., and Wiernik, P. H. (1973). *Fed. Proc. Fed. Am. Soc. Exp. Biol.* **58,** 790.

Lichtenfeld, J. L., Desner, M. R., Wiernik, P. H., Moore, S., and Mardiney, M. R., Jr. (1975). *In* "Modulation of Host Immune Resistance in the Prevention or Treatment of Induced Neoplasia" (M. A. Chirigos, ed.). Fogarty Int. Center Proc., No 28. US Govt. Printing Office, Washington, D.C.

Lieberman, R., and Mae-Hsu (1975). *In* "Modulation of Host Immune Resistance in the Prevention or Treatment of Induced Neoplasia" (M. A. Chirigos, ed.). Fogarty Int. Center Proc., No. 28. US Govt. Printing Office, Washington, D.C.

Likhite, V. V. (1974). *Int. J. Cancer* **14,** 684–690.

Mackaness, G. B., Auclair, D. J., and Lagrange, P. H. (1973). *J. Natl. Cancer Inst.* **51,** 1655–1667.

Mackaness, G. B., Lagrange, P. H., and Ishibashi, T. (1974). *J. Exp. Med.* **139,** 1540–1545.

MacLennan, I. C. M., and Harding, B. (1973). *Br. J. Cancer* **28,** 7–10.

Maeda, Y. Y., and Chihara, G. (1971). *Nature (London)* **229,** 634.

Marchalonis, J. J., Cone, R. E., and Rolley, R. T. (1973). *J. Immunol.* **110,** 561–567.

Mastrangelo, M. J., Kim, Y. H., Bornstein, R. S., Chee, D. O., Sulit, H. L., and Yarbro, J. W. (1974). *J. Natl. Cancer Inst.* **52,** 19–24.

Mathé, G. (1969). *Hosp. Pract.* **6,** 43–51.

Mathé, G., Hayat, M., Sakouhi, M., and Choay, J. (1971). *C. R. Acad. Sci., Ser. D* **272,** 170–173.

Mathé, G., Halle-Pannenko, O., and Bourut, C. (1973). *Natl. Cancer Inst. Monogr.* **39,** 107–112.

Megel, H., Raychaudhuri, A., Goldstein, S., Kinsolving, C. R., *et al.* (1974). *Proc. Soc. Exp. Biol. Med.* **145,** 513–518.

Migliore-Samour, D., Korontzis, M., and Jolles, P. (1974). *Immunol. Commun.* **3,** 593–603.

Milas, L., Hunter, H., Basic, I., and Withers, H. R. (1974). *J. Natl. Cancer Inst.* **52,** 1875–1880.

Minden, P., Wainberg, M., and Weiss, D. W. (1974). *J. Natl. Cancer Inst.* **52,** 1643–1645.

Mitchell, M. S., Kirkpatrick, D., Mokyr, M. B., and Gery, I. (1973). *Nature (London) New Biol.* **243,** 216–217.

Mitchell, M. S., Mokyr, M. B., and Kahane, I. (1975a). *In* "Modulation of Host Immune Resistance in the Prevention or Treatment of Induced Neoplasia" (M. A. Chirigos, ed.). Fogarty Int. Center Proc., No. 28. US Govt. Printing Office, Washington, D.C.

Mitchell, M. S., Mokyr, M. B., and Goldwater, D. J. (1975b). *Cancer Res.* **35,** 1121–1127.
Modolell, M., Luckenbach, G. A., Parant, M., and Munder, P. G. (1974). *J. Immunol.* **113,** 395–403.
Moore, M., Nisbet, N. W., and Haigh, M. V., eds. (1973). *Br. J. Cancer, Suppl.* **1**.
Morahan, P. S., Munson, J. A., Baird, L. G., *et al.* (1974). *Cancer Res.* **34,** 506–514.
Mota, I., Perini, A., and Trinidade, V. S. (1974). *Int. Arch. Allergy Appl. Immunol.* **47,** 425–432.
Munson, A. E., Munson, J. A., Regelson, W., and Wampler, G. L. (1974). *Cancer Res.* **32,** 1397–1403.
Newburger, P. E., Hamaoka, T., and Katz, D. H. (1974). *J. Immunol.* **113,** 824–829.
Ohno, R., Esaki, K., Kodera, Y., Shiku, H., and Yamada, K. (1973). *Ann. N. Y. Acad. Sci.* **207,** 430–441.
Old, L. J., Clarke, D. A., and Benacerraf, B. (1959). *Nature (London)* **184,** 291–292.
Old, L. J., Benacerraf, B., Clarke, D. A., *et al.* (1961). *Cancer Res.* **21,** 1281–1301.
Oliveira-Lima, A., Javierre, M. Q., Dias da Silva, W., and Sette-Camara, D. (1974). *Experientia* **30,** 945–946.
Olivotto, M., and Bomford, R. (1974). *Int. J. Cancer* **13,** 478–488.
O'Neill, G. J., Henderson, D. C., and White, R. G. (1973). *Immunology* **24,** 977–995.
Pearson, J. W., Turner, W., Ebert, P. S., and Chirigos, M. A. (1969). *Appl. Microbiol.* **18,** 474–478.
Pearson, J. W., Pearson, G. R., Gibson, W. T., Chermann, J. C., and Chirigos, M. A. (1972). *Cancer Res.* **32,** 904–907.
Pearson, J. W., Chaparas, S. D., and Chirigos, M. A. (1973). *Cancer Res.* **33,** 1845–1848.
Pearson, J. W., Chirigos, M. A., Chaparas, S. D., and Sher, N. A. (1974). *J. Natl. Cancer Inst.* **52,** 463–468.
Pearson, J. W., Perk, K., Chirigos, M. A., Pryor, J. W., and Fuhrman, F. S. (1975). *Int. J. Cancer* **16,** 142–152.
Piessens, W. F., Lachapelle, F. L., Legras, N., and Henson, J. C. (1970). *Nature (London)* **228,** 1210–1212.
Pilch, Y. H., and Ramming, K. P. (1970). *Cancer* **26,** 630.
Pilch, Y. H., and Ramming, K. P. (1971). *Transplantation* **11,** 10–19.
Pilch, Y. H., Veltman, L. L., and Kern, D. H. (1974). *Surgery* **76,** 23–34.
Pilch, Y. H., Myers, G. H., Sparks, F. C., *et al.* (1975). *Curr. Probl. Surg.* **2,** 1–61.
Pimm, M. V., and Baldwin, R. W. (1975). *Nature (London)* **254,** 77–78.
Potmesil, M., and Goldfeder, A. (1972). *Proc. Soc. Exp. Biol. Med.* **139,** 1392–1397.
Ralph, P., Nakoinz, I., and Raschke, W. C. (1974). *Biochem. Biophys. Res. Commun.* **61,** 1268–1275.
Regelson, W. (1967). *Adv. Exp. Med. Biol.* **1,** 315–332.
Regelson, W., Munson, A. E., Wooles, W. R., Lawrence, W., Jr., and Levy, H. (1970). *In* "Colloque Institut National de la Santé et Recherche Medicale," No. 6, p. 381.
Remold-O'Donnell, E., and Remold, H. G. (1974). *J. Biol. Chem.* **249,** 3622–3627.
Renoux, G., and Renoux, M. (1971). *C. R. Acad. Sci. Ser. D* **272,** 349–350.
Rhim, J. S., and Huebner, R. J. (1971). *Proc. Soc. Exp. Biol. Med.* **136,** 524–529.
Ruhl, H., Vogt, W., Bochert, G., and Diamantstein, T. (1974). *Immunology* **26,** 937–941.
Sandberg, J., and Goldin, A. (1971). *Cancer Chemother. Rep., Part 1* **55,** 233–238.
Schaffer, M. P., Chirigos, M. A., and Papas, T. S. (1974). *Cancer Chemother. Rep., Part 1* **58,** 821–827.
Scher, I., Strong, D. M., Ahmed, A., Knudsen, R. C., and Sell, K. W. (1973). *J. Exp. Med.* **138,** 1545–1563.

Schlager, S. T., Paque, R. E., and Dray, S. (1975). *Cancer Res.* **35,** 1907–1914.
Schmidtke, J. R., and Johnson, A. G. (1971). *J. Immunol.* **106,** 1191–1200.
Schuller, G. B., Morahan, P. S., and Snodgrass, M. (1975). *Cancer Res.* **55,** 1915–1920.
Scott, M. T. (1974). *In* "Seminars in Oncology" (J. W. Yarbro, R. S. Bornstein, and M. J. Mastrangelo, eds.), Vol. 1, pp. 367–368. Grune & Stratton, New York.
Seyberth, H. W., Schmidt-Gayk, H., Jakobs, K. H., and Hackenthal, E. (1973). *J. Cell Biol.* **57,** 567–571.
Sharma, B., Kohasi, O., Mickey, M. R., and Terasaki, P. I. (1975). *Cancer Res.* **35,** 666–669.
Sinkovics, J. G., Ahearn, M. J., Shirato, E., and Shullenberger, C. C. (1970). *J. Reticuloendothel. Soc.* **8,** 474–492.
Skidmore, B. J., Chiller, J. M., Morrison, O. C., and Weigle, W. O. (1975). *J. Immunol.* **114,** 770–775.
Smith, L. H., and Woodruff, M. F. A. (1968). *Nature (London)* **219,** 197–198.
Snodgrass, M. J., and Hanna, M. G. (1973). *Cancer Res.* **33,** 701–716.
Sparks, F. C., Silverstein, M. J., Hunt, J. S., *et al.* (1973). *N. Engl. J. Med.* **289,** 827–830.
Spitler, L. E., Glogau, R., Nelms, D., Silverman, S., Olson, J., O'Connor, R., Ostler, H., Smolin, G., Basch, K., Wong, P., Engleman, E. P., and Brugmans J. (1975). *In* "Modulation of Host Immune Resistance in the Prevention or Treatment of Induced Neoplasia" (M. A. Chirigos, ed.). Fogarty Int. Center Proc., No. 28. US Govt. Printing Office, Washington, D.C.
Steinkuller, C. B., Krigbaum, L. G., and Weiss, D. W. (1969). *Immunology* **16,** 255–275.
Stjernsward, J. (1966). *Cancer Res.* **26,** 1591–1594.
Strausser, H. R., and Bober, L. A. (1972). *Cancer Res.* **32,** 2156–2159.
Strom, T. B., Carpenter, C. B., Garovoy, M. R., Austen, K. R., *et al.* (1973). *J. Exp. Med.* **138,** 381–393.
Sunshine, G., Lopez-Corrales, E. J., Hadden, E. M., Coffey, R. G., *et al.* (1975). *In* "Modulation of Host Immune Resistance in the Prevention or Treatment of Induced Neoplasia" (M. A. Chirigos, ed.). Fogarty Int. Center Proc. No. 28. US Govt. Printing Office, Washington, D.C.
Suter, E., and White, R. G. (1954). *Am. Rev. Tuberc.* **70,** 783–805.
Teng, C. T., Chen, M. C., and Hamilton, L. O. (1973). *Proc. Natl. Acad. Sci., U. S. A.* **70,** 3904–3908.
Tennant, R. W., Hanna, M. G., and Farrelly, J. G. (1974). *Proc. Natl. Acad. Sci., U. S. A.* **71,** 3167–3171.
Ter-Grigorov, V. S., and Drlin, I. S. (1968). *Int. J. Cancer* **3,** 760–764.
Thor, D. E., and Dray, S. (1973). *Ann. N. Y. Acad. Sci.* **207,** 355–368.
Toy, S. T., Weislow, O. S., and Wheelock, E. F. (1973). *Proc. Soc. Exp. Biol. Med.* **143,** 726–732.
Tripodi, D., Parks, L. C., and Brugmans, J. (1973). *N. Engl. J. Med.* **289,** 354–358.
Turner, W., Chen, J. P., and Chirigos, M. A. (1970). *Proc. Soc. Exp. Biol. Med.* **133,** 334–338.
Vilkas, E., Amar, C., Markovits, J., *et al.* (1973). *Biochim. Biophys. Acta* **297,** 423–435.
Vogt, W., Ruhl, H., Wagner, B., and Diamantstein, T. (1973). *Eur. J. Immunol.* **3,** 493–496.
Wagner, H., and Cone, R. E. (1974). *Cell Immunol.* **10,** 394–403.
Watanabe, T. (1969). *Jpn. J. Exp. Med.* **39,** 631–647.
Watson, J., Epstein, R., and Cohn, M. (1973). *Nature (London)* **246,** 405–409.
Weislow, O. S., and Wheelock, E. F. (1975a). *J. Immunol.* **114,** 211–215.
Weislow, O. S., and Wheelock, E. F. (1975b). *Infect. Immun.* **11,** 129–136.

Weislow, O. S., Friedman, H., and Wheelock, E. F. (1973). *Proc. Soc. Exp. Biol. Med.* **142,** 401–405.
Weiss, D. W. (1972). *Natl. Cancer Inst. Monogr.* **35,** 157–171.
Weiss, D. W., Bonhag, R. S., and DeOme, K. B. (1961). *Nature (London)* **190,** 889–891.
Weiss, D. W., Bonhag, R. S., and Leslie, P. (1966). *J. Exp. Med.* **124,** 1039–1065.
Werner, G. H., Maral, R., Floch, F., and Migliore-Samour, D. (1974). *C. R. Acad. Sci., Ser. D* **278,** 789–792.
Wheelock, E. F. (1967). *Proc. Soc. Exp. Biol. Med.* **124,** 855–858.
Wheelock, E. F. (1975). *In* "Modulation of Host Immune Resistance in the Prevention or Treatment of Induced Neoplasia" (M. A. Chirigos, ed.). Fogarty Int. Center Proc. No. 28. US Govt. Printing Office, Washington, D.C.
Wheelock, E. F., Caroline, N. L., and Moore, R. D. (1969). *J. Virol.* **4,** 1–6.
Wheelock, E. F., Toy, S. T., Sibal, L. R., Fink, M. A., Beverly, P., and Allison, A. C. (1972). *J. Natl. Cancer Inst.* **48,** 665–674.
Wheelock, E. F., Weislow, O. S., and Toy, S. T. (1973). *In* "Virus Tumorigenesis and Immunogenesis" (W. S. Ceglowski and H. Friedman, eds.), p. 351. Academic Press, New York.
Wheelock, E. F., Toy, S. T., Weislow, O. S., and Levy, M. H. (1975). *Prog. Exp. Tumor Res.* **19,** 369–389.
Wilkinson, P. C., O'Niell, G. J., and Wapshaw, K. G. (1973). *Immunology* **24,** 997–1006.
Wittmann, G., Dietzschold, B., and Bauer, K. (1975). *Arch. Virol.* **47,** 225–235.
Wolmark, N. and Fisher, B. (1974). *Cancer Res.* **34,** 2869–2872.
Woods, W. A., Siegel, M. J., and Chirigos, M. A. (1974). *Cell Immunol.* **14,** 327–331.
Woods, W. A., Fliegelman, M. J., and Chirigos, M. A. (1975a). *Cancer Chemother. Rep., Part 1* **59,** 531–536.
Woods, W. A., Fliegelman, M. J., and Chirigos, M. A. (1975b). *Proc. Soc. Exp. Biol. Med.* **148,** 1048–1050.
Woods, W. A., Papas, T. S., and Chirigos, M. A. (1975c). *In* "Modulation of Host Immune Resistance in the Prevention or Treatment of Induced Neoplasia" (M. A. Chirigos, ed.). Fogarty Int. Center Proc. No. 28. US Govt. Printing Office, Washington, D.C.
Yarbro, J. W., Bornstein, R. S., and Mastrangelo, M. S., eds. (1974). *Semin. Immunol.* **1** .
Yashphe, D. J. (1971). *In* "Immunological Parameters of Host Tumor Relationships" (D. W. Weiss, ed.), pp. 90–107. NY Acad. Sci., New York.
Yron, I., Weiss, D. W., Robinson, E., *et al.* (1973). *Natl. Cancer Inst. Monogr.* **39,** 33–55.
Yron, I., Cohen, O., Robinson, E., Haber, M., and Weiss, D. W. (1975). *Cancer Res.* **35,** 1779–1790.
Zbar, B., and Tanaka, T. (1971). *Science* **172,** 271–273.
Zbar, B., Bernstein, I. D., and Rapp, H. J. (1971). *J. Natl. Cancer Inst.* **46,** 831–839.
Zbar, B., Bernstein, I. D., Bartlett, G. L., *et al.* (1972). *J. Natl. Cancer Inst.* **49,** 119–130.
Zenser, T. V., and Metzger, J. F. (1974). *Infect. Immun.* **10,** 503–509.

# Persorption of Particles: Physiology and Pharmacology

GERHARD VOLKHEIMER

*Bayerischer Platz 9*
*Berlin, West Germany*

I. Introduction . . . . . 163
A. Absorption—Persorption . . . . . 163
B. Initial Studies . . . . . 164
C. General Methods . . . . . 164
II. Mechanism of Persorption . . . . . 165
A. Model Substances . . . . . 165
B. Methods and Results . . . . . 165
C. Further Transport of Persorbed Particles . . . . . 166
D. Persorbability of Particles . . . . . 166
E. Persorbable Particles . . . . . 166
III. Determination of the Rate of Persorption . . . . . 167
A. Methods . . . . . 167
B. Persorption Rates in Animals . . . . . 168
C. Persorption Rates in Man . . . . . 170
IV. Modification of Persorption Rates . . . . . 175
A. Effect of Drugs on Persorption Rates . . . . . 175
B. Effects of Coffee Drinking and Smoking . . . . . 176
V. Excretion of Persorbed Particles . . . . . 178
A. Urinary Excretion . . . . . 178
B. Biliary Excretion . . . . . 181
C. Other Excretory Routes . . . . . 181
VI. Breakdown of Persorbed Particles . . . . . 182
A. Enzymic Breakdown . . . . . 182
B. Phagocytosis . . . . . 183
VII. Discussion . . . . . 184
VIII. Future Developments . . . . . 186
IX. Conclusion . . . . . 186
References . . . . . 187

## I. Introduction

### A. ABSORPTION—PERSORPTION

In the molecular form, i.e., in solution, substances are transported through the epithelial enterocytes of the small intestine. Very small particles in the nanometer size range can also be transported through the enterocytes by way of pinocytosis. Earlier, however, it was considered impossible for large solid particles in the micrometer size range to cross the barrier of the intestinal mucosa—despite the observation made long ago that large, solid, insoluble, nondeformable particles somehow succeed in passing from the digestive tract into the bloodstream. The earliest reports that orally ingested particles could be detected in the blood were made by Herbst (1844), Oesterlen (1846), Marfels and Moleschott (1854), Hirsch (1906), and Verzar (1911), but these findings were assumed to be either misapprehensions or the result of impurities in the materials used. This phenomenon, to which the name *persorption* has now been given, has been the subject of a thorough and systematic investigation by the present author (Volkheimer, 1964, 1968, 1972, 1974).

## B. Initial Studies

In a long series of preliminary studies (Volkheimer, 1964), it was found that the oral application of native starch was followed after only a few minutes by the appearance in the blood and urine of starch granules of the same kind as those ingested. Special precautions were taken to exclude any possibility of contamination of the material examined by carrying out a large number of control tests. The specific microscopical structure of the starch granules made it impossible for any error or misapprehension to occur. The same phenomenon was observed when polyvinyl chloride (PVC) particles were used as the model substance.

## C. General Methods

### 1. *Model Substances*

The experimental work to be described in this review is limited to the persorption of starch granules of various diameters, such as cornstarch (3–25 $\mu$m), potato starch (5–110 $\mu$m), and rice starch (3–10 $\mu$m) granules. Other particles, e.g., diatoms (5–150 $\mu$m), pollen (10–120 $\mu$m), PVC (5–100 $\mu$m), and other particulate matter have been used successfully (see Section II,E).

### 2. *Vehicles*

Homogeneous suspensions of 200 gm have been prepared in water, cold tea, or buttermilk for consumption by human volunteers. Dogs took doses of 50–250 gm of starch particles in water, but preferred cream, although this vehicle owing to its fat content increases the persorption during the first 90 minutes. In humans this increase is delayed (Volkheimer, 1972).

### 3. *Administration*

Small animals, e.g., chickens, were treated with 20 gm cornstarch by gastric intubation; rats, mice, or guinea pigs were used for special studies of phagocytosis and received starch granula by either oral or rectal administration. Human subjects and dogs consumed the particle suspensions by drinking.

It is important that no particle residues are in the system of the test animals or humans. The experiments were, therefore, carried out in animals after 24–36 hours fasting, in human volunteers after 3 days of starch-free diet.

Further details of the test procedures, particularly the counting of particles in the blood, are described in the following sections. It may be mentioned, however, that particles in other body fluids, such as urine, cerebrospinal fluid, bile, and chyle, are also demonstrated and counted in the centrifuged sediment, occasionally (bile, chyle) with dilution of viscous specimens in water.

## II. Mechanism of Persorption

The mechanism by which particles pass through the epithelial cell layer was studied on the rat intestine.

### A. Model Substances

Starch granules are a suitable model substance for studying the mechanism of persorption in the wall of the intestine since they are readily identifiable in body fluids and tissue sections.

### B. Methods and Results

When rats have been fed with starch, tissue sections prepared from the wall of the digestive tract reveal the presence of occasional starch granules in between the epithelial cells. Others are seen in the subepithelial region and in the lumen of lymph and blood vessels. These findings demonstrate that paracellular passage through the epithelial cell layer is the persorption route for such large, solid, nondeformable particles. This is possible where the intestinal mucosa is covered by a single layer of epithelium. Mechanical factors are mainly responsible for the persorption process. Movements of the structures in the digestive tract as well as the vascular pulsations transmitted to the mucosa play an important part in the transepithelial passage of the particles.

## C. Further Transport of Persorbed Particles

The further transport of persorbed particles takes place via both the chyle and the portal circulation.

### 1. *Transport by Chyle*

That starch granules are transported by the chyle is shown by the observation that they are found only in the lymphatics of those segments of the digestive tract containing starch. Lymphatics of segments free of starch contain no starch granules.

### 2. *Portal Transport*

Portal transport of starch granules is demonstrated by a quantitative comparison of the numbers of granules in blood samples taken simultaneously from mesenteric veins and from the aorta of dogs fed with starch. The mesenteric venous blood from segments of the digestive tract in which starch is present contains significantly more starch granules than arterial blood. Control observation: rather fewer starch granules are found in the mesenteric venous blood from starch-free intestinal segments than in the arterial blood.

## D. Persorbability of Particles

The persorbability of particles is limited by their size and hardness. For experimental observations, hard particles with a diameter between 7 and 70 $\mu$m give the best results.

For PVC particles and rounded quartz particles, the upper size limit for persorbability has been found to be 150 $\mu$m. When fed to dogs, such large particles were, however, found only very rarely in the chyle. Particles with a diameter of 70 $\mu$m are regularly found in this fluid.

Using smaller particles, the lower size limit for persorbability has also been studied. Paracellular transport of particles about 5 $\mu$m in diameter was observed. This is also possible, however, for even smaller particles, as is evidenced particularly by the passage of yeast cells and bacteria through the mucosa.

## E. Persorbable Particles

1. Observations of persorption *in man* have been made by the author on himself using various model substances. After enteral application (oral, rectal), diatoms, pollen, spores, cellulose particles, plant cells, and

starch granules were regularly demonstrable in the body fluids (blood, urine) (Volkheimer, 1964).

2. *Experimental animals* (mainly dogs) were fed the same substances as in the foregoing observation and also colored particles obtained by grinding crab and lobster shells, fish meal and bone meal, PVC and other plastic particles, metallic iron powder, parasite eggs, asbestos fibers, fragments of animal hairs, powdered industrial diamonds, silicates, crystals, etc. All these particles could be demonstrated in the body fluids. Examination of the chyle from the thoracic duct of dogs constitutes the simplest method of detecting such particles (Volkheimer, 1964).

## III. Determination of the Rate of Persorption

The rate of persorption depends on several factors. In addition to the amount of the substance present, an important role is played by the motion of the mucosa of the digestive tract, particularly that of the muscularis mucosae.

The rate of persorption can be measured quantitatively. Reproducible results are given by the methods described in the following, for which starch granules are again a very suitable material.

### A. Methods

After hemolysis, the blood sample is centrifuged several times. The sediment obtained is then mounted between slides and examined under the microscope. The various kinds of particles present are counted separately. Starch granules are identified under polarized light. Reproducible results are obtained only when the whole sediment is thoroughly examined, an excessively time-consuming procedure. Apart from this, very special precautions must be taken to exclude any possibility of contamination. Here again a great deal of time is taken up by the necessary control tests.

When starch granules are used as the model in these quantitative tests, it is absolutely essential that the bloodstream be free from nutritional starch granules before tests are started. To attain this end, it is sufficient to avoid the ingestion of any food containing starch for 3 days. Granule size distribution and particle counts obtained in tests carried out mainly with cornstarch and potato starch are shown in Table I and Fig. 1.

TABLE I

DIAMETER AND NUMBER OF STARCH GRANULES IN CORNSTARCH AND POTATO STARCH

| Starch variety | Granule diameter ($\mu$m) | No. granules in 1 gm | No. granules in 200 gm |
|---|---|---|---|
| Cornstarch | 3–25 | $240 \times 10^6$ | $48 \times 10^9$ |
| Potato starch | 5–110 | $12 \times 10^6$ | $2.4 \times 10^9$ |

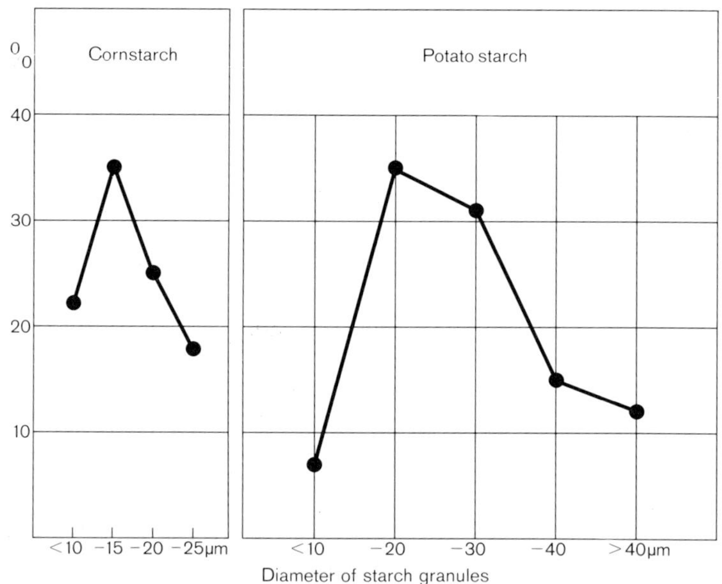


FIG. 1. Size distribution of cornstarch and potato-starch granules.

## B. PERSORPTION RATES IN ANIMALS

Starch grains can always be found in the venous blood of animals fed with cereals. The granules disappear from the blood only after 3 days on a starch-free diet.

### 1. *Detection of Persorbed Starch Granules in Chickens*

*a*. Chickens ($n = 4$) were kept for 3 days on a starch-free diet, after which starch granules were no longer present in the venous blood. Then, using gastric intubation, 20 gm cornstarch (= $4.8 \times 10^9$ starch granules) was applied orally. This was followed by taking 1-ml blood samples from the wing veins at 0.5-hour intervals. Cornstarch granules were found to be present in all the samples. The mean values are shown in Fig. 2A. The peak value was reached after 60 minutes.

*b*. Chickens ($n = 4$) were fed cereals, the last feed being given on the evening prior to the test. In the morning, a 1-ml venous blood sample was taken, followed by the application of 20 gm cornstarch by stomach tube. Further 1-ml venous blood samples were then taken at 0.5-hour intervals. Starch granules were found in all the samples. The mean values are shown in Fig. 2B. The peak value was reached after 60 minutes.

*c*. Chickens ($n = 4$) were fed cereals and a 1-ml venous blood sample taken shortly after feeding. This was followed by the application of 20 gm cornstarch by gastric tube, after which 1-ml venous blood samples were taken at 0.5-hour intervals. Starch granules were present in all the samples. The mean values are shown in Fig. 2C. The peak value was reached after 60 minutes.

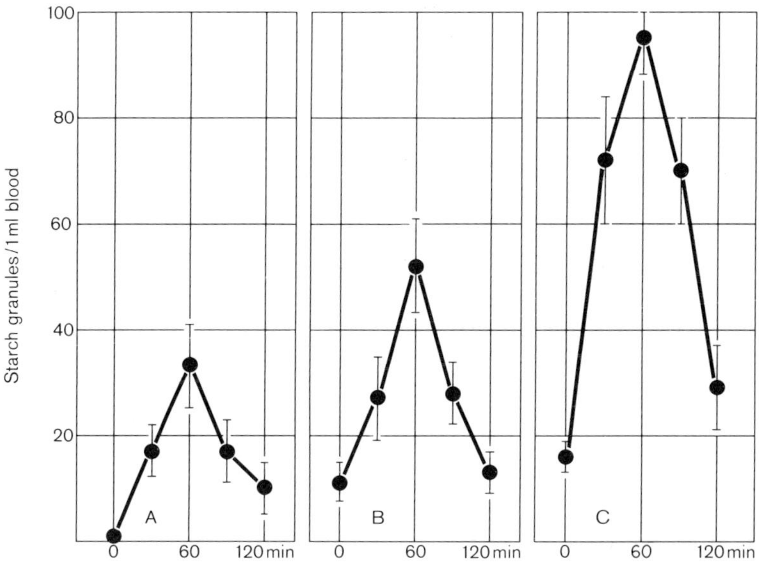


FIG. 2. Starch granules in the venous blood of chickens after oral application of 20 gm cornstarch: (A) starch-free feed for 3 days prior to the test; (B) cereal feed 8 hours before the test; (C) cereal feed immediately prior to the test.

### 2. *Detection of Persorbed Starch Granules in the Venous Blood of Dogs*

*a. Detection of Persorbed Cornstarch Granules.* Medium-sized dogs ($n = 4$) were fed 200 gm cornstarch ($= 48 \times 10^9$ starch granules), after which 10-ml venous blood samples were taken at 0.5-hour intervals. Cornstarch granules were detected in all the samples. The mean values are shown in Fig. 3A. The peak value was reached after 2 hours.

*b. Detection of Persorbed Potato-Starch Granules in the Venous Blood of Dogs.* Medium-sized dogs ($n = 4$) were fed 200 gm potato starch ($= 2.4 \times 10^9$ starch granules) mixed with cream, after which 10-ml venous blood samples were taken at 0.5-hour intervals. Potato-starch granules were detected in all the samples. The mean values are shown in Fig. 3B. The peak value was reached after 1 hour.

## C. Persorption Rates in Man

Persorption rates were investigated by means of self-testing with the aid of a large team of medical students of both sexes from the Humbolt University, Berlin. The most important results obtained are described below.

### 1. *Detection of Persorbed Cornstarch Granules in the Blood*

*a.* Young (22–26 years of age) test subjects of both sexes ($n = 4$) drank a suspension of 200 gm cornstarch ($= 48 \times 10^9$ starch granules) in buttermilk, after which 10-ml venous blood samples were taken from them at 2-minute intervals, time being reckoned from the first swallowing. Cornstarch granules were detected in all the samples. The mean values are shown in Fig. 4A. The peak value was reached after 6 minutes.

*b.* Young test subjects ($n = 4$) drank a suspension of 200 gm cornstarch, after which 10-ml venous blood samples were taken at 0.5-hour intervals. Cornstarch granules were found in all samples. The mean values are shown in Fig. 4B. The peak value was reached after 90 minutes.

*c.* Young test subjects ($n = 4$) drank a suspension of 200 gm cornstarch, after which 10-ml venous blood samples were taken at intervals of 4 hours. Cornstarch granules were found in all samples. The mean values are shown in Fig. 4C. The starch granules had almost completely disappeared from the blood after 24 hours.

### 2. *Detection of Persorbed Potato-Starch Granules in the Blood*

*a.* Young test subjects ($n = 4$) drank a suspension of 200 gm potato starch ($= 2.4 \times 10^9$ starch granules) in buttermilk, after which 10-ml

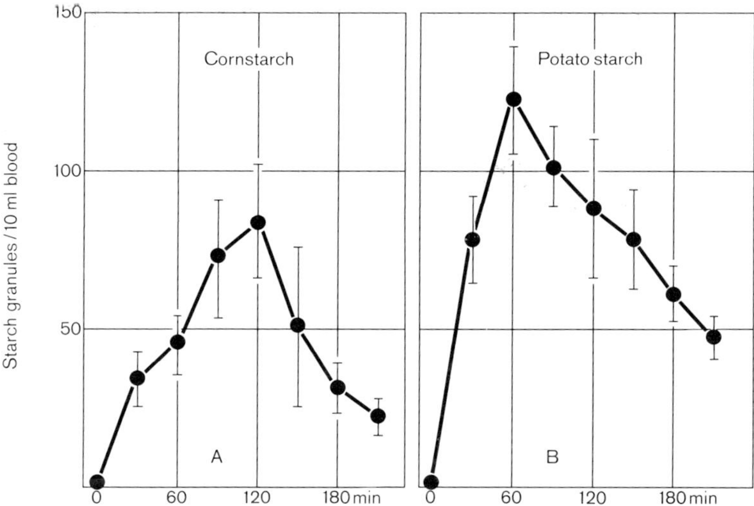


FIG. 3. Starch granules in the venous blood of dogs after a meal of starch: (A) after 200 gm cornstarch ($48 \times 10^9$ starch granules); (B) after 200 gm potato starch ($2.4 \times 10^9$ starch granules).

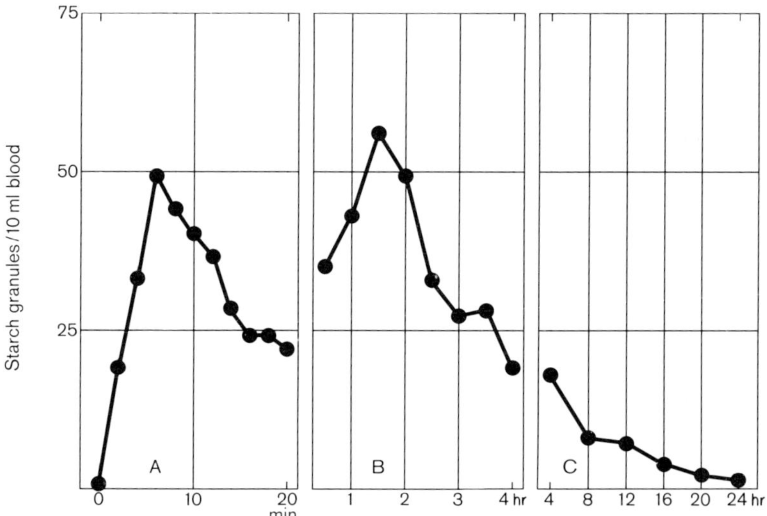


FIG. 4. Cornstarch granules in the venous blood of young test subjects after ingestion of 200 gm cornstarch. A first peak appears 6 minutes after ingestion (A), a second after 90 minutes (B). Only a few isolated starch granules remain in the blood 24 hours after ingestion (C).

blood samples were taken at 5-minute intervals. Potato-starch granules were found in all the samples. The mean values are shown in Fig. 5A. The peak value was reached after 10 minutes.

*b*. Young test subjects ($n = 4$) drank a suspension of 200 gm potato starch, after which 10-ml venous blood samples were taken at 0.5-hour intervals. Potato-starch granules were present in all samples. The mean values are shown in Fig. 5B. The peak value was reached after 90 minutes.

### 3. *Persorption Rates Following Ingestion of Different Numbers of Particles*

*a. Cornstarch Granules*. Young test subjects ($n = 4$) drank successive, increasing amounts (50, 100, 200, and 300 gm; 100 gm = $24 \times 10^9$ starch granules) of cornstarch in suspension at intervals of 1 week. In the time interval 60–150 minutes after each intake, 10-ml venous blood samples were taken at 0.5-hour intervals. The greater the amount of starch ingested, the larger was the number of cornstarch granules in the blood (Fig. 6A).

*b. Potato-Starch Granules*. Young test subjects ($n = 4$) drank successive, increasing amounts (50, 100, 200, and 300 gm; 100 gm = $1.2 \times 10^9$

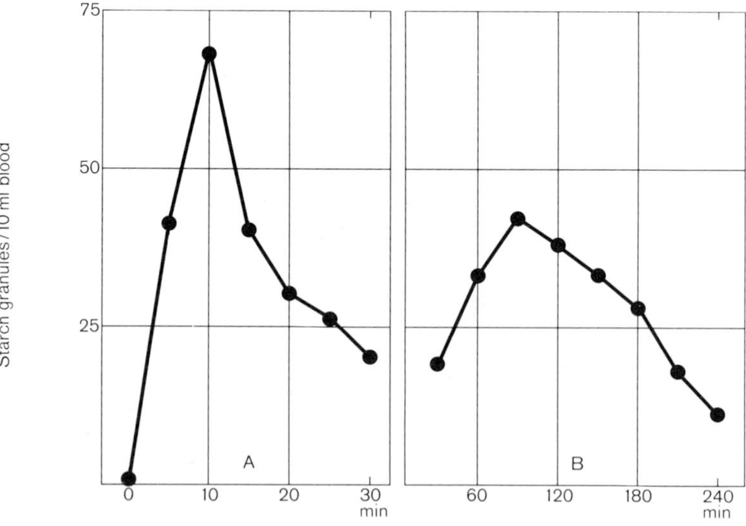


FIG. 5. Potato-starch granules in the venous blood of young test subjects after ingestion of 200 gm potato starch. A first peak appears 10 minutes after ingestion (A), a second after 90 minutes (B).

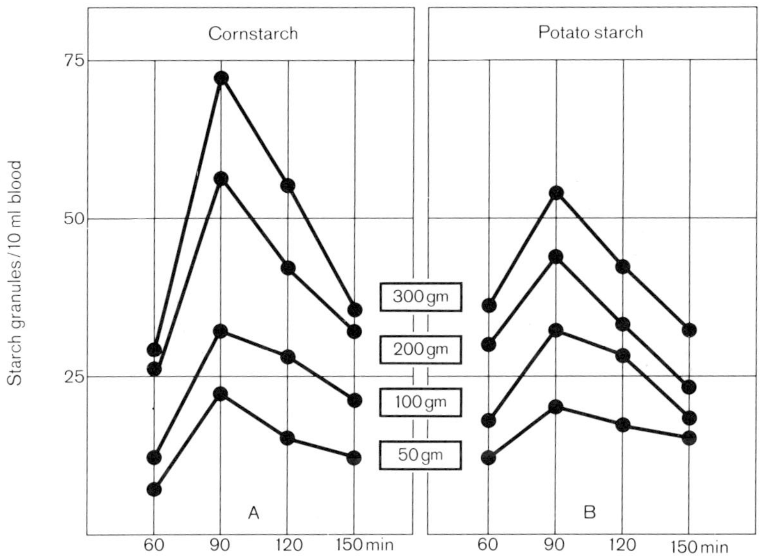


FIG. 6. Starch granules in the venous blood of young test subjects after ingestion of various amounts of starch: (A) after 50, 100, 200, and 300 gm cornstarch; (B) after 50, 100, 200, and 300 gm potato starch.

starch granules) of potato starch in suspension at intervals of 1 week. In the time interval 60–150 minutes after each intake, 10-ml venous blood samples were taken at 0.5-hour intervals. The greater the amount of starch ingested, the larger was the number of potato-starch granules in the blood (Fig. 6B).

### 4. *Age Differences*

*a. In Rate of Persorption of Cornstarch Granules.* Young test subjects ($n$ = 4) with an average age of 24 years, together with elderly test subjects ($n$ = 4) with an average age of 72 years, each drank a suspension of 200 gm cornstarch. From 1 to 3 hours after the intake, 10-ml venous blood samples were taken at 0.5-hour intervals. The number of cornstarch granules in the blood was higher in the younger than in the older subjects (Fig. 7A).

*b. In Rate of Persorption of Potato-Starch Granules.* Young test subjects ($n$ = 4) with an average age of 24 years, together with elderly test subjects ($n$ = 4) with an average age of 72 years, each drank a suspension of 200 gm potato starch. From 1 to 3 hours after the intake, 10-ml venous blood samples were taken at 0.5-hour intervals. The

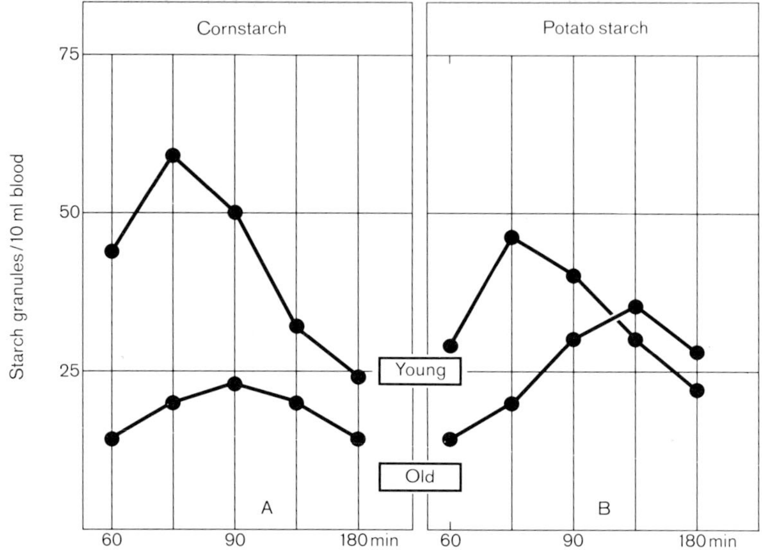


FIG. 7. Comparison of persorption rates in young and old test subjects after ingestion of 200 gm cornstarch (A) and after ingestion of 200 gm potato starch (B).

number of potato-starch granules in the blood was at first higher in the younger than in the older subjects. (Fig. 7B). This relationship was, however, reversed at 120 minutes after intake.

## 5. *Persorption during Sleep*

*a*. Young test subjects ($n = 4$) drank a suspension of 200 gm cornstarch during the morning, after which 10-ml venous blood samples were taken at 1-hour intervals. One week later the test was repeated during physiological night sleep after the subjects had taken the same amount of starch late in the evening before going to bed. A cannula had previously been inserted in the cubital vein. During sleep, the subject's partner took 10-ml venous blood samples at 1-hour intervals. The mean values of the numbers of starch granules found are shown in Fig. 8A. The number of persorbed starch granules in the blood is noticeably higher during sleep than during the day.

*b*. Young test subjects ($n = 4$) carried out the same test using 200 gm potato starch. The mean values of the numbers of starch granules (Fig. 8B) likewise revealed a noticeably higher rate of persorption during sleep.

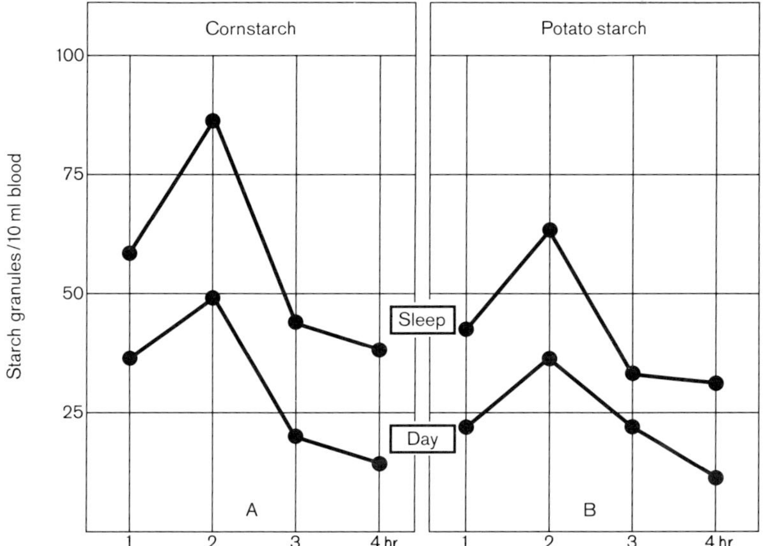


FIG. 8. Comparison of persorption rates during the day and during sleep after ingestion of 200 gm cornstarch (A) and after ingestion of 200 gm potato starch (B).

## IV. Modification of Persorption Rates

### A. EFFECT OF DRUGS ON PERSORPTION RATES

#### 1. *Increase in the Persorption Rate*

*a. Effect of Neostigmine.* As in the tests already described, young test subjects ($n = 4$) drank a suspension of 200 gm cornstarch. One week later the test was repeated with the simultaneous application of 0.5 mg neostigmine by subcutaneous injection. The rate of persorption was noticeably higher under neostigmine (Fig. 9A).

*b. Effect of Caffeine.* As in the tests already described, young test subjects ($n = 4$) drank a suspension of 200 gm cornstarch. One week later the test was repeated with the simultaneous application of 200 mg caffeine by subcutaneous injection. The rate of persorption was noticeably higher under caffeine (Fig. 9B).

*c. Other Drugs.* Similar tests to the foregoing demonstrated a noticeable increase in the persorption rate after application of the following drugs: metoclopramide, 10 mg by intramuscular injection; papaverine,

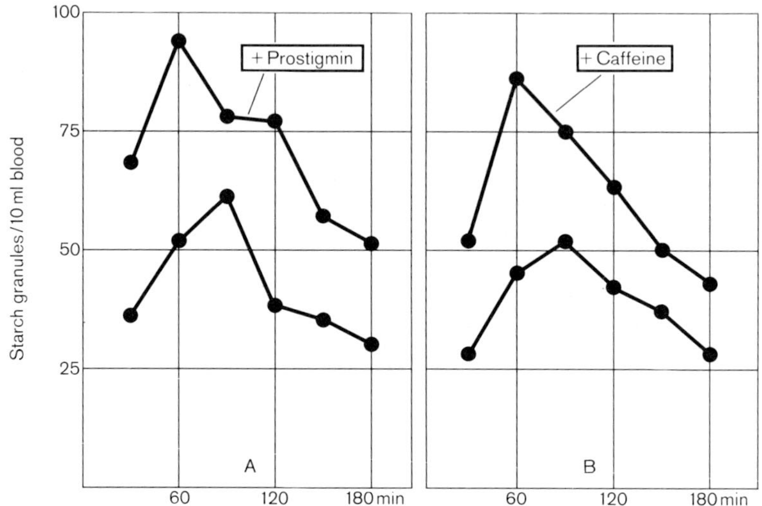


FIG. 9. Effect of drugs on the persorption rate: both (A) neostigmine (Prostigmin) and (B) caffeine increase the rate.

100 mg by intramuscular injection; castor oil, 20 gm per os; polygalacturonic acid, per os (30 gm Solcoray; Solco Basel, AG).

### 2. *Decrease in the Persorption Rate*

*a. Effect of Atropine.* Young test subjects ($n = 4$) drank a suspension of 200 gm cornstarch. One week later the test was repeated with the simultaneous application of atropine (0.01 mg/kg body weight). The rate of persorption was noticeably lower under atropine (Fig. 10A).

*b. Effect of Barbituric Acid.* Young test subjects ($n = 4$) drank a suspension of 200 gm cornstarch. One week later the test was repeated with the simultaneous application of barbituric acid (250 mg per os). The rate of persorption was noticeably lower under barbituric acid (Fig. 10B).

*c. Effect of Detergents.* A marked reduction in the rate of persorption was also observed when 10 gm of Tween 20 was added to the starch suspension. This effect was even greater when Tween 80 was added.

## B. EFFECTS OF COFFEE DRINKING AND SMOKING

### 1. *Effect of Coffee on Persorption of Cornstarch Granules*

Young test subjects ($n = 4$) drank a suspension of 200 gm cornstarch immediately after consuming coffee prepared in the usual way from 20

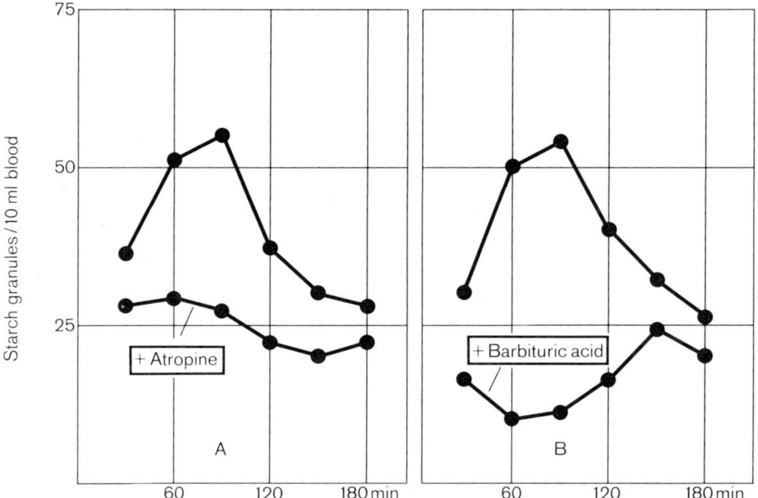


FIG. 10. Effect of drugs on the persorption rate: both (A) atropine and (B) barbituric acid reduce the rate.

gm ground coffee beans (caffeine content 228 mg). Then, 10-ml venous blood samples were taken at 0.5-hour intervals. For comparison, the test was repeated after 1 week without the consumption of coffee. The mean values for persorbed starch granules (Fig. 11A) revealed a marked increase in the rate of persorption under the action of coffee.

## 2. *Effect of Coffee on Persorption of Potato-Starch Granules*

In similar tests in which young subjects ($n = 4$) drank a suspension of 200 gm potato starch, the simultaneous consumption of coffee (20 gm, caffeine content 228 mg) was again seen to cause a marked increase in the rate of persorption (Fig. 11B).

## 3. *Caffeine-Free Coffee*

Further tests similar to the foregoing showed that caffeine-free coffee did not cause any increase in the rate of persorption of starch granules.

## 4. *Nicotine*

A large number of comparative tests were carried out to investigate the effect of nicotine on the rate of persorption. It was found that continuous cigarette smoking increased the rate of persorption on the average by 30%.

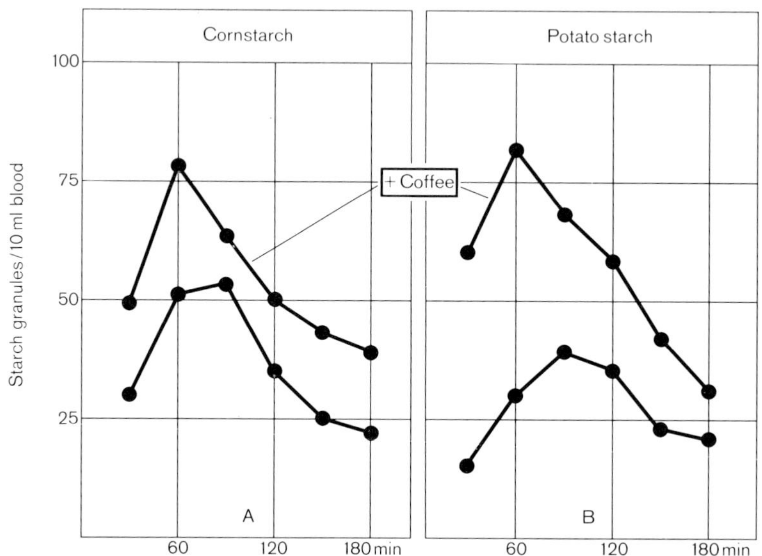


FIG. 11. Effect of coffee on the persorption rate. Simultaneous drinking of coffee (caffeine content 228 mg) increases the rate. Observations were made following ingestion of 200 gm cornstarch (A) and of 200 gm potato starch (B).

## V. Excretion of Persorbed Particles

Several factors are involved in the elimination of particles from the blood circulation. One of these is the temporary embolism of smaller vessels prior to removal of the particles from the vascular system [see Volkheimer (1972), pp. 61 and 70].

### A. URINARY EXCRETION

#### 1. *Quantitative Tests*

*a. Excretion of Cornstarch Granules.* Young tests subjects ($n = 4$) drank a suspension of 200 gm cornstarch, after which each of them emptied the urinary bladder completely at 1, 2, 3, 4, and 8 hours. The average number of cornstarch granules excreted during this 8-hour period was 124. The percentage distribution of the separate fractions is shown in Fig. 12A.

*b. Excretion of Potato-Starch Granules.* Young tests subjects ($n = 4$) drank a suspension of 200 gm potato starch, after which each of them

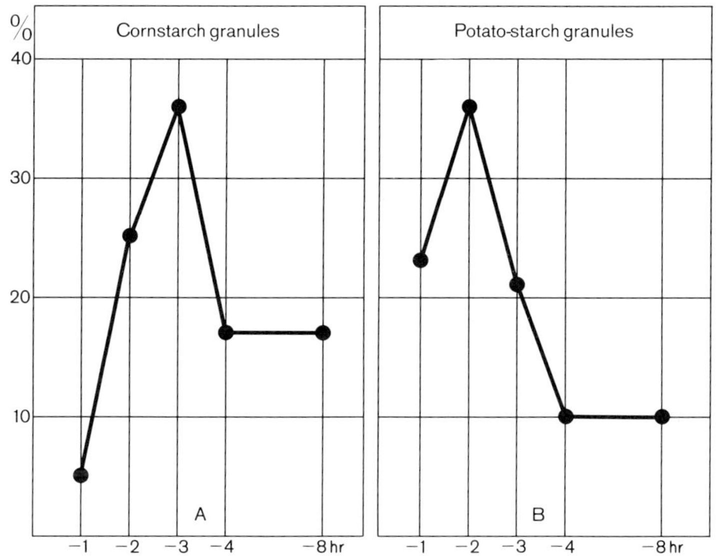


FIG. 12. Excretion (%) of persorbed starch granules in the urine after ingestion of 200 gm cornstarch (A) and of 200 gm potato starch (B). Urinary fractions collected at 1, 2, 3, 4, and 8 hours after ingestion were examined.

emptied the urinary bladder completely at 1, 2, 3, 4, and 8 hours. The average number of potato-starch granules excreted during this 8-hour period was 79. The percentage distribution of the separate fractions is shown in Fig. 12B.

### 2. *Granule Size Distribution*

*a. Cornstarch Granules (diameter 3–25 μm).* Young test subjects ($n$ = 4) drank a suspension of 200 gm cornstarch, after which a venous blood sample was taken every hour for 3 hours, hemolyzed, and centrifuged. At the same time the urine spontaneously discharged at hourly intervals was collected and centrifuged. The sizes of the cornstarch granules in the blood and urine were measured and compared with those of the native starch granules as shown in Fig. 13.

*b. Potato-Starch Granules (5–110 μm).* Young test subjects ($n$ = 4) drank a suspension of 200 gm potato starch, after which a venous blood sample was taken every hour for 3 hours, hemolyzed, and centrifuged. At the same time the urine passed spontaneously at hourly intervals was collected and centrifuged. The sizes of the potato-starch granules in the blood and urine were measured and compared with those of the native starch granules (see Fig. 14).

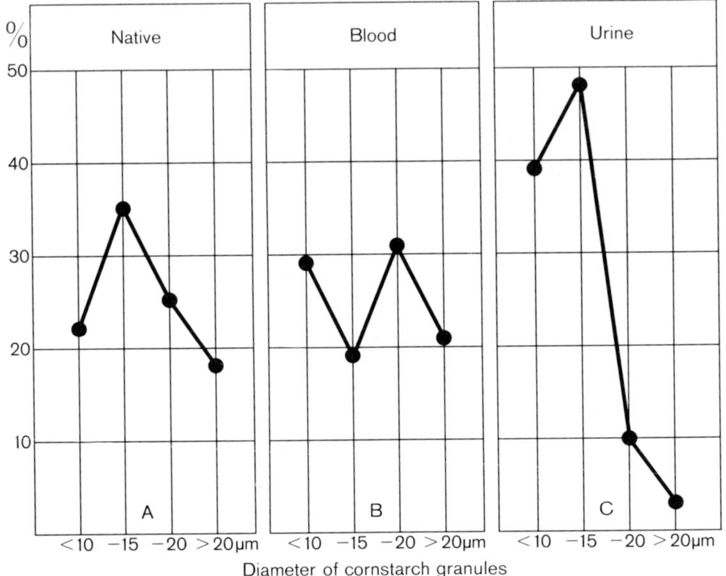


FIG. 13. Size distribution (%) of cornstarch granules in blood and urine compared with that of native starch.

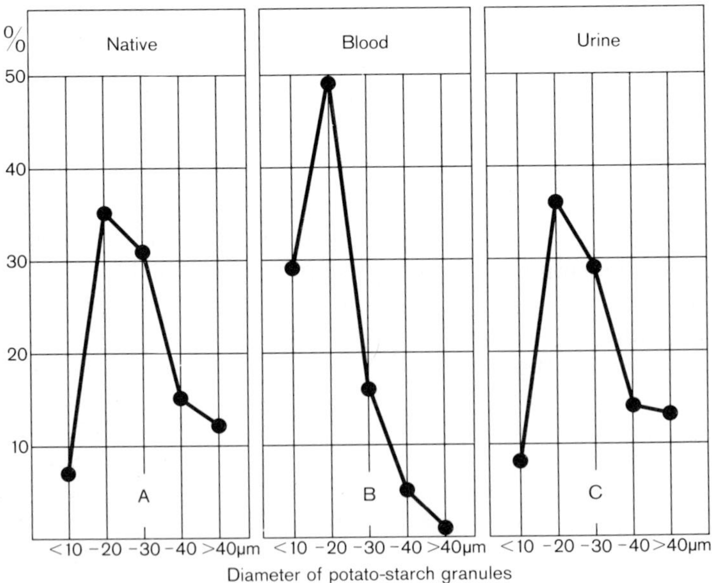


FIG. 14. Size distribution (%) of potato-starch granules in blood and urine compared with that of native starch.

### 3. *Effect of Drugs*

*a. Caffeine.* Young test subjects ($n = 4$) drank a suspension of 200 gm potato starch. In the 8-hour urine subsequently collected, the average number of potato-starch granules counted was 66. One week later the test was repeated with the simultaneous application of 200 mg caffeine per os. The average number of potato-starch granules in the subsequent 8-hour urine was 178.

*b. Diuretics.* Comparative observations made under the simultaneous action of furosemide (40 mg given intravenously) and, in separate tests, of hydrochlorothiazide (75 mg per os) revealed a considerable increase in the amount of urine passed but no significant change in the rate of excretion of the persorbed starch granules.

## B. Biliary Excretion

### 1. *Cornstarch Granules*

A few days after cholecystectomy—with T-drain *in situ*—cooperative cholecystectomized patients ($n = 4$) drank a suspension of 200 gm cornstarch in cold tea. The bile discharged via the T-drain was then collected in 10-minute fractions for 1 hour. The number of cornstarch granules in the bile was counted and the average number per 1 ml bile calculated. The results are shown in Fig. 15A. By means of X-ray film tests, the bile was shown to be free of trypsin, i.e., there was no reflux discharge from the duodenum.

### 2. *Potato-Starch Granules*

A few days after cholecystectomy—with T-drain *in situ*—cooperative cholecystectomized patients ($n = 4$) drank a suspension of 200 gm potato starch. The bile discharged via the T-drain was then collected in 10-minute fractions for 1 hour. The number of potato-starch granules in the bile was counted and the average number per 1 ml bile calculated. The values are shown in Fig. 15B.

## C. Other Excretory Routes

Similar tests were carried out to study the elimination of persorbed particles in breast milk and cerebrospinal fluid as well as their diaplacental passage. Quantitative measurements of these routes were also made. The mechanism by which persorbed particles pass from the pulmonary vessels into the alveolar lumen was investigated with the aid of histological sections (Volkheimer, 1972, p. 65).

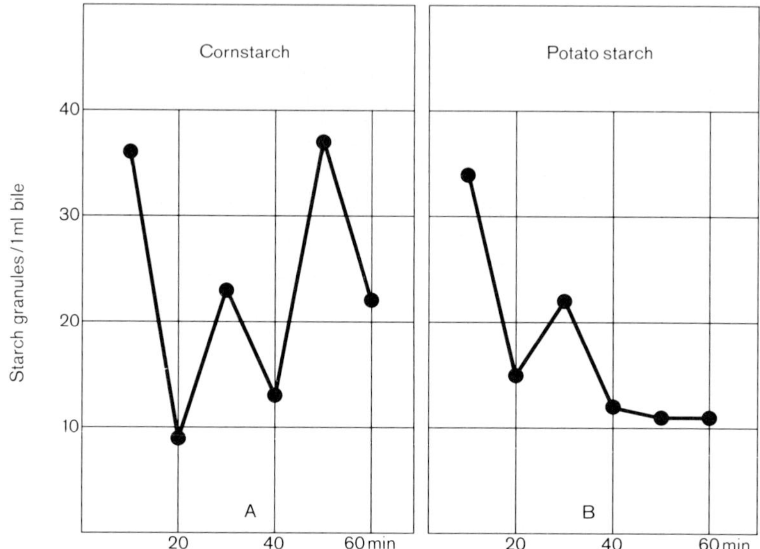


FIG. 15. Excretion of persorbed starch granules in the bile after ingestion of 200 gm cornstarch (A) and of 200 gm potato starch (B).

## VI. Breakdown of Persorbed Particles

The relatively rapid clearance of persorbed particles from the blood cannot be explained solely by their elimination from the vascular system. A further factor involved in the disappearance of particles from the circulation and other organs is their breakdown, a process in which both enzymes and phagocytosis play an important part.

### A. ENZYMIC BREAKDOWN

Favorable sites for observing the enzymic breakdown of particles are the serous cavities of the body.

#### 1. *Enzymic Breakdown in the Peritoneal Cavity*

Considerable structural changes were shown by some of the starch granules present in fluid used to rinse out the peritoneal cavity of laboratory animals fed potato starch. These changes are of the same kind as those seen in starch grains introduced directly into the peritoneal cavity. Larger potato-starch granules undergo more rapid breakdown than smaller ones.

### 2. *Enzymic Breakdown in the Cerebrospinal Fluid*

*a. In Dogs.* Twenty-four hours after feeding potato starch to dogs, potato-starch granules showing considerable structural changes could be seen in the cerebrospinal fluid. The structural changes were of the kind occurring in enzymic breakdown of starch granules.

*b. In Man.* Volunteer patients in whom lumbar puncture had to be carried out for diagnostic reasons drank a suspension of potato starch 24 hours beforehand. Some of the potato-starch granules found in the cerebrospinal fluid sediment showed marked structural changes similar to those occurring in enzymic breakdown.

## B. Phagocytosis

### 1. *Model Substance*

Rice-starch granules, which have a diameter of 2 to 10 $\mu$m, are very suitable for phagocytosis tests.

### 2. *Phagocytosis in the Spleen*

Dogs fed rice starch were subjected to splenectomy at varying intervals after feeding. Smears were prepared from the cut surface of the spleen and stained. A few phagocytized rice-starch granules were visible in macrophages and microphages (Volkheimer, 1972, 1974).

### 3. *Phagocytosis in the Liver*

Small laboratory animals were given potato starch by the enteral route. At varying intervals the liver was excised and examined histologically. A few potato-starch granules surrounded by phagocytizing cells could be seen in the sinusoids and interlobular veins.

### 4. *Effect of Aristolochic Acid*

Aristolochic acid is used therapeutically as an activator of phagocytosis. Young tests subjects ($n = 4$) drank a suspension of 200 gm rice starch ($= 160 \times 10^9$ starch granules), after which 1-ml venous blood samples were taken at 0.5-hour intervals and the number of rice-starch granules counted. The test was repeated after 1 week when the subjects had been under medication with aristolochic acid for 3 days at an oral dosage of 0.45 mg/day. Ninety minutes after ingestion of the rice starch, the average numbers of rice-starch granules in the blood in the two sets of tests differed significantly (Fig. 16). No differences were detectable among the blood samples taken at other times.

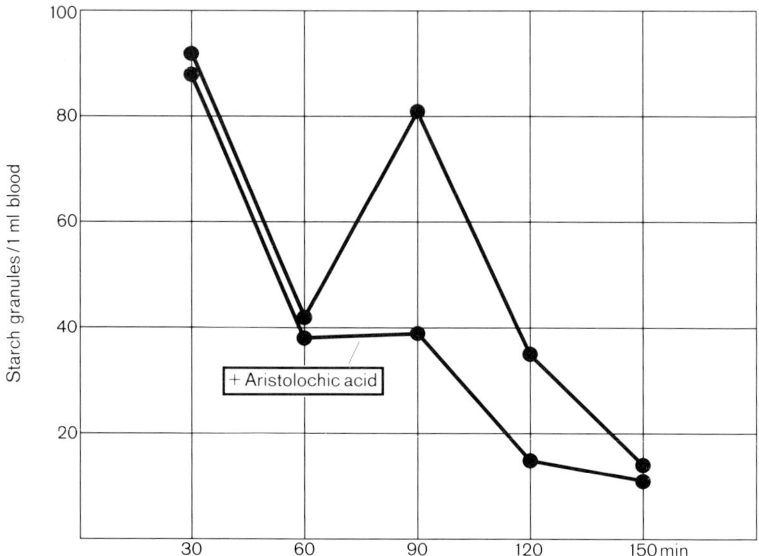


FIG. 16. Rice-starch granules in the venous blood of young test subjects after ingestion of 200 gm rice starch ($160 \times 10^9$ rice-starch granules). Premedication with aristolochic acid suppresses the second rise in the number of granules at 90 minutes after ingestion.

## VII. Discussion

Persorption of solid particles in the micrometer size range is a fact. The observations described in this review effectively disposed of any doubt that such large particles were capable of passing through the intestinal mucosa. The question whether persorption is a "physiological" or "pathological" process remains a purely academic one.

Absorption of a particle of this size by the enterocyte body can be ruled out: many of the persorbed particles have a far larger diameter than the frontal aspect of the enterocyte that is directed toward the lumen. Paracellular passage between the enterocytes has been demonstrated as the mechanism of persorption.

Actually, the closely interlocked enterocyte layer (the so-called tight junction) forms a fairly impenetrable barrier to passage of particles in this way. The only interruption in this network of tight junctions is that due to goblet cells. In fact, as examination under the electron scanning microscope reveals, a loosening of the tight junctions of the intestinal mucosa occurs in the immediate neighborhood of the goblet cells. Spontaneous loosening is also possible as a result of cell desquamation.

Histological sections studied in our laboratory have often revealed the passage of particles through the mucosa in a desquamation zone, namely at the tips of the intestinal villi (Volkheimer, 1972). A further possibility for the passage of particles is offered by mechanical lesions of the tight junctions around the bases of the tightly packed villi due to the entry between them of large particles. The result is a mechanical loosening of the tight junctions that is exacerbated by two factors: (*1*) the rhythmic contraction of the villi and (*2*) the rhythmic hammering action of the vascular pulsation, which is transmitted to the mucosa.

The assumption that mechanical factors are responsible for the "kneading" of particles through the epithelial cell layer finds support in the observation that the rate of persorption is affected by changes in the movements of the villi brought about by drugs. When the movements of the villi are stimulated by neostigmine or caffeine, the rate of persorption increases, but when it is slowed down by atropine or barbituric acid, the rate decreases. In the case of caffeine, there is also the possibility that the increase in the rate of persorption is potentiated by the intensification of vascular pulsation induced by this substance.

*Primary removal* of persorbed particles from the mucosa occurs by two routes—via the chyle and via the portal circulation. The proportions transported in these two ways have not so far been determined, although it seems likely that smaller particles are carried mainly by the portal circulation, and larger ones mainly by the chyle. Particles transported by the *chyle* first pass via the thoracic duct into the pulmonary circulation, where they may cause temporary embolism of small pulmonary vessels. After a short time they are eliminated by passage into the alveolar lumina (Volkheimer, 1972). Many particles, including larger ones, also reach the pulmonary circulation, however, via vascular anastomoses. Particles transported by the *portal circulation* may bring about temporary embolism of hepatic vessels (Volkheimer, 1972). The excretion of particles in the bile can be measured quantitatively.

The *rate of persorption*, which is derived from the number of particles counted in the peripheral blood, furnishes only a *relative* measure of the actual number of persorbed particles. Many of the factors here involved must first be disregarded since neither their quantitative effect nor chronological course is determinable. Account must also be taken of the very extensive surface area—extending from the cardia to the rectum—over which persorption occurs. Among the nonquantifiable factors involved are temporary embolisms and the breakdown, phagocytosis, distribution, and excretion of the particles.

No automatic method of counting persorbed particles in the blood has yet been devised. The method of counting used in these studies is not only very tedious but excessively time-consuming. To count the particles in 10 ml of blood, a fairly experienced operator requires about 5 hours. It is essential that the whole of the sediment is examined if important findings are not to be missed: a superficial examination reveals nothing. In the studies reported here, a standard amount of 200 gm starch was adopted. Clearly, however, 100 gm would also be adequate to give valid results.

The *persorption ratio* can be roughly estimated at 1:50,000 (±50%). This means that 1 out of about every 50,000 ingested particles capable of persorption will be persorbed. In spite of this low ratio, an astonishingly large number of persorbed particles circulate in the blood. Here the decisive factor is the enormous quantity of persorbable particles made available by conventional foodstuffs (Volkheimer, 1972).

In the experiments carried out to measure the rate of persorption, it was noticeable that the first particles appeared in the peripheral blood only a few seconds after ingestion of the test substance. The number of particles in the blood attains a first maximum after a few minutes. It then falls, only to rise again after a short time to a second peak value at about 100 minutes after ingestion. In many other tests, a third maximum was observed at about 210 minutes after ingestion. The precise causes of these two or even three peaks in the numbers of particles are unknown.

## VIII. Future Developments

The immunological significance of the persorption phenomenon is obvious. Preliminary studies in the microangiological and experimental gerontological fields have yielded interesting results, in particular the destruction of small vascular areas in the region of the CNS as a result of embolism by persorbed particles. Since PVC particles and asbestos fibers undergo persorption in the small intestine, the phenomenon acquires importance in the field of environmental protection. Its heuristic possibilities are still, however, a long way from being exhausted.

## IX. Conclusion

Persorption is an extremely interesting phenomenon whose full implications will be revealed only when much further work on the problem has been done. The aim of this brief review of the fundamental studies so far undertaken has been to make it known to a wider scientific circle and to stimulate interest in further research.

## References

Herbst, G. (1844). "Das Lymphgefäss-System," pp. 333–337. Vandenhoeck & Ruprecht, Göttingen.
Hirsch, R. (1906). *Z. Exp. Pathol. Ther.* **3,** 390.
Marfels, F., and Moleschott, J. (1854). *Wien. Med. Wochenschr.* **4,** 817.
Oesterlen, F. (1846). *Z. Rat. Med.* **5,** 434.
Verzár, F. (1911). *Biochem. Z.* **34,** 86.
Volkheimer, G. (1964). *Z. Gastroent.* **2,** 57.
Volkheimer, G. (1968). *Z. Geront.* **1,** 360.
Volkheimer, G. (1972). "Persorption." Thieme, Stuttgart.
Volkheimer, G. (1974), *Environ, Health Perspect.* **9,** 215.

# Pharmacological Control of the Synthesis and Metabolism of Cyclic Nucleotides

BENJAMIN WEISS AND RICHARD FERTEL*

*Department of Pharmacology*
*Medical College of Pennsylvania*
*Philadelphia, Pennsylvania*

I. Introduction . . . . . . . . . . . . . . . . . . . . . 189
II. Adenylate Cyclase . . . . . . . . . . . . . . . . . . . 191
A. Distribution and Properties of Adenylate Cyclase . . . . . . 191
B. Modulation of Adenylate Cyclase . . . . . . . . . . . . 194
C. Chronic Factors Influencing the Activity of Adenylate Cyclase . . 209
III. Guanylate Cyclase . . . . . . . . . . . . . . . . . . 221
A. Tissue Distribution. . . . . . . . . . . . . . . . . . 221
B. Cellular and Subcellular Distribution . . . . . . . . . . 221
C. Multiple Forms of Guanylate Cyclase . . . . . . . . . . 222
D. Effect of Ions on Guanylate Cyclase Activity . . . . . . . 222
E. Activation of Guanylate Cyclase . . . . . . . . . . . . 224
F. Inhibition of Guanylate Cyclase . . . . . . . . . . . . 225
G. Conclusions . . . . . . . . . . . . . . . . . . . . 226
IV. Cyclic Nucleotide Phosphodiesterases . . . . . . . . . . . 226
A. Discovery and Characterization of Cyclic Nucleotide Phosphodiesterase . . . . . . . . . . . . . . . . . 226
B. Distribution of Cyclic Nucleotide Phosphodiesterase . . . . . 226
C. Properties of Cyclic Nucleotide Phosphodiesterase . . . . . . 227
D. Multiple Forms of Phosphodiesterase . . . . . . . . . . 228
E. Regulation of Phosphodiesterase Activity . . . . . . . . . 233
F. Effect of Pharmacological Agents on the Multiple Forms of Phosphodiesterase . . . . . . . . . . . . . . . . . 257
V. Transport of Cyclic AMP . . . . . . . . . . . . . . . . 262
VI. Inhibition of Action of Cyclic AMP . . . . . . . . . . . . 262
VII. Directions of Future Research in Pharmacological Control of Cyclic Nucleotides . . . . . . . . . . . . . . . . . . . 263
VIII. Clinical Implications . . . . . . . . . . . . . . . . . 264
IX. Concluding Remarks . . . . . . . . . . . . . . . . . . 265
References . . . . . . . . . . . . . . . . . . . . . 266

## I. Introduction

The past two decades have witnessed the birth of a new era in biology. What began in 1958 with the discovery by Sutherland and Rall

* Present address: Department of Pharmacology, Ohio State University School of Medicine, Columbus, Ohio 43210.

of a cyclic nucleotide that mediates the epinephrine-induced activation of liver phosphorylase has developed into a broad and novel concept touching every facet of biological control mechanisms. Adenosine 3′,5′-monophosphate (cyclic AMP) and other cyclic nucleotides have now been demonstrated not only to mediate the effects of most hormones and neurotransmitters but also to be involved in scores of biochemical and physiological events (for reviews, see Haynes *et al.,* 1960; Rall and Sutherland, 1961; Haugaard and Hess, 1965; Sutherland and Robison, 1966; Sutherland *et al.,* 1968; Robison *et al.,* 1968; Exton and Park, 1968; Weiss and Kidman, 1969; Rall *et al.,* 1969; Weiss, 1970; Greengard and Costa, 1970; Weiss and Crayton, 1970a; Bonner, 1971; Robison *et al.,* 1971a,b; Hardman *et al.,* 1971; Weiss, 1971a; Hittleman and Butcher, 1972; Greengard *et al.,* 1972; Rall, 1972; Bitensky and Gorman, 1973; Kahn and Lands, 1973; Greengard and Robison, 1973, 1974; Burkard, 1975; Drummond *et al.,* 1975; Weiss, 1975a).

The evidence that cyclic nucleotides influence the function of normal cells suggests that any abnormal alteration in the concentration of these compounds may be responsible for abnormal cell function, that is, a diseased state. Indeed, several lines of investigation indicate that cyclic nucleotides may be involved in a variety of clinical conditions ranging from cancer to cardiovascular disease to mental illness (Levine, 1970; Uzunov and Weiss, 1972a; Murad, 1973; Kahn and Lands, 1973; Schultz and Gratzner, 1973; Weiss, 1975a).

Most of the studies performed during the past several years have dealt with the role of endogenous hormones and neurotransmitters in controlling the intracellular concentration of these cyclic nucleotides. More recently, investigators have turned their attention to the possibility of manipulating the concentrations of these nucleotides by pharmacological means (for recent reviews, see Breckenridge, 1970; Amer and McKinney, 1973; Amer and Kreighbaum, 1975). The pharmacological alteration of cyclic nucleotides in specific cells may provide the route for directing basic preclinical knowledge into practical clinical application.

If cyclic AMP is involved in so many processes and has so many actions, then the question arises, How can drugs that act by changing the concentration of cyclic AMP produce a specific effect? The answer to this question is provided by the evidence that the enzymes responsible for the biosynthesis (nucleotide cyclases) and hydrolysis (cyclic nucleotide phosphodiesterases) of cyclic nucleotides are not simple molecular entities but, rather, are complex enzyme systems existing in multiple molecular forms. These enzyme systems are unequally distributed in the different tissues and cell types and may be differentially activated and inhibited by endogenous and exogenous chemicals. Accordingly, one may be able to develop pharmacological agents that will selectively change the activity of the form of the enzyme that is contained in a certain type of cell. This would result in a selective alteration of the intracellular concentration of a cyclic nucleotide in that cell and, thereby, cause a selective modulation in the function of that cell.

Our purpose here will be to review the general properties of these nucleotide cyclases and cyclic nucleotide phosphodiesterase systems and to examine the evidence suggesting that the intracellular concentrations of cyclic nucleotides in discrete cell types may be selectively modified with specific pharmacological agents acting on one of these complex enzyme systems.

## II. Adenylate Cyclase

### A. Distribution and Properties of Adenylate Cyclase

The distribution and properties of adenylate cyclase have been reviewed by several authors over the past few years (see Rall, 1969; Weiss, 1970; Robison *et al.*, 1971a; Perkins, 1973), and the reader should consult these papers for more detailed information. What follows is a brief summary of this topic.

#### 1. *Chemistry*

Adenylate cyclase, the enzyme that catalyzes the conversion of ATP to cyclic AMP, was originally described by Sutherland *et al.*, in 1962. Although substantial advances have since been made in determining the effects of cyclic AMP on biological systems, relatively little progress has been made to clarify the structure of this enzyme.

Robison *et al.* (1967) hypothesized that the adenylate cyclase system is located in the cell membrane and consists of a catalytic subunit facing the interior of the cell and one or more receptive structures in contact with the extracellular fluid. This basic model of adenylate cyclase has been subsequently modified (Birnbaumer *et al.*, 1970; Perkins, 1973) but has not been changed significantly from that originally proposed. There is general agreement that the catalytic portion of the enzyme system is similar in all of the adenylate cyclases, but the receptive portion of the enzyme system is not. Sodium fluoride, which activates all the mammalian adenylate cyclases, apparently acts at the catalytic portion of the enzyme system. Hormones and neurotransmitters, on the other hand, are thought to interact with the receptor portion of the enzyme system, causing a conformational change at the catalytic site, thereby increasing enzyme activity.

This concept gains support from studies showing that hormones and sodium fluoride act at separate sites on the adenylate cyclase system (Oye and Sutherland, 1966; Weiss, 1969a; Birnbaumer *et al.*, 1969, 1971; Burke, 1970a; Menon *et al.*, 1973). The hypothesis that there is a separate receptor moiety of adenylate cyclase is supported by studies showing that a given hormone activates only the adenylate cyclase contained in the tissue in which that hormone exerts a physiological action (Haynes, 1958; Mansour *et al.*, 1960; Marsh *et al.*, 1966; Grahame-Smith *et al.*, 1967; Pastan and Katzen, 1967; Gilman and Rall, 1968; Chase and Aurbach, 1968; Weiss and Costa, 1968; Zor *et al.*, 1969; Pohl *et al.*, 1969; Chase *et al.*, 1969; Bitensky *et al.*, 1970; Birnbaumer and Pohl, 1973; Huang *et al.*, 1973a). In tissues that are acted upon by more than one hormone, each hormone apparently acts on a distinct receptor associated with an identical adenylate cyclase catalytic unit (Bitensky *et al.*, 1968; Bar and Hechter, 1969a; Rodbell *et al.*, 1970; Bourne and Melmon, 1971). (See also reviews by Robison *et al.*, 1969; Weiss, 1970; Braun and Hechter, 1970; Wolff and Jones, 1971; Birnbaumer, 1973; Perkins, 1973.) Variations in the properties of this receptor element apparently are responsible for the specificity with which different hormones can activate the various adenylate cyclases.

The receptor component has been studied by several investigators. Klein *et al.* (1973), for example, have presented evidence that a dissociable receptor site for glucagon exists on the myocardial adenylate cyclase system. Using rat liver plasma membranes, Tomasi *et al.* (1970) also showed that the hormone receptor proteins are separate from adenylate cyclase. More recent studies (Bilezikian and Aurbach, 1973a,b) have shown that the catecholamine receptor on adenylate cyclase could be solubilized and separated from erythrocyte adenylate cyclase by treatment with a detergent. This receptor component may be related to a phospholipid since the norepinephrine responsiveness of myocardial adenylate cyclase, which is lost after solubilization, can be partially restored by the addition of phosphatidylinositol to the enzyme preparation (Levey, 1970), and the glucagon responsiveness of solubilized myocardial adenylate cyclase can be restored by the addition of phosphatidylserine (Levey, 1971a,b).

Other lines of evidence support the suggestion that the receptor may be associated with a phospholipid. For example, phospholipase decreases the response of adenylate cyclase systems that are sensitive to thyroid-stimulating hormone (Yamashita and Field, 1973), catecholamines (Bilezikian and Aurbach, 1973a,b), and glucagon Birnbaumer *et al.*, 1971; Rethy *et al.*, 1972; Rubalcava and Rodbell, 1973). The sensitivity of these receptors was at least partially restored by the addition of specific phospholipids. In addition, von Hungen and Roberts (1973) showed that the addition of phospholipids to preparations of brain enhanced the catecholamine-induced stimulation of adenylate cyclase.

Another way of studying the nature of the receptor moiety of adenylate cyclase is to study the structure–activity relationships between agonist and enzyme activity. The relationship between chemical structure of several phenylethylamines and their ability to activate adenylate cyclase of frog erythrocytes has been investigated by Rosen and her colleagues (Rosen *et al.*, 1970; Grunfeld *et al.*, 1974). They have found that agonists must have two functional groups on the phenyl ring. A functional group other than a hydroxyl can be substituted but only at position 3. An amino and a hydroxyl group at the $\beta$-carbon increase the activity of the compound although neither is essential for adenylate cyclase activity. These studies have not only added to our understanding of the receptor moiety of adenylate cyclase but have also shown that the general structural requirements of the phenylethylamines for activating adenylate cyclase are similar to those necessary for their pharmacological activity.

2. *Species and Tissue Distribution*

With the exception of certain microorganisms (Sahyoun and Durr, 1972; Uno and Ishikawa, 1973), adenylate cyclase activity has been detected in virtually every living cell and is unequally distributed among the various tissues of an organism (Weiss and Costa, 1968b; Rall *et al.*, 1969; Weiss, 1970; Robison *et al.*, 1971a).

3. *Cellular Location*

Within a given tissue, the hormone-sensitive adenylate cyclase appears to be concentrated in specific cell types or on specific sites on the cell. The following findings support this notion: Sweat and Hupka (1971) and Christoffersen *et al.* (1972a) have reported that the glucagon-sensitive adenylate cyclase is found in much higher concentrations in the parenchymal cells of liver than in the reticuloendothelial cells; Jande and Robert (1974) have shown that a parathyroid-sensitive adenylate cyclase is localized on the brush border of cells found in the proximal tubules of kidney, and in the pineal gland the norepinephrine-sensitive adenylate cyclase system appears to be located in the pinealocytes rather than in the nerves innervating these cells (Weiss and Costa, 1967; Weiss, 1969b; Strada and Weiss, 1974). In studies of the sciatic nerve, Bray *et al.* (1971) showed that adenylate cyclase activity is present in axons and that this enzyme migrates down the axonal membrane. These experiments suggest that adenylate cyclase is located in nerve terminals. In agreement with this is the study of Johnson *et al.* (1973) showing a high specific activity of cyclic AMP in the synaptic vesicles of presynaptic nerve endings.

### 4. *Subcellular Distribution*

In certain bacteria (Hirata and Hayaishi, 1967; Ide, 1969, 1971; Khandelwal and Hamilton, 1971; Chiang and Cheung, 1973), adenylate cyclase is found in the soluble supernatant fraction. However, the adenylate cyclases of all animal tissues, from *Amoeba* to man, are bound to particulate material (Sutherland *et al.,* 1962). The enzyme has been demonstrated in a variety of subcellular structures: it has been detected in the plasma membranes of erythrocytes, liver, thyroid, corpus luteum, kidney, heart, and fat cells (Davoren and Sutherland, 1963a; Rosen and Rosen, 1968; Pohl *et al.,* 1969; Wolff and Jones, 1971; Wollenberger *et al.,* 1973, Bockaert *et al.,* 1973; Menon and Kiburz, 1974; Rodbell *et al.,* 1971a,b,c); it is found in subcellular fractions associated with the synaptic elements of nervous tissue (DeRobertis *et al.,* 1967; Weiss and Costa, 1968b; Chlapowski and Butcher, 1973); it has been localized in fractions of mitochondria, microsomes, sarcolemma, and sarcoplasmic reticulum of skeletal and cardiac muscle (Rabinowitz *et al.,* 1965; Entman *et al.,* 1969a; Katz *et al.,* 1974; Sulakhe and Dhalla, 1973); and it has been found in nuclei of prostate and liver (Liao *et al.,* 1971; Soifer and Hechter, 1971).

## B. Modulation of Adenylate Cyclase

### 1. *Endogenous Activators of Adenylate Cyclase*

The activation of adenylate cyclase by hormones and neurotransmitters was originally reported by Sutherland, Rall, and their co-workers (Rall and Sutherland, 1958; Sutherland *et al.,* 1962; Rall and Sutherland, 1962; Murad *et al.,* 1962; Klainer *et al.,* 1962). These observations, which have revolutionized our concept concerning the biochemical mechanism of hormone action, have since been confirmed and extended by scores of research workers (for reviews, see Rall *et al.,* 1969; Weiss, 1970; Robison *et al.,* 1971a; Perkins, 1973).

A partial listing of some of the biological agents that alter adenylate cyclase activity of various tissue appears in Table I. Only studies in which adenylate cyclase was measured directly are included in this table. It does not include studies in which the accumulation of cyclic AMP was measured or those studies in which radiolabeled cyclic AMP was determined following a prelabeling of the nucleotide pools with radiolabeled adenine or adenosine.

Although there is usually good agreement between the results obtained using these latter techniques to estimate the rate of formation of cyclic AMP and the results obtained when adenylate cyclase activity is measured directly, one should bear in mind that in whole tissues or in tissue slices many factors besides adenylate cyclase activity (including changes in phosphodiesterase activity or changes in the concentration of the precursor) might influence the accumulation of cyclic AMP in tissues. For this reason, the results of experiments in which accumulation of cyclic AMP is measured do not always correspond with the results of experiments in which adenylate cyclase is measured. For example, adenosine has been reported to inhibit adenylate cyclase activity of particulate fractions of brain homogenates (McKenzie and Bar, 1973) but to increase the concentration of cyclic AMP in brain slices (Sattin and Rall, 1970; Huang *et al.,* 1971). Other examples in which measurement of cyclic AMP concentration did not correlate with adenylate cyclase activity are studies of the effects of menadione and prostaglandin. Menadione increased the accumulation of cyclic AMP in fat cells but inhibited the norepinephrine-induced activation of adenylate cyclase in fat cell "ghosts" (Fain, 1971). Prostaglandin $E_1$ activated adenylate cyclase (see Table II), but antagonized the elevation of cyclic AMP induced by catecholamines, ACTH, glucagon, or thyroid-stimulating hormone (TSH) (Butcher and Baird, 1968).

Besides hormones, several other endogenous factors alter enzyme activity. A divalent cation, such as $Mg^{2+}$ or $Mn^{2+}$, is required for enzyme activity. Certain other divalent cations, although not required for enzyme activity per se, are necessary for the hormonal stimulation of adenylate cyclase activity. Thus, Bar and Hechter (1969b) showed that calcium was needed for the ACTH-induced activation of adenylate cyclase of adipose tissue, a finding that might explain the requirement of calcium for the lipolytic effects of ACTH (Lopez *et al.,* 1959). In addition, Bockaert *et al.* (1972) reported that low concentrations of calcium (1 $\mu M$) were required for the oxytocin-induced stimulation of adenylate cyclase. Bradham (1972) and Johnson and Sutherland (1973) also came to the conclusion that adenylate cyclase of brain requires calcium, in addition to magnesium, for the full expression of enzyme

TABLE I

EFFECT OF VARIOUS ENDOGENOUSLY OCCURRING BIOLOGICAL AGENTS ON ADENYLATE CYCLASE ACTIVITY

| Tissue | Agent | Effect | Reference |
|---|---|---|---|
| Adipose tissue | ACTH | Activation | Rodbell (1967) |
| | ACTH | Activation | Birnbaumer *et al.* (1969) |
| | ACTH | Activation | Braun and Hechter (1970) |
| | ACTH | Activation | Bar and Hechter (1969a,b) |
| | ACTH | Activation | Birnbaumer and Rodbell (1969) |
| | ACTH | Activation | Vaughan and Murad (1969) |
| | Catecholamines | Activation | Vaughan and Murad (1969) |
| | Catecholamines | Activation | Forn *et al.* (1970) |
| | Epinephrine | Activation | Bar and Hechter (1969a) |
| | Epinephrine | Activation | Birnbaumer and Rodbell (1969) |
| | Epinephrine | Activation | Braun and Hechter (1970) |
| | Glucagon | Activation | Manganiello and Vaughan (1972a) |
| | GTP | Inhibition | Harwood *et al.* (1973) |
| | Insulin | Inhibition | Jungas (1966) |
| | Insulin | Inhibition | Ho *et al.* (1967) |
| | Luteinizing hormone | Activation | Birnbaumer and Rodbell (1969) |
| | Norepinephrine | Activation | Therriault *et al.* (1969) |
| | Nucleotides | Inhibition | Cryer *et al.* (1969) |
| | Secretin | Activation | Rodbell *et al.* (1970) |
| | Thyroid-stimulating hormone | Activation | Birnbaumer and Rodbell, (1969) |
| Adrenal cortex | ACTH | Activation | Taunton *et al.* (1967, 1969) |
| | ACTH | Activation | Hechter *et al.* (1969) |
| | ACTH | Activation | Shima *et al.* (1971) |
| | ACTH | Activation | Pastan *et al.* (1970) |
| | ACTH | Activation | Ide *et al.* (1972) |
| | GTP | Activation | Glossmann and Gips (1974) |

| | | | |
|---|---|---|---|
| Bladder | Neurohypophyseal hormones | Activation | Roy *et al.* (19 73) |
| | Neurohypophyseal hormones | Activation | Bar *et al.* (1970) |
| | Neurohypophyseal hormones | Activation | Hynie and Sharpe (1971) |
| | Vasopressin | Activation | Walter *et al.* (1972a) |
| | Vasopressin | Activation | Walter *et al.* (1972b) |
| | Vasotocin | Activation | Walter *et al.* (1972b), Dousa (1974b) |
| Brain | Adenosine | Inhibition | McKenzie and Bar (1973) |
| | Catecholamines | Activation | von Hungen and Roberts (1973) |
| | Catecholamines | Activation | Walker and Walker (1973) |
| | Catecholamines | Activation | Chou *et al.* (1971) |
| | Dopamine | Activation | Von Voightlander *et al.* (1973) |
| | Epinephrine | Activation | Klainer *et al.* (1962) |
| Caudate nucleus | Dopamine | Activation | Kebabian *et al* (1972) |
| | Dopamine | Activation | Kebabian and Greengard (1971) |
| Corpus luteum | Luteinizing hormone | Activation | Marsh (1970) |
| *Escherichia coli* | Glucose | Activation | Abou-Sabe and Nardi (1973) |
| | Oxalacetate | Inhibition | Ide (1969) |
| | Pyridoxal phosphate | Inhibition | Ide (1969) |
| | Pyrophosphate | Inhibition | Tao and Lippman (1969) |
| Epidermis | β-Ecdysone | Activation | Applebaum and Gilbert (1972) |
| | Epinephrine | Activation | Marks and Rebien (1972) |
| | Isoproterenol | Activation | Duell *et al.* (1971) |
| | Isoproterenol | Activation | Marks and Rebien (1972) |
| | Isoproterenol | Inhibition | Marks and Rebien (1972) |

*(Continued)*

TABLE I—*Continued*

| Tissue | Agent | Effect | Reference |
| --- | --- | --- | --- |
| Erythrocytes | Catecholamines | Activation | Davoren and Sutherland (1963b) |
| | Catecholamines | Activation | Rosen *et al.* (1971) |
| | Catecholamines | Activation | Rosen and Rosen (1968, 1969) |
| | Catecholamines | Activation | Sheppard and Burghardt (1970) |
| | Clostridial neuraminadase | Activation | Rosen and Rosen (1970) |
| | Epinephrine | Activation | Oye and Sutherland (1966) |
| | Epinephrine | Activation | Schramm *et al.* (1972) |
| | Prostaglandin $E_2$ | Activation | Sheppard and Burghardt (1970) |
| | Serotonin | Inhibition | Davoren and Sutherland (1963b) |
| Fibroblasts | Epinephrine | Activation | Makman (1970) |
| | Prostaglandin $E_1$ | Activation | Peery *et al.* (1971) |
| Ganglia | Dopamine | Activation | Nathanson and Greengard (1973) |
| | Octopamine | Activation | Nathanson and Greengard (1973) |
| Gastric mucosa | Histamine | Activation | Nakajima *et al.* (1971) |
| | Pentagastrin | Activation | Nakajima *et al.* (1971) |
| Glial cells | Epinephrine | Activation | Schimmer (1971) |
| Hair follicles | Estrone | Activation | Adachi and Kano (1970) |
| Heart | Catecholamines | Activation | Sobel *et al.* (1968) |
| | Catecholamines | Activation | Entman *et al.* (1969a,b) |
| | Catecholamines | Activation | Murad and Vaughan (1969) |
| | Catecholamines | Activation | Murad *et al.* (1962) |
| | Catecholamines | Activation | Burges and Blackburn (1972) |

| | | | |
|---|---|---|---|
| | Epinephrine | Activation | Drummond *et al.* (1971) |
| | Epinephrine | Activation | Sobel *et al.* (1969) |
| | Epinephrine | Activation | McNeill and Muschek (1972a) |
| | Glucagon | Activation | Drummond *et al.* (1971) |
| | Glucagon | Activation | Levey and Epstein (1969) |
| | Glucagon | Activation | Murad and Vaughan (1969) |
| | Glucagon | Activation | Levey (1971a) |
| | Histamine | Activation | Wollenberger *et al.* (1973) |
| | Histamine | Activation | McNeill and Muschek (1972b) |
| | Norepinephrine | Activation | Brus and Hess (1973) |
| | Norepinephrine | Activation | Levey (1971b) |
| | Norepinephrine | Activation | Levey *et al.* (1969) |
| | Prostaglandin $E_1$ | Activation | Klein and Levey (1971) |
| | Prostaglandins | Activation | Levey and Klein (1973) |
| | Thyroid hormone | Activation | Klein *et al.* (1971) |
| | Thyroid hormone | Activation | Levey and Epstein (1968) |
| HeLa cells | Epinephrine | Activation | Makman (1970, 1971) |
| | Glucagon | Activation | Makman (1971) |
| | Prostaglandin $E_1$ | Activation | Makman (1971) |
| Hepatoma | Epinephrine | Activation | Pennington *et al.* (1970) |
| | Epinephrine | Activation | Brown *et al.* (1970) |
| | Epinephrine | Activation | Emmelot and Bos (1971) |
| | Glucagon | Activation | Emmelot and Bos (1971) |
| Hybrid cells | Isoproterenol | Activation | Benda *et al.* (1972) |
| Kidney | Adenosine | Inhibition | McKenzie and Bar (1973) |
| | Parathyroid hormone | Activation | Melson *et al.* (1970) |
| | Parathyroid hormone | Activation | Streeto (1969) |

*(Continued)*

TABLE I—*Continued*

| Tissue | Agent | Effect | Reference |
|---|---|---|---|
| Kidney | Parathyroid hormone | Activation | Gengler and Forte (1972) |
| | Parathyroid hormone | Activation | Dousa and Rychlik (1968) |
| | Vasopressin | Activation | Dousa and Hechter (1970) |
| | Vasopressin | Activation | Ohsawa and Endo (1972) |
| | Vasopressin | Activation | Gengler and Forte (1972) |
| | Vasotocin | Activation | Dousa (1974b) |
| Kidney cortex | Parathyroid hormone | Activation | Chase and Aurbach (1968) |
| | Parathyroid hormone | Activation | Marcus and Aurbach (1969) |
| Kidney medulla | Vasopressin | Activation | Chase and Aurbach (1968) |
| Leukocytes | Cholera enterotoxin | Activation | Bourne *et al.* (1973a) |
| | Catecholamines | Activation | Bourne and Melmon (1971) |
| | Prostaglandin $E_1$ | Activation | Bourne and Melmon (1971) |
| | Phytohemagglutinin | Activation | Krishnaraj and Talwar (1974) |
| Liver | Adenosine | Inhibition | McKenzie and Bar (1973) |
| | Glucagon | Activation | Christofferson *et al.* (1972a) |
| | Glucagon | Activation | Spiegel and Bitensky (1969) |
| | Glucagon | Activation | Pohl *et al.* (1969) |
| | Glucagon | Activation | Becker and Bitensky (1969) |
| | Glucagon | Activation | Marinetti *et al.* (1969) |
| | Glucagon | Activation | Sweat and Hypka (1971) |
| | Glucagon | Activation | Makman and Sutherland (1964) |
| | Glucagon | Activation | Birnbaumer *et al.* (1971) |
| | Glucagon | Activation | Ray *et al.* (1970) |
| | Glucagon | Activation | Rall *et al.* (1957) |

| | | | |
|---|---|---|---|
| | Glucagon | Activation | Rall and Sutherland (1958) |
| | Glucagon | Activation | Soifer and Hechter (1971) |
| | Glucagon | Activation | Bar and Hahn (1971) |
| | Glucagon | Activation | Bitensky *et al.* (1968) |
| | Glucagon | Activation | Rethy *et al.* (1972) |
| | Glucagon | Activation | Rubalcava and Rodbell (1973) |
| | Glucagon | Activation | Birnbaumer *et al.* (1971) |
| | Glucagon | Activation | Emmelot and Bos (1971) |
| | Glucagon | Activation | Rosselin and Freychot (1973) |
| | Glucagon | Activation | Hepp *et al.* (1970) |
| | Epinephrine | Activation | Becker and Bitensky (1969) |
| | Epinephrine | Activation | Ray *et al.* (1970) |
| | Epinephrine | Activation | Rall *et al.* (1957) |
| | Epinephrine | Activation | Rall and Sutherland (1958) |
| | Epinephrine | Activation | Bar and Hahn (1971) |
| | Epinephrine | Activation | Bitensky *et al.* (1968) |
| | Epinephrine | Activation | Rethy *et al.* (1972) |
| | Epinephrine | Activation | Marinetti *et al.* (1969) |
| | Epinephrine | Activation | Makman (1970) |
| | Insulin | Inhibition | Ray *et al.* (1970) |
| | Purine nucleotides | Activation | Rodbell *et al.* (1971c) |
| | Purine nucleotides | Activation | Leray *et al.* (1972) |
| | Purine nucleotides | Activation | Swislocki *et al.* (1973) |
| Liver cells | Epinephrine | Activation | Makman (1970) |
| | Epinephrine | Activation | Makman and Klein (1972) |
| Lung | Catecholamines | Activation | Burges and Blackburn (1972) |
| | Catecholamines | Activation | Weinryb *et al.* (1973) |
| | Glucagon | Activation | Weinryb *et al.* (1973) |
| | Histamine | Activation | Weinryb *et al.* (1973) |
| | Prostaglandins | Activation | Weinryb *et al.* (1973) |

*(Continued)*

TABLE I—*Continued*

| Tissue | Agent | Effect | Reference |
|---|---|---|---|
| Lymphocytes | Prostaglandin $E_1$ | Activation | Polgar *et al.* (1973) |
| | Prostaglandin $E_2$ | Activation | Polgar *et al.* (1973) |
| | Prostaglandin $F_{2\alpha}$ | Activation | Polgar *et al.* (1973) |
| Melanoma | Prostaglandin $E_1$ | Activation | Kreiner *et al.* (1973) |
| Ovary | Follicle-stimulating hormone | Activation | Kolena and Channing (1971) |
| | Follicle-stimulating hormone | Activation | Fontaine *et al.* (1973) |
| | Gonadotropins | Activation | Fontaine *et al.* (1972) |
| | Luteinizing hormone | Activation | Smith and Major (1971) |
| | Luteinizing hormone | Activation | Kolena and Channing (1971) |
| | Luteinizing hormone | Activation | Fontaine *et al.* (1973) |
| Oviduct | Progesterone | Activation | Kissel *et al.* (1970) |
| | Prostaglandins | Activation | Lerner *et al.* (1973) |
| Pancreas | Acetylcholine | Activation | Kuo *et al.* (1973) |
| | Glucagon | Activation | Kuo *et al.* (1973) |
| | Glucagon | Activation | Levey *et al.* (1972) |
| | GTP | Activation | Johnson *et al.* (1974) |
| | Insulin | Inhibition | Kuo *et al.* (1973) |
| | Pancreozymin | Activation | Kuo *et al.* (1973) |
| | Prostaglandin $E_1$ | Activation | Johnson *et al.* (1974) |
| | Prostaglandins | Activation | Kuo *et al.* (1973) |
| | Secretin | Activation | Kuo *et al.* (1973) |
| Parathyroid | Epinephrine | Activation | Matsuzaki and Dumont (1972) |

| Parotid gland | Isoproterenol | Activation | Malamud (1969) |
|---|---|---|---|
| | Isoproterenol | Activation | Malamud (1969) |
| | Norepinephrine | Activation | Schramm and Naim (1970) |
| Pineal gland | Catecholamines | Activation | Weiss and Costa (1967, 1968a) |
| | Catecholamines | Activation | Weiss (1969a,b) |
| | Catecholamines | Activation | Weiss and Crayton (1970a,b) |
| | Catecholamines | Activation | Weiss (1971a, 1971b) |
| | Purines | Inhibition | Weiss (1970) |
| Pituitary (anterior) | Hypothalamic extract | Activation | Zor *et al.* (1969) |
| | Prostaglandin $E_1$ | Activation | Zor *et al.* (1969) |
| Placenta | Gonadotropin | Activation | Menon and Jaffe (1973) |
| Platelets | Catecholamines | Inhibition | Zieve and Greenough (1969) |
| | Prostaglandin $E_1$ | Activation | Wolfe and Shulman (1969) |
| | Prostaglandin $E_1$ | Activation | Zieve and Greenough (1969) |
| Prostate | ACTH | Activation | Liao *et al.* (1971) |
| | Epinephrine | Activation | Liao *et al.* (1971) |
| | Glucagon | Activation | Liao *et al.* (1971) |
| Reticulocytes | Isoproterenol | Activation | Gauger *et al.* (1973) |
| Retina | Catecholamines | Activation | Brown and Makman (1972) |
| Skeletal muscle | Catecholamines | Activation | Severson *et al.* (1972) |
| | Parathyroid hormone | Activation | Chase *et al.* (1969) |
| | Pyrophosphate | Inhibition | Severson *et al.* (1972) |

(*Continued*)

TABLE I—*Continued*

| Tissue | Agent | Effect | Reference |
|---|---|---|---|
| Small intestine | Cholera toxin | Activation | Sharp *et al.* (1973) |
| | Estrogens | Activation | Stifel *et al.* (1971) |
| Spermatozoa | Thyroxine | Activation | Casillas and Hoskins (1970) |
| | Triiodothyronine | Activation | Casillas and Hoskins (1970) |
| Spleen | Phytohemagglutinin | Activation | Winchurch *et al.* (1971) |
| | Oligo- and polynucleotides | Activation | Winchurch *et al.* (1971) |
| Stomach | Gastrin pentapeptide | Activation | Bersimbaev *et al.* (1971) |
| | Histamine | Activation | Bersimbaev *et al.* (1971) |
| Submaxillary gland | Isoproterenol | Activation | Barka and Van der Noen (1974) |
| Synovial membrane | Thyroid-stimulating hormone | Activation | Newcombe *et al.* (1972) |
| Testes | ACTH | Activation | Murad *et al.* (1969a) |
| | Epinephrine | Activation | Murad *et al.* (1969a) |
| | Follicle-stimulating hormone | Activation | Kuehl *et al.* (1970) |
| | Gonadotropins | Activation | Murad *et al.* (1969a) |
| | Interstitial cell-stimulating hormone | Activation | Murad *et al.* (1969a) |
| | Luteinizing hormone | Activation | Kuehl *et al.* (1970) |
| Thymus and thymic lymphocytes | Catecholamines | Activation | Huang *et al.* (1973b) |
| | Catecholamines | Activation | Makman (1971) |
| | Epinephrine | Activation | MacManus *et al.* (1971) |
| | Prostaglandins | Activation | Franks *et al.* (1971) |
| | Prostaglandins | Activation | Huang *et al.* (1973) |

| | | | |
|---|---|---|---|
| Thyroid | Long-acting thyroid stimulator | Activation | Levey and Pastan (1970) |
| | Prostaglandin $E_1$ | Activation | Burke (1973) |
| | Prostaglandin $E_1$ | Activation | Mashiter *et al.* (1974) |
| | Purine nucleotides | Activation | Wolff and Cook (1973) |
| | Thyroid-stimulating hormone | Activation | Yamashita and Field (1970) |
| | Thyroid-stimulating hormone | Activation | Wolff *et al.* (1970) |
| | Thyroid-stimulating hormone | Activation | Wolff and Jones (1971) |
| | Thyroid-stimulating hormone | Activation | Burke (1970a) |
| | Thyroid-stimulating hormone | Activation | Zor *et al.* (1969) |
| | Thyroid-stimulating hormone | Activation | Yamashita and Field (1973) |
| | Thyroid-stimulating hormone | Activation | Mashiter *et al.* (1974) |
| | Thyroid-stimulating hormone | Activation | Pastan and Katzen (1967) |
| Uterus | Catecholamines | Activation | Triner *et al.* (1970) |
| | Epinephrine | Activation | Beatty *et al.* (1973) |
| | Estrogen | Activation | Rosenfeld and O'Malley (1970) |
| | Isoproterenol | Activation | Lerner *et al.* (1973) |
| | Oxytocin | Inhibition | Lerner *et al.* (1973) |
| | Oxytocin | Activation | Beatty *et al.* (1973) |
| | Prostaglandins | Activation | Lerner *et al.* (1973) |

activity. It should be noted, however, that relatively high concentrations of calcium (1 m*M*) can inhibit adenylate cyclase activity (Streeto, 1969; Jakobs *et al.,* 1972).

In contrast to the divalent cations, certain monovalent cations, such as lithium, inhibit the stimulatory effects of several hormones on adenylate cyclase (Birnbaumer *et al.,* 1969; Dousa and Hechter, 1970; Burke, 1970b; Forn and Valdecasas, 1971; Uzunov and Weiss, 1972a; Wang *et al.,* 1974).

There are other endogenous materials that also stimulate adenylate cyclase activity. Early studies of Hirata and Hayaishi (1965; 1967) showed that pyruvate increased the activity of adenylate cyclase of *Brevibacterium liquifaciens.* This effect of pyruvate on adenylate cyclase activity, however, has never been demonstrated for the adenylate cyclase obtained from mammalian tissue.

Of the other endogenous compounds that have been reported to enhance adenylate cyclase activity, the most notable are the guanine nucleotides, particularly GTP. The influence of guanine nucleotides on adenylate cyclase activity is quite complex. Thus, GTP and ITP increase the activity of a solubilized adenylate cyclase prepared from liver (Swislocki *et al.,* 1973), and several reports show that the presence of GTP is obligatory for the hormonal activation of adenylate cyclase (Rodbell *et al.,* 1971c; Krishna *et al.,* 1972; Leray *et al.,* 1972; Harwood *et al.,* 1973; Bilezikian and Aurbach, 1974). On the other hand, guanyl nucleotides have also been shown to inhibit both basal (Harwood *et al.,* 1973) and fluoride-stimulated adenylate cyclase activity (Rodbell *et al.,* 1971c).

### 2. *Endogenous Inhibitors of Adenylate Cyclase*

Several naturally occurring substances have been reported to inhibit the activity of adenylate cyclase. The following are examples: ADP inhibits adenylate cyclase of pineal gland (Weiss, 1970); adenosine inhibits adenylate cyclase of brain, kidney, and liver (McKenzie and Bar, 1973), and guanine, cytidine, and uridine nucleotides inhibit adenylate cyclase of fat cells (Cryer *et al.,* 1969). Pyrophosphate, one of the products of adenylate cyclase activity, also inhibits the activity of adenylate cyclase (Tao and Lipmann, 1969; Severson *et al.,* 1972), as does cyclic AMP itself (Weiss and Costa, 1968a). Thus, several metabolic products of ATP metabolism, including cyclic AMP, adenosine, ADP, and pyrophosphate, all reduced adenylate cyclase activity, suggesting that this enzyme may be regulated by a feedback control mechanism.

One precaution that should be observed when studying the effects of purine derivatives on adenylate cyclase deserves emphasis. Given the right conditions, virtually all purines may eventually be converted to ATP. Should this occur, the specific activity of radioactive ATP (the substrate for the reaction) would be reduced, causing an apparent decrease in cyclic AMP formation. Therefore, in all studies of this type, the investigator should determine the specific activity of ATP in the absence and presence of the purine derivative (see Weiss, 1970).

In addition to the purine and pyrimidine derivatives, other endogenously occurring compounds have also been shown to inhibit adenylate cyclase; for example, oxalacetate and pyridoxal phosphate inhibit adenylate cyclase of *Escherichia coli* (Ide, 1969).

Finally, the report of Ho and Sutherland (1971) suggested that there is an endogenous inhibitor of adenylate cyclase in adipose tissue. Their conclusion is based on evidence that glucagon, epinephrine, and ACTH promote the formation of a substance that antagonizes the elevation of cyclic AMP in adipose tissue. However, whether this material was, in fact, blocking adenylate cyclase activity or was preventing the accumulation of cyclic AMP by some other mechanism is still an open question.

### 3. *Exogenous Activators of Adenylate Cyclase*

Sodium fluoride is the most potent, most studied, and least specific activator of adenylate cyclase. Its ability to activate the adenylate cyclase of liver was originally reported by Rall and Sutherland in 1958. Since then it has been shown to increase adenylate cyclase activity in virtually every tissue and species examined with the exception of certain bacteria (Ide, 1971).

Table II compares the effects of sodium fluoride and norepinephrine on adenylate cyclase of several tissues of the rat. These experiments demonstrate the relative specificity of norepinephrine in activating adenylate cyclase compared with the nonspecific and, in general, more pronounced stimulatory effects of sodium fluoride. It should be noted, however, that under certain experimental conditions fluoride appears to inhibit the basal (Tao and Lipmann, 1969) or hormone-stimulated (Harwood and Rodbell, 1973) adenylate cyclase.

Although the effect of fluoride on adenylate cyclase activity has been studied in various laboratories, no universally accepted hypothesis for its mechanism of action has emerged. For a more detailed discussion of the effect of fluoride, see the recent review of Perkins, 1973 (see also, Weiss, 1969a; Drummond and Duncan, 1970; Hepp *et al.*, 1970; Khandelwal and Hamilton, 1971).

TABLE II

COMPARISON OF THE EFFECTS OF NOREPINEPHRINE (NE) AND SODIUM FLUORIDE ON ADENYLATE CYCLASE ACTIVITY OF VARIOUS TISSUES OF THE RAT[a]

| Tissue | Cyclic 3′,5′-AMP formed (pmole/mg protein/min) | | |
|---|---|---|---|
| | Control | NE($10^{-4}$ *M*) | NaF($10^{-2}$ *M*) |
| Pancreas | 1.0 ± 0.3 | 2.0 ± 0.9 | 14 ± 4[c] |
| Thyroid | 1.1 ± 0.4 | 1.3 ± 0.3 | 18 ± 2[c] |
| Spleen | 1.9 ± 0.4 | 3.7 ± 0.1[b] | 43 ± 2[c] |
| Liver | 2.9 ± 0.3 | 4.5 ± 0.5 | 18 ± 2[c] |
| Submaxillary gland | 3.0 ± 0.4 | 6.0 ± 1.3[b] | 85 ± 11[c] |
| Adrenal gland | 4.4 ± 0.6 | 5.9 ± 0.8 | 108 ± 16[c] |
| Lung | 12 ± 3 | 17 ± 4 | 142 ± 38[c] |
| Pineal gland | 111 ± 3 | 288 ± 4[c] | 399 ± 6[c] |

[a] Adenylate cyclase activity was determined according to the method of Krishna *et al.*, (1968a), using ATP-$^{14}$C as substrate. Each incubation vessel contained an equivalent of about 500 μg protein for liver, pancreas, lung, and spleen, and about 100 μg protein for the other tissues. Values presented are the mean ± S.E. of 3 to 6 experiments.

[b] $p < 0.05$ compared with paired control values.

[c] $p < 0.001$ compared with paired control values.

## 4. *Exogenous Inhibitors of Adenylate Cyclase*

The agents that have been shown to inhibit adenylate cyclase activity may be divided into two general categories: those that inhibit the basal activity, i.e., activity in the absence of any added hormonal activator, and those that do not alter adenylate cyclase activity directly but modify the response of the enzyme to hormonal stimulation (see Table III). Compounds in the former category include reagents that interfere with the sulfhydryl groups of tissue proteins, including presumably adenylate cyclase. Among these are ethacrynic acid and dithiobisnitrobenzoic acid. Agents such as the purine nucleotides may alter the binding of substrate (i.e., ATP) to the catalytic moiety of the enzyme. These compounds would also be expected to reduce the basal activity.

There are other groups of compounds that appear to be more specific for the receptor moiety of adenylate cyclase. These compounds probably act by competing with the hormonal agonist for the receptor portion of the adenylate cyclase system. Compounds in this group include the adrenergic blocking agents and phenothiazine tranquilizers, which interfere specifically with the catecholamine-induced activation of adenylate cyclase, and analogs of ACTH and oxytocin, which interfere specifically with the ACTH- or neurohypophyseal hormone-induced activation of adenylate cyclase. The action of the antibiotics and the various other compounds shown in Table III is more difficult to interpret on the basis of their ability to compete with either the agonist or the substrate for adenylate cyclase.

With the possible exception of the β-adrenergic blocking agents, the purine nucleotides, or the analogs of the polypeptide hormones, there are no specific and potent inhibitors of adenylate cyclase available. This has severely limited the application of adenylate cyclase inhibitors to clinical therapy. The further development of analogs of the various cyclic nucleotides or hormonal agonists may provide the basis for a new class of effective and specific therapeutic agents.

In addition to compounds that have been shown to alter adenylate cyclase (Tables I and III), many agents have been reported to prevent the accumulation of cyclic AMP in whole cells or in tissue slices: α- and β-adrenergic blocking agents prevent the increased concentration of cyclic AMP induced by catecholamines in a variety of tissues (Kakiuchi and Rall, 1968; Chasin *et al.*, 1971; Schultz and Daly, 1973; Strada *et al.*, 1972); several psychotropic drugs, including the phenothiazine tranquilizers, butyrophenones, thioxanthenes, and lithium, prevent the catecholamine-induced increase in the concentration of cyclic AMP of brain (Kakiuchi and Rall, 1968; Uzunov and Weiss, 1971, 1972a; Walker and Walker, 1973; Weiss and Greenberg, 1975); numerous other centrally acting compounds (Paul *et al.*, 1970; Palmer, 1973; Schmidt *et al.*, 1972), histamine analogs (Shimizu *et al.*, 1970a), and depolarizing agents (Shimizu *et al.*, 1970b,c; Huang *et al.*, 1971) also increase the concentration of cyclic AMP in brain. A group of miscellaneous agents that have been reported to inhibit the hormone-induced elevation of cyclic AMP in tissue include *p*-chlorophenoxyisobutyrate (Weis *et al.*, 1973), dicyclohexylcarbodiimide, antimycin, and piericidin (Dorigo *et al.*, 1973 a,b).

### C. Chronic Factors Influencing the Activity of Adenylate Cyclase

The studies discussed thus far have dealt with the acute or immediate effects of drugs and hormones on the formation of cyclic AMP. However, it is probable that the degree to which receptors respond to hormones in an acute experiment may be influenced by the prior state of the organism. The question to which we now address ourselves, therefore, is How do the environment and other factors influence the

TABLE III

EFFECT OF VARIOUS PHARMACOLOGICAL AGENTS ON ADENYLATE CYCLASE ACTIVITY

| Agent | Tissue | Basal activity | Hormone-stimulated activity[a] | Reference |
|---|---|---|---|---|
| ACTH analog | Adipose | — | Inhibition (ACTH) | Ramachandran and Lee (1970) |
| | Adipose | — | Inhibition (ACTH) | Birnbaumer and Rodbell (1969) |
| Adenosine | Brain | — | Inhibition (gluc, ACTH, epi) | McKenzie and Bar (1973) |
| | Kidney | — | Inhibition (gluc, ACTH, epi) | McKenzie and Bar (1973) |
| | Liver | — | Inhibition (gluc, ACTH, epi) | McKenzie and Bar (1973) |
| | Platelets | Activation | Inhibition (PGE) | Haslam and Lynham (1972) |
| 2-Chloroadenosine | Platelets | Activation | Inhibition (PGE) | Haslam and Lynham (1972) |
| Alloxan | Brain | Inhibition | — | Cohen and Bitensky (1969) |
| | Heart | Inhibition | — | Cohen and Bitensky (1969) |
| | Kidney | Inhibition | — | Cohen and Bitensky (1969) |
| | Liver | Inhibition | — | Cohen and Bitensky (1969) |
| Amphetamine | Heart | — | Inhibition (epi) | McNeill and Muschek (1972a) |
| Antibiotics | Adipose | Inhibition | Inhibition (NE) | Dorigo *et al.* (1973a,b) |
| | Adipose | Inhibition | Inhibition (NE, gluc) | Counis *et al.* (1973) |
| | Adipose | Activation | Inhibition (NE) | Fain and Loken (1971) |
| | Thyroid | Inhibition | Inhibition (TSH) | Butcher and Serif (1969) |
| $\alpha$-Adrenergic blockers | Erythrocytes | — | Inhibition (NE) | Sheppard and Burghardt (1970, 1971) |
| | Thyroid | — | Inhibition (TSH) | Burke (1970a) |
| | Retina | — | Inhibition (Dm) | Brown and Makman (1973) |

| | | | | |
|---|---|---|---|---|
| Apomorphine | Caudate nucleus | Activation | — | Kebabian *et al.* (1972) |
| | Retina | Activation | — | Brown and Makman (1973) |
| $\beta$-Adrenergic blockers | Adipose | — | Inhibition (epi) | Birnbaumer and Rodbell (1969) |
| | Erythrocytes | — | Inhibition (NE) | Sheppard and Burghardt (1970, 1971) |
| | Erythrocytes | — | Inhibition (NE) | Bilezikian and Aurbach (1973a) |
| | Heart | Inhibition | — | Rabinowitz *et al.* (1973) |
| | Heart | — | Inhibition (NE) | Mayer (1972) |
| | Heart | — | Inhibition (ISO) | Vatner and Lefkowitz (1974) |
| | Brain | — | Inhibition | von Hungen and Roberts (1973) |
| | Liver | — | Inhibition (ISO, epi) | Newton and Hornbrook (1972) |
| | Liver | — | Inhibition (NE) | Mayer (1972) |
| | Pineal | — | Inhibition (NE) | Weiss (1969a) |
| | Pineal | — | Inhibition (NE) | Weiss and Costa (1968a) |
| $\beta$-Adrenergic agonists | Erythrocytes | Activation | — | Grunfeld *et al.* (1974) |
| | Erythrocytes | Activation | — | Rosen *et al.* (1970) |
| | Erythrocytes | — | Inhibition (ISO) | Rosen *et al.* (1970) |
| | Heart | — | Inhibition (epi) | McNeill *et al.* (1970) |
| | Lung | Activation | — | Burges and Blackburn (1972) |
| | Thyroid | — | Inhibition (TSH) | Burke (1970a) |
| Bax 439 (2-amino-4,5-diphenylthiazole) | Kidney | — | Inhibition (ADH) | Dousa *et al.* (1973) |
| Betazole | Heart | Activation | Inhibition (hist) | McNeill and Muschek, (1972b) |
| Butaclamol | Olfactory tubercle | — | Inhibition (Dm) | Lippmann *et al.* (1975) |
| Chelators | Brain | Inhibition | — | Bradham *et al.* (1970) |
| | Brain | Inhibition | — | Bradham (1972) |

*(Continued)*

TABLE III—*Continued*

| Agent | Tissue | Basal activity | Hormone-stimulated activity[a] | Reference |
|---|---|---|---|---|
| Cholinomimetics | Gastric mucosa | Inhibition | — | Nakajima *et al.* (1971) |
| Endotoxin | Liver | — | Potentiation (epi) | Bitensky *et al.* (1971) |
| Ethanol | Kidney | Activation | — | Mashiter *et al.* (1974) |
| | Liver | Activation | — | Mashiter *et al.* (1974) |
| | Pancreas | Activation | — | Kuo *et al.* (1973) |
| Ecdysterone | Brain | Inhibition | — | Rojakovick and March (1972) |
| Glucagon analog | Liver | — | Inhibition (gluc) | Birnbaumer and Pohl (1973) |
| Haloperidol | Caudate nucleus | — | Inhibition (Dm) | Kebabian *et al.* (1972) |
| | Brain | — | Inhibition (Dm) | von Hungen and Roberts (1973) |
| | Erythrocytes | — | Inhibition (NE) | Sheppard and Burghardt (1971) |
| | Heart | — | Inhibition (ISO) | Vatner and Lefkowitz (1974) |
| | Retina | — | Inhibition (Dm) | Brown and Makman (1973) |
| Dihydrotestosterone | Hair follicles | Inhibition | — | Adachi and Kano (1970) |
| Insecticides | Kidney | Activation | — | Kacew and Singhal (1974) |
| Insulin | Adipose tissue | — | Inhibition (gluc, CA) | Butcher *et al.* (1966) |
| | | | | Illiano and Cautrecasas (1972) |
| | | | | Hepp and Renner (1972) |

| | | | | |
|---|---|---|---|---|
| Lithium | Brain | — | Inhibition (F) | Forn and Valdecasas (1971) |
| | Thyroid | — | Inhibition (TSH) | Burke (1970b) |
| | | | | Wolff *et al.* (1970) |
| Morphine | Caudate nucleus | Activation | — | Puri *et al.* (1975) |
| Nicotinic acid | Adipose tissue | Inhibition | — | Skidmore *et al.* (1972) |
| Ouabain | Thyroid | — | Inhibition (TSH) | Burke (1970b) |
| Oxytocin analogs | Bladder | — | Inhibition (VT) | Walter *et al.* (1972a) |
| | Bladder | — | Inhibition (ADH) | Walter *et al.* (1972a) |
| | Kidney | — | Inhibition (VT, ADH) | Walter *et al.* (1972b) |
| Phenothiazines | Adrenal | — | Inhibition (ACTH) | Wolff and Jones (1970) |
| | Caudate | — | Inhibition (Dm) | Kebabian *et al.* (1972) |
| | Erythrocytes | — | Inhibition (NE) | Sheppard and Burghardt (1971) |
| | Heart | — | Inhibition (ISO) | Vatner and Lefkowitz (1974) |
| | Liver | — | Inhibition (epi, gluc) | Wolff and Jones (1970) |
| | Pineal | — | Inhibition (NE) | Weiss and Kidman (1969) |
| | Retina | — | Inhibition (Dm) | Brown and Makman (1973) |
| | Thyroid | — | Inhibition (TSH, $PGE_1$) | Wolff and Jones (1970, 1971) |
| Purine nucleotides | Adipose | Inhibition | — | Cryer *et al.* (1969) |
| | Erythrocytes | — | Potentiation (CA) | Bilezikian and Aurbach (1974) |
| | Liver | — | Potentiation (gluc) | Rodbell *et al.* (1971c) |
| | Lung | Inhibition | — | Weinryb *et al.* (1973) |
| Pyrophosphate | Skeletal muscle | Inhibition | — | Severson *et al.* (1972) |
| 3-Pyridylacetic acid | Adipose | Inhibition | — | Skidmore *et al.* (1972) |

*(Continued)*

TABLE III—*Continued*

| Agent | Tissue | Basal activity | Hormone-stimulated activity[a] | Reference |
|---|---|---|---|---|
| Somatomedin | Adipose | Inhibition | Inhibition (epi) | Tell *et al.* (1973) |
| | Cartilage | Inhibition | Inhibition (PTH) | Tell *et al.* (1973) |
| | Liver | Inhibition | Inhibition ($PGE_2$) | Tell *et al.* (1973) |
| | Lymphocytes | Inhibition | Inhibition (epi) | Tell *et al.* (1973) |
| Serotonin | Erythrocytes | — | Inhibition (NE) | Sheppard and Burghardt (1970, 1971) |
| | Pineal | — | Inhibition (NE) | Weiss and Costa (1968a) |
| Sulfhydryl reagents | Brain | Inhibition | — | Ferrendelli *et al.* (1973) |
| | Kidney | Inhibition | Inhibition (PTH) | Jakobs *et al.* (1972) |
| | Kidney | Inhibition | Inhibition (ADH) | Jakobs *et al.* (1972) |
| | Liver | Inhibition | — | Pohl *et al.* (1971) |
| | *Streptococcus salivarius* | Inhibition | — | Khandelwal and Hamilton (1971) |
| | Sea anemone | Activation | — | Gentleman and Mansour (1974) |
| | Thyroid | — | Inhibition (TSH) | Wolff and Jones (1971) |
| Tolbutamide | Pancreas | Activation | — | Kuo *et al.* (1973) |
| | Pancreas | Activation | — | Levey *et al.* (1972) |
| Triiodothyronine | Adipose tissue | — | Potentiation (epi) | Challoner and Allen (1970) |

[a] Hormonal agonists are shown in parentheses.

Abbreviations: ACTH = adrenocorticotropic hormone; ADH = antidiuretic hormone; gluc = glucagon; hist = histamine; PTH = parathyroid hormone; epi = epinephrine; NE = norepinephrine; Dm = dopamine; ISO = isoproterenol; $PGE_1$ = prostaglandin $E_1$; CA = catecholamines; TSH = thyroid-stimulating hormone; VT = vasotocin; F = fluoride.

responsiveness of the organism to these drugs and hormones? Although much less information is available to answer this question, sufficient studies have been performed to indicate that the previous condition of the organism can, in fact, substantially alter the response of adenylate cyclase to hormones and pharmacological agents (Table IV). For example, the species and age of the organism, hormonal and neuronal factors, and chronic drug treatment all have been shown to have pronounced effects on the degree to which adenylate cyclase can respond to subsequent hormonal stimuli.

1. *Species*

Several species differences were noted in the selectivity with which hormones activate adenylate cyclase. For example, Dousa (1974a) reported that vasotocin activated adenylate cyclase from kidneys of certain species (bullfrogs and toads) but not that from other species (pigeon, chicken, alligator, and goldfish). He also showed that this polypeptide hormone activated adenylate cyclase of amphibian urinary bladders but not that from rat urinary bladders.

2. *Age*

The age of the animal influences the degree to which adenylate cyclase is activated by hormones. Cyclic AMP and the enzymes responsible for its biosynthesis and degradation are present in all tissues at all stages of their development. However, the rate at which these enzymes develop varies with the tissue and species. Moreover, the rate at which the hormone-sensitive adenylate cyclase system develops does not necessarily coincide with the development of the basal or fluoride-stimulatable enzyme. For example, the responsiveness to catecholamines of rat pineal adenylate cyclase increases markedly during the first few postnatal days (Weiss, 1971b), This hormone-sensitive adenylate cyclase system increased at a greater rate than the hormone-insensitive enzyme system. A similar age-related increase in adenylate cyclase activity or an increase in its responsiveness to hormones is also seen in insects (Castillon *et al.,* 1973) and tadpole erythrocytes (Rosen and Erlichman, 1969) as well as in mammalian tissues such as brain (Schmidt *et al.,* 1970; Kohrman, 1973; Perkins and Moore, 1973), heart (Brus and Hess, 1973; Williams and Thompson, 1973; Clark *et al.*, 1973), testis (Hollinger, 1970), adipose tissue (Skala *et al.,* 1972), and skeletal muscle (Williams and Thompson, 1973). By contrast, adenylate cyclase activity of several other tissues, such as liver (Bitensky *et al.,* .1970; Bar and Hahn, 1971; Kohrman, 1973), submaxillary gland (Barka and Van der

TABLE IV

CHRONIC FACTORS THAT ALTER ADENYLATE CYCLASE ACTIVITY OR ITS SENSITIVITY TO HORMONES

| Agent or factor | Tissue | Effect on adenylate cyclase activity | | References |
|---|---|---|---|---|
| | | Basal activity | Hormone-stimulated activity[a] | |
| Acetylphenylhydrazine | Erythrocytes | Increase | — | Gauger *et al.* (1973) |
| 2-Acetylaminofluorene | Liver | — | Increase (epi) | Christoffersen *et al.* (1972b) |
| Adrenalectomy | Adipocytes | — | Decrease (NE) | Schonhofer *et al.* (1972) |
| Adrenalectomy | Adipose | — | Decrease (ACTH) | Allen and Beck (1972) |
| Adrenalectomy | Adipocyte | — | Decrease (ACTH) | Braun and Hechter (1970) |
| Adrenalectomy | Liver | — | Increase (epi) | Leray *et al.* (1972)<br>Bitensky *et al.* (1970) |
| Age | (see text) | | | |
| Cold exposure | Adipose tissue | Increase | — | Kuriyama and Israel (1973) |
| Cortisone | Liver | — | Decrease (epi) | Leray *et al.* (1972) |
| Cholera toxin | Mucosa | Increase | Inhibit (CA) | Sharp *et al.* (1973) |
| Denervation | Pineal | — | Increase (NE) | Weiss and Costa (1967)<br>Weiss (1969b, 1970)<br>Weiss and Kidman (1969)<br>Deguchi and Axelrod (1973a,b)<br>Strada and Weiss (1974) |

| | | | | |
|---|---|---|---|---|
| Dexamethasone | Adipocyte | — | Increase (ACTH) | Braun and Hechter (1970) |
| Estradiol | Pineal | Decrease | Decrease (NE) | Weiss and Crayton (1970a,b) |
| Ethanol | Brain | Increase | — | Kuriyama and Israel (1973) |
| Fasting | Adipose tissue | — | Increase (NE) | Therriault *et al.* (1969) |
| Fasting | Pancreas | Decrease | Decrease (gluc) | Howell *et al.* (1973) |
| Hypophysectomy | Adipocyte | — | Decrease (ACTH) | Braun and Hechter (1970) |
| 6-Hydroxydopamine | Brain | — | Increase (NE) | Weiss and Strada (1972) |
| | | | | Palmer (1972) |
| | | | | Huang *et al.* (1973a) |
| | | | | Kalisker *et al.* (1973) |
| | | | | Dismukes and Daly (1974) |
| Immunosympathectomy | Pineal | — | Increase (NE) | Weiss (1970b) |
| Light | Pineal | — | Increase (NE) | Weiss (1969b) |
| Light | Cerebellum | Increase | — | Weiss and Strada (1972) |
| Morphine | Brain | Decrease | — | Chou *et al.* (1971) |
| Morphine | Brain | Increase | — | Naito and Kuriyama (1973) |
| Orchidectomy | Prostate | Decrease | — | Sutherland and Singhal (1974) |
| Orchidectomy | Seminal vesicles | Decrease | — | Thomas and Singhal (1973) |
| Testosterone | Seminal vesicles | Increase | — | Thomas and Singhal (1973) |
| Thyroxine | Adipose tissue | Increase | — | Brodie *et al.* (1966) |
| | | | | Krishna *et al.* (1968b) |

[a] Hormonal agonists are shown in parentheses.

Abbreviations: epi = epinephrine; NE = norepinephrine; ACTH = adrenocorticotropic hormone; CA = catecholamines; gluc = glucagon.

Noen, 1974), kidney (Gengler and Forte, 1972), and ovary (Smith and Major, 1971), show a reduced responsiveness to catecholamine stimulation during the first few weeks of postnatal life. In other studies of the ovary, Fontaine *et al.* (1973) showed that hormonal responsiveness of adenylate cyclase reaches a peak at about 20 days of age, and then declines.

### 3. *Hormonal Factors*

A pronounced effect of gonadal hormones was demonstrated in the adenylate cyclase system of rat pineal gland (Weiss and Crayton, 1970 a,b). These studies showed that norepinephrine stimulates the adenylate cyclase activity of male rat pineal glands to a greater extent than that of female rat pineals. This decreased sensitivity of adenylate cyclase apparently was due to an inhibitory action of the female sex hormones since ovariectomy increased the stimulatory actions of norepinephrine, and this effect, in turn, was antagonized by estradiol treatment. Orchiectomy or testosterone treatment, on the other hand, failed to alter pineal adenylate cyclase activity. The physiological significance of these studies was demonstrated by the data showing that norepinephrine failed to activate pineal adenylate cyclase when rats were in proestrus, a stage of the estrus cycle characterized by high plasma levels of estrogen. This work suggests that the concentration of gonadal hormones in plasma plays an important role in the responsiveness of a hormone-sensitive adenylate cyclase system in a distal target tissue.

The report of Sayers and Beall (1973) supports the hypothesis that one endocrine gland can influence the adenylate cyclase system of another endocrine gland. They found that the adrenals of hypophysectomized rats exhibited a greater rate of formation of cyclic AMP in response in ACTH than in that of control animals. An analogous study was reported by Kuehl *et al.* (1970) who showed that rat testicular adenylate cyclase was sensitive to follicle-stimulating hormone (FSH) only in immature rats, i.e., only in those rats that previously had been exposed to low concentrations of FSH.

### 4. *Neuronal Factors: Denervation Supersensitivity and Subsensitivity*

The pharmacological consequences of prolonged denervation of sympathetically innervated structures have been known for almost a century (Lewandowsky, 1899), and in the intervening years this phenomenon has been studied extensively by many investigators (see Emmelin, 1961; Trendelenburg, 1963, 1966; Fleming *et al.*, 1973). Studies in our laboratory have suggested a biochemical explanation for the slowly developing, postjunctional denervation supersensitivity. We have found that reducing the sympathetic input to a structure causes an enhanced responsiveness of adenylate cyclase to catecholamines and a greater increase in the catecholamine-induced elevation of cyclic AMP. Conversely, increasing the sympathetic input reduced the norepinephrine-induced formation of cyclic AMP. This was demonstrated originally in rat pineal glands that had been sympathetically denervated by bilateral removal of the superior cervical ganglia (Weiss and Costa, 1967). In these experiments, adenylate cyclase of rat pineal gland was assayed after all sympathetic nerves had degenerated. Although denervation did not cause any loss of the basal enzyme activity, it did cause a marked increase in the sensitivity of the adenylate cyclase system to norepinephrine. These results have been subsequently confirmed using a variety of techniques, all of which reduce the neuronal input to the pineal gland; namely, surgical denervation of the pineal gland or decentralization of the superior cervical ganglia (Weiss, 1969b; Weiss and Kidman, 1969; Strada and Weiss, 1974), chemical sympathectomy with 6-hydroxydopamine (Weiss and Strada, 1972; Strada and Weiss, 1974, and immunosympathectomy (Weiss, 1970). Chronic exposure of rats to light, which also reduces the neuronal input to the pineal gland, similarly increased the neurohormonal responsiveness of the adenylate cyclase system (Weiss, 1969b). Maintaining rats in darkness, on the other hand, which increases sympathetic input to the pineal gland, reduced the norepinephrine-induced formation of cyclic AMP (Strada and Weiss, 1972).

Experiments with 6-hydroxydopamine allowed us to extend these studies to other tissues as well. Thus, treatment of rats with 6-hydroxydopamine, which destroys sympathetic nerve endings in brain, produced an increased responsiveness to norepinephrine of the cyclic AMP system of brain (Weiss and Strada, 1972).

By using similar techniques, other investigators have recently confirmed these findings and have also reached the conclusion that increased sympathetic activity causes a reduction in the responsiveness (subsensitivity) of the adrenergic receptor (i.e., a portion of the adenylate cyclase system) to catecholamine stimulation (Palmer, 1972; Huang *et al.*, 1973a; Kalisker *et al.*, 1973; Deguchi and Axelrod, 1973a,b; Dismukes and Daly, 1974).

The mechanism of this biochemical denervation supersensitivity is still unclear. However, there is evidence that the increased responsiveness of adenylate cyclase may be due to a reduced interaction of the neurotransmitters with adenylate cyclase, since chronic administration of norepinephrine prevented the development of supersensitivity to catecholamines on the cyclic AMP system (Strada and Weiss, 1974).

These results are supported by the recent finding of Mukherjee *et al.* (1975), who showed that the number of adenylate cyclase receptor sites on the cell is increased in the absence of catecholamines and is decreased by an excess of catecholamines.

### 5. *Chronic Drug Treatment*

Several pharmacological agents, such as cholera toxin, morphine, ethanol, and the chemical carcinogen, 2-acetylaminofluorene have been shown to alter adenylate cyclase activity or its responsiveness to hormonal stimulation. Some studies, however, offer conflicting evidence. Chou *et al.* (1971) reported that acute injections of morphine enhanced adenylate cyclase activity of mouse brain, but chronic administration of morphine caused a reduction in adenylate cyclase activity. Naito and Kuriyama (1973), on the other hand, reported an increase in adenylate cyclase activity of brain following chronic administration of morphine.

### 6. *Conclusions*

The following conclusions may be drawn from these studies of the chronic factors influencing adenylate cyclase activity:

1. The basal activity of adenylate cyclase and the sensitivity of adenylate cyclase to hormonal stimulation develop ontogenetically at different rates, suggesting that the receptor portion and the catalytic moiety of the adenylate cyclase system can develop independently.
2. Different tissues develop their hormonal sensitivity at different rates, suggesting that each cell type is independently programmed to synthesize its specific, hormone-sensitive adenylate cyclase system.
3. The hormonal sensitivity of adenylate cyclase is altered by certain endocrine factors as well as by chronic drug treatment.
4. The hormonal sensitivity is also related to the degree to which the tissue has been previously exposed to the hormonal stimulator, that is, repeated or prolonged exposure of a hormone-sensitive adenylate cyclase to its agonist may reduce its responsiveness to the subsequent addition of its agonist. This latter effect may constitute a feedback control mechanism which would tend to reduce the effects of prolonged or excessive hormonal stimulation.
5. These long-term or chronic effects on adenylate cyclase must be considered when examining the influence of pharmacological agents on this system.

## III. Guanylate Cyclase

In the past several years, the physiological and biochemical function of guanosine 3′,5′-cyclic monophosphate (cyclic GMP) has been examined by a number of investigators. Although cyclic AMP and cyclic GMP affect similar physiological processes, there is evidence suggesting that these two cyclic nucleotides may have opposing roles in many biological systems (for a review of cyclic GMP, see Goldberg *et al.*, 1973, 1975).

Cyclic GMP is formed from GTP by guanylate cyclase, in a reaction analogous to the adenylate cyclase reaction that forms cyclic AMP from ATP. The existence of guanylate cyclase was postulated (Price *et al.*, 1967) to explain the existence of cyclic GMP in urine, a phenomenon first observed by Ashman *et al.* (1963). The presence of guanylate cyclase activity in tissue was demonstrated soon thereafter (White and Aurbach, 1969; Hardman and Sutherland, 1969; Schultz *et al.*, 1969). Its distribution and properties, described in the following sections, have since been investigated by a number of other workers.

### A. Tissue Distribution

Several groups of investigators have studied the tissue distribution of guanylate cyclase (Hardman and Sutherland, 1969; White and Aurbach, 1969; Bohme, 1970; Bensinger *et al.*, 1974a; Thompson *et al.*, 1974; Kimura and Murad, 1974; Nakazawa and Sano, 1974). Of the tissues studied, lung has the highest specific activity and skeletal muscle and adipose tissue have the lowest specific activity of guanylate cyclase. Iris and retina, in particular the outer rod segment fraction, also have high specific activities of guanylate cyclase (Goridis *et al.*, 1973; Pannbacker, 1973, 1974; Bensinger *et al.*, 1974 a,b; Thompson *et al.*, 1974).

Nakazawa and Sano (1974), who studied the regional distribution of this enzyme in rat brain, found that the telencephalon had the highest specific activity of guanylate cyclase and spinal cord the lowest.

### B. Cellular and Subcellular Distribution

Although the results of studies on the subcellular localization of guanylate cyclase are influenced by the methods used to disrupt the cells and the subsequent treatment of the subcellular fractions (Kimura and Murad, 1974), experiments in which both adenylate cyclase and guanylate cyclase activities were determined in the same subcellular fractions showed clearly that these two enzymes have different subcellular distributions. Thus, adenylate cyclase is found predominantly in the particulate fraction of tissue homogenates (see above), but guanylate cyclase is found mainly in the soluble fraction (Hardman and Sutherland, 1969; Schultz *et al.*, 1969; White and Aurbach, 1969; Bohme, 1970; Marks, 1973; Chrisman *et al.*, 1975; Kimura and Murad, 1974). However, significant amounts of the total guanylate cyclase activity are associated with particulate subcellular fractions as well (Hardman and Sutherland, 1969; Goridis *et al.*, 1973; Bensinger, 1974 a,b; Kimura and Murad, 1974; Rudland *et al.*, 1974; Nakazawa and Sano, 1974).

The use of more complex subcellular fractionation procedures led Goridis and Morgan (1973) to conclude that the specific activity of guanylate cyclase of rat brain was high in both the soluble and particulate fractions of synaptosomes. A subsequent study (Goridis *et al.*, 1974) was carried out in dissociated chick brain cell cultures containing different ratios of neuronal and glial elements. Cultures containing pure glial cells had no guanylate cyclase activity, whereas those with a high proportion of neuronal cells had correspondingly higher levels of guanylate cyclase. These studies suggest that, in the brain, guanylate cyclase is of neuronal rather than of glial or meningeal cell origin and that it is located primarily in neuronal synaptosomes.

### C. Multiple Forms of Guanylate Cyclase

Kimura and Murad (1974) in studies of the rat heart and Chrisman *et al.* (1975) working with rat lung have postulated that the guanylate cyclase found in the soluble and particulate fractions are, in fact, different enzymes. The major evidence in support of this conclusion was their data showing that gel chromatography of a homogenate of rat heart resolved two peaks of guanylate cyclase activity (Kimura and Murad, 1974) and that the guanylate cyclase activity of a homogenate, soluble and of a solubilized particulate enzyme preparation of lung migrate at different rates on gel filtration columns (Chrisman *et al.*, 1975). In addition, the different responses of the soluble and particulate enzymes to detergents, ions, and gel chromatography indicate that the soluble enzyme has a lower molecular weight, is activated to a lesser extent by detergent and to a greater extent by $Ca^{2+}$, and is less sensitive to inhibition by excess $Mn^{2+}$ than is the particulate enzyme.

### D. Effect of Ions on Guanylate Cyclase Activity

Manganese is required for the activity of guanylate cyclase in all tissues studied (Schultz *et al.*, 1969; White and Aurbach, 1969; Hardman and Sutherland, 1969; Marks, 1973; Kimura and Murad, 1974;

Nakazawa and Sano, 1974; Chrisman *et al.,* 1975). In the absence of $Mn^{2+}$, generally little or no enzyme activity was seen (Bohme, 1970; Marks, 1973; Kimura and Murad, 1974; Bensinger *et al.,* 1974 a,b; Chrisman *et al.,* 1975). Other divalent cations can substitute for manganese, but they are much less effective. In some preparations, $Ca^{2+}$ has a slight stimulatory effect on guanylate cyclase (Schultz *et al.,* 1969; White and Aurbach, 1969; Hardman and Sutherland, 1969; Bohme, 1970; Hardman *et al.,* 1972; Marks, 1973; Pannbacker, 1973, 1974; Kimura and Murad, 1974; Nakazawa and Sano, 1974), as does $Fe^{2+}$ (Marks, 1973). Other cations studied have variable effects on the guanylate cyclase: $Ba^{2+}$ has no effect, and $Zn^{2+}$ inhibits the guanylate cyclase of rat kidney supernatant fraction (Bohme, 1970); $Ba^{2+}$ and $Sr^{2+}$ stimulate the soluble, but not the particulate, fraction from rat lung (Chrisman *et al.,* 1975); $Ba^{2+}$, $Co^{2+}$, and $Ni^{2+}$ do not stimulate the enzyme of sea urchin sperm (Hardman *et al.,* 1972); $Cd^{2+}$, $Zn^{2+}$, and $Hg^{2+}$ inhibit the lung enzyme (Hardman and Sutherland, 1969); and $Co^{2+}$ and $Zn^{2+}$ inhibit the enzyme from mouse epidermis (Marks, 1973).

There are several differences between the ionic requirements for guanylate cyclase and adenylate cyclase. Fluoride, for example, which markedly activates adenylate cyclase (see above), has little or no effect on guanylate cyclase activity (Hardman and Sutherland, 1969; White and Aurbach, 1969; Bohme, 1970; Sung *et al.,* 1973; Kimura and Murad, 1974). Moreover, in contrast to adenylate cyclase, which requires $Mg^{2+}$ for optimum activity, guanylate cyclase is activated much more readily by $Mn^{2+}$ than by $Mg^{2+}$ (Hardman and Sutherland, 1969; Schultz *et al.,* 1969; White and Aurbach, 1969; Bohme, 1970; Marks, 1973; Chrisman *et al.,* 1975). This evidence, combined with the data showing that the two enzymes are not found in the same subcellular fractions, are not stimulated by the same hormones, and have different substrate specificities, strongly support the assumption that the two enzyme systems are distinctly different.

Studies of the kinetic properties of guanylate cyclase in different tissues suggest that different forms of the enzyme may exist. Thus, rat lung guanylate cyclase has an apparent Michaelis constant ($K_m$) value between 10 and 100 $\mu M$ (Hardman and Sutherland, 1969), bovine lung has a $K_m$ of about 300 $\mu M$ (White and Aurbach, 1969), rat kidney has a $K_m$ of about 400 $\mu M$ (Bohme, 1970), rat liver has a $K_m$ of about 50 $\mu M$ (Thompson *et al.,* 1973 a,b), and rat retina has a $K_m$ of about 270 $\mu M$ (Nakazawa and Sano, 1974). Moreover, the kinetic properties of the soluble and particulate guanylate cyclases appear to be different. The soluble fraction apparently has a single $K_m$ value of 12 $\mu M$ for the enzyme from rat heart (Kimura and Nurad, 1974), and 65 $\mu M$ for the enzyme from rat lung (Chrisman *et al.,* 1975). The guanylate cyclase from the particulate fraction of both tissues had nonlinear kinetics, once more suggesting that this enzyme may exist in multiple forms.

The requirement of guanylate cyclase for both $Mn^{2+}$ and GTP has prompted an investigation of the interaction among ion, substrate, and enzyme (Kimura and Murad, 1974; Chrisman *et al.,* 1975). There are apparently two binding sites for $Mn^{2+}$ on both the soluble and particulate guanylate cyclases from rat heart (Kimura and Murad, 1974). In rat lung, an $Mn^{2+}$–GTP complex and free $Mn^{2+}$ were both required for activity (Chrisman *et al.,* 1975).

Apparently, guanylate cyclase can use only GTP as substrate, since ATP inhibits guanylate cyclase activity (Hardman and Sutherland, 1969; White and Aurbach, 1969; Thompson *et al.,* 1973a). Several other nucleotides are also inhibitory (Hardman and Sutherland, 1969; White and Aurbach, 1969).

#### *pH Optimum of Guanylate Cyclase*

The pH optimum for guanylate cyclase is about 7.4 to 8.0 (Hardman and Sutherland, 1969; White and Aurbach, 1969; Nakazawa and Sano, 1974; Kimura and Murad, 1974).

### E. Activation of Guanylate Cyclase

In contrast to adenylate cyclase, which can be stimulated by a wide variety of humoral and neurohumoral agents (see above), there is relatively little direct evidence that guanylate cyclase can be activated. However, recent studies suggest that, under the appropriate conditions, guanylate cyclase can be stimulated *in vitro,* and there is substantial evidence indicating that pharmacological and physiological agents can increase the tissue concentration of cyclic GMP. Thus, George *et al.* (1970) demonstrated that acetylcholine elevated cyclic GMP in the perfused rat heart, and Stoner *et al.* (1974) found that a variety of cholinergic agents increased the concentration of cyclic GMP in rat lung slices but did not activate guanylate cyclase. Similarly, although carbamylcholine increased cyclic GMP of rat liver (Thompson *et al.,* 1973a) and acetylcholine increased cyclic GMP of mouse epidermis (Marks, 1973), neither compound activated guanylate cyclase activity of these tissues. Other agents that have been examined for their effect on guanylate cyclase activity *in vitro* and have been found to have little or no effect include: glucagon (Hardman and Sutherland, 1969; Thompson *et al;* 1973a); epinephrine (Hardman and Sutherland, 1969); catecholamines, thyroxin, somatotropin, and epidermal chalones (Marks, 1973);

histamine (Sung *et al.,* 1973; Thompson *et al.,* 1973a); pentagastrin (Sung *et al.,* 1973); carbachol, insulin, hydrocortisone, methoxamine, and pancreozymin (Thompson *et al.,* 1973a); and serotonin (Marks, 1973; Thompson *et al.,* 1973a).

Thompson *et al.* (1973b), however, did find that secretin is capable of activating a supernatant fraction of guanylate cyclase of rat liver more than ten-fold. The maximum velocity of the enzyme was increased; no effect on its Michaelis constant was seen. In a more recent study, Thompson *et al.* (1974) found that secretin activated the guanylate cyclase of several other tissues, as well as one of three human islet cell carcinomas. In addition, Rudland *et al.* (1974) found that fibroblast growth factor activated a microsomal guanylate cyclase from fibroblasts but had no effect on a soluble fraction from these cells.

## F. Inhibition of Guanylate Cyclase

### 1. *Endogenous Factors*

One of the most interesting phenomena associated with guanylate cyclase is the ability of light to inhibit the enzyme in segments of retinal photoreceptors. Bensinger *et al.* (1974b) found that segments exposed to light had lower guanylate cyclase activity than segments kept in darkness, a result similar to that found earlier by Pannbacker (1973). This effect, however, is contradicted by the results of Goridis *et al.* (1973) who found that exposure of bovine retinas to light did not affect their guanylate cyclase activity. There is no apparent explanation for these differences. The effects of other endogenous agents, predominantly purine nucleotides, are discussed above.

### 2. *Exogenous Factors*

Because the exogenous factors that have been shown to inhibit guanylate cyclase *in vetro* are all highly reactive agents, they would be expected to inhibit a number of enzymes. Thus, alloxan inhibits the guanylate cyclase activity of rat lung (Keirns *et al.*, 1974b), and parachloromercuriphenylsulfonate inhibits the enzyme from rat liver, an effect that is reversed by dithiothreitol (Thompson *et al.*, 1973b), suggesting that this action is due to a nonspecific alteration of sulfhydryl groups. The involvement of sulfhydryl groups in the activity of guanylate cyclase is supported by the report that *N*-ethylmaleimide inhibits guanylate cyclase activity (Garbers and Hardman, 1975). Future investigations should be directed toward the search for more specific agents that inhibit guanylate cyclase activity.

### G. Conclusions

Relative to the information concerning adenylate cyclase, current knowledge of guanylate cyclase is limited. For example, it is unclear how the activity of this apparently soluble enzyme is altered by physiological agents. In fact, few of the physiological factors that act on guanylate cyclase have been identified. Recent investigations of more purified guanylate cyclases demonstrated the ability of cholinergic agents to increase the concentration of cyclic GMP and may provide a starting point for developing pharmacological means for controlling the activity of this enzyme and therefore, the means of regulating the intracellular concentration of its product.

## IV. Cyclic Nucleotide Phosphodiesterases

### A. Discovery and Characterization of Cyclic Nucleotide Phosphodiesterase

In 1957, Rall, Sutherland, and Berthet found that the activity of a heat-stable substance was rapidly lost during incubation with extracts of heart, liver, and brain. This factor, which was subsequently identified as cyclic AMP, was shown to be hydrolyzed to 5′-AMP by an enzyme found in the heart (Sutherland and Rall, 1958). Since these studies, this enzyme, cyclic nucleotide phosphodiesterase, has been extensively characterized by numerous investigators. The early work of Drummond and Perrot-Yee (1961) described its distribution in rabbit tissues, its cation dependence, and its substrate specificities. This work was confirmed and extended by Butcher and Sutherland (1962). A number of investigators have subsequently studied cyclic nucleotide phosphodiesterase, and their results are summarized below.

### B. Distribution of Cyclic Nucleotide Phosphodiesterase

#### 1. *Subcellular Distribution*

Cyclic AMP phosphodiesterase is found predominantly in the 100,000*g* supernatant fraction of mammalian cells (Nair, 1966; Weiss and Costa, 1968b; Menahan *et al.,* 1969; Jard and Bernard, 1970; Sams and Montague, 1972; Campbell and Oliver, 1972; Beavo *et al.,* 1970a; Sakai *et al.,* 1974; Fertel and Weiss, 1974). Its subcellular distribution apparently varies with the tissue studied. For example, there is a relatively high level of phosphodiesterase associated with the mitochondrial fraction of neural tissue, in particular with the synaptic elements (Weiss and

Costa, 1968b; Campbell and Oliver, 1972; DeRobertis *et al.*, 1967; Johnson *et al.*, 1973). In cardiac tissue, on the other hand, a high specific activity was found in the nuclear fraction (Nair, 1966; Campbell and Oliver, 1972; Beavo *et al.*, 1970a); the microsomal fraction has a uniformly low activity of phosphodiesterase. Beavo *et al.* (1970a) and Fertel and Weiss (1974) studied the distribution of cyclic GMP phosphodiesterase and found that it closely parallels that of the cyclic AMP phosphodiesterase. However, there is some evidence that the enzymes hydrolyzing cyclic AMP and cyclic GMP are not the same. For example, in cardiac tissue, cyclic AMP phosphodiesterase is higher in the nuclear fraction, and cyclic GMP phosphodiesterase is higher in the supernatant fraction (Beavo *et al.*, 1970a). In addition, Russell and Pastan (1973), using chick embryo fibroblasts, have found a cyclic AMP phosphodiesterase associated with the cell membrane and a cyclic GMP phosphodiesterase associated with the soluble fraction. Other investigators have also found evidence for the association of a low $K_m$, cyclic AMP phosphodiesterase with the cell membrane fraction (Amer and Mayol, 1973; Thompson and Appleman, 1971a; Thompson *et al.*, 1973c).

### 2. *Regional Distribution*

The distribution of phosphodiesterase in different tissues has been studied in several laboratories (Drummond and Perrot-Yee, 1961; Butcher and Sutherland, 1962; Campbell and Oliver, 1972; Beavo *et al.*, 1970a; Fertel and Weiss, 1974). It has been found in all tissues examined including blood (Hemington *et al.*, 1973) where most of the activity appears to be in the platelets (Song and Cheung, 1971). The distribution of cyclic GMP phosphodiesterase closely follows the distribution of cyclic AMP phosphodiesterase (Beavo *et al.*, 1970a; Fertel and Weiss, 1974). There is general agreement that the central nervous system and, particularly, the cerebral cortex, has the highest phosphodiesterase activity. Other areas of the brain, such as the hippocampus and caudate nucleus, also have relatively high activities, whereas the spinal cord has low activity (Weiss and Costa, 1968b; Breckenridge and Johnson, 1969; Williams *et al.*, 1969; Dalton *et al.*, 1974).

## C. Properties of Cyclic Nucleotide Phosphodiesterase

### 1. *pH Dependence*

The pH optimum for phosphodiesterase is between 7.5 and 9.0 (Drummond and Perrot-Yee, 1961; Nair, 1966; Menahan *et al.*, 1969;

Weiss *et al.*, 1972; Schroeder and Rickenberg, 1973; Cheung, 1971a; Szabo and Burke, 1972; Rosen, 1970a; Song and Cheung, 1971; Huang and Kemp, 1971; Goren and Rosen, 1972a; Rutten *et al.*, 1973).

### 2. *Ion Dependence*

Phosphodiesterase has an absolute requirement for $Mg^{2+}$, and under certain assay conditions calcium has been shown to be required for enzyme activity (Butcher and Sutherland, 1962; Kakiuchi *et al.*, 1971, 1972, 1973; Cheung, 1971a; Teo and Wang, 1973). For a detailed description of the effects of other divalent cations on phosphodiesterase activity, the reader should refer to the papers of Drummond and Perrot-Yee (1961), Nair (1966), Song and Cheung (1971), Cheung (1971a), Huang and Kemp (1971), Goren and Rosen (1972a), Kakiuchi *et al.* (1972), Teo and Wang (1973), and Fertel and Weiss (1974).

### 3. *Substrate Specificity*

Unpurified phosphodiesterase can hydrolyze not only cyclic AMP, but also cyclic GMP and a number of other cyclic nucleotides (Brooker *et al.*, 1968; Rosen, 1970a,b; Beavo *et al.*, 1970a; Thompson and Appleman, 1971b; Song and Cheung, 1971; Beavo *et al.*, 1970a; 1971a; Sung *et al.*, 1972; Klotz *et al.*, 1972; Campbell and Oliver, 1972; Szabo and Burke, 1972; Goren and Rosen, 1972a; Michal *et al.*, 1974; Harris *et al.*, 1973; Russell *et al.*, 1973; Amer and Mayol, 1973; Miller *et al.*, 1973a,b,c).

## D. Multiple Forms of Phosphodiesterase

Kinetic studies of phosphodiesterase activity in a number of tissues have suggested the existence of at least two forms of phosphodiesterase, one having a relatively high affinity (low $K_m$) for cyclic AMP and another having a low affinity (high $K_m$) (Senft *et al.*, 1968a; Brooker *et al.*, 1968; Jard and Bernard, 1970; Loten and Sneyd, 1970; Song and Cheung, 1971; Thompson and Appleman, 1971b; Szabo and Burke, 1972; Klotz *et al.*, 1972; Ashcroft *et al.*, 1972; Weiss *et al.*, 1972; Weiss and Strada, 1972; Sung *et al.*, 1972; Schonhofer *et al.*, 1972; Sams and Montague, 1972; Amer and Mayol, 1973; Weiss and Strada, 1973; Uzunov *et al.*, 1974; Strada *et al.*, 1974). An alternative possibility is that the two $K_m$'s may be an expression of one enzyme that has negative cooperativity (Russell *et al.*, 1972).

Chromatographic analysis of preparations containing phosphodiesterase activity indicate that there are a number of forms of phosphodiesterase which may, in fact, represent different enzymes. For example, Monn and Christiansen (1971) analyzed several different rat and rabbit tissues by starch gel electrophoresis and have identified seven different bands of cyclic AMP phosphodiesterase activity. Studies using polyacrylamide gel electrophoresis to separate the phosphodiesterase isoenzymes have demonstrated six forms of the enzyme in rat cerebellum (Uzunov and Weiss, 1972b; Strada *et al.*, 1974), four forms in rat (Uzunov *et al.*, 1974) and beef (Weiss, 1975b) cerebrum, and two forms in rat caudate nucleus (Fertel and Weiss, 1974). Other chromatographic analyses also indicate the existence of multiple forms of phosphodiesterase in a variety of tissues (Senft *et al.*, 1968a; Cheung, 1969; Jard and Bernard, 1970; Thompson and Appleman, 1971 a,b,c; Goren *et al.*, 1971; Hrapchak and Rasmussen, 1972; Klotz and Stock, 1972; Schroeder and Rickenberg, 1973; Hemington *et al.*, 1973; Pichard *et al.*, 1973; Kakiuchi *et al.*, 1972; Amer and Mayol, 1973; Russell *et al.*, 1973; Pledger *et al.*, 1974; Strada and Pledger, 1975).

### 1. *Tissue and Cellular Distribution*

Work from several different laboratories has now established that the pattern and ratio of the different molecular forms of phosphodiesterase are unique to each tissue and perhaps to each cell type. For example, studies of the phosphodiesterases of brain have shown that the cerebrum (Uzunov *et al.*, 1974) has a ratio of the multiple forms of cyclic AMP phosphodiesterases that differs markedly from that of the cerebellum (Uzunov and Weiss, 1972b) or caudate nucleus (Fertel and Weiss, 1974). Studies of cloned cell types grown in tissue culture showed that individual cells possess phosphodiesterases that are similar to those of whole brain but in an entirely different ratio and pattern. Thus, a C21 astrocytoma cell line had only two forms of cyclic AMP phosphodiesterase, corresponding to peaks I and IV of rat brain (Uzunov *et al.*, 1974); a C6 cell line, on the other hand, had three forms of phosphodiesterase (Uzunov *et al.*, 1974). Both of these astrocytoma cell lines had a very large Peak I phosphodiesterase, a peak that constitutes only a very small percentage of the total phosphodiesterase in rat brain. By contrast, clones of two different neuroblastoma cell lines showed only a single major form of phosphodiesterase, corresponding to Peak III of rat brain (Uzunov *et al.*, 1974.)

Figure 1 shows the electrophoretic pattern of cyclic AMP phosphodiesterase of rat pancreas. Two major peaks of activity were seen. Based on their electrophoretic mobility and their response to a series of

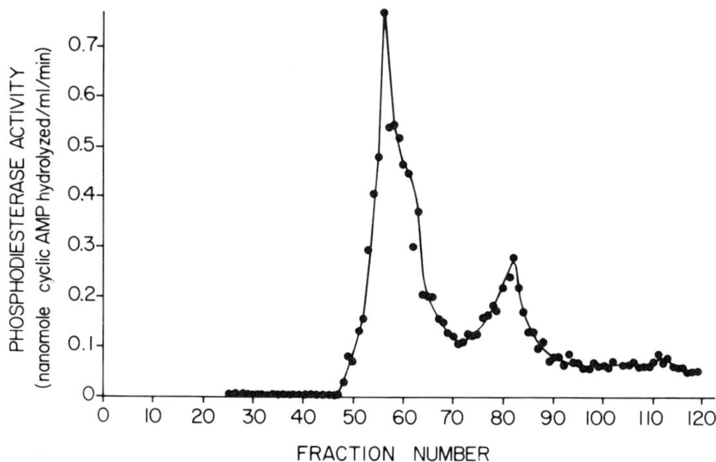


FIG. 1. Multiple forms of cyclic AMP phosphodiesterase of rat pancreas. A 250-gm male rat was decapitated, and the pancreas was rapidly removed, washed in buffer, and weighed. It was homogenized in 4 volumes of 0.32 *M* sucrose and centrifuged at 100,000*g* for 60 minutes. Two milliliters of the supernatant fraction were removed and placed on a preparative gel electrophoresis column, as described by Uzunov and Weiss (1972b). The eluted fractions were collected and analyzed for cyclic AMP phosphodiesterase activity by the method of Weiss *et al.* (1972) at a substrate concentration of 200 $\mu M$.

inhibitors and an activator, these peaks correspond to Peaks I and II of a similarly prepared rat cerebrum (Uzunov *et al.,* 1974).

These and other studies indicate that there are not only quantitative differences in the relative amounts or ratios of phosphodiesterase in each tissue and cell type but there may be qualitative differences in the patterns of the isoenzymes as well. Therefore, if one could selectively inhibit the activity of each of these forms of phosphodiesterase, one may be able to alter selectively the intracellular concentrations of cyclic AMP in discrete cells. This possibility is considered more fully in a subsequent section of this paper (p. 259).

## 2. *Properties of Phosphodiesterase Isozymes*

*a. Stability.* The chromatographically separated forms of phosphodiesterase have markedly different stabilities. Of the six peaks isolated from rat cerebellum, four lost 50% of their activity in 1 day or less, whereas the two remaining peaks retained most of their activity even after 7 to 14 days. The addition of bovine serum albumin increased the half-time for each of the less stable peaks to at least 10 days. Dithiothreitol stabilized one of the peaks of activity but labilized another form of the enzyme

(Uzunov and Weiss, 1972b; Uzunov *et al.,* 1974). Schroeder and Rickenberg (1973) also found that dithiothreitol or other reducing agents, as well as albumin, could stabilize the enzyme forms separated from bovine liver. Similarly, Hrapchak and Rasmussen (1972) found that dithiothreitol was necessary to maintain the activity of isozymes separated from beef heart. Jard and Bernard (1970) found that of the two phosphodiesterase isozymes from rat kidney and frog bladder, one was stable for long periods when stored at -20°C, whereas the other had a half-time of only 7 days. Kakiuchi *et al.* (1971) found that of two fractions separated from rat brain, one was very labile, losing 40% of its activity after 2 hours at 30°C. This fraction was also labile to freeze–thawing and storage at 4°C. Pichard *et al.* (1973) found that one of the phosphodiesterase components of human platelets was stable at 50°C, and one was labile under the same conditions. Finally, Goren and Rosen (1972a) found that both phosphodiesterase components isolated from beef heart were inactivated by heating at 55°C for 5 minutes.

The conclusions to be drawn from these studies are that most tissues contain both labile and stable phosphodiesterase isozymes and that bovine serum albumin and a sulfhydryl reagent appear to be stabilizing factors for most of the labile isozymes. The problem of the differential stability of the isoenzymes is extremely important and may account for some of the discrepancies in the studies of phosphodiesterase from different laboratories. Moreover, the possibility that the various enzyme forms are interconvertible (Chassy, 1972) compounds the complexity of studying the multiple forms of phosphodiesterase.

*b. Molecular Weights.* A number of laboratories have estimated the molecular weight of the phosphodiesterase isozymes. The results of these studies are as follows: Thompson and Appleman (1971a) separated the phosphodiesterase of several tissues of the rat and found three phosphodiesterase activities, one with a very high molecular weight and others with molecular weights of 200,000 and 400,000; Schroeder and Rickenberg (1973) found three fractions of phosphodiesterase in bovine liver, with molecular weights of 120,000, 240,000, and 360,000; Russell *et al.* (1973), on the other hand, found that in rat liver all three fractions had a molecular weight of 400,000; Hemington *et al.* (1973) found that cyclic AMP phosphodiesterase of rat plasma had a molecular weight of 500,000 and cyclic GMP phosphodiesterase had a molecular weight of 700,000, but cyclic AMP phosphodiesterase of erythrocytes had a molecular weight of 400,000 and cyclic GMP phosphodiesterase had a molecular weight of 200,000; Goren and Rosen (1972a) estimated molecular weights of 125,000 and 170,000 for the isozymes from bovine heart; Klotz and Stock (1972) found three peaks of phosphodiesterase in adipose tissue with molecular weights of >1 million, of 400,000 and of <400,000; Jard and Bernard (1970) estimated molecular weights of about 40,000 and 80,000 for isozymes separated from rat kidney and frog epithelium; and Hrapchak and Rasmussen (1972) calculated a molecular weight of about 120,000 for an isozyme obtained from beef heart.

The discrepancies between the reported molecular weights may result from several factors: (*1*) it is possible that the isozymes of different tissues have different molecular weights; (*2*) if the enzymes exist as multiple subunits, the method of isolation may cause dissociation of the subunits leading to spurious molecular weight determinations, and, in addition, the presence or absence of cations may affect subunit dissociation (Schroeder and Rickenberg, 1973); (*3*) different methods of determining molecular weight may lead to estimates that differ (Teo *et al.*, 1973).

*c. Kinetic Properties*. The kinetic properties of the phosphodiesterase isozymes are extremely complex. There are indications that in some preparations the phosphodiesterases may have more than one $K_m$ value. This tends to support the contention, first suggested by Thompson and Appleman (1971b) and advanced by Russell *et al.* (1972), that phosphodiesterase has negatively cooperative kinetics. However, in other studies (Uzunov *et al.*, 1974) it was shown that, for tissues with more than one form of phosphodiesterase, kinetic results indicated more than one form of the enzyme, whereas in tissue preparations (cloned neuroblastoma cells, for example) that contain only a single form of phosphodiesterase, linear kinetics were found. Uzunov *et al.* (1974) found that the purified phosphodiesterases gave kinetic evidence of a single form of phosphodiesterase in all cases. That certain purified preparations of phosphodiesterase show linear kinetics whereas others show evidence for both a high and low $K_m$ phosphodiesterase may be explained by the differences in purity of the enzyme preparations and the conditions of assay since these factors can have a significant effect on the kinetic measurements (Russell *et al.*, 1973).

Several investigators have compared the relative affinities of the phosphodiesterase isoenzymes for cyclic AMP and cyclic GMP. There is general agreement that in most tissues the phosphodiesterase hydrolyzing cyclic GMP has a lower $K_m$ for cyclic GMP than for cyclic AMP (see Amer and Kreighbaum, 1975).

*d. Ionic Requirements*. In general, the phosphodiesterase isozymes reflect the magnesium ion requirement of the homogenate phosphodiesterase (Schroeder and Rickenberg, 1973; Jard and Bernard, 1970; Goren and Rosen, 1972a; Kakiuchi *et al.*, 1972). However, there is a phosphodiesterase isozyme described by Kakiuchi *et al.* (1972), which is also dependent on calcium ion. This calcium activation occurs in only one of the phosphodiesterase isozymes isolated from rat brain and may be related to the phosphodiesterase activator fraction (see below). In confirmation of this, Uzunov and Weiss (1972b) found that the activity of a phosphodiesterase isozyme from rat brain which can be increased by the protein activator is also enhanced by calcium. Moreover, Teo *et al.* (1973) found that calcium is required for the increase in phosphodiesterase activity stimulated by the activator.

Goren and Rosen (1972a) found that a low molecular weight phosphodiesterase isozyme was inhibited by several divalent cations, including $Zn^{2+}$, $Fe^{2+}$, and $Cu^{2+}$.

The ability of the different molecular forms of phosphodiesterase to be selectively activated and inhibited are considered in the succeeding sections of this paper.

## E. Regulation of Phosphodiesterase Activity

### 1. *Stimulation of Phosphodiesterase Activity by Endogenous Mechanisms*

*a. Phosphodiesterase Development and Induction.* It has been established that, in general, the activity of phosphodiesterase in the rat brain increases as the animal reaches maturity (Weiss, 1971b; Weiss and Strada, 1973; Strada *et al.*, 1974) and decreases thereafter (Williams and Thompson, 1973; Gaballah and Popoff, 1971; Kauffman *et al.*, 1972; Dail and Palmer, 1972; Gengler and Forte, 1972; Forn *et al.*, 1970). Although the mechanism of the control of phosphodiesterase in development has not been established, the induction of phosphodiesterase in cell cultures has been demonstrated by several investigators.

Phosphodiesterase activity increases in HeLa and fibroblast cells that are contact-inhibited (Heidrick and Ryan, 1971; D'Armiento *et al.*, 1972). This correlates with the increased level of cyclic AMP in these cells (Otten *et al.*, 1972) and is probably a result of this increased intracellular concentration of cyclic AMP. In fact, there is also an increase in phosphodiesterase activity when these cells are treated with dibutyryl cyclic AMP. This increase is enhanced by the addition of a phosphodiesterase inhibitor and is completely blocked by protein synthesis inhibitors (D'Armiento *et al.*, 1972). A similar induction of phosphodiesterase has been shown for other fibroblast strains in which cyclic AMP levels are increased by prostaglandin $E_1$ (Manganiello and Vaughan, 1972b).

There is also evidence that a given stimulus may have a selective effect on the induction of specific phosphodiesterase isozymes. For example, Uzunov *et al.* (1973) found that norepinephrine, which increases cyclic AMP in astrocytoma cells (Clark and Perkins, 1971; Gilman and Nirenberg, 1971), increases only one of the two chromatographically separable molecular forms of cyclic AMP phosphodiesterase. This effect could be blocked by a $\beta$-adrenergic blocking agent or by an inhibitor of protein synthesis.

The induction of phosphodiesterase by cyclic AMP is probably mediated by a cyclic AMP-dependent protein kinase. Evidence for this is provided by experiments with two cultured lymphoma cell lines, one of which is deficient in cyclic AMP-activated protein kinase. Either isoproterenol (which stimulates cyclic AMP production in these cells) or dibutyryl cyclic AMP and theophylline can induce cyclic AMP phosphodiesterase formation in the cell line with the protein kinase, but not in the cell line without protein kinase (Bourne *et al.*, 1973b).

Cyclic AMP may activate phosphodiesterase on a short-term basis as well. Pawlson *et al.* (1974) found that increasing the concentration of cyclic AMP causes a rapid increase in the activity of a low $K_m$, particulate cyclic AMP phosphodiesterase of adipose cells.

Recently attempts have been made to explain the actions of certain hormones on the basis of changing either the activity or the actual amounts of specific phosphodiesterases. Van Inwegen *et al.* (1975) found that the adipose cells of hypothyroid rats have an increased activity of a low $K_m$ cyclic nucleotide phosphodiesterase. This activity returned to normal after treatment with triiodothyronine.

*b. The Endogenous Activator.* In the course of purifying cyclic AMP phosphodiesterase from bovine cerebra, Cheung (1970 a,b) found that the phosphodiesterase activity in a purified fraction had a lower specific activity than the less pure preparation. This suggested to him that there might be some factor in brain that increased the phosphodiesterase activity and was removed from the phosphodiesterase upon purification. This proved to be the case since adding this factor to the purified phosphodiesterase increased its activity. No preincubation with the factor was necessary for activation of the enzyme, and the degree of activation was proportional to the amount of factor added to the enzyme. This factor has subsequently been studied in a number of laboratories, and several of its characteristics (summarized in the following) have been elucidated (Kakiuchi *et al.*, 1970; Goren and Rosen, 1971; Uzunov and Weiss, 1972b; Teo *et al.*, 1973; Teo and Wang, 1973; Wolff and Brostrom, 1974; Lin *et al.*, 1974; Teshima and Kakiuchi, 1974; Strada *et al.*, 1974; Weiss *et al.*, 1974; Wickson *et al.*, 1975). (See also Fig. 2.)

*i. Heat stability.* Cheung (1970b) initially observed that the activating

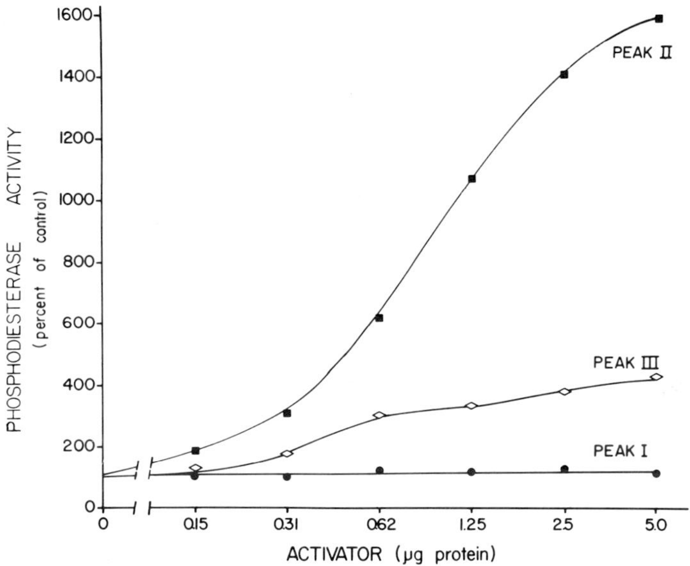


FIG. 2. Effect of phosphodiesterase activator on purified peaks of cyclic AMP phosphodiesterase of beef cerebrum. The soluble supernatant fraction of beef cerebral homogenates was subjected to polyacrylamide gel electrophoresis according to the procedure of Uzunov and Weiss (1972b), and the cyclic AMP phosphodiesterase activity was determined as described by Weiss *et al.* (1972). The activator was prepared as described by Cheung (1971b). (Data taken from Weiss, 1975b.)

factor was stable to boiling at low pH. Subsequent investigators have confirmed this observation (Kakiuchi *et al.*, 1970; Goren and Rosen, 1971; Uzunov and Weiss, 1972b; Wolff and Brostrom, 1974; Wickson *et al.*, 1975).

*ii. Molecular weight.* Cheung (1971b) initially estimated the molecular weight of the activator from bovine brain to be 40,000. Subsequent estimates from the same laboratory indicated a molecular weight of 15,000 (Lin *et al.*, 1974). Other laboratories have reported molecular weights varying from 11,500 to 28,000: Teshima and Kakiuchi found a molecular weight of 28,000 for the activator from rat cerebrum; Teo *et al.* (1973), using bovine heart, obtained molecular weight estimates of 19,200 or 17,000, depending on the method of determination; and Wolff and Siegel (1972) estimated the molecular weight of a calcium-binding protein from pig brain (later shown to be a phosphodiesterase activator) to be 11,500.

*iii. Distribution.* Smoake *et al.* (1974) examined the tissue and subcellular distribution of the activator and found that the amount of activator in a given tissue and the phosphodiesterase activity in that tissue did not always correspond. Moreover, they found that developmental changes of the activator in a given tissue do not change in proportion to the increase in phosphodiesterase activity: the activator generally shows much less of a change in specific activity during development. Their analysis of the subcellular distribution of phosphodiesterase and activator in parenchymal cells indicated that both are found primarily in the supernatant fraction and are distributed in an equivalent manner in the other subcellular fractions. The authors note that any parallel between activator and phosphodiesterase may be an artifact due to the preparation procedure. In addition, they state that the variable tissue ratio may be explained either on the basis of cellular heterogeneity or the existence of multiple forms of phosphodiesterase. Our own data favor this second possibility (see below).

Strada *et al.* (1974) isolated the activator from several areas of adult and neonatal rats and determined their effect on phosphodiesterase activity. They found that there was a significant difference in the activator isolated from several brain areas of newborn rats, but that this difference was not seen in the activator from adult rats. They concluded that the activator found in different brain areas may be formed at different rates during development.

More recent data from our laboratory indicate that there maybe tissues containing activator but little or no activatable phosphodiesterase (Fertel and Weiss, 1976; Hait and Weiss, 1976). For example, rat lung contains an activator fraction that is capable of stimulating the cyclic AMP phosphodiesterase from a supernatant fraction of rat cerebrum, but this same activator has little or no effect on phosphodiesterase activity of rat lung (Fig. 3). The activator isolated from rat cerebrum behaves in a similar fashion: it stimulates phosphodiesterase from cerebrum but not that from lung. The existence of a phosphodiesterase activator in a tissue that has no activatable enzymes suggests that the activator may have a function in cells other than that of activating phosphodiesterase. In fact, recent studies indicate that this activator of phosphodiesterase also increases the activity of adenylate cyclase (Brostrom *et al.*, 1975; Cheung *et al.*, 1975).

*iv. Ion requirements.* The relationship between the activator and calcium ions has been firmly established by a number of laboratories. The initial observation was by Kakiuchi and co-workers (Kakiuchi and Yamazaki, 1970; Kakiuchi *et al.*, 1971) who found a calcium ion-dependent phosphodiesterase. This calcium-stimulated phosphodiesterase may be similar to that found by Uzunov and Weiss (1972b) who showed that calcium stimulated only one of several phosphodiesterase

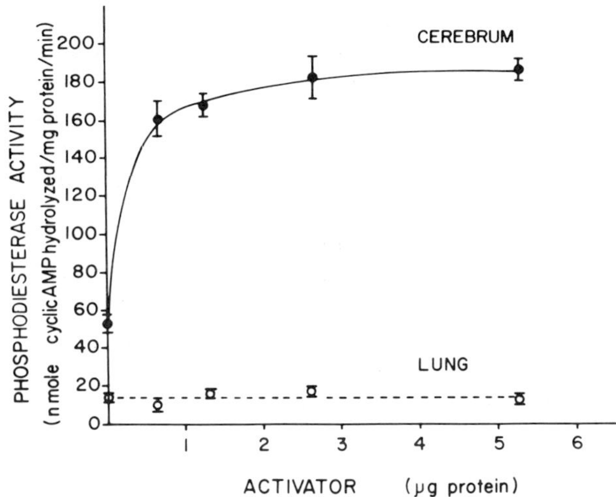


FIG. 3. Effect of activator on cyclic AMP phosphodiesterase activity of rat lung and rat cerebrum. The rat cerebrum and rat lung were homogenized in 0.32 *M* sucrose and centrifuged at 100,000*g* for 60 minutes. Cyclic AMP phosphodiesterase activity in the soluble supernatant fraction was determined as described by Weiss *et al.* (1972), using 400 $\mu M$ cyclic AMP as substrate, 40 $\mu M$ calcium, and varying quantities of a phosphodiesterase activator. The activator was prepared from lung according to Cheung (1971b). Each point represents the mean of five determinations; horizontal bars indicate the standard error. (Taken from Fertel and Weiss, 1976.)

isozymes found in rat cerebellum; this same form of phosphodiesterase was also activated by the heat-stable activator. Subsequent work by Kakiuchi *et al.* (1973) confirmed that the activity of a calcium-dependent phosphodiesterase isozyme is increased by activator.

Teo and Wang (1973) demonstrated that stimulation of bovine heart phosphodiesterase by an activator required low concentrations of calcium ion. Their binding studies indicated that the activator had two binding sites for calcium and gave half-maximal activation at a calcium ion concentration of 2.3 $\mu M$. On the basis of this work, they suggested that a $Ca^{2+}$–activator complex was the activator for cyclic AMP phosphodiesterase. A number of laboratories have subsequently studied the role of $Ca^{2+}$ in activation. Kakiuchi *et al.* (1973) demonstrated that at least 2 $\mu M$ $Ca^{2+}$ was necessary for activation of rat cerebral cortex phosphodiesterase, and Teshima and Kakiuchi (1974) showed that ethylene glycol bis($\beta$-aminoethyl ether)-*N*,*N'*-tetraacetic acid) (EGTA), which preferentially chelates calcium ions, inhibited activation. Teo and Wang (1973) showed that $Ca^{2+}$ was specifically bound at three or four sites to an activator fraction isolated from bovine brain, and a concentration of 2 $\mu M$ was necessary to give half-maximal activation. Wolff and Brostrom (1974) found half-maximal stimulation of an activator from pig brain at 4 $\mu M$ $Ca^{2+}$ and complete inhibition of activation by EGTA. More recently, Wickson *et al.* (1975) found stimulation of a phosphodiesterase from bovine cortex by an activator fraction and $Ca^{2+}$. This stimulation also was reversed by EGTA.

*v. Mechanism of activation.* Studies on the mechanism by which the activator–calcium complex enhances phosphodiesterase activity revealed the complexity of this interaction. Cheung (1971b) found, as did Goren and Rosen (1971), that the activator increased the $V_{max}$ and decreased the $K_m$ of bovine brain phosphodiesterase. By contrast, Weiss *et al.* (1974) found that activator increased the $V_{max}$ but not the $K_m$ of rat cerebrum. This result was supported by Wickson *et al.* (1975) who found that activator increased $V_{max}$ of cyclic GMP phosphodiesterase from bovine cerebrum but had no effect on the $K_m$ of the enzyme. The discrepancy in results of the effect of activator on the $K_m$ may be explained by the data of Teo *et al.* (1973), who found that at relatively low levels the activator increases the $V_{max}$ of phosphodiesterase, but does not affect the $K_m$. At higher levels, both the $K_m$ and $V_{max}$ are altered. However, it is apparent that the kinetic mechanism is dependent not only on substrate and activator concentrations but also on calcium concentrations. On this basis a kinetic model for the interaction between the phosphodiesterase and the enzyme–$Ca^{2+}$–activator complex has been devised (see Wickson *et al.*, 1975).

There are several possible temporal sequences by which the activator-calcium–phosphodiesterase complex can occur: an activator–phosphodiesterase complex can form which is then activated by calcium; a calcium–phosphodiesterase complex can form which is subsequently activated by the protein activator; or a Ca–activator complex can form which then binds to and activates the phosphodiesterase. Most of the evidence (Teo and Wang, 1973; Wolff and Brostrom, 1974) favors the hypothesis that calcium interacts first with the activator rather than with the phosphodiesterase. The activator–calcium complex then reacts with the phosphodiesterase causing the activation of the enzyme.

*vi. Effect of activator on phosphodiesterase isozymes.* Evidence that the activator has differential effects on the phosphodiesterase isoenzymes is well documented. Kakiuchi *et al.* (1971) separated the cyclic AMP phosphodiesterase of rat cerebral cortex on a Sepharose column, and found two peaks of activity, only one of which was stimulated by the activator fraction (Kakiuchi *et al.*, 1972). Other studies indicate that the activator exerts a differential effect on the isozymes of phosphodiesterase from several tissues. For example, activator stimulates only two peaks from adult (Uzunov and Weiss, 1972b) or newborn (Strada *et al.*, 1974) rat cerebellum and preferentially activates only one form of phosphodiesterase from rat cerebrum (Weiss *et al.*, 1974). It is tempting to speculate that the physiological role of the phosphodiesterase activator is based on this interaction with the specific isozymes of phosphodiesterase found in cells (see Fig 2 ).

*c. Other Activators. i. Insulin and glucagon.* Several lines of evidence suggests that insulin can activate a low $K_m$, membrane-bound cyclic AMP phosphodiesterase. Such an effect would be responsible for the decreases in cyclic AMP following the addition of insulin to adipose tissue (Butcher *et al*: 1968), liver (Jefferson *et al.*, 1968; Exton *et al.*, 1966), and cardiac muscle (Das and Chain, 1972). The initial studies, however, provided conflicting evidence for the possibility that insulin affected phosphodiesterase activity. Senft *et al.* (1968b), using 80 $\mu M$ cyclic AMP and the 1000 *g* supernatant fractions of rat liver, skeletal muscle, adipose tissue, and kidney, found that insulin increased phosphodiesterase activity of all but the kidney enzyme. By contrast, the phosphodiesterase of the 2000 *g* supernatant and sediment fraction of rat adipose tissue at high (500 $\mu M$) substrate concentration (Blecher *et al.*, 1968) and the 100,000 *g* supernatant phosphodiesterase of rat liver cells (Menahan *et al.*, 1969) were not activated by insulin. Subsequent workers have found that insulin stimulated the phosphodiesterase of adipose tissue homogenates at low substrate concentrations (Loten and Sneyd, 1970; Zinman and Hollenberg, 1974) and increased phosphodiesterase in membrane fractions of rat liver (House *et al.*, 1972; Thompson *et al.*, 1973c), skeletal muscle (Woo and Manery, 1973), and rat ventricle (Das, 1973). On the basis of this work, one can conclude that insulin probably stimulates a membrane-bound, low $K_m$ phosphodiesterase.

Recently, Allan and Sneyd (1975) presented evidence that glucagon activates a low $K_m$, cyclic AMP phosphodiesterase of rat hepatocytes. It is possible that this effect is caused by an increased concentration of cyclic AMP at the cell membrane which, in turn, activates phosphodiesterase (Pawlson *et al.*, 1974).

*ii. Cyclic GMP and other cyclic nucleotides.* Several investigators have recently demonstrated that cyclic GMP can stimulate the hydrolysis of cyclic AMP. Beavo *et al.* (1970a) found that cyclic GMP increased the activity of the cyclic AMP phosphodiesterase in a 20,000 *g* supernatant fraction of rat liver and in a subsequent publication (Beavo *et al.*, 1971a) demonstrated that 2 $\mu M$ cyclic GMP stimulated cyclic AMP phosphodiesterase (at substrate concentrations of 1 $\mu M$) in the 20,000*g* particulate fraction of liver, brain, heart, kidney, and thymus. Russell *et al.* (1973) observed a similar activation in a 100,000*g* supernatant fraction of rat liver. Other studies (Franks and MacManus, 1971) indicate that particulate cyclic AMP phosphodiesterase from thymic lymphocytes is maximally stimulated by 0.5–5 $\mu M$ cyclic GMP. Sakai *et al.* (1974) found that 0.2–2 $\mu M$ cyclic GMP stimulated hydrolysis of cyclic AMP (10 $\mu M$) by a soluble fraction of phosphodiesterase from rat adipose tissue but had no effect on the cyclic AMP phosphodiesterase in a particulate fraction.

The stimulation of cyclic AMP phosphodiesterase by cyclic GMP has been shown in partially purified phosphodiesterase preparations as well. Klotz and Stock (1972) separated a 100,000 *g* supernatant fraction of rat adipose tissue into three peaks of phosphodiesterase, all of which were stimulated by cyclic GMP, and Bevers *et al.* (1974) found that the high $K_m$ enzyme of rat liver was preferentially stimulated by cyclic GMP.

Both Beavo *et al.* (1971a) and Klotz and Stock (1972) found that cyclic IMP gave similar, but less potent, stimulation of cyclic AMP phosphodiesterase. In addition, Michal *et al.* (1974) found that a number of 8-substituted nucleotide analogs were able to activate cyclic AMP phosphodiesterase from several sources.

The mechanism by which cyclic GMP stimulates cyclic AMP phosphodiesterase and the physiological significance of these findings have not been established, but the effect is probably direct and not due to metabolites of the activating nucleotides (Klotz and Stock, 1972).

Although cyclic GMP can activate cyclic AMP phosphodiesterase, cyclic AMP is apparently unable to activate cyclic GMP phosphodiesterase (Klotz and Stock, 1972). Cyclic AMP and other nucleotides can, however, inhibit cyclic GMP phosphodiesterase. These effects are discussed in the following sections.

*iii. Naturally occurring lipids*. Bublitz (1973) studied a number of lipids for their effect on the activity of a soluble cyclic AMP phosphodiesterase obtained from rat brain. At low concentrations, lysolecithin, bovine lecithin, phosphatidylinositol, sphingomyelin, phosphatidylethanolamine, and phosphatidylserine all stimulated phosphodiesterase activity. These effects were not seen when several synthetic detergents were examined. The lipids even showed some specificity for the individual phosphodiesterases. Lysolecithin inhibited one peak of phosphodiesterase isolated from brain but stimulated both the cyclic AMP and cyclic GMP phosphodiesterase activity of the other two peaks. The mechanism by which these lipids stimulate or inhibit the phosphodiesterases is still unclear. It is worth noting that phospholipids have also been shown to stimulate adinylate cyclase activity (see Section II,A,1).

### 2. *Stimulation of Phosphodiesterase by Exogenous Agents*

Relatively few agents have been shown to stimulate the activity of phosphodiesterase. The first demonstration of such an activator was by Butcher and Sutherland (1962) who found that imidazole stimulated cyclic AMP phosphodiesterase of beef heart. A number of investigators have since confirmed this observation with other phosphodiesterase preparations (Cheung, 1971a; Ashcroft *et al.*, 1972; Amer and McKinney, 1972; Miki and Yoshida, 1972; McNeill *et al.*, 1972). The mechanism of this activation has not been established, but Huang and Kemp (1971) have shown that imidazole can increase the $V_{max}$ of phosphodiesterase from rabbit skeletal muscle. It also decreases the pH optimum of the enzyme.

Another group of agents that stimulate activity are the proteolytic enzymes. Cheung (1967) found that snake venom stimulated the activity of a partially purified phosphodiesterase from bovine brain. The factor in venom that caused stimulation was labile to heat and was not dialyzable. On the basis of subsequent studies (Cheung, 1969), the activating factor in venom was identified as a proteolytic enzyme. Such an effect on phosphodiesterase has also been shown for other proteolytic enzymes (Cheung, 1967; Cheung and Jenkins, 1969). By contrast, Russell and Pastan (1973) found that trypsin inhibits a cyclic AMP phosphodiesterase in the particulate fraction of chick embryo fibroblasts.

Several other miscellaneous factors have been shown to enhance phosphodiesterase activity: McNeill *et al.* (1972) found that high (10 m*M*) levels of histamine and a triazole derivative (3-amino-1,2,4-triazole) stimulated phosphodiesterase from rat brain; Amer and McKinney (1972) reported that cholecystokinin and other small polypeptides stimulated cyclic AMP phosphodiesterase from a number of rabbit tissues; Sullivan and Parker (1973) demonstrated that compound 48/80, a high molecular weight polyamine, stimulated a high $K_m$ phosphodiesterase from rat mast cells in a dose-dependent fashion; and Price (1973) has proposed that bitter taste stimuli enhance the phosphodiesterase activity of tongue epithelium. This last report has been disputed, however (Kurihara, 1972).

### 3. *Inhibition of Phosphodiesterase by Endogenous Factors*

*a. Product Inhibition.* The products of the cyclic AMP phosphodiesterase reaction are inorganic phosphate and 5′-AMP. Both have been reported to inhibit phosphodiesterase under certain conditions (Shimoyama *et al.*, 1972a; Gulyassy, 1971; Gulyassy and Oken, 1970). Metabolites of 5′-AMP, such as adenosine and adenine and naturally occurring adenine analogs, including ATP, ADP, and inosine, have also been found to inhibit phosphodiesterase activity (Cheung, 1966). In most instances the inhibitory effect may be attributed to the $Mg^{2+}$ chelating ability of these compounds, but the effect of adenosine is independent of $Mg^{2+}$ levels (Gulyassy, 1971; Cheung, 1966). In a comprehensive study of adipose tissue phosphodiesterase, Davies (1968) found that several naturally occurring nucleosides slightly inhibited phosphodiesterase activity.

*b. Other Endogenous Inhibitors.* Citrate and other carboxylic acids that are products of intermediate metabolism inhibit phosphodiesterase, probably through their metal chelating abilities (Cheung, 1967); pyrophosphate inhibits phosphodiesterase by a similar mechanism (Gulyassy, 1971; Cheung, 1966).

Shimoyama *et al.* (1972b) have reported that nicotinamide is a competitive inhibitor of cyclic AMP phosphodiesterase from rat liver. However, the concentrations required for significant inhibition are clearly nonphysiological. Nicotinic acid and NAD or NADP had little or no effect on the enzyme. The lack of effect of nicotinic acid was also reported by Therriault and Winters (1970).

Cyclic nucleotides such as cyclic GMP have also been shown to inhibit cyclic AMP phosphodiesterase, probably by competitively binding to a substrate site (Nair, 1966; Beavo *et al.*, 1970a; Rosen, 1970b; Song and Cheung, 1971; Franks and MacManus, 1971; Klotz and Stock, 1972). The effect of cyclic nucleotides and their analogs will be discussed in a subsequent section (p. 245).

### 4. *Inhibition of Phosphodiesterase by Exogenous Agents*

The effect of any inhibitor on a given enzyme system is usually expressed either as the dissociation constant of the inhibitor–enzyme complex ($K_i$) or as the concentration of inhibitor causing 50% inhibition of enzyme activity at a given substrate concentration ($I_{50}$). These two factors are equal only under certain kinetic conditions (Cheng and Prusoff, 1973). Since there is a differential distribution of phosphodiesterase isoenzymes according to tissue and cell type (Uzunov *et al.*, 1974) and since these isozymes have a differential response to inhibitors (Weiss *et al.*, 1974), a comparison of the effect of phosphodiesterase inhibitors based on studies using different phosphodiesterase sources is difficult. Moreover, many investigators have studied the effects of phosphodiesterase inhibitors in the presence of high concentrations of substrate. Under these assay conditions the total phosphodiesterase activity will reflect both the high $K_m$ and low $K_m$ enzyme. Having given this caveat, we will consider the structure–activity relationship of several classes of phosphodiesterase inhibitors, give comparable inhibitor potencies wherever possible, and discuss the differential inhibition of the phosphodiesterase isozymes.

*a. Structural Classes. i. Xanthine analogs.* Analogs of xanthine were the first pharmacological agents found to inhibit phosphodiesterase (Butcher and Sutherland, 1962). In order of decreasing inhibitory activity, they were theophylline (1,3-dimethylxanthine), caffeine (1,3,7-trimethylxanthine), and theobromine (3,7-dimethylxanthine). Although other xanthine derivatives have been found to be more potent phosphodiesterase inhibitors, theophylline has been the most widely used xanthine analog. The information obtained by using theophylline as a phosphodiesterase inhibitor is valuable because theophylline is the only inhibitory agent whose use is common to phosphodiesterases isolated from a wide variety of tissue sources. However, it should be noted that there is substantial evidence suggesting that the physiological effect of theophylline may be due to properties other than its ability to inhibit phosphodiesterase. For example, the effect of theophylline on the contractile force of cardiac muscle can be explained, in part, by its effects on $Ca^{2+}$ levels in the cell (McNeill *et al.*, 1969), and the potent lipolytic effect of theophylline (Vaughan and Steinberg, 1963; Weiss *et al.*, 1966) has been separated, to some extent, from its ability to inhibit adipose tissue phosphodiesterase (Dalton *et al.*, 1970; Allen *et al.*, 1973). Therefore, although some of the pharmacological actions of phosphodiesterase inhibitors may be explained by their ability to inhibit phosphodiesterase activity (Weinryb *et al.*, 1972), other biochemical effects of these agents should not be ignored.

In a study of a series of xanthine analogs, Beavo *et al.* (1970b, 1971b) found a fair correlation between the ability of these agents to inhibit phosphodiesterase and their lipolytic activity. As the authors point out, however, this close correlation between phosphodiesterase inhibition and lipolysis may have been caused by other factors.

Goodsell *et al.* (1971) tested a series of 8-substituted theophylline derivatives for their effect on beef heart phosphodiesterase. On the basis of the relationship that they found between the structure of these compounds and their phosphodiesterase inhibitory activity, they concluded that the partition coefficient of the compounds may be an important factor in their effects on phosphodiesterase. Mizon *et al.* (1971) studied the inhibitory effects of several theophylline analogs on bovine brain phosphodiesterase and found that most of these compounds were less effective inhibitors than theophylline itself. On the other hand, Goren and Rosen (1972b) studied several xanthine analogs, including theophylline, for their effect on partially purified, bovine heart phosphodiesterase and found that certain substitutions enhanced phosphodiesterase inhibitory activity. The addition of alkyl groups at the 1 and 3 positions led to increased phosphodiesterase inhibition, the amount of inhibition increasing as substituent size increased. They also found that an ethyl group at N-7 further increased the potency of N-1, N-3 disubstituted xanthines. On the basis of these studies, they concluded that the addition of alkyl groups at positions 1,3, and 8 may enhance inhibitory activity, whereas substitution at position 7 alone may decrease the activity of xanthine analogs.

*ii. Papaverine and its analogs.* Muscle relaxation is associated with an increase in the concentration of cyclic AMP (Bueding and Bulbring, 1964) and can be induced with exogenously added dibutyryl cyclic AMP (Moore *et al.,* 1968). Therefore, it was not surprising to find that papaverine and other muscle relaxants inhibited cyclic AMP phosphodiesterase activity of myocardium, coronary arteries (Kukovetz *et al.,* 1969a,b; Kukovetz and Poch, 1970; Poch and Kukovetz, 1972; Hanna *et al.,* 1972; Lugnier *et al.,* 1972; Toson and Carpenedo, 1972), other smooth muscle (Triner *et al.,* 1970), and other tissue such as platelets (Markwardt and Hoffman, 1970; Vigdahl *et al.,* 1971) and rat ventricles (Lugnier and Stoclet, 1974). Papaverine also inhibits the phosphodiesterase activity of a variety of other tissues (Poch and Kukovetz, 1971). In these systems, papaverine and its derivatives were consistently more potent inhibitors of phosphodiesterase than theophylline. For example, on the basis of their $K_i$ values, papaverine is 10 times more potent (23 vs 230 $\mu M$) an inhibitor of beef heart phosphodiesterase (Kukovetz and Poch, 1970), 20 times more potent (6 vs 130 $\mu M$) an inhibitor of coronary artery phosphodiesterase (Poch, 1971), 15 times more potent an inhibitor of rat aorta phosphodiesterase (Lugnier *et al.,* 1972), and 10 times more potent an inhibitor of rat lung phosphodiesterase (Fertel and Weiss, 1976) than theophylline. A number of papaverine analogs are also more potent than theophylline (Lugnier *et al.,* 1972; Kukovetz and Poch, 1970).

Knowledge of the structure–activity relationships for this series of compounds is limited. However, based on the inhibition of beef heart phosphodiesterase by a number of papaverine analogs, Hanna *et al.* (1972) have concluded that (*a*) methoxy or ethoxy groups are important for inhibition, (*b*) the 6- and 7-position substituents are apparently more important than the 3′,4′-positions, (*c*) the dimethoxy isoquinoline moiety itself has some inhibitory action, and (*d*) in general, reduction of the isoquinoline ring leads to decreased activity. Thus, 1-benzylisoquinoline, or papaverine with no methoxy groups, had no activity under the test conditions, which is a result similar to that found by Belpaire and Bogaert (1973). Furlanut *et al.* (1973) have also studied the effects of a number of isoquinoline compounds and their derivatives on cyclic AMP phosphodiesterase activity of guinea pig brain. Their findings indicate that isoquinoline compounds and pyridylmethylisoquinoline derivatives are ineffective at concentrations up to 10 m*M*, but that the benzylisoquinoline derivatives (such as papaverine) are effective inhibitors at concentrations three orders of magnitude lower. Their observation that dihydrogenation of papaverine (3,4-dihydropapaverine) leads to complete loss of activity is in agreement with the study of Hanna *et al.* (1972).

In summary, a nonhydrogenated isoquinoline ring structure with ether groups at 6,7 positions is required for phosphodiesterase inhibition, and substitution with a benzene ring at the C-1 position leads to an enhanced activity.

*iii. Cyclic nucleotides and their analogs.* The effects of the naturally occurring cyclic nucleotide, cyclic GMP, on cyclic AMP phosphodiesterase have been studied extensively. Following the demonstration that cyclic GMP is present in mammalian urine and tissues (Goldberg *et al.*, 1969; Ishikawa *et al.*, 1969; Hardman *et al.*, 1966), the possibility was raised that one biochemical role of cyclic GMP might be to regulate the intracellular concentration of cyclic AMP. One mechanism by which cyclic GMP could control cyclic AMP is by stimulating cyclic AMP phosphodiesterase, a possibility discussed previously. In addition, a number of investigators have demonstrated that cyclic GMP is a potent inhibitor of cyclic AMP phosphodiesterase, with a $K_i$ of 0.53–40 $\mu M$, depending on the tissue source and method of preparing the phosphodiesterase (Beavo *et al.*, 1970a; Rosen, 1970a,b; Murad *et al.*, 1970; Thompson and Appleman, 1971b; O'Dea *et al.*, 1971; Franks and MacManus, 1971; Goren and Rosen, 1971, 1972a; Klotz *et al.*, 1972; Ashcroft *et al.*, 1972; Klotz and Stock, 1972; Harris *et al.*, 1973; Russell *et al.*, 1973; Michal *et al.*, 1974).

Cyclic GMP phosphodiesterase is inhibited by cyclic AMP in some systems (Beavo *et al.*, 1970a; Russell *et al.*, 1973; Thompson and Appleman, 1971b; O'Dea *et al.*, 1971; Miller *et al.*, 1973b) but not in others (Rosen, 1970b). In general, cyclic GMP is a better inhibitor of the cyclic AMP phosphodiesterase from a given tissue than is cyclic AMP an inhibitor of the cyclic GMP phosphodiesterase.

Another unmodified cyclic nucleotide that has been shown to inhibit phosphodiesterase is cyclic inosine monophosphate (IMP), which, like cyclic AMP and cyclic GMP, has a purine nucleus. Although it is generally a less potent inhibitor of cyclic AMP phosphodiesterase than is cyclic GMP, it is still quite effective, with $K_i$ values ranging from 1.8 to 940 $\mu M$, depending on the tissue source (Rosen, 1970b; Beavo *et al.*, 1971a; Song and Cheung, 1970; Szabo and Burke, 1972; Goren and Rosen, 1972a; Klotz and Stock, 1972; Harris *et al.*, 1973; Shuman *et al.*, 1973). Cyclic xanthosine monophosphate (XMP) may also have a slight inhibitory effect on phlsphodiesterase (Miller *et al.*, 1973b; Rosen, 1970a).

In contrast to the purine cyclic nucleotides, the pyrimidine cyclic nucleotides [cyclic uridine monophosphate (UMP), cyclic cytidine monophosphate (CNP), cyclic thymidine monophosphate (TMP), and their analogs] have little or no effect on cyclic AMP phosphodiesterase (Rosen, 1970b; Song and Cheung, 1971; Beavo *et al.*, 1971a; Szabo and Burke, 1972; Goren and Rosen, 1972a; Klotz and Stock, 1972; Harris *et al.*, 1973; Miller *et al.*, 1973b).

Although a large number of substituted derivatives of cyclic AMP and other cyclic nucleotides have been synthesized (Posternak and Cehovic, 1971; Posternak, 1974), only a few laboratories have investigated the effect of these analogs on cyclic AMP phosphodiesterase.

*Dibutyryl cyclic AMP.* $N^6$-2′-*O*-Dibutyryl cyclic AMP has been the most extensively studied analog of cyclic AMP. It has been widely used to simulate the action of cyclic AMP in experimental systems, presumably because it is transported through the cell membrane, whereas cyclic AMP itself is not. Although the mechanism of action of dibutyryl cyclic AMP is unknown, it is clearly capable of inhibiting cyclic AMP phosphodiesterase (Cheung, 1970b; Heersche *et al.*, 1971; Szabo and Burke, 1972; Harris *et al.*, 1973; Anisuzzaman *et al.*, 1973; Miller *et al.*, 1973a). In some tissues, dibutyryl cyclic AMP is a more potent inhibitor of phosphodiesterase than theophylline (Miller *et al.*, 1973a). Dibutyryl cyclic AMP can be hydrolyzed to one of two monobutyryl derivatives, $N^Y$-butyryl cyclic AMP or 2′-*O*-butyryl cyclic AMP. Of the two products, $N^6$-butyryl cyclic AMP is less susceptible to hydrolysis by phosphodiesterase and is a better stimulator of protein kinase (Miller *et al.*, 1973a; Neelon and Birch, 1973). However, both of these derivatives are better inhibitors of cyclic AMP phosphodiesterase than dibutyryl cyclic AMP itself (Szabo and Burke, 1972; Miller *et al.*, 1973a). It is probable, therefore, that the pharmacological effects of dibutyryl cyclic AMP are a result of the actions of the monobutyryl derivatives as well as of the parent molecule.

*2′ Derivatives.* Miller *et al.* (1973c) studied the effects of several 2′ derivatives of cyclic AMP on phosphodiesterase activity and found that 2′-substituted derivatives and 2′-deoxy cyclic AMP were good substrates as well as good inhibitors of cyclic AMP phosphodiesterase. Rabbit lung and beef heart enzymes were inhibited to a greater extent by the less bulky 2′-*O* substituents, whereas beef brain and rabbit kidney were inhibited to a greater extent by the bulkier substituents. In general, the 2′-substituted derivatives were better enzyme inhibitors than theophylline at both high and low substrate levels. The ability to inhibit phosphodiesterase did not always correlate with the ability to act as a substrate for phosphodiesterase. Thus, $N^6$-2′-*O*-dibutyryl cyclic AMP and 2′-*O*-(2,4-dinitrophenyl) cyclic AMP were poor substrates but good inhibitors, whereas 2′-deoxy cyclic AMP was a good substrate but a poor inhibitor of cyclic AMP phosphodiesterase.

*4′-Thio derivatives.* Anisuzzaman *et al.* (1973), using beef heart phosphodiesterase, showed that substitution of cyclic AMP, $N^6$-2′-*O*-dibutyryl cyclic AMP, or $N^6$-(*n*-butyl) cyclic AMP to form their 4′-thioether derivatives produced compounds that inhibited the hydrolysis of cyclic AMP. 4′-Cyclic AMP probably prevented cyclic AMP hydrolysis by serving as an alternate substrate with equivalent binding to phosphodiesterase, but the other two analogs were not well hydrolyzed by phosphodiesterase.

*5′-Thiophosphates.* A study of 5′-thio cyclic IMP and 5′-thio cyclic AMP on phosphodiesterase activity of a variety of tissues showed that these compounds had a wide range of inhibitory activity toward the phosphodiesterases but were more potent than theophylline in each case (Shuman *et al.*, 1973). The $K_i$ value for 5′-thio cyclic AMP was 3.5 $\mu M$ for rabbit lung and 15 $\mu M$ for beef heart phosphodiesterase. By contrast, 5′-thio cyclic IMP had a $K_i$ value of 120 $\mu M$ for rabbit lung and 2.6 $\mu M$ for beef heart phosphodiesterase. 5′-Thio cyclic AMP was a substrate for phosphodiesterase, but 5′-thio cyclic IMP was not; both derivatives were competitive inhibitors of phosphodiesterase. The authors concluded that the $N^6$-amino and 5′-oxygen of cyclic AMP are necessary for the hydrolysis by phosphodiesterase but not for the binding to the phosphodiesterase molecule.

*7-Substituted derivatives of cyclic AMP.* Miller *et al.* (1973a) substituted carbon for the nitrogen in the 7-position of cyclic AMP to form tubercidin 3′,5′-cyclic phosphate, and substituted either a cyanide (CN) to form toyocamycin 3′,5′-cyclic phosphate or a carbamyl ($CHNH_2$) to form sangivimycin 3′,5′-cyclic phosphate. The corresponding nucleotides, nucleosides, and free bases were also synthesized. The three cyclic phosphates were all good inhibitors of phosphodiesterase from rabbit lung and beef heart, with $I_{50}$ values from 2 to 20 $\mu M$. Their nucleotides and nucleosides were much less effective, with $I_{50}$ values from 170 $\mu M$ to more than 2 m*M*. However, the heterocyclic bases, especially toyocamycin and sangivimycin, were good inhibitors, with $I_{50}$

values between 10 and 60 $\mu M$. The cyclic nucleotides were competitive inhibitors, and the heterocyclic bases show mixed inhibition. In a prior study, Blecher *et al.* (1971) found that tubercidin was a mixed inhibitor of rat epididymal adipose tissue phosphodiesterase.

*8-Substituted derivatives of cyclic AMP.* In a study of a number of 8-substituted cyclic AMP derivatives on phosphodiesterase from cat heart and rat brain, Harris *et al.* (1973) found that, in general, the cat heart phosphodiesterase was more sensitive to inhibition than was the rat brain. The most effective inhibitors examined were those with a sulfur substituent at C-8. With few exceptions, the potency of these compounds as inhibitors of both enzymes increased as the size of the side chain increased. However, as the length of the *N*-substituted side chain increased, the inhibition of phosphodiesterase decreased. Derivatives with a nitrogen-containing substitution were less potent than the sulfur-containing derivatives. 8-Bromo cyclic AMP was a potent competitive inhibitor of both phosphodiesterases, with a $K_i$ value of 20 $\mu M$ for cat heart phosphodiesterase. Muneyama *et al.* (1971) also reported that the 8-substituted cyclic AMP analogs were potent inhibitors of phosphodiesterase and found, in addition, that they were capable of activating bovine brain protein kinase.

Miller *et al.* (1973b) have reported extensive studies with several 8-substituted cyclic nucleotides, including cyclic AMP, cyclic GMP, cyclic IMP, and cyclic XMP. They found that, with the exception of 8-amino cyclic AMP, all the 8-substituted cyclic nucleotide derivatives were not good substrates of rabbit lung or beef heart phosphodiesterase. The hydrolysis of cyclic GMP was preferentially inhibited by cyclic AMP and cyclic IMP derivatives with aromatic groups in the 8 position, although these compounds were not potent inhibitors of cyclic AMP phosphodiesterase. Their results agree with those of Harris *et al.* (1973) in that the sulfur-containing substituents are more potent inhibitors than the nitrogen-containing substituents and an increase in the size of the substituent groups leads to an increase in inhibitory effect. In contrast to the results of Harris *et al.*, however, there is apparently no decrease in potency as the length of the N-substituent chain increases. This discrepancy may be explained by the difference in the source of phosphodiesterase.

Michal *et al.* (1974) studied a wide variety of 8-substituted cyclic nucleotide analogs for their effect on beef heart phosphodiesterase. They found that among the best inhibitors of phosphodiesterase were 8-bromo, 8-methylmercapto, and 8-benzylamino cyclic AMP, 8-bromo and 8-benzylamino cyclic IMP, and 8-bromo, 8-mercapto, and 8-methylmercapto cyclic GMP.

*Other analogs.* Several 5′ derivatives of cyclic AMP were examined as inhibitors of cyclic AMP phosphodiesterase of *Dictyostelium* (Malchow *et al.,* 1973). The 5′-NH cyclic AMP derivative was the most potent inhibitor, followed by 5′-$CH_2$ cyclic AMP, 5′-$NCH_3$ cyclic AMP, and 5′-*N*-$C_8H_{17}$ cyclic AMP. The 3′-$CH_2$ cyclic AMP was the least potent analog examined. They also concluded that 6-substituted derivatives of cyclic AMP were more potent inhibitors than the 8-substituted derivatives.

In a study of purine nucleotide derivatives, Michal *et al.* (1974) reported that 6-piperidinopurine riboside-3′5′-cyclophosphate and 6-(4-methylbenzylamino)purine riboside-3′,5′-cyclophosphate inhibited the phosphodiesterase of beef heart.

The cytokinins, a group of naturally occurring $N^6$-substituted purine derivatives that promote cell growth and division in plants (Skoog *et al.,* 1965), have been shown to be competitive inhibitors of the high (200 $\mu M$) $K_m$ cyclic AMP phosphodiesterase of beef heart (Hecht *et al.,* 1974).

*iv. Imidazolidinone derivatives.* Several investigators (Sheppard and Wiggan, 1971; Sheppard *et al.,* 1972; Pettinger *et al.,* 1973) have examined the structure–activity relationship of substituted 2-imidazolidinones as inhibitors of phosphodiesterase from rat erythrocyte. The parent compound of the series studied was 4-(3,4-dimethoxybenzyl) 2-imidazolidinone. An increase in the size of the alkyl group attached to the oxygen at the 3-position increased the potency of these compounds, whereas an increase in the size of the alkyl group attached to the oxygen at the 4-position decreased the inhibitory effect. The absence of alkyl groups resulted in a completely inactive compound. The most potent inhibitor was the 3-butoxy-4-methoxy derivative (RO-20-1724). These compounds were much less effective against the phosphodiesterase from other tissue sources, including that from several arteries and veins of the dog and dog cerebral cortex.

*v. Pyrazolo and pyridine derivatives.* Chasin *et al.* (1972) demonstrated that 1-ethyl-4-(isopropylidene hydrazino)-1*H*-pyrazolo-(3,4-6)-pyridine-5-carboxylic acid, ethyl ester, hydrochloride (SQ 20009) was capable of inhibiting phosphodiesterase from several tissue sources. They showed that, at a substrate concentration of 0.17 $\mu M$, this agent was a competitive inhibitor of rat brain phosphodiesterase with an $I_{50}$ of 2$\mu M$. By comparison, theophylline had an $I_{50}$ of 120 $\mu M$ under the same conditions. The $K_i$ for cyclic GMP phosphodiesterase in this tissue was 24 $\mu M$. However, the compound was a noncompetitive inhibitor of cat heart cyclic AMP phosphodiesterase, with a $K_i$ value of 64 $\mu M$. It was also a noncompetitive inhibitor of cyclic GMP phosphodiesterase of cat heart, with a $K_i$ of 30 $\mu M$; by contrast, cyclic AMP phosphodiesterase of beef heart was competitively inhibited with a $K_i$ of 95 $\mu M$.

*vi. Substituted imidazopyrazines.* The effect of substituted imidazopyrazines on cyclic AMP phosphodiesterase from several tissue sources was studied by Mandel (1971) who showed that 5-chloro-6-(ethylamino)-1,3-dihydro-2*H*-imidazo-(4,5-*b*)-pyrazin-2-one (CEIP) was a potent competitive inhibitor of phosphodiesterase from bovine heart or pancreas, rabbit uterus, and rat heart or lung.

*vii. Substituted pyrroles, triazines, and pyridazines.* Kupiecki (1973) reported that three lipolytic agents, 2,5-bis-(2-chlorethyl-1-sulfonyl)pyrrole-3,4-dicarbonitrile, 2,4-diamino-6-butoxy-3-triazine, and 2,3-dihydro-5,6-dimethyl-3-oxo-4-pyridazine carbonitrile, all inhibited phosphodiesterase activity of rat epididymal fat pad.

*viii. Substituted quinazolines.* Amer and Browder (1970) found that quazodine (6,7-dimethoxy-4-ethyl quinazoline) noncompetitively inhibited cyclic AMP phosphodiesterase from a variety of sources. The $K_i$ values ranged from 118 $\mu M$ for bovine brain to 1.54 $\mu M$ for rabbit spleen. In all cases it was a more effective inhibitor than theophylline.

*ix. Imidazoline derivatives.* The imidazoline derivatives, phentolamine and tolazoline, inhibited cyclic AMP phosphodiesterase activity of rat brain (McNeill *et al.*, 1972), but fairly high concentrations, particularly of tolazoline, were required to demonstrate this effect.

*x. Semicarbazones.* Webb *et al.* (1974) have found that *N*-methylisatin $\beta$-semicarbazone (Me-IBT), an inhibitor of viral replication, was capable of raising the level of cyclic AMP in human peripheral blood lymphocytes. This effect apparently was due to inhibition of the cyclic AMP phosphodiesterase of these cells by Me-IBT and not to the semicarbazide portion of the Me-IBT molecule. A particularly intriguing finding was that the Me-IBT had no effect on phosphodiesterase activity of mouse lymphoma cells.

*xi. Phenethylamines.* Epinephrine and other 3,4-dihydroxyphenylethylamines are noncompetitive inhibitors of cyclic AMP and cyclic GMP phosphodiesterase of beef heart (Goren and Rosen, 1972b). Although nitrogen and $\beta$-carbon substituents could be changed without altering inhibitory activity, modification of the 3,4-dihydroxyphenyl moiety decreased the inhibitory effects. The amine moiety was not absolutely required for the inhibitory effects, but it did enhance the inhibitory potency. Alpha- and beta-blocking agents had no effect on phosphodiesterase activity and did not affect the inhibition of phosphodiesterase induced by the catecholamines.

A study of the effect of adrenergic agents on cyclic AMP phosphodiesterase from guinea pig lung (Hitchcock, 1973) showed that isoproterenol and epinephrine were equipotent inhibitors of the high $K_m$ enzyme, followed in potency by norepinephrine and methoxamine. Only norepinephrine inhibited the low $K_m$ enzyme. Butoxamine, propranolol, and phentolamine had no effect on the high $K_m$ enzyme, and propranolol did not reverse the inhibitory effect of isoproterenol and epinephrine. Phentolamine did not alter inhibition by epinephrine hydrochloride but did reverse the inhibition due to epinephrine bitartrate.

*xii. Ergot alkaloids and lysergic acid derivatives.* Poch and Kukovetz, in 1969, reported that bromolysergic acid inhibited the phosphodiesterase of guinea pig heart. Subsequent work by Iwangoff and Enz (1971, 1972) demonstrated inhibition of cat brain phosphodiesterase by dihydroergotamine analogs. The inhibitory potency of these compounds was of the same order of magnitude as theophylline. These agents evidenced some specificity in that they were more effective in inhibiting phosphodiesterase of brain than that of heart, lung, liver, or kidney (Iwangoff and Enz, 1973). Dihydroergotamine also has been reported to inhibit phosphodiesterase of fat cells (Ward and Fain, 1971).

*xiii. Reserpine and reserpine analogs.* Reserpine and its diethylamino analog were reported to inhibit phosphodiesterase activity of brain (Honda and Imamura, 1968). In a more recent study, Beer *et al.* (1972) showed that not only reserpine but a wide variety of centrally active agents also inhibited phosphodiesterase of brain.

*xiv. Phenothiazines.* Honda and Imamura (1968) reported that certain phenothiazine derivatives inhibited the cyclic AMP phosphodiesterase of beef heart and rabbit cerebral cortex. Substitution of a halogen atom in the 2-position of the phenothiazines increased their activity. In their system, theophylline was a competitive inhibitor of both brain and heart phosphodiesterase, with a $K_i$ of 110 $\mu M$, and perphenazine was noncompetitive, with a $K_i$ of 20 $\mu M$. In agreement with this, Horlington and Watson (1970) found that promethazine had 3 times the potency of theophylline as an inhibitor of beef heart phosphodiesterase, and chlorpromazine had 6 times the effect. Beer *et al.* (1972) found that the major tranquilizers, including reserpine and the phenothiazines, inhibited rat brain phosphodiesterase and Berndt and Schwabe (1973) found that chlorpromazine, triflupromazine, and chlorprothixene were noncompetitive inhibitors of rat brain phosphodiesterase, with $K_i$ values of 80, 130, and 170 $\mu M$, respectively.

Our own studies on the influence of phenothiazine derivatives on phosphodiesterase activity of brain (Uzunov and Weiss, 1971, 1972a; Weiss *et al.*, 1974; Weiss, 1975b) showed that trifluoperazine is a potent inhibitor of rat brain phosphodiesterase with a $K_i$ value of 10 $\mu M$ (Peak II; activated) compared to a $K_i$ value of 350 $\mu M$ for theophylline. Its metabolite, trifluoperazine sulfoxide, and the antihistaminic phenothiazine, promethazine, which have little central psychotropic activity, were both less effective inhibitors of rat brain phosphodiesterase (Weiss *et al.*, 1974).

*xv. Benzodiazepines.* In addition to the centrally active phenothiazine derivatives, several benzodiazepines were also shown to inhibit cyclic AMP phosphodiesterase of rat brain (Beer *et al.* 1972) and beef brain (Levin and Weiss, 1976). Diazepam was found to be more potent than chlordiazepoxide. Dalton *et al.* (1974) in a study of the effects of a series of benzodiazepines on the cyclic AMP phosphodiesterase of several areas of cat brain found that, although the effects varied with tissue area, diazepam was, in general, the most potent agent, followed by *N*-methyl oxazepam, *N*-dimethyl diazepam, chlordiazepoxide, and oxazepam.

*xvi. Dibenzazepines.* The possibility that the tricyclic antidepressants could inhibit phosphodiesterase was first suggested by Abdallah and Hamadah (1970), Ramsden (1970), and McNeill and Muschek (1970). Subsequently, Muschek and McNeill (1971) studied a series of dibenzazepines for their effect on cyclic AMP phosphodiesterase of rat brain. They found that all of the agents were more potent inhibitors than theophylline. Other studies confirmed the observation that dibenzazepines can competitively inhibit cyclic AMP phosphodiesterase activity of rat brain (Beer *et al.*, 1972; Berndt and Schwabe, 1973) and human brain (Pichard *et al.*, 1972).

*xvii. Sulfonylureas.* Several of the sulfonylurea oral hypoglycemic agents have been examined for their effect on phosphodiesterase from the kidney (Senft *et al.*, 1968a), islets of Langerhans and other tissues. There is general agreement that these agents are effective but not very potent. Thus, Goldfine *et al.* (1971) found that tolbutamide and 1-butyl-3-(acetylphenyl) sulfonylurea were effective inhibitors of pancreatic islet cell tumor of the hamster but not as active as either theophylline or caffeine. In addition, they showed that tolbutamide was capable of inhibiting phosphodiesterase from several rat tissues; Rosen *et al.* (1971) reported that chlorpropamide inhibited both the cyclic AMP and cyclic GMP phosphodiesterase from hamster islet cell tumor, but was less effective than theophylline; Ashcroft *et al.* (1972) found that glibenclamide was an inhibitor of mouse islet cyclic AMP phosphodiesterase; Sams and Montague (1972) showed that both tolbutamide and glibenclamide inhibited the cyclic AMP phosphodiesterase of guinea pig islets of Langerhans but they were less potent than either theophylline or caffeine; and finally Brooker and Fichman (1971) found that chlorpropamide and tolbutamide inhibited phosphodiesterase of rat kidney, but both sulfonylureas were less effective than caffeine.

*xviii. Steroids.* It is well known that steroids can alter the response of a tissue to another hormone. This response has been characterized as a "permissive" effect of steroids on a cyclic AMP-mediated process. The possibility that this effect is due to the interaction of cyclic AMP phosphodiesterase with the steroid has been studied in several laboratories with mixed results. Vernikos-Danellis and Harris (1968), for example, found that hydrocortisone and dexamethasone produced little alteration of phosphodiesterase activity in several tissues, and Higazi and Kvinnsland (1974), in studies of the effect of estradiol on the cervicovaginal epithelium of neonatal mice, also found little effect of the steroid on phosphodiesterase activity. By contrast, Manganiello and Vaughan (1972c) showed that dexamethasone inhibited the cyclic AMP phosphodiesterase of HTC hepatoma cells, Senft *et al.* (1968c) demonstrated that 6-α methylprednisolone had a similar inhibitory effect on beef heart phosphodiesterase, and Stoff *et al.* (1973) found that aldosterone inhibited the cyclic AMP phosphodiesterase of toad bladder cells. This effect of dexamethasone was not seen when the steroid was added *in vitro*. One possible explanation is that the dexamethasone acts only in a complete cell system to cause the synthesis of a phosphodiesterase inhibitor. It is also conceivable that the dexamethasone prevents the activation of phosphodiesterase, either by inhibiting the synthesis or the effect of an endogenous activator of phosphodiesterase.

*xix. Cardiac glycosides.* Lippmann (1974) demonstrated that certain analogs of cardiac glycosides, such as 3β-14-dihydroxy-21-oxo-23 desoxo-5β-card-20(22)-enolide 3-acetate, an isomer with the steroid nucleus attached to the α- rather than to the β-carbon of the α-β unsaturated lactone ring, is more potent than theophylline in inhibiting phosphodiesterase of beef heart. Other isomers were less potent than theophylline, as was the naturally occurring cardiac glycoside, digitoxin.

*xx. α-Tocopherol and analogs.* Analogs of α-tocopherol (vitamin E) that lack its lipophilic side chain, but not α-tocopherol itself, are more potent inhibitors of cyclic AMP phosphodiesterase of beef liver than is theophylline (Schroeder, 1974). Interestingly, they are apparently less effective as inhibitors of cyclic GMP phosphodiesterase than of cyclic AMP phosphodiesterase.

*xxi. Disodium cromoglycate.* Roy and Warren (1974) reported that the antiasthmatic agent, disodium cromoglycate (DSCG) is an inhibitor of cyclic AMP phosphodiesterase with an activity slightly greater than that of theophylline. As with so many other studies, however, comparing the effectiveness of agents with theophylline may be misleading since theophylline, although historically an important prototype, is a relatively ineffective inhibitor of phosphodiesterase activity.

*xxii. Triiodothyronine and thyroxine.* An early publication by Mandel and Kuehl (1967) showed that high concentrations of L-triiodothyronine inhibited phosphodiesterase of beef heart and rat adipose tissue. By contrast, L-thyroxine, D-triiodothyronine, diiodothyronine, thyronine, and D-thyroxine were relatively ineffective inhibitors. They calculated the $K_i$ of triiodothyronine for the beef heart enzyme to be about 400 $\mu M$.

Rosen (1970a), using a phosphodiesterase from frog erythrocytes, found that triiodothyronine was a more potent inhibitor than thyroxine. However, the D-isomer, which is not physiologically active, had a similar effect on the enzyme, and both compounds were inhibitory only at concentrations well above their normal physiological concentrations.

More recently, Thannassi and Newcombe (1974), working with phosphodiesterase from a soluble fraction of chicken epiphyseal cartilage, confirmed the inhibitory effects of L-triiodothyronine. They also noted that D-triiodothyronine and L- and D-thyroxine were less potent inhibitors of this enzyme. Similarly, Marcus (1974) found that thyroxine and its analogs were competitive inhibitors of both the high and low $K_m$ phosphodiesterases prepared from rat calvaria. In this system, tetraiodothyronine and its analogs were more effective inhibitors than triiodothyronine and its analogs.

*xxiii. Eritadenine.* The isopentyl ester derivative of eritadenine [2(*R*)-dihydroxy-4-(9-adenyl)butyric acid], a potent hypolipidemic agent, has been shown by Iwai (1974) to inhibit cyclic AMP phosphodiesterase of adipose tissue. In both cases, the eritadenine isoamyl ester had slightly less inhibitory activity than theophylline.

*xxiv. Ascorbic and dehydroascorbic acid.* Tisdale (1975) found that ascorbic acid was a noncompetitive inhibitor of a low $K_m$, soluble phosphodiesterase from Walker carcinoma cells grown *in vivo,* with a $K_i$ of 3.75 m$M$. The same cells were competitively inhibited by dehydroascorbic acid with a $K_i$ of 1.95 m$M$. These values are comparable to that for theophylline (2.34 m$M$). At higher substrate levels, both agents were competitive inhibitors, with $K_i$ values of 900 $\mu M$ for ascorbate and 1.43 m$M$ for dehydroascorbate. Both inhibitors were reversible.

*xxv. Acid mucopolysaccharides.* A series of acid mucopolysaccharides, including heparin, chondroitin sulfate, and hyaluronic acid, were shown to inhibit the activity of bovine heart phosphodiesterase *in vitro* (Stefanovich, 1974a). The inhibitory activity of these agents generally paralleled their sulfate group content, with the exception of hyaluronic acid, which has no sulfates but has inhibitory activity. None of these compounds were very potent. The $K_i$ value for heparin, the most active of these agents, was 12 m$M$. A series of sulfopolysaccharides was somewhat more potent. The $K_i$ for the most active of these agents, sulfoenervan, was 1.5 m$M$.

*xxvi. Flavoxate.* Conti and Setnikar (1975) have shown that both flavoxate, a direct-acting smooth muscle antispasmodic agent, and its primary metabolite were competitive inhibitors of beef heart phosphodiesterases with $K_i$ values of 147 and 688 $\mu M$, respectively. The $K_i$ value for theophylline under the same conditions was about 3 m$M$.

*xxvii. Benzopyran derivatives.* Nitz *et al.* (1968) found that the coronary vasodilator chromonar, a benzopyran derivative, was a more potent inhibitor of the cyclic AMP phosphodiesterase from rat heart than was theophylline.

*xxviii. Miscellaneous pharmacological agents. Diuretics.* Schultz *et al.* (1966) published an early report that diazoxide, a benzothiadiazine derivative, inhibited phosphodiesterase. This report was confirmed by Moore (1968) who calculated the relative potency of several benzothiadiazines as inhibitors of beef heart phosphodiesterase. All of the agents examined had inhibitory activity, the most effective being polythiazide. Gadd *et al.* (1973) studied several mercurial diuretics for their effect on guinea pig heart phosphodiesterase. The most potent inhibitor was phenylmercuric acetate, but all the agents were more inhibitory than equimolar concentrations of theophylline. The effect of these agents was only partially decreased by the addition of the sulfhydryl-containing reagent, dithiothreitol, which suggests that the mechanism of action of these agents was more than simple enzyme inactivation due to reaction of the mercurial compounds with sulfhydryl groups on the enzymes. Other studies of the influence of diuretics on phosphodiesterase activity showed that furosemide and bendroflumethiazide, but not acetazolamide, inhibited rat brain phosphodiesterase (Weinryb *et al.*, 1972) and that ethacrynic acid, chlorthalidon, and acetazolamide inhibited phosphodiesterase of beef heart, acetazolamide being the least potent of these three compounds (Senft *et al.*, 1968a).

*Metabolic inhibitors.* Most of the studies using metabolic inhibitors were designed to determine whether these compounds can prevent the induction of phosphodiesterase rather than inhibit its activity per se. For example, Uzunov *et al.* (1973) showed that cycloheximide can prevent the norepinephrine-induced elevation of phosphodiesterase in astrocytoma cells. Similarly, D'Armiento *et al.* (1972) found that both cycloheximide and actinomycin D prevent the induction of cyclic AMP phosphodiesterase activity in 3T3 fibroblasts, and Prasad and Kumar (1972), using cultured neuroblastoma cells, found that treatment with cycloheximide for 6 hours decreased the activity of phosphodiesterase. By contrast, actinomycin D treatment had no such effect. In a study in which puromycin was added acutely to a phosphodiesterase prepared from rat diaphragm, Appleman and Kemp (1966) found that this protein-synthesis inhibitor competitively blocked the activity of phosphodiesterase. Later studies confirmed that other inhibitors of protein synthesis were also able to prevent the induction as well as the activity of phosphodiesterase. Thus, there is no doubt that phosphodiesterase can be induced *in vitro* and that this induction can be blocked by inhibitors of protein synthesis. The work of Appleman and Kemp suggests, however, that these compounds may have additional effects on cyclic nucleotide metabolism independent of their protein-synthesis inhibitory activity.

*Alkylating agents.* Tisdale and Phillips (1975) studied the effect of several antitumor alkylating agents on the cyclic AMP phosphodiesterases of Walker carcinoma cells, which are either sensitive or resistant to the effect of alkylating agents. Neither the high $K_m$ nor the low $K_m$ phosphodiesterases of the resistant cells was affected by the difunctional aklylating agent, chlorambucil, in concentrations of up to 5 $\mu$g/ml. By contrast, the low, but not the high $K_m$ enzyme from the sensitive cells was inhibited. This effect on phosphodiesterase does not occur with monofunctional alkylating agents.

*Bitter taste stimuli.* Kurihara (1972) found that the cyclic AMP phosphodiesterase of bovine taste papillae was inhibited by several bitter taste stimuli. Their effect on the phosphodiesterase correlated with the taste threshold of each compound. However, Price (1973) found that these stimuli activated the phosphodiesterase of bovine epithelium. Although this controversy has not been resolved, the results suggest the possibility that the cyclic AMP system is, in some way, an integral part of the taste chemoreceptor system.

*Anti-inflammatory agents.* A series of anti-inflammatory agents was examined by Newcombe *et al.* (1974) for their ability to inhibit phosphodiesterase of chicken epiphyseal and articular cartilage. Indomethacin and several of its analogs were the most potent of the inhibitors studied. Similar inhibitory effects on phosphodiesterase were obtained with arylacetic acid and mefenemic acid. Quinoline compounds and pyrazolones were less effective, whereas salicylic acid and gold-containing compounds had relatively little effect. When several of the more potent inhibitors were tested against cyclic GMP phosphodiesterase, the results were similar to those obtained with the same compounds on cyclic AMP phosphodiesterase.

Stefanovich (1974b) also tested a series of anti-inflammatory agents for their effect on bovine heart phosphodiesterase. The most potent of these was mefenamic acid ($K_i$=68 $\mu M$), followed by flufenamic acid ($K_i$=82 $\mu M$) and indomethacin ($K_i$=93 $\mu M$). All three of these agents were noncompetitive inhibitors of phosphodiesterase. Indomethacin has also been shown to inhibit phosphodiesterase activity of bovine heart, human lung (Roy and Warren, 1974), and toad bladder (Flores and Sharp, 1972). Other anti-inflammatory and antihistaminic agents, such as salicylates, phenylbutazone, and mepyramine, however, had no inhibitory effects on phosphodiesterase (Roy and Warren, 1974).

*b. Summary.* In spite of the large number of agents that have been shown to inhibit phosphodiesterase and the structure–activity relationships obtained with some of these agents, it is not currently possible to predict the effect of a given new pharmacological agent on the enzyme. This may be due, in part, to the existence of multiple forms of phosphodiesterase (which were unrecognized at the time of the initial structure–activity studies) that can be differentially altered by pharmacological agents. Future studies on the relationship between the structure of phosphodiesterase inhibitors and their inhibitory effects on each isozyme of phosphodiesterase may provide the information required to design specific agents that will selectively alter the cyclic nucleotide levels in discrete cells.

## F. Effect of Pharmacological Agents on the Multiple Forms of Phosphodiesterase

The existence of multiple forms of cyclic AMP phosphodiesterase and cyclic GMP phosphodiesterase has been demonstrated in various tissues (see Section IV,D), and their properties have been extensively studied. Our objective has been to determine the response of the multiple forms to endogenous and pharmacological agents, with the aim of identifying compounds that are capable of selectively inhibiting or activating a specific isozyme of phosphodiesterase. To this end, we have studied the effect of the endogenous heat-stable phosphodiesterase activator and a series of structurally unrelated pharmacological agents on phosphodiesterase isozymes from several tissue sources. Our results, discussed below, show that there is a marked difference in the specificity by which the different forms of phosphodiesterase can be inhibited by drugs (Uzunov *et al.*, 1974; Weiss *et al.*, 1974; Weiss, 1975b; Fertel and Weiss, 1976). This suggests that one might be able to inhibit specifically the form of phosphodiesterase found in certain cell types and thereby specifically to alter the intracellular concentration of cyclic nucleotides in these cells. The selective regulation of cyclic nucleotides in discrete cell types would not only provide the means of clarifying the physiological role of cyclic nucleotides in these cells but could have revolutionary clinical implications as well.

### 1. *Effect of Activator on Phosphodiesterase Isoenzymes*

The endogenous activator shows a striking specificity for one of the isozymes of phosphodiesterase found in the cerebrum (Peak II, Fig. 2). A similar specificity exists for the Peak II isozyme in cerebellum (Uzunov and Weiss, 1972b). By contrast, the lung, which has no Peak II isozyme, is not activatable (Fig. 3). The demonstration that $Ca^{2+}$ is required for the activation of phosphodiesterase (Teo and Wang, 1973; Kakiuchi *et al.*, 1973; Teshima and Kakiuchi, 1974; Wolff and Brostrom, 1974; Wickson *et al.*, 1975) is in accord with the observation that only Peak II is activated by $Ca^{2+}$ (Uzunov and Weiss, 1972b). The specificity with which the activator increased the activity of one form of phosphodiesterase suggested the possibility that there may be pharmacological agents that could specifically inhibit this activated enzyme. Recent studies from our laboratory show that this is, in fact, the case (see below).

### 2. *Effect of Pharmacological Agents on Activation of Phosphodiesterase*

Studies (Weiss *et al.*, 1974; Weiss, 1975b; Levin and Weiss, 1976) on the interaction between the activator of phosphodiesterase and pharmacological agents may provide one basis for the differential control of the activity of the phosphodiesterase isozymes. The initial results, which involved the separation of the phosphodiesterase isozymes by preparative polyacrylamide gel electrophoresis (Uzunov and Weiss, 1972b), indicated that the phenothiazine tranquilizer, trifluoperazine, had a much greater effect on Peak II isolated from rat cerebrum than on any of the other peaks of phosphodiesterase.

Other studies (Weiss *et al.*, 1974) showed that trifluoperazine was more effective in inhibiting the activated form of Peak II than the same peak in its unactivated state. Figure 4, for example, shows the specificity with which the activator and trifluoperazine alter the activity of the different forms of phosphodiesterase isolated from rat cerebrum. As can be seen, the activator increased the phosphodiesterase activity of Peak II more than ten-fold but had no effect on Peak I phosphodiesterase. Trifluoperazine (25 $\mu M$) had essentially no effect on Peak I but almost completely blocked the activation of Peak II phosphodiesterase. On the other hand, trifluoperazine sulfoxide and promethazine, analogs of

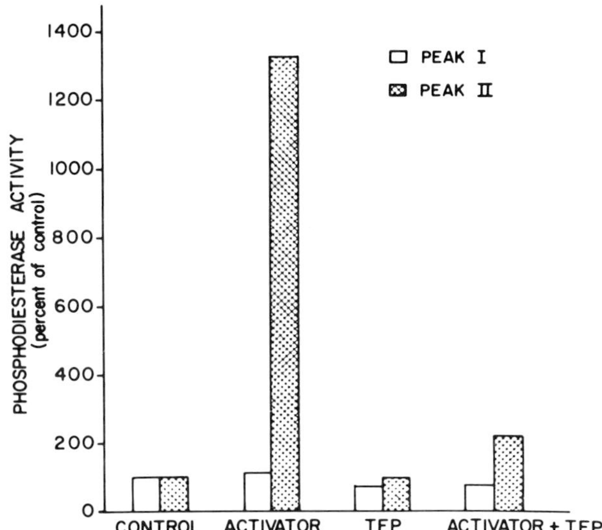


FIG. 4. Effects of trifluoperazine and activator on Peak I and Peak II phosphodiesterase activity of rat cerebrum. Each purified peak of phosphodiesterase was assayed for cyclic AMP phosphodiesterase activity in the absence and presence of activator and trifluoperazine (TFP) (25 $\mu M$). The activator was added in amounts that produced a maximum increase in enzyme activity. (Taken from Weiss and Greenberg, 1975. © 1975 University Park Press, Baltimore.)

trifluoperazine that have little or no physiological effect on the central nervous system, were less potent inhibitors of any of the isozymes and showed little specificity for the activated form of Peak II. Two other phosphodiesterase inhibitors, papaverine and theophylline, inhibited the activated and nonactivated enzymes to an equal extent (Weiss *et al.*, 1974). In agreement with these results, Lin *et al.* (1974) found that another methylxanthine, caffeine, also inhibited the activity of both the activated and unactivated phosphodiesterase from bovine brain.

Further studies on the interaction between activator and trifluoperazine demonstrated that the effect of trifluoperazine on the isozyme could be overcome by the addition of activator, and the effect of activator could be overcome by the addition of trifluoperazine (Weiss *et al.*, 1974). More recent studies from our laboratory (Levin and Weiss, 1976) have confirmed these observations with other phenothiazine tranquilizers and have shown further that a variety of antipsychotic agents with diverse chemical structures all have the common ability to inhibit selectively the activation of phosphodiesterase.

The effect of activator on trifluoperazine inhibition could not be altered by the addition of exogenous protein, suggesting that the added activator did not serve as an alternate source of protein to bind the inhibitor. Moreover, the addition of excess calcium did not alter the effect of the inhibitor, suggesting that the phenothiazine does not prevent activation by chelating calcium (Levin and Weiss, 1976). The evidence indicates that the selective inhibition of the activatable phosphodiesterase isozyme by trifluoperazine is a result of the ability of trifluoperazine to prevent the interaction of this specific isozyme of phosphodiesterase with the activator. Since several other antipsychotic agents—but not other structurally related derivatives that are pharmacologically inactive—share this property with trifluoperazine, one is tempted to speculate that the selective inhibition of a specific activatable form of phosphodiesterase in discrete brain areas may help explain some of the diverse pharmacological actions of the neuroleptics on the central nervous system.

### 3. *Effect of Pharmacological Agents on Other Phosphodiesterase Isozymes*

That pharmacological agents can differentially inhibit the various isozymes of phosphodiesterase has now been documented in several studies (Uzunov *et al.*, 1974; Weiss *et al.*, 1974; Weiss, 1975b; Fertel and Weiss, 1976). In general, of the several peaks of phosphodiesterase that could be isolated from brain and other tissue, Peak I phosphodies-

TABLE V

$K_i$ VALUES OF INHIBITORS FOR CYCLIC NUCLEOTIDE PHOSPHODIESTERASE ISOZYMES OF RAT LUNG[a]

| Inhibitor | Cyclic AMP phosphodiesterase Peak I ($\mu M$) | Cyclic AMP phosphodiesterase Peak III ($\mu M$) | Cyclic GMP phosphodiesterase Peak III ($\mu M$) |
|---|---|---|---|
| Theophylline | 1190 | 410 | 210 |
| Trifluoperazine | 890 | 52 | 32 |
| Papaverine | 170 | 29 | 42 |
| SQ 20009 | 550 | 16 | 27 |
| Cyclic GMP | 980 | 88 | — |

[a] The soluble supernatant fraction of rat lung was subjected to polyacrylamide gel electrophoresis. Peak I was assayed for cyclic AMP phosphodiesterase and Peak III was assayed for cyclic AMP phosphodiesterase and cyclic GMP phosphodiesterase in the absence and presence of various concentrations of inhibitors. The $K_i$ values were calculated according to the method of Dixon (1953). (Taken from Fertel and Weiss, 1976.)

terase is the most resistant to inhibition. For example, based on work done with the phosphodiesterase forms isolated from rat lung, Peak I cyclic AMP phosphodiesterase was several-fold less sensitive to inhibition by a wide variety of phosphodiesterase inhibitors than was Peak III phosphodiesterase when cyclic AMP or cyclic GMP was used as substrate (Table V).

The ability of papaverine to inhibit differentially the peaks of phosphodiesterase isolated from rat cerebrum is shown in Fig. 5. As can be seen, there is a marked difference in the degree to which the different isozymes of phosphodiesterase are inhibited.

The results presented in the foregoing serve as clear examples that the different isozymes of phosphodiesterase can be differentially inhibited by drugs. These findings suggest that an inhibitor with a given isozyme specificity and potency can be used to inhibit selectively the isozymes of a given tissue and thereby raise the intracellular concentrations of cyclic AMP in those tissues.

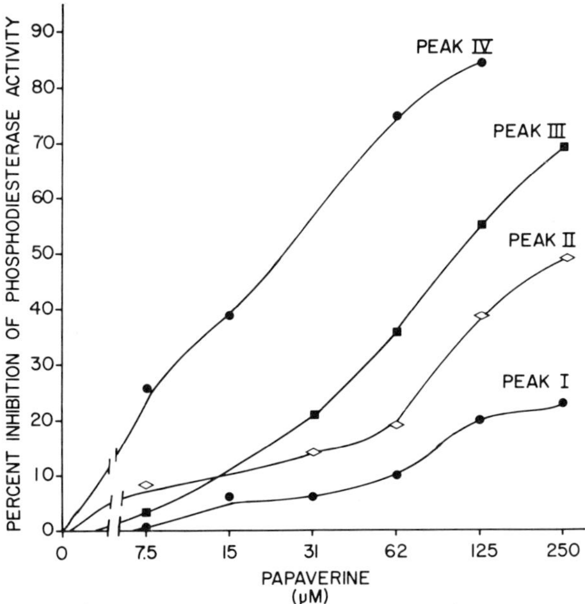


FIG. 5. Inhibition by papaverine of the multiple forms of phosphodiesterase of rat cerebrum. The 100,000*g* soluble supernatant fraction of rat cerebral homogenates was subjected to polyacrylamide gel electrophoresis, and the fractions were analyzed for phosphodiesterase activity in the presence of varying concentrations of papaverine. (Taken from Weiss, 1975b.)

## V. Transport of Cyclic AMP

Another factor governing the intracellular concentration of cyclic AMP is the transport of the cyclic nucleotide from within the cell to the extracellular fluid. Although this problem has received relatively little attention, there is evidence that cyclic AMP is secreted by cells (Davoren and Sutherland, 1963b) and that this process may involve an active transport. For example, Penit *et al.* (1974) reported that glial cells growing in culture secrete cyclic AMP into the external medium, a process that was blocked by probenecid. More examples of drugs acting by blocking the transport of cyclic AMP will surely be forthcoming.

## VI. Inhibition of Action of Cyclic AMP

Besides acting on the nucleotide cyclases or phosphodiesterases, pharmacological agents could also alter the effects of cyclic AMP by preventing the interaction of cyclic AMP with its receptor. Since cyclic AMP appears to exert most of its effects by activating protein kinase (Langan, 1973), it may be possible to alter the physiological effects of the nucleotide by blocking the activation of this enzyme.

As early as 1962 it was reported that heated extracts of several tissues of the rat contain a substance that inhibits the cyclic AMP-dependent activation of liver phosphorylase (Murad *et al.,* 1962; Murad *et al.,* 1969b). This endogenous material apparently is formed when ATP is incubated with adenylate cyclase preparations. Whether this inhibitor blocks phosphorylase directly or acts at a previous step (e.g., protein kinase) is still uncertain.

Meyer and Miller (1974) recently reviewed evidence showing that a large number of analogs of cyclic AMP and cyclic GMP can activate their respective protein kinases. The relative activities of these cyclic nucleotide analogs on the protein kinases was not necessarily related to their ability to be hydrolyzed by phosphodiesterase. Their results suggest the possibility that one may be able to develop specific activators of protein kinase that are resistant to hydrolysis by the cyclic nucleotide phosphodiesterase.

An endogenous substance that inhibits cyclic AMP binding and protein kinase activity has been reported by several laboratories (Walsh *et al.,* 1971; Ashby and Walsh, 1972, 1973; Tsung and Weissman, 1973). The only study reported thus far on an exogenous inhibitor is that of Wray and Harris (1973) who showed that tolbutamide inhibits the cyclic

AMP-dependent protein kinase of adipose tissue. Since protein kinase may exist in several different molecular forms (Reimann *et al.,* 1971; Rubin *et al.,* 1972; Labrie *et al.,* 1971), is is possible that different agents may be found which selectively inhibit the activity of each form of the enzyme, as has been shown for the different phosphodiesterases (see previous section). This area of research is ripe for exploitation.

## VII. Directions of Future Research in Pharmacological Control of Cyclic Nucleotides

Our present knowledge of the interaction between phosphodiesterase isozymes and pharmacological agents is limited, as is our information about the distribution of isozymes in tissues and cell types. It is probable, for example, that there are distinct phosphodiesterase isozymes associated with a particulate cell fraction (Thompson *et al.,* 1973c; Russell *et al.,* 1972), and it is possible that these isozymes are also differentially responsive to phosphodiesterase effectors. The number of agents that have been examined for their interaction with the isozymes is also limited. It is almost certain that the ability to discriminate between phosphodiesterase isozymes with drugs will increase with the number of drugs studied.

A role for cyclic GMP in physiological and biochemical events has now been established, and knowledge of the existence of cyclic GMP phosphodiesterase has been steadily growing. Our own information about cyclic GMP phosphodiesterase is based on experimental evidence obtained working with rat lung phosphodiesterase, which apparently has two cyclic AMP phosphodiesterases and one cyclic GMP phosphodiesterase that coincides with the cyclic AMP phosphodiesterase. Although our inhibitor data suggest that the cyclic GMP phosphodiesterase in this tissue is identical to the cyclic AMP phosphodiesterase, there is information indicating that some tissues have separate phosphodiesterases for the hydrolysis of cyclic AMP and cyclic GMP (Russell *et al.,* 1972).

The existence of phosphodiesterase isozymes that are differentially distributed by tissue and cell type, coupled with the selective activation and inhibition of these isozymes, may provide a mechanism by which pharmacological agents can be selectively used to control cyclic nucleotide levels in discrete cell types. The wide number of disease processes that may be associated with abnormal cyclic nucleotide levels or metabolism (see Weiss, 1975a) suggests that the control of cyclic nucleotide levels is a goal of vast clinical importance. The discovery of phosphodiesterase isozymes and the demonstration that certain drugs can selectively alter the activity of these isozymes brings us one step closer to achieving that goal.

## VIII. Clinical Implications

Since cyclic AMP has so many effects on biological systems, it is not too great an extrapolation to predict that an alteration of the intracellular concentration of cyclic AMP may either be responsible for clinical diseases or may change the course of a disease process that already exists (for a recent monograph on this subject, see Weiss, 1975a). In fact, there have been several studies suggesting the involvement of cyclic AMP in such diverse conditions as hypertension (Amer, 1975), asthma (Sheppard, 1973), heart failure (Sobel *et al.,* 1969; Gold *et al.,* 1970; Goldstein *et al.,* 1971; Schreiber *et al.,* 1971; Sulakhe and Dhalla, 1972; Levey, 1975), myasthenia gravis (Hopkanen *et al.,* 1972), psoriasis (Voorhees *et al.,* 1975), immunological reactions (Ignarro, 1975), cancer (Johnson, 1975; Prasad, *et al.,* 1975), diabetes (Kupiecki, 1969; Bell *et al.,* 1974; Kuo *et al.,* 1975), and certain diseases of the central nervous system (Paul *et al.,* 1971a,b; Cramer *et al.,* 1972a,b; Uzunov and Weiss, 1971, 1972a; Sproles, 1973; Weiss and Greenberg, 1975). As an example, it has been shown that transformation of hamster astrocytoma cells with SV40 virus causes a marked reduction in adenylate cyclase activity (Weiss *et al.,* 1971). Other types of cancer cells also showed a reduction in adenylate cyclase activity or a reduction in its hormonal responsiveness (Burk, 1968; Allen *et al.,* 1971; Schorr and Ney, 1971; Macchia *et al.,* 1972; Raska, 1973; Polgar *et al.,* 1973; Anderson *et al.,* 1973).

There is also evidence that certain diseases may be associated with an alteration of phosphodiesterase activity. Kupiecki (1969) found that phosphodiesterase activity in the pancreas and adipose tissue of a spontaneously diabetic mouse was lower than in the same tissue of normal mice. Other investigators have shown a reduction of phosphodiesterase activity in heart (Das, 1973) and plasma (Hemington *et al.,* 1973) of diabetic rats. Moreover, mice with an inherited retinal degeneration also showed an alteration in the phosphodiesterase activity of the retina (Schmidt and Lolley, 1973; Farber and Lolley, 1973). Certain types of cancer cells also may have an altered phosphodiesterase activity (Rhoads *et al.*, 1972; Sharma, 1972; Schroeder and Plagemann, 1972; Clark *et al.*, 1973). Studies in our own laboratory (Hait and Weiss, 1976), for example, showed that the activity of phosphodiesterase in leukemic lymphocytes was markedly greater than that of normal lymphocytes. Since cyclic AMP inhibits the growth of malignant cells and induces morphological differentiation of these cells (Ryan and Heidrick, 1968; Hsie and Puck, 1971), a selective inhibition of phosphodiesterase in these cells may provide a new approach toward the treatment of certain types of cancer. These studies on phosphodiesterase are particularly exciting because, if the activity or the pattern of phosphodiesterases in neoplastic cells is different from that of normal cells, one may be able to design drugs that will specifically inhibit the phosphodiesterase activity of only those cells and, therefore, increase the intracellular concentration of cyclic AMP in the cancer cells specifically.

## IX. Concluding Remarks

The nucleotide cyclases and the cyclic nucleotide phosphodiesterases are complex enzyme systems having multiple receptor sites or multiple molecular forms. The various forms of these enzyme systems exist in specific cell types and can be differentially activated and inhibited by several endogenous and exogenous compounds. This selective alteration of specific forms of the nucleotide cyclases and cyclic nucleotide phosphodiesterases by pharmacological agents suggests the possibility of modulating the activity of these enzymes in individual cell types, resulting in a specific alteration of the cyclic nucleotide concentration in certain cells. This evidence, taken together with the evidence that cyclic nucleotides have profound biological effects and may be involved in certain disease states, suggests that one may be able to develop a new class of drugs whose pharmacological action is based on the specific alteration of the intracellular concentration of cyclic nucleotides in discrete cell types.

ACKNOWLEDGMENTS

This work was supported in part by grants from The Benevolent Foundation of Scottish Rite Freemasonry, Northern Jurisdiction, U.S.A., and from the United States Public Health Service, National Cancer Institute (Grant CA 15883).

## References


Abdallah, Y. H., and Hamadah, K. (1970). *Lancet* **21,** 378–381.

Abou-Sabe, M., and Nardi, R. (1973). *Biochem. Biophys. Res. Commun.* **51,** 551–557.

Adachi, K., and Kano, A. (1970). *Biochem. Biophys. Res. Commun.* **41,** 884–890.

Allan, E. H., and Sneyd, J. G. T. (1975). *Biochem. Biophys. Res. Commun.* **62,** 594–601.

Allen, D. F., Clark, J. F., and Ashmore, J. (1973). *J. Pharmacol. Exp. Ther.* **185,** 379–385.

Allen, D. O., and Beck, R. P. (1972). *Endocrinology* **91,** 504–510.

Allen, D. O., Munshower, J., Morris, H. P., and Weber, G. (1971). *Cancer Res.* **31,** 557–560.

Amer, M. S. (1975). *In* "Cyclic Nucleotides in Disease" (B. Weiss, ed.), pp. 133–156. Univ. Park Press, Baltimore, Md.

Amer, M. S., and Browder, H. P. (1970). *Proc. Soc. Exp. Biol. Med.* **136,** 750–752.

Amer, M. S., and Kreighbaum, W. E. (1975). *J. Pharm. Sci.* **64,** 1–37.

Amer, M. S., and McKinney, G. R. (1972). *J. Pharmacol. Exp. Ther.* **183,** 535–548.

Amer, M. S., and McKinney, G. R. (1973). *Life Sci.* **13,** 753–767.

Amer, M. S., and Mayol, R. F. (1973). *Biochim. Biophys. Acta* **309,** 149–156.

Anderson, W. B., Russell, T. R., Carchman, R. A., and Pastan, I. (1973). *Proc. Natl. Acad. Sci. U.S.A.* **70,** 3802–3805.

Anisuzzaman, A. K. M., Lake, W. C., and Whistler, R. L. (1973). *Biochemistry* **12,** 2041–2045.

Applebaum, S. W., and Gilbert, L. I. (1972). *Dev. Biol.* **27,** 165–175.

Appleman, M. M., and Kemp, R. G. (1966). *Biochem. Biophys. Res. Commun.* **24,** 564–568.

Ashby, C. D., and Walsh, D. A. (1972). *J. Biol. Chem.* **247,** 6637–6642.

Ashby, C. D., and Walsh, D. A. (1973). *J. Biol. Chem.* **248,** 1255–1261.

Ashcroft, S. J. H., Randle, P. J., and Taljedal, I-B. (1972). *FEBS Lett.* **20,** 263–265.

Ashman, D. F., Lipton, R., Melicow, M. M., and Price, T. D. (1963). *Biochem. Biophys. Res. Commun.* **11,** 330–334.

Bar, H. P., and Hahn, P. (1971). *Can. J. Biochem.* **49,** 85–89.

Bar, H. P., and Hechter, O. (1969a). *Proc. Natl. Acad. Sci. U.S.A.* **63,** 350–356.

Bar, H. P., and Hechter, O. (1969b). *Biochem. Biophys. Res. Commun.* **35,** 681–686.

Bar, H. P., Hechter, O., Schwartz, I. L., and Walter, R. (1970). *Proc. Natl. Acad. Sci. U.S.A.* **67,** 7–12.

Barka, T., and Van der Noen, H. (1974). *Life Sci.* **14,** 267–280.

Beatty, C. H., Bocek, R. M., and Young, M. K. (1973). *Horm. Metab. Res.* **5,** 213–215.

Beavo, J. A., Hardman, J. G., and Sutherland, E. W. (1970a). *J. Biol. Chem.* **245,** 5649–5655.

Beavo, J. A., Rogers, N-L., Crofford, O. B., Hardman, J. G., Sutherland, E. W., and Newman, E. V. (1970b). *Mol. Pharmacol.* **6,** 597–603.

Beavo, J. A., Hardman, J. G., and Sutherland, E. W. (1971a). *J. Biol. Chem.* **246,** 3841–3846.

Beavo, J. A., Rogers, N-L., Crofford, O. B., Baird, E. D., Hardman, J. G., Sutherland, E. W., and Newman, E. V. (1971b). *Ann. N. Y. Acad. Sci.* **185,** 129–136.

Becker, F. F., and Bitensky, M. W. (1969). *Proc. Soc. Exp. Biol. Med.* **130,** 983–986.

Beer, B., Chasin, M., Clody, D. E., Vogel, J. R., and Horovitz, Z. P. (1972). *Science* **176,** 428–430.

Bell, N. H., Clark, C. M., Avery, S., Sinha, T., Trygstad, C. W., and Allen, D. O. (1974). *Pediatr. Res.* **8,** 223–230.

Belpaire, F. M., and Bogaert, M. G. (1973). *Arch. Int. Pharmacodyn. Ther.* **203,** 388–390.
Benda, P., Premont, J., and Jard, S. (1972). *C.R. Acad. Sci., Ser. D* **275,** 1303–1306.
Bensinger, R. E., Fletcher, R. T., and Chader, G. J. (1974a). *J. Neurochem.* **22,** 1131–1134.
Bensinger, R. E., Fletcher, R. T., and Chader, G. J. (1974b). *Science* **183,** 86–87.
Berndt, S., and Schwabe, U. (1973). *Brain Res.* **63,** 303–312.
Bersimbaev, R. I., Argutinskaya, S. V., and Salganik, R. I. (1971). *Experientia* **27,** 1389–1390.
Bevers, M. M., Smits, R. A. E., Van Rijn, J., and Van Wijk, R. (1974). *Biochim. Biophys. Acta* **341,** 120–128.
Bilezikian, J. P., and Aurbach, G. D. (1973a). *J. Biol. Chem.* **248,** 5584–5589.
Bilezikian, J. P., and Aurbach, G. D. (1973b). *J. Biol. Chem.* **248,** 5575–5583.
Bielzikian, J. P., and Aurbach, G. D. (1974). *J. Biol. Chem.* **249,** 157–161.
Birnbaumer, L. (1973). *Biochim. Biophys. Acta* **300,** 129–158.
Birnbaumer, L., and Pohl, S. L. (1973). *J. Biol. Chem.* **248,** 2056–2061.
Birnbaumer, L., and Rodbell, M. (1969). *J. Biol. Chem.* **244,** 3477–3482.
Birnbaumer, L., Pohl, S. L., and Rodbell, M. (1969). *J. Biol. Chem.* **244,** 3468–3476.
Birnbaumer, L., Pohl, S. L., Michiel, H., Kraus, J., and Rodbell, M. (1970). *Adv. Biochem. Psychopharmacol.* **3,** 185–208.
Birnbaumer, L., Pohl, S., and Rodbell, M. (1971). *J. Biol. Chem.* **246,** 1857–1860.
Bitensky, M. W., and Gorman, R. E. (1973). *Prog. Biophys. Mol. Biol.* **26,** 411–461.
Bitensky, M. W., Russell, V., and Robertson, W. (1968). *Biochem. Biophys. Res. Commun.* **31,** 706–712.
Bitensky, M. W., Russell, V., and Blanco, M. (1970). *Endocrinology* **86,** 154–159.
Bitensky, M. W., Gorman, R. E., and Thomas, L. (1971). *Proc. Soc. Exp. Biol. Med.* **138,** 773–775.
Blecher, M., Merlino, N. S., and RoAne, J. T. (1968). *J. Biol. Chem.* **243,** 3973–3977.
Blecher, M., Ro'Ane, J. T., and Flynn, P. D. (1971). *Biochem. Pharmacol.* **20,** 249–257.
Bockaert, J., Roy, C., and Jard, S. (1972). *J. Biol. Chem.* **247,** 7073–7081.
Bockaert, J., Roy, C., Rajerison, R., and Jard, S. (1973). *J. Biol. Chem.* **248,** 5922–5931.
Bohme, E. (1970). *Eur. J. Biochem.* **14,** 422–429.
Bonner, J. T. (1971). *Annu. Rev. Microbiol.* **25,** 75–92.
Bourne, H. R., and Melmon, K. L. (1971). *J. Pharmacol. Exp. Ther.* **178,** 1–7.
Bourne, H. R., Lehrer, R. I., Lichtenstein, L. M., Weissmann, G., and Zurier, R. (1973a). *J. Clin. Invest.* **52,** 698–708.
Bourne, H. R., Tompkins, G. M., and Dion, S. (1973b). *Science* **181,** 952–954.
Bradham, L. S. (1972). *Biochim. Biophys. Acta* **276,** 434–443.
Bradham, L. S., Holt, D. A., and Sims, M. (1970). *Biochim. Biophys. Acta* **201,** 250–260.
Braun, T., and Hechter, O. (1970). *Proc. Natl. Acad. Sci. U.S.A.* **66,** 995–1001.
Bray, J. J., Kon, C. M., and Breckenridge, B. McL. (1971). *Brain Res.* **26,** 385–394.
Breckenridge, B. McL. (1970). *Annu. Rev. Pharmacol.* **10,** 19–34.
Breckenridge, B. McL., and Johnston, R. E. (1969). *J. Histochem. Cytochem.* **17,** 505–511.
Brodie, B. B., Davies, J. I., Hynie, S., Krishna, G., and Weiss, B. (1966). *Pharmacol. Rev.* **18,** 273–289.
Brooker, G., and Fichman, M. (1971). *Biochem. Biophys. Res. Commun.* **42,** 824–828.
Brooker, G., Thomas, L. J., Jr., and Appleman, M. M. (1968). *Biochemistry* **7,** 4177–4181.
Brostrom, C. O., Huang, Y-C., Breckenridge, B. McL., and Wolff, D. J. (1975). *Proc. Natl. Acad. Sci. U.S.A.* **72,** 64–68.

Brown, H. D., Chattopadhyay, S. K., Morris, H. P., and Pennington, S. N. (1970). *Cancer Res.* **30,** 123–126.
Brown, J. H., and Makman, M. H. (1972). *Proc. Natl. Acad. Sci. U.S.A.* **69,** 539–543.
Brown, J. H., and Makman, M. H. (1973). *J. Neurochem.* **21,** 477–479.
Brus, R., and Hess, M. E. (1973). *Endocrinology* **93,** 982–984.
Bublitz, C. (1973). *Biochem. Biophys. Res. Commun.* **52,** 173–180.
Bueding, E., and Bulbring, E. (1964). *In* "Pharmacology of Smooth Muscle (E. Bulbring, ed.), pp. 37–56. Pergamon, Oxford.
Burges, R. A., and Blackburn, K. L. (1972). *Nature (London) New Biol.* **235,** 249–250.
Burk, R. R. (1968). *Nature (London)* **219,** 1272–1275.
Burkard, W. P. (1975). *Prog. Neurobiol. (Oxford)* **4,** 241–267.
Burke, G. (1970a). *Endocrinology* **86,** 346–352.
Burke, G. (1970b). *Biochim. Biophys. Acta* **220,** 30–41.
Burke, G. (1973). *Prostaglandins* **3,** 537–540.
Butcher, F. R., and Serif, G. S. (1969). *Biochim. Biophys. Acta* **192,** 409–419.
Butcher, R. W., and Baird, C. E. (1968). *J. Biol. Chem.* **243,** 1713–1717.
Butcher, R. W., and Sutherland, E. W. (1962). *J. Biol. Chem.* **237,** 1244–1250.
Butcher, R. W., Sneyd, J. G. T., Park, C. R., and Sutherland, E. W., Jr. (1966). *J. Biol. Chem.* **241,** 1651–1653.
Butcher, R. W., Baird, C. E., and Sutherland, E. W. (1968). *J. Biol. Chem.* **243,** 1705–1712.
Campbell, M. T., and Oliver, I. T. (1972). *Eur. J. Biochem.* **28,** 30–37.
Casillas, E. R., and Hoskins, D. D. (1970). *Biochem. Biophys. Res. Commun.* **40,** 255–262.
Castillon, M. P., Catalan, R. E., and Municio, A. M. (1973). *FEBS Lett.* **32,** 113–115.
Challoner, D. R., and Allen, D. O. (1970). *Metab., Clin. Exp.* **19,** 480–487.
Chase, L. R., and Aurbach, G. D. (1968). *Science* **159,** 545–547.
Chase, L. R., Fedak, S. A., and Aurbach, G. D. (1969). *Endocrinology* **84,** 761–768.
Chasin, M., Rivkin, I., Mamrak, F., Samaniego, S. G. and Hess, S. M. (1971). *J. Biol. Chem.* **246,** 3037–3041.
Chasin, M., Harris, D. N., Phillips, M. B., and Hess, S. M. (1972). *Biochem. Pharmacol.* **21,** 2443–2450.
Chassy, B. M. (1972). *Science* **175,** 1016–1018.
Cheng, Y., and Prusoff, W. H. (1973). *Biochem. Pharmacol.* **22,** 3099–3108.
Cheung, W. Y. (1966). *Biochem. Biophys. Res. Commun.* **23,** 214–220.
Cheung, W. Y. (1967). *Biochem. Biophys. Res. Commun.* **29,** 478–482.
Cheung, W. Y. (1969). *Biochim. Biophys. Acta* **191,** 303–315.
Cheung, W. Y. (1970a). *Adv. Biochem. Psychopharmacol.* **3,** 51–65.
Cheung, W. Y. (1970b). *Biochem. Biophys. Res. Commun.* **38,** 533–538.
Cheung, W. Y. (1971a). *Biochim. Biophys. Acta* **242,** 395–409.
Cheung, W. Y. (1971b). *J. Biol. Chem.* **246,** 2859–2869.
Cheung, W. Y., and Jenkins, A. (1969). *Fed. Proc., Fed. Am. Soc. Exp. Biol.* **28,** 473.
Cheung, W. Y., Bradham, L. S., Lynch, T. J., Lin, Y. M., and Tallant, E. A. (1975). *Biochem. Biophys. Res. Commun.* **66,** 1055–1062.
Chiang, M. H., and Cheung, W. Y. (1973). *Biochem. Biophys. Res. Commun.* **55,** 187–192.
Chlapowski, F. J., and Butcher, R. W. (1973). *Biochim. Biophys. Acta* **309,** 138–148.
Chou, W. S., Ho, A. K. S., and Loh, H. H. (1971). *Proc. West. Pharmacol. Soc.* **14,** 42–46.

Chrisman, T. D., Garbers, D. L., Parks, M. A., and Hardman, J. G. (1975). *J. Biol. Chem.* **250,** 374–381.
Christoffersen, T., Morland, J., Osnes, J. B., Berg, T., Boman, D., and Seglen, P. O. (1972a). *Arch. Biochem. Biophys.* **150,** 807–809.
Christoffersen, T., Morland, J., Osnes, J. B., and Elgjo, K. (1972b). *Biochim. Biophys. Acta* **279,** 363–366.
Clark, C. M., Jr., Beatty, B., and Allen, D. O. (1973). *J. Clin. Invest.* **52,** 1018–1025.
Clark, R. B., and Perkins, J. P. (1971). *Proc. Natl. Acad. Sci. U.S.A.* **68,** 2757–2760.
Cohen, K. L., and Bitensky, M. W. (1969). *J. Pharmacol. Exp. Ther.* **169,** 80–86.
Conti, M., and Setnikar, I. (1975). *Arch. Int. Pharmacodyn. Ther.* **213,** 186–189.
Counis, R., Koumanov, K., Raulin, J., and Infante, R. (1973). *Eur. J. Biochem.* **37,** 244–247.
Cramer, H., Goodwin, F. K., Post, R. M., and Bunney, W. E., Jr. (1972a). *Lancet* **1,** 1346–1347.
Cramer, H., Ng, L. K. Y., and Chase, T. N. (1972b). *J. Neurochem.* **19,** 1601–1602.
Cryer, P. E., Jarett, L., and Kipnis, D. M. (1969). *Biochim. Biophys. Acta* **177,** 586–590.
Dail, W. J., Jr., and Palmer, G. C. (1972). *Anat. Rec.* **177,** 265–288.
Dalton, C., Quinn, J. B., Burghardt, C. R., and Sheppard, H. (1970). *J. Pharmacol. Exp. Ther.* **173,** 270–276.
Dalton, C., Crowley, H. J., Sheppard, H., and Schallek, W. (1974). *Proc. Soc. Exp. Biol. Med.* **145,** 407–410.
D'Armiento, M., Johnson, G. S., and Pastan, I. (1972). *Proc. Natl. Acad. Sci. U.S.A.* **69,** 459–462.
Das, I. (1973). *Horm. Metab. Res.* **5,** 330–333.
Das, I., and Chain, E. B. (1972). *Biochem. J.* **128,** 95–96.
Davies, J. I. (1968). *Nature (London)* **218,** 349–352.
Davoren, P. R., and Sutherland, E. W. (1963a). *J. Biol. Chem.* **238,** 3016–3023.
Davoren, P. R., and Sutherland, E. W. (1963b). *J. Biol. Chem.* **238,** 3009–3015.
Deguchi, T., and Axelrod, J. (1973a). *Mol. Pharmacol.* **9,** 612–618.
Deguchi, T., and Axelrod, J. (1973b). *Proc. Natl. Acad. Sci. U.S.A.* **8,** 2411–2414.
DeRobertis, E. D., Arnaiz, G. R. D. L., Alberici, M., Butcher, R. W., and Sutherland, E. W. (1967). *J. Biol. Chem.* **242,** 3487–3493.
Dismukes, K., and Daly, J. W. (1974). *Mol. Pharmacol.* **10,** 933–940.
Dixon, M. (1953). *Biochem. J.* **55,** 170–171.
Dorigo, P., Gaion, R. M., Toth, E., and Fassina, G. (1973a). *Biochem. Pharmacol.* **22,** 1949–1956.
Dorigo, P., Visco, L., Fiandini, G., and Fassina, G. (1973b). *Biochem. Pharmacol.* **22,** 1957–1964.
Dousa, T., and Hechter, O. (1970). *Life Sci.* **9,** 765–770.
Dousa, T., and Rychlik, I. (1968). *Biochim. Biophys. Acta* **158,** 484–486.
Dousa, T. P. (1974a). *Am. J. Physiol.* **226,** 1193–1197.
Dousa, T. P. (1974b). *Endocrinology* **95,** 1359–1366.
Dousa, T. P., Rowland, R. G., and Carone, F. A. (1973). *Proc. Soc. Exp. Biol. Med.* **142,** 720–722.
Drummond, G. I., and Duncan, L. (1970). *J. Biol. Chem.* **245,** 976–983.
Drummond, G. I., and Perrot-Yee, S. (1961). *J. Biol. Chem.* **236,** 1126–1129.
Drummond, G. I., Severson, D. L., and Duncan, L. (1971). *J. Biol. Chem.* **246,** 4166–4173.

Drummond, G. I., Greengard, P., and Robison, G. A., eds. (1975). *Adv. Cyclic Nucleotide Res.* **5,** 1–872.

Duell, E. A., Voorhees, J. J., Kelsey, W. H., and Hayes, E. (1971). *Arch. Dermatol.* **104,** 601–610.

Emmelin, N. (1961). *Pharmacol. Rev.* **13,** 17–37.

Emmelot, P., and Bos, J. (1971). *Biochim. Biophys. Acta* **249,** 285–292.

Entman, M. L., Levey, G. S., and Epstein, S. E. (1969a). *Biochem. Biophys. Res. Commun.* **35,** 728–733.

Entman, M. L., Levey, G. S., and Epstein, S. E. (1969b). *Circ. Res.* **25,** 429–438.

Exton, J. H., and Park, C. R. (1968). *Adv. Enzyme Regul.* **5,** 391–407.

Exton, J. H., Jefferson, L. S., Jr., Butcher, R. W., and Park, C. R. (1966). *Am. J. Med.* **40,** 709–715.

Fain, J. N. (1971). *Mol. Pharmacol.* **7,** 465–479.

Fain, J. N., and Loken, S. C. (1971). *Mol. Pharmacol.* **7,** 455–464.

Farber, D. B., and Lolley, R. N. (1973). *J. Neurochem.* **21,** 817–828.

Ferrendelli, J. A., Johnson, E. M., Jr., Chang, M. M., and Needleman, P. (1973). *Biochem. Pharmacol.* **22,** 3133–3135.

Fertel, R., and Weiss, B. (1974). *Anal. Biochem.* **59,** 386–398.

Fertel, R., and Weiss, B. (1976). *Mol. Pharmacol.* **12,** 678–687.

Fleming, W. W., McPhillips, J. J., and Westfall, D. P. (1973). *Ergeb. Physiol., Biol. Chem. Exp. Pharmakol.* **68,** 1–65.

Flores, A. G. A., and Sharp, G. W. G. (1972). *Am. J. Physiol.* **233,** 1392–1397.

Fontaine, Y. A., Salmon, C., Fontaine-Bertrand, E., Burzawa-Gerard, E., and Donaldson, E. M. (1972). *Can. J. Zool.* **50,** 1673–1676.

Fontaine, Y. A., Salmon, C., Fontaine-Bertrand, E., and Delerue-Le Belle, N. (1973). *Horm. Metab. Res.* **5,** 376–380.

Forn, J., and Valdecasas, F. G. (1971). *Biochem. Pharmacol.* **20,** 2773–2779.

Forn, J., Schonhofer, P. S., Skidmore, I. F., and Krishna, G. (1970). *Biochim. Biophys. Acta* **208,** 304–309.

Franks, D. J., and MacManus, J. P. (1971). *Biochem. Biophys. Res. Commun.* **42,** 844–849.

Franks, D. J., MacManus, J. P., and Whitfield, J. F. (1971). *Biochem. Biophys. Res. Commun.* **44,** 1177–1183.

Furlanut, M., Carpenedo, F., and Ferrari, M. (1973). *Biochem. Pharmacol.* **22,** 2642–2644.

Gaballah, S., and Popoff, C. (1971). *Brain Res.* **25,** 220–222.

Gadd, R. E. A., Clayman, S., and Hebert, D. (1973). *Experientia* **29,** 1217–1219.

Garbers, D. L., and Hardman, J. G. (1975). *J. Biol. Chem.* **250,** 2482–2486.

Gauger, D., Palm, D., Kaiser, G., and Quiring, K. (1973). *Life Sci.* **13,** 31–40.

Gengler, W. R., and Forte, L. R. (1972). *Biochim. Biophys. Acta* **279,** 367–372.

Gentleman, S., and Mansour, T. E. (1974). *Biochim. Biophys. Acta* **343,** 469–479.

George, W. J., Polson, J. B., O'Toole, A. G., and Goldberg, N. D. (1970). *Proc. Natl. Acad. Sci. U.S.A.* **66,** 398–403.

Gilman, A. G., and Nirenberg, M. (1971). *Proc. Natl. Acad. Sci. U.S.A.* **68,** 2165–2168.

Gilman, A. G., and Rall, T. W. (1968). *J. Biol. Chem.* **243,** 5867–5871.

Glossmann, H., and Gips, H. (1974). *Naunyn-Schmiedeberg's Arch. Pharmacol.* **286,** 239–249.

Gold, H. K., Prindle, K. H., Levey, G. S., and Epstein, S. E. (1970). *J. Clin. Invest.* **49,** 999–1006.

Goldberg, N. D., Dretz, S. B., and O'Toole, A. G. (1969). *J. Biol. Chem.* **244,** 4458–4466.
Goldberg, N. D., O'Dea, R. F., and Haddox, M. K. (1973). *Adv. Cyclic Nucleotide Res.* **3,** 156–221.
Goldberg, N. D., Haddox, M. K., Nicol, S. E., Glass, D. B., Sanford, C. H., Kuehl, F. A., Jr., and Estenson, R. (1975). *Adv. Cyclic Nucleotide Res.* **5,** 307–330.
Goldfine, I. D., Perlman, R., and Roth, J. (1971). *Nature (London)* **234,** 295–297.
Goldstein, R. E., Skelton, C. L., Levey, G. S., Glancy, D. L., Beiser, G. D., and Epstein, S. E. (1971). *Circulation* **44,** 638–647.
Goodsell, E. B., Stein, H. H., and Wenzke, K. J. (1971). *J. Med. Chem.* **14,** 1202–1205.
Goren, E. N., and Rosen, O. M. (1971). *Arch. Biochem. Biophys.* **142,** 720–723.
Goren, E. N., and Rosen, O. M. (1972a). *Arch. Biochem. Biophys.* **153,** 384–397.
Goren, E. N., and Rosen, O. M. (1972b). *Mol. Pharmacol.* **8,** 380–384.
Goren, E. N., Hirsch, A. H., and Rosen, O. M. (1971). *Anal. Biochem.* **43,** 156–161.
Goridis, C., and Morgan, I. G. (1973). *FEBS Lett.* **34,** 71–73.
Goridis, C., Virmaux, N., Urban, P. F., and Mandel, P. (1973). *FEBS Lett.* **30,** 163–166.
Goridis, C., Massarelli, R., Sensenbrenner, M., and Mandel, P. (1974). *J. Neurochem.* **23,** 135–138.
Grahame-Smith, D. G., Butcher, R. W., Ney, R. L., and Sutherland, E. W. (1967). *J. Biol. Chem.* **242,** 5535–5541.
Greengard, P., and Costa, E., eds. (1970). *Adv. Biochem. Psychopharmacol.* **3,** 11–381.
Greengard, P., and Robison, G. A., eds. (1973). *Adv. Cyclic Nucleotide Res.* **3,** 1–406.
Greengard, P., and Robison, G. A., eds. (1974). *Adv. Cyclic Nucleotide Res.* **4,** 1–488.
Greengard, P., Paoletti, R., and Robison, G. A., eds. (1972). *Adv. Cyclic Nucleotide Res.* **1,** 7–610.
Grunfeld, C., Grollman, A. P., and Rosen, O. M. (1974). *Mol. Pharmacol.* **10,** 605–614.
Gulyassy, P. F. (1971). *Life Sci.* **10,** 451–461.
Gulyassy, P. F., and Oken, R. L. (1970). *Proc. Soc. Exp. Biol. Med.* **137,** 361–365.
Hait, W. N., and Weiss, B. (1976). *Nature (London)* **259,** 321–323.
Hanna, P. E., O'Dea, R. F., and Goldberg, N. D. (1972). *Biochem. Pharmacol.* **21,** 2266–2268.
Hardman, J. G., and Sutherland, E. W. (1969). *J. Biol. Chem.* **244,** 6363–6370.
Hardman, J. G., Davis, J. W., and Sutherland, E. W. (1966). *J. Biol. Chem.* **241,** 4812–4815.
Hardman, J. G., Robison, G. A., and Sutherland, E. W. (1971). *Annu. Rev. Physiol.* **33,** 311–336.
Hardman, J. G., Chrisman, T. D., Gray, J. P., Suddath, J. L., and Sutherland, E. W. (1972). *Int. Congr. Pharmacol., 5th,* pp. 227–228. (Abstracts of invited presentations.)
Harris, D. N., Chasin, M., Phillips, M. B., Goldenberg, H., Samaniego, S., and Hess, S. M. (1973). *Biochem. Pharmacol.* **22,** 221–228.
Harwood, J. P., and Rodbell, M. (1973). *J. Biol. Chem.* **248,** 4901–4904.
Harwood, J. P., Low, H., and Rodbell, M. (1973). *J. Biol. Chem.* **248,** 6239–6245.
Haslam, R. J., and Lynham, J. A. (1972). *Life Sci.* **11,** 1143–1154.
Haugaard, N., and Hess, M. E. (1965). *Pharmacol. Rev.* **17,** 27–69.
Haynes, R. C., Jr. (1958). *J. Biol. Chem.* **233,** 1220–1222.
Haynes, R. C., Jr., Sutherland, E. W., and Rall, T. W. (1960). *Recent Prog. Horm. Res.* **16,** 121–133.
Hecht, S. M., Faulkner, R. D., and Hawrelak, S. D. (1974). *Proc. Natl. Acad. Sci. U.S.A.* **71,** 4670–4674.

Hechter, O., Bar, H. P., Matsuba, M., and Soifer, D. (1969). *Life Sci.* **8,** 935–942.
Heersche, J. N. M., Fedak, S. A., and Aurbach, G. D. (1971). *J. Biol. Chem.* **246,** 6770–6775.
Heidrick, M. L., and Ryan, W. L. (1971). *Cancer Res.* **31,** 1313–1315.
Hemington, J. G., Chenowith, M., and Dunn, A. (1973). *Biochim. Biophys. Acta* **304,** 552–559.
Hepp, K. D., Edel, R., and Wieland, O. (1970). *Eur. J. Biochem.* **17,** 171–177.
Higazi, M. G., and Kvinnsland, S. (1974). *J. Reprod. Fertil.* **36,** 135–139.
Hirata, M., and Hayaishi, O. (1965). *Biochem. Biophys. Res. Commun.* **21,** 361–365.
Hirata, M., and Hayaishi, O. (1967). *Biochim. Biophys. Acta* **149,** 1–11.
Hitchcock, M. (1973). *Biochem. Pharmacol.* **22,** 959–969.
Hittleman, K. J., and Butcher, R. W. (1972). *In* "Effects of Drugs on Cellular Control Mechanisms" (B. R. Rabin and R. B. Freedman, eds.), pp. 153–174. Univ. Park Press, Baltimore, Md.
Ho, R. J., and Sutherland, E. W. (1971). *J. Biol. Chem.* **246,** 6822–6827.
Ho, R. J., Jeanrenaud, B., Posternak, T., and Renold, A. E. (1967). *Biochim. Biophys. Acta* **144,** 74–82.
Hollinger, M. A. (1970). *Life Sci.* **9,** 533–540.
Honda, F., and Imamura, H. (1968). *Biochim. Biophys. Acta* **161,** 267–269.
Hopkanen, E., Vapaatolo, H., and Antilla, P. (1972). *Acta Neurol. Scand.* **51,** 375–376.
Horlington, M., and Watson, P. A. (1970). *Biochem. Pharmacol.* **19,** 955–956.
House, P. D. R., Poulis, P., and Weidemann, M. J. (1972). *Eur. J. Biochem.* **24,** 429–437.
Howell, S. L., Green, J. C., and Montague, W. (1973). *Biochem. J.* **136,** 343–349.
Hrapchak, R. J., and Rasmussen, H. (1972). *Biochemistry* **11,** 4458–4465.
Hsie, A. W., and Puck, T. T. (1971). *Proc. Natl. Acad. Sci. U.S.A.* **68,** 358–361.
Huang, M., Shimizu, H., and Daly, J. (1971). *Mol. Pharmacol.* **7,** 155–162.
Huang, M., Ho, A. K. S., and Daly, J. W. (1973a). *Mol. Pharmacol.* **9,** 711–717.
Huang, Y. C., and Kemp, R. G. (1971). *Biochemistry* **10,** 2278–2283.
Huang, Y. C., Duquesnoy, R. J., and Kemp, R. G. (1973b). *Int. J. Biochem.* **4,** 79–88.
Hynie, S., and Sharp, G. W. G. (1971). *Biochim. Biophys. Acta* **230,** 40–51.
Ide, M. (1969). *Biochem. Biophys. Res. Commun.* **36,** 42–46.
Ide, M. (1971). *Arch. Biochem. Biophys.* **144,** 262–268.
Ide, M., Tanaka, A., and Nakamura, M. (1972). *Arch. Biochem. Biophys.* **149,** 189–196.
Ignarro, L. J. (1975). *In* "Cyclic Nucleotides in Disease" (B. Weiss, ed.), pp. 184–210. Univ. Park Press, Baltimore, Md.
Illiano, G., and Cuatrecasas, P. (1972). *Science* **175,** 906–908.
Ishikawa, E., Ishikawa, S., Davis, J. W., and Sutherland, E. W. (1969). *J. Biol. Chem.* **244,** 6371–6376.
Iwai, H. (1974). *J. Biochem.* **76,** 419–429.
Iwangoff, P., and Enz, A. (1971). *Experientia* **27,** 1258–1259.
Iwangoff, P., and Enz, A. (1972). *Agents Actions* **2,** 223–229.
Iwangoff, P., and Enz, A. (1973). *Experientia* **29,** 1067–1069.
Jakobs, K. H., Schultz, K., and Schultz, G. (1972). *Naunyn-Schmiedeberg's Arch. Pharmacol.* **273,** 248–266.
Jande, S. S., and Robert, P. (1974). *Histochemistry* **40,** 323–327.
Jard, S., and Bernard, M. (1970). *Biochem. Biophys. Res. Commun.* **41,** 781–788.
Jefferson, L. S., Exton, J. H., Butcher, R. W., Sutherland, E. W., and Park, C. R. (1968). *J. Biol. Chem.* **243,** 1031–1038.
Johnson, D. G., Thompson, W. J., and Williams, R. H. (1974). *Biochemistry* **13,** 1920–1924.

Johnson, G. A., Boukma, S. J., Lahti, R. A., and Matthews, J. (1973). *J. Neurochem.* **20,** 1387–1392.
Johnson, G. S. (1975). *In* "Cyclic Nucleotides in Disease" (B. Weiss, ed.), pp. 35–44. Univ. Park Press, Baltimore, Md.
Johnson, R., and Sutherland, E. W. (1973). *J. Biol. Chem.* **248,** 5114–5121.
Jungas, R. L. (1966). *Proc. Natl. Acad. Sci. U.S.A.* **56,** 757–763.
Kacew, S., and Singhal, R. L. (1974). *J. Pharmacol. Exp. Ther.* **188,** 265–276.
Kahn, R. H., and Lands, W. E. M., eds. (1973). "Prostaglandins and Cyclic AMP: Biological Actions and Clinical Applications." Academic Press, New York.
Kakiuchi, S., and Rall, T. W. (1968). *Mol. Pharmacol.* **4,** 367–378.
Kakiuchi, S., and Yamazaki, R. (1970). *Biochem. Biophys. Res. Commun.* **41,** 1104–1110.
Kakiuchi, S., Yamazaki, R., and Nakajima, H. (1970). *Proc. Jpn. Acad.* **46,** 587–592.
Kakiuchi, S., Yamazaki, R., and Teshima, Y. (1971). *Biochem. Biophys. Res. Commun.* **42,** 968–974.
Kakiuchi, S., Yamazaki, R., and Teshima, Y. (1972). *Adv. Cyclic Nucleotide Res.* **1,** 455–472.
Kakiuchi, S., Yamazaki, R., Teshima, Y., and Uenishi, K. (1973). *Proc. Natl. Acad. Sci. U.S.A.* **70,** 3526–3530.
Kalisker, A., Rutledge, C. O., and Perkins, J. P. (1973). *Mol. Pharmacol.* **9,** 619–629.
Katz, A. M., Tada, M., Repke, D. I., Iorio, J. M., and Kirchberger, M. A. (1974). *J. Mol. Cell. Cardiol.* **6,** 73–78.
Kauffman, F. C., Harkonen, M. H. A., and Johnson, E. C. (1972). *Life Sci.* **11,** 613–621.
Kebabian, J. W., and Greengard, P. (1971). *Science* **174,** 1346–1349.
Kebabian, J. W., Petzold, G. L., and Greengard, P. (1972). *Proc. Natl. Acad. Sci. U.S.A.* **69,** 2145–2149.
Keirns, J. J., Wheeler, M. A., and Bitensky, M. W. (1974). *Anal. Biochem.* **61,** 336–348.
Khandelwal, R. L., and Hamilton, I. R. (1971). *J. Biol. Chem.* **246,** 3297–3304.
Kimura, H., and Murad, F. (1974). *J. Biol. Chem.* **249,** 6910–6116.
Kissel, J. H., Rosenfeld, M. G., Chase, L. R., and O'Malley, B. W. (1970). *Endocrinology* **86,** 1019–1023.
Klainer, L. M., Chi, Y-M., Friedberg, S. L., Rall, T. W., and Sutherland, E. W. (1962). *J. Biol. Chem.* **237,** 1239–1243.
Klein, I., and Levey, G. S. (1971). *Metab. Clin. Exp.* **20,** 890–896.
Klein, I., Levey, G. S., and Epstein, S. E. (1971). *Proc. Soc. Exp. Biol. Med.* **137,** 366–369.
Klein, I., Fletcher, M., and Levey, G. S. (1973). *J. Biol. Chem.* **248,** 5552–5554.
Klotz, U., and Stock, K. (1972). *Naunyn-Schmiedeberg's Arch. Pharmacol.* **274,** 54–62.
Klotz, U., Berndt, S., and Stock, K. (1972). *Life Sci.* **11,** 7–17.
Kohrman, A. F. (1973). *Pediatr. Res.* **7,** 575–581.
Kolena, J., and Channing, C. P. (1971). *Biochim. Biophys. Acta* **252,** 601–606.
Kreiner, P. W., Gold, C. J., Keirns, J. J., Brock, W. A., and Bitensky, M. W. (1973). *Yale J. Biol. Med.* **46,** 583–591.
Krishna, G., Weiss, B., and Brodie, B. B. (1968a). *J. Pharmacol. Exp. Ther.* **163,** 379–385.
Krishna, G., Hynie, S., and Brodie, B. B. (1968b). *Proc. Natl. Acad. Sci. U.S.A.* **59,** 884–889.
Krishna, G., Harwood, J. P., Barber, A. J., and Jamieson, G. A. (1972). *J. Biol. Chem.* **247,** 2253–2254.
Krishnaraj, R., and Talwar, G. P. (1974). *J. Immunol.* **111,** 1010–1017.
Kuehl, F. A., Jr., Patanelli, D. J., Tarnoff, J., and Humes, J. L. (1970). *Biol. Reprod.* **2,** 154–163.

Kukovetz, W. R., and Poch, G. (1970). *Naunyn-Schmiedeberg's Arch. Pharmacol.* **267,** 189–194.
Kukovetz, W. R., Juan, H., and Poch, G. (1969a). *Naunyn Schmiedberg's Arch. Pharmacol.* **264,** 262–264.
Kukovetz, W. R., Poch, G., and Juan, H. (1969b). *In* "Abstract of the Fourth International Congress on Pharmacology," p. 170. Schwabe, Basel.
Kuo, J. F., Kuo, W-N., and Hodgins, D. S. (1975). *In* "Cyclic Nucleotides in Disease" (B. Weiss, ed.), pp. 211–226. Univ. Park Press, Baltimore, Md.
Kuo, W. N., Hodgins, D. S., and Kuo, J. F. (1973). *J. Biol. Chem.* **248,** 2705–2711.
Kupiecki, F. P. (1969). *Life Sci.* **8,** 645–649.
Kupiecki, F. P. (1973). *J. Lipid Res.* **14,** 250–254.
Kurihara, K. (1972). *FEBS Lett.* **27,** 279–281.
Kuriyama, K., and Israel, M. A. (1973). *Biochem. Pharmacol.* **22,** 2119–2922.
Labrie, F., Lemaire, S., and Courte, C. (1971). *J. Biol. Chem.* **246,** 7293–7302.
Langan, T. A. (1973). *Adv. Cyclic Nucleotide Res.* **3,** 99–153.
Leray, F., Chambaut, M., and Hanoune, J. (1972). *Biochem. Biophys. Res. Commun.* **48,** 1385–1391.
Lerner, L. J., Carminati, P., and Rubin, B. L. (1973). *Proc. Soc. Exp. Biol. Med.* **143,** 536–539.
Levey, G. S. (1970). *Biochem. Biophys. Res. Commun.* **38,** 86–92.
Levey, G. S. (1971a). *J. Biol. Chem.* **246,** 7405–7410.
Levey, G. S. (1971b). *Biochem. Biophys. Res. Commun.* **43,** 108–113.
Levey, G. S. (1975). *In* "Cyclic Nucleotides in Disease" (B. Weiss, ed.), pp. 157–164. Univ. Park Press, Baltimore, Md.
Levey. G. S., Skeleton, C. L., and Epstein, S. E. (1969). *Endocrinology* **85,** 1004–1009.
Levey, G. S., and Epstein, S. E. (1968). *Biochem. Biophys. Res. Commun.* **33,** 990–995.
Levey, G. S., and Epstein. S. E. (1969). *Circ. Res.* **24,** 151–156.
Levey, G. S., and Klein, I. (1973). *Life Sci.* **13,** 41–46.
Levey, G. S., and Pastan, I. (1970). *Life Sci.* **9,** 67–73.
Levey, G. S., Schmidt, W. M., and Mintz, D. H. (1972). *Metab. Clin. Exp.* **21,** 93–98.
Levin, R. M., and Weiss, B. (1976). *Mol. Pharmacol.* **12,** 581–589.
Levine, R. A. (1970). *Gastroenterology* **59,** 280–300.
Lewandowsky, M. (1899). *Arch. Anat. Physiol., Physiol. Abt.* 360–366.
Liao, S., Lin, A. H., and Tomoczko, J. L. (1971). *Biochim. Biophys. Acta.* **230,** 535–538.
Lin, Y. M., Liu, Y. P., and Cheung, W. Y. (1974). *J. Biol. Chem.* **249,** 4943–4954.
Lippmann, W. (1974). *Experientia* **30,** 237–239.
Lippmann, W., Pugsley, T., and Merker, J. (1975). *Life Sci.* **16,** 213–224.
Lopez, E., White, J. E., and Engel, F. L. (1959). *J. Biol. Chem.* **234,** 2254–2258.
Loten, E. G., and Sneyd, J. G. T. (1970). *Biochem. J.* **120,** 187–193.
Lugnier, C., and Stoclet, J. C. (1974). *Biochem. Pharmacol.* **23,** 3071–3074.
Lugnier, C., Bertrand, Y., and Stoclet, J. C. (1972). *Eur. J. Pharmacol.* **19,** 134–136.
Macchia, V., Meldolesi, M. F., and Chiariello, M. (1972). *Endocrinology* **90,** 1483–1491.
McKenzie, S. G., and Bar, H. P. (1973). *Can. J. Physiol. Pharmacol.* **51,** 190–196.
MacManus, J. P., Whitfield, J. F., and Youdale, T. (1971). *J. Cell. Physiol.* **77,** 103–116.
McNeill, J. H., and Muschek, L. D. (1970). *Clin. Res.* **18,** 625.
McNeill. J. H., and Muschek, L. D. (1972a). *Arch. Int. Pharmacodyn. Ther.* **197,** 236–244.
McNeill, J. H., and Muschek, L. D. (1972b). *J. Mol. Cell. Cardiol.* **4,** 611–624.
McNeill, J. H., Nassar, M., and Brody, T. M. (1969). *J. Pharmacol. Exp. Ther.* **165,** 234–241.

McNeill, J. H., Muschek, L. D., and Commarato, M. A. (1970). *Eur. J. Pharmacol.* **10,** 145–150.
McNeill, J. H., Lee, C. Y., and Muschek, L. D. (1972). *Can. J. Physiol. Pharmacol.* **50,** 840–844.
Makman, M. H. (1970). *Science* **170,** 1421–1423.
Makman, M. H. (1971). *Proc. Natl. Acad. Sci. U.S.A.* **68,** 885–889.
Makman, M. H., and Klein, M. I. (1972). *Proc. Natl. Acad. Sci. U.S.A.* **69,** 456–458.
Makman, M. H., and Sutherland, E. W., Jr. (1964). *Endocrinology* **75,** 127–134.
Malamud, D. (1969). *Biochem. Biophys. Res. Commun.* **35,** 754–758.
Malchow, D., Fuchila, J., and Jastorff, B. (1973). *FEBS Lett.* **34,** 5–9.
Mandel, L. R. (1971). *Biochem. Pharmacol.* **20,** 3413–3421.
Mandel, L. R., and Kuehl, F. A., Jr. (1967). *Biochem. Biophys. Res. Commun.* **28,** 13–18.
Manganiello, V., and Vaughan, M. (1972a). *J. Lipid Res.* **13,** 12–16.
Manganiello, V., and Vaughan, M. (1972b). *Proc. Natl. Acad. Sci. U.S.A.* **69,** 269–273.
Manganiello, V., and Vaughan, M. (1972c). *J. Clin. Invest.* **51,** 2763–2767.
Mansour, T. E., Sutherland, E. W., Rall, T. W., and Bueding. E. (1960). *J. Biol. Chem.* **235,** 466–470.
Marcus, R. (1974). *Endocrinology* **96,** 400–408.
Marcus, R., and Aurbach, G. D. (1969). *Endocrinology* **85,** 801–810.
Marinetti, G. V., Ray, T. K., and Tomasi, V. (1969). *Biochem. Biophys. Res. Commun.* **36,** 185–193.
Marks, F. (1973). *Biochim. Biophys. Acta* **309,** 349–356.
Marks, F., and Rebien, W. (1972). *Biochim. Biophys. Acta* **284,** 556–567.
Markwardt, F., and Hoffmann, A. (1970). *Biochem. Pharmacol.* **19,** 2519–2520.
Marsh, J. M. (1970). *J. Biol. Chem.* **245,** 1596–1603.
Marsh, J. M., Butcher, R. W., Savard, K., and Sutherland, E. W. (1966). *J. Biol. Chem.* **241,** 5436–5440.
Mashiter, K., Mashiter, G. D., and Field, J. B. (1974). *Endocrinology* **94,** 370–376.
Matsuzaki, S., and Dumont, J. E. (1972). *Biochim. Biophys. Acta* **284,** 227–234.
Mayer, S. E. (1972). *J. Pharmacol. Exp. Ther.* **181,** 116–125.
Melson, G. L., Chase, L. R., and Aurbach, C. D. (1970). *Endocrinology* **86,** 511–518.
Menahan, L. A., Hepp, K. D., and Wieland, O. (1969). *Eur. J. Biochem.* **8,** 435–443.
Menon, K. M. J., and Jaffe, R. B. (1973). *J. Clin. Endocrinol. Metab.* **36,** 1104–1109.
Menon, K. M. J., and Kiburz, J. (1974). *Biochem. Biophys. Res. Commun.* **56,** 363–371.
Menon, K. M. J., Giese, S., and Jaffe, R. B. (1973). *Biochim. Biophys. Acta* **304,** 203–209.
Meyer, R. B., Jr., and Miller, J. P. (1974). *Life Sci.* **14,** 1019–1040.
Michal, G., Muhlegger, K., Nelboeck, M., Thiessen, C., and Wermann, G. (1974). *Pharmacol. Res. Commun.* **6,** 203–252.
Miki, N., and Yoshida, H. (1972). *Biochim. Biophys. Acta* **268,** 166–174.
Miller, J. P., Boswell, K. H., Muneyama, K., Tolman, R. L., Scholten, M. B., Robins, R. K., Simon, L. N., and Shuman, D. A. (1973a). *Biochem. Biophys. Res. Commun.* **55,** 843–849.
Miller, J. P., Boswell, K. H., Muneyama, K., Simon, L. N., Robins, R. K., and Shuman, D. A. (1973b). *Biochemistry* **12,** 5310–5319.
Miller, J. P., Shuman, D. A., Scholten, M. B., Drimmitt, M. K., Stewart, C. M., Khwaja, T. A., Robins, R. K., and Simon, L. N. (1973c). *Biochemistry* **12,** 1010–1016.
Mizon, J., Skandrani, E., and Mizon, C. (1971). *Therapie* **36,** 911–917.
Monn, E., and Christiansen, R. O. (1971). *Science* **173,** 540–542.
Moore, P. F. (1968). *Ann. N. Y. Acad. Sci.* **150,** 256–260.

Moore, P. F., Iorio, L. C., and McManus, J. M. (1968). *J. Pharm. Pharmacol.* **20,** 368–372.
Mukherjee, C., Caron, M. G., and Lefkowitz, R. J. (1975). *Proc. Natl. Acad. Sci. U.S.A.* **72,** 1945–1949.
Muneyama, K., Bauer, R. J., Shuman, D. A., Robins, R. K., and Simon, L. N. (1971). *Biochemistry* **10,** 2390–2395.
Murad, F. (1973). *Adv. Cyclic Nucleotide Res.* **3,** 355–383.
Murad, F., and Vaughan, M. (1969). *Biochem. Pharmacol.* **18,** 1053–1059.
Murad, F., Chi, Y. M., Rall, T. W., and Sutherland, E. W. (1062). *J. Biol. Chem.* **237,** 1233–1238.
Murad, F., Strauch, B. S., and Vaughan, M. (1969a). *Biochim. Biophys. Acta* **177,** 591–598.
Murad, F., Rall, T. W., and Vaughan, M. (1969b). *Biochim. Biophys. Acta* **192,** 430–445.
Murad, F., Manganiello, V., and Vaughan, M. (1970). *J. Biol. Chem.* **245,** 3352–3360.
Muschek, L. D., and McNeill, J. H. (1971). *Fed. Proc., Fed. Am. Soc. Exp. Biol.* **30,** 330.
Nair, K. G. (1966). *Biochemistry* **5,** 150–157.
Naito, K., and Kuriyama, K. (1973). *Jpn. J. Pharmacol.* **23,** 274–276.
Nakajima, S., Hirschowitz, B. I., and Sachs, G. (1971). *Arch. Biochem. Biophys.* **143,** 123–126.
Nakazawa, S., and Sano, M. (1974). *J. Biol. Chem.* **249,** 4207–4211.
Nathanson, J. A., and Greengard, P. (1973). *Science* **180,** 308–310.
Neelon, F. A., and Birch, B. M. (1973). *J. Biol. Chem.* **248,** 8361–8365.
Newcombe, D. S., Ortel, R. W., and Levey, G. S. (1972). *Biochem. Biophys. Res. Commun.* **48,** 201–204.
Newcombe, D. S., Thanassi, N. M., and Ciosek, C. P., Jr. (1974). *Life Sci.* **14,** 505–519.
Newton, N. E., and Hornbrook, K. R. (1972). *J. Pharmacol. Exp. Ther.* **181,** 479.
O'Dea, R. F., Haddox, M. K., and Goldberg, N. D. (1971). *J. Biol. Chem.* **246,** 6183–6190.
Ohsawa, M., and Endo, H. (1972). *Endocrinol. Jpn.* **19,** 251–257.
Otten, J., Johnson, G. S., and Pastan, I. (1972). *J. Biol. Chem.* **247,** 7082–7087.
Oye, I., Sutherland, E. W. (1966). *Biochim. Biophys. Acta* **127,** 347–354.
Palmer, G. C. (1972). *Neuropharmacology* **11,** 145–149.
Palmer, G. C. (1973). *Life Sci.* **12,** 345–355.
Pannbacker, R. G. (1973). *Science* **182,** 1138–1140.
Pannbacker, R. G. (1974). *Invest. Ophthalmol.* **13,** 535–538.
Pastan, I., and Katzen. R., (1967). *Biochem. Biophys. Res. Commun.* **29,** 792–798.
Pastan, I., Pricer, W., and Blanchette-Mackie, J. (1970). *Metab. Clin. Exp.* **19,** 809–817.
Paul, M. I., Pauk, G. L., and Ditzion, B. R. (1970). *Pharmacology* **3,** 148–154.
Paul, M. I., Cramer, H., and Bunney, W. E., Jr. (1971a). *Science* **171,** 300–303.
Paul, M. I., Kvetnansky, R., Cramer, H., Silbergeld, S., and Kopin, I. J. (1971b). *Endocrinology* **88,** 338–344.
Pawlson, L. G., Lovell-Smith, C. J., Manganiello, V. C., and Vaughan, M. (1974). *Proc. Natl. Acad. Sci. U.S.A.* **71,** 1639–1642.
Peery, C. V., Johnson, G. S., and Pastan, I. (1971). *J. Biol. Chem.* **246,** 5785–5790.
Penit, J., Jard, S., and Benda, P. (1974). *FEBS Lett.* **41,** 156–160.
Pennington, S. N., Brown, H. D., Chattopadhyay, S., Conaway, C., and Morris, H. P. (1970). *Experientia* **26,** 139–140.
Perkins, J. P. (1973). *Adv. Cyclic Nucleotide Res.* **3,** 1–64.
Perkins, J. P., and Moore, M. M. (1973). *J. Pharmacol. Exp. Ther.* **185,** 371–378.
Pettinger, W., Sheppard, H., Palkoski, Z., and Renyi, E. (1973). *Life Sci.* **12,** 49–62.

Pichard, A-L., Hanoune, J., and Kaplan, J-C. (1972). *Biochim. Biophys. Acta* **279,** 217–220.

Pichard, A-L., Hanoune, J., and Kaplan, J-C. (1973). *Biochim. Biophys. Acta* **315,** 370–377.

Pledger, W. J., Stancel, G. M., Thompson, W. J., and Strada, S. J. (1974). *Biochim. Biophys. Acta* **370,** 242–248.

Poch, G. (1971). *Naunyn-Schmiedeberg's Arch. Pharmacol.* **268,** 272–299.

Poch, G., and Kukovetz, W. R. (1969). *Naunyn-Schmiedeberg's Arch. Pharmacol.* **263,** 244–245.

Poch, G., and Kukovetz, W. R. (1971). *Life Sci.* **10,** 133–144.

Poch, G., and Kukovetz, W. R. (1972). *Adv. Cyclic Nucleotide Res.* **1,** 195–211.

Pohl, S. L., Birnbaumer, L., and Rodbell, M. (1969). *Science* **164,** 566–567.

Pohl, S. L., Birnbaumer, L., and Rodbell, M. (1971). *J. Biol. Chem.* **246,** 1849–1856.

Polgar, P., Vera, J. C., Kelley, P. R., and Rutenburg, A. M. (1973). *Biochim. Biophys. Acta* **297,** 378–383.

Posternak, T. (1974). *Annu. Rev. Pharmacol.* **14,** 23–33.

Posternak, T., and Cehovic, G. (1971). *Ann. N.Y. Acad. Sci.* **185,** 42–49.

Prasad, K. N., and Kumar, S. (1972). *Proc. Soc. Exp. Biol. Med.* **142,** 406–409.

Prasad, K. N., Kumar, S., Becker, G., and Sahu, S. K. (1975). *In* "Cyclic Nucleotides in Disease" (B. Weiss, ed.), pp. 45–66. Univ. Park Press, Baltimore, Md.

Price, S. (1973). *Nature (London)* **241,** 54–55.

Price, T. D., Ashman, D. F., and Melicow, M. M. (1967). *Biochim. Biophys. Acta* **138,** 452–465.

Puri, S. K., Cochin, J., and Volicer, L. (1975). *Life Sci.* **16,** 759–768.

Rabinowitz, B., Parmley, W. W., and Bonnoris, G. (1973). *Proc. Soc. Exp. Biol. Med.* **143,** 1072–1076.

Rabinowitz, M., DeSalles, L., Meisler, J., and Lorand, L. (1965). *Biochim. Biophys. Acta* **97,** 29–36.

Rall, T. W. (1969). *In* "The Role of Adenyl Cyclase and Cyclic 3′,5′-AMP in Biological Systems" (T. W. Rall, M. Rodbell, and P. Condliffe, eds.) Nat. Inst. Health, Bethesda, Md.

Rall, T. W. (1972). *Pharmacol. Rev.* **24,** 399–409.

Rall, T. W., and Sutherland, E. W. (1958). *J. Biol. Chem.* **232,** 1065–1076.

Rall, T. W., and Sutherland, E. W. (1961). *Cold Spring Harbor Symp. Quant. Biol.* **26,** 347–354.

Rall, T. W., and Sutherland, E. W. (1962). *J. Biol. Chem.* **237,** 1228–1232.

Rall, T. W., Rodbell, M., and Condliffe, P., eds. (1969). "The Role of Adenyl Cyclase and Cyclic 3′,5′-AMP in Biological Systems," pp. 7–15. Nat. Inst. Health, Bethesda, Md.

Rall, T. W., Sutherland, E. W., and Berthet, J. (1957). *J. Biol. Chem.* **224,** 463–475.

Ramachandran, J., and Lee, V. (1970). *Biochem. Biophys. Res. Commun.* **41,** 358–366.

Ramsden, E. N. (1970). *Lancet* **1,** 108.

Raska, K., Jr. (1973). *Biochem. Biophys. Res. Commun.* **50,** 35–41.

Ray, T. K., Tomasi, V., and Marinetti, G. V. (1970). *Biochim. Biophys. Acta* **211,** 20–30.

Reimann, E. M., Walsh, D. A., and Krebs, E. G. (1971). *J. Biol. Chem.* **246,** 1986–1995.

Rethy, A., Tomasi, V., Trevisani, A., and Barnabei, O. (1972). *Biochim. Biophys. Acta* **290,** 58–69.

Rhoads, A. R., Morris, H. P., and West, W. L. (1972). *Cancer Res.* **32,** 2651–2655.

Robison, G. A., Butcher, R. W., and Sutherland, E. W. (1967). *Ann. N.Y. Acad. Sci.* **139,** 703–723.

Robison, G. A., Butcher, R. W., and Sutherland, E. W. (1968). *Annu. Rev. Biochem.* **37,** 149–174.

Robison, G. A., Butcher, R. W., and Sutherland, E. W. (1969). *In* "Fundamental Concepts in Drug-Receptor Interactions" (J. F. Danielli, J. F. Moran, and D. F. Triggle, eds.), pp. 59–91. Academic Press, New York.

Robison, G. A., Butcher, R. W., and Sutherland, E. W. (1971a). "Cyclic AMP." Academic Press, New York.

Robison, G. A., Nahas, G. G. and Triner, L., eds. (1971b). *Ann. N.Y. Acad. Sci.* **185,** 1–556.

Rodbell, M. (1967). *J. Biol. Chem.* **242,** 5744–5750.

Rodbell, M., Birnbaumer, L., and Pohl, S. L. (1970). *J. Biol. Chem.* **245,** 718–722.

Rodbell, M., Krans, H. M. J., Pohl, S. L., and Birnbaumer, L. (1971a). *J. Biol. Chem.* **246,** 1872–1876.

Rodbell, M., Krans, H. M. J., Pohl, S. L., and Birnbaumer, L. (1971b). *J. Biol. Chem.* **246,** 1861–1871.

Rodbell, M., Birnbaumer, L., Pohl, S. L., and Krans, H. M. J. (1971c). *J. Biol. Chem.* **246,** 1877–1882.

Rojakovick, A. S., and March, R. B. (1972). *Comp. Biochem. Physiol. B* **43,** 209–215.

Rosen, O. M. (1970a). *Arch. Biochem. Biophys.* **137,** 435–441.

Rosen, O. M. (1970b). *Arch. Biochem. Biophys.* **139,** 447–449.

Rosen, O. M., and Erlichman, J. (1969). *Arch. Biochem. Biophys.* **133,** 171–177.

Rosen, O. M., and Rosen, S. M. (1968). *Biochem. Biophys. Res. Commun.* **31,** 82–91.

Rosen, O. M., and Rosen, S. M. (1969). *Arch. Biochem. Biophys.* **131,** 449–456.

Rosen, O. M., and Rosen, S. M. (1970). *Arch. Biochem. Biophys.* **141,** 346–352.

Rosen, O. M., Erlichman, J., and Rosen, S. M. (1970). *Mol. Pharmacol.* **6,** 524–531.

Rosen, O. M., Hirsch, A. H., and Goren, E. N. (1971). *Arch. Biochem. Biophys.* **146,** 660–663.

Rosenfeld, M. G., and O'Malley, B. W. (1970). *Science* **168,** 253–255.

Rosselin, G., and Freychet, P. (1973). *Biochim. Biophys. Acta* **304,** 541–551.

Roy, A. C., and Warren, B. T. (1974). *Biochem. Pharmacol.* **23,** 917–920.

Roy, C., Bockaert, J., Rajerison, R., and Jard, S. (1973). *FEBS Lett.* **30,** 329–334.

Rubalcava, B., and Rodbell, M. (1973). *J. Biol. Chem.* **248,** 3831–3837.

Rubin, C. S., Erlichman, J., and Rosen, O. M. (1972). *J. Biol. Chem.* **247,** 6135–6139.

Rudland, P. S., Gospodarowicz, D., and Seifert, W. (1974). *Nature (London)* **250,** 771–774.

Russell, T. R., and Pastan, I. (1973). *J. Biol. Chem.* **248,** 5835–5840.

Russell, T. R., Thompson, W. J., Schneider, F. W., and Appleman, M. M. (1972). *Proc. Natl. Acad. Sci. U.S.A.* **69,** 1791–1795.

Russell, T. R., Terasaki, W. L., and Appleman, M. M. (1973). *J. Biol. Chem.* **248,** 1334–1340.

Rutten, W. J., Schoot, B. M., DePont, J. J. H. H. M., and Bonting, S. L. (1973). *Biochim. Biophys. Acta* **315,** 384–393.

Ryan, W. L., and Heidrick, M. L. (1968). *Science* **162,** 1484–1485.

Sahyoun, N., and Durr, I. F. (1972). *J. Bacteriol.* **112,** 421–426.

Sakai, T., Thompson, W. J., Lavis, V. R., and Williams, R. W. (1974). *Arch. Biochem. Biophys.* **162,** 331–339.

Sams, D. J., and Montague, W. (1972). *Biochem. J.* **129,** 945–952.

Sattin, A., and Rall, T. W. (1970). *Mol. Pharmacol.* **6,** 13–23.

Sayers, G., and Beall, R. J. (1973). *Science* **179,** 1330–1331.

Schimmer, B. P. (1971). *Biochim. Biophys. Acta* **252,** 567–573.
Schmidt, M. J., Palmer, E. C., Dettbarn, W. D., and Robison, G. A. (1970). *Dev. Psychobiol.* **3,** 53–67.
Schmidt, M. J., Hopkins, J. T., Schmidt, D. E., and Robison, G. A. (1972). *Brain Res.* **42,** 465–477.
Schmidt, S. Y., and Lolley, R. N. (1973). *J. Cell. Biol.* **57,** 117–123.
Schonhofer, P. S., Skidmore, I. F., Bourne, H. R., and Krishna, G. (1972). *Pharmacology* **7,** 65–77.
Schorr, I., and Ney, R. L. (1971). *J. Clin. Invest.* **50,** 1295–1299.
Schramm, M., and Naim, E. (1970). *J. Biol. Chem.* **245,** 3225–3231.
Schramm, M., Feinstein, H., Naim, E., Lang, M., and Lasser, M. (1972). *Proc. Natl. Acad. Sci. U.S.A.* **69,** 523–527.
Schreiber, S. S., Klein, I. L., Oratz, M., and Rothschild, M. S. (1971). *J. Mol. Cell. Cardiol.* **2,** 55–65.
Schroeder, J. (1974). *Biochim. Biophys. Acta* **343,** 173–181.
Schroeder, J., and Plagemann, P. G. W. (1972). *Cancer Res.* **32,** 1082–1087.
Schroeder, J., and Rickenberg, H. V. (1973). *Biochim. Biophys. Acta* **302,** 50–63.
Schultz, G., Senft, G., Losert, W., and Sitt, R. (1966). *Naunyn-Schmiedeberg's Arch. Pharmacol.* **253,** 372.
Schultz, G., Bohme, E., and Munske, K. (1969). *Life Sci.* **8,** 1323–1332.
Schultz, J., and Daly, J. W. (1973). *J. Neurochem.* **21,** 573–579.
Schultz, J., and Gratzner, H. G., eds. (1973). "The Role of Cyclic Nucleotides in Carcinogenesis." Academic Press, New York.
Senft, G., Munske, K., Schultz, G., and Hoffman, M. (1968a). *Naunyn-Schmiedeberg's Arch. Pharmacol.* **259,** 344–359.
Senft, G., Schultz, G., Munske, K., and Hoffmann, M. (1968b). *Diabetologia* **4,** 322–329.
Senft, G., Schultz, G., Munske, K., and Hoffmann, M. (1968c). *Diabetologia* **4,** 330–335.
Severson, D. L., Drummond, G. I., and Sulakhe, P. V. (1972). *J. Biol. Chem.* **247,** 2949–2958.
Sharma, R. (1972). *Cancer Res.* **32,** 1734.
Sharp, G. W. G., Heinie, S., Ebel, H., Parkinson, and Witkum, P. (1973). *Biochim. Biophys. Acta* **309,** 339–348.
Sheppard, H. (1973). *In* "Asthma Physiology, Immunopharmacology and Treatment" (K. F. Austen and L. M. Lichtenstein, eds.). Academic Press, New York.
Sheppard, H., and Burghardt, C. R. (1970). *Mol. Pharmacol.* **6,** 425–429.
Sheppard, H., and Burghardt, C. R. (1971). *Mol. Pharmacol.* **7,** 1–7.
Sheppard, H., and Wiggan, G. (1971). *Mol. Pharmacol.* **7,** 111–115.
Sheppard, H., Wiggan, G., and Tsien, W. (1972). *Adv. Cyclic Nucleotide Res.* **1,** 103–112.
Shima, S., Mitsunaga, M., and Nakao, T. (1971). *Endocrinology* **88,** 465–469.
Shimizu, H., Creveling, C. R., and Daly, J. W. (1970a). *J. Neurochem.* **17,** 441–444.
Shimizu, H., Creveling, C. R., and Daly, J. W. (1970b). *Mol. Pharmacol.* **6,** 184–188.
Shimizu, H., Creveling, C. R., and Daly, J. (1970c). *Proc. Natl. Acad. Sci. U.S.A.* **65,** 1033–1040.
Shimoyama, M., Sakamoto, M., Nasu, S., Shigehisa, S., and Ueda, I. (1972a). *Biochem. Biophys. Res. Commun.* **48,** 235–241.
Shimoyama, M., Kawai, M., Hosin, Y., and Ueda, I. (1972b). *Biochem. Biophys. Res. Commun.* **49,** 1137–1141.
Shuman, D. A., Miller, J. P., Scholten, M. B., Simon, L. N., and Robins, R. K. (1973). *Biochemistry* **12,** 2781–2786.

Skala, J., Novak, E., Hahn, P., and Drummond, G. I. (1972). *Int. J. Biochem.* **3,** 229.
Skidmore, I. F., Schonhofer, P. S., and Kritchevsky, D. (1972). *Pharmacology* **6,** 330–338.
Skoog, F., Strong, F. M., and Miller, C. O. (1965). *Science* **148,** 532–533.
Smith, B. M., and Major, P. W. (1971). *Life Sci.* **10,** 1433–1439.
Smoake, J. A., Song, S. Y., and Cheung, W. Y. (1974). *Biochim. Biophys. Acta* **341,** 402–411.
Sobel, B. E., Dempsey, P. J., and Cooper, T. (1968). *Biochem. Biophys. Res. Commun.* **33,** 758–762.
Sobel, B. E., Henry, P. D., Robison, A., Bloor, C., and Ross, J., Jr. (1969). *Circ. Res.* **24,** 507–512.
Soifer, D., and Hechter, O. (1971). *Biochim. Biophys. Acta* **230,** 539–542.
Song, S. Y., and Cheung, W. Y. (1971). *Biochim. Biophys. Acta* **242,** 593–605.
Spiegel, A. M., and Bitensky, M. W. (1969). *Endocrinology* **85,** 638–643.
Sproles, A. C. (1973). *J. Dent. Res.* **52,** 915–917.
Stefanovich, V. (1974a). *Res. Commun. Chem. Path. Pharmacol.* **7,** 557–572.
Stefanovich, V. (1974b). *Res. Commun. Chem. Path. Pharmacol.* **7,** 573–582.
Stifel, F. B., Greene, H. L., and Herman, R. H. (1971). *Endocrinology* **89,** 896–897.
Stoff, J. S., Handler, J. S., Preston, A. S., and Orloff, J. (1973). *Life Sci.* **13,** 545–552.
Stoner, J., Manganiello, V. C., and Vaughan, M. (1974). *Mol. Pharmacol.* **10,** 155–161.
Strada, S. J., and Pledger, W. J. (1975). *In* "Cyclic Nucleotides in Disease" (B. Weiss, ed.), pp. 3–34. Univ. Park Press, Baltimore, Md.
Strada, S. J., and Weiss, B. (1972). *Soc. Neurosci.* **2,** 229.
Strada, S. J., and Weiss, B. (1974). *Arch. Biochem. Biophys.* **160,** 197–204.
Strada, S. J., Klein, D. C., Weller, J., and Weiss, B. (1972). *Endocrinology* **90,** 1470–1475.
Strada, S. J., Uzunov, P., and Weiss, B. (1974). *J. Neurochem.* **23,** 1097–1103.
Streeto, J. M. (1969). *Metab. Clin. Exp.* **18,** 968–973.
Sulakhe, P. V., and Dhalla, N. S. (1972). *Biochem. Med.* **6,** 471–482.
Sulakhe, P. V., and Dhalla, N. S. (1973). *Biochim. Biophys. Acta* **293,** 379–396.
Sullivan, T. J., and Parker, C. W. (1973). *Biochem. Biophys. Res. Commun.* **55,** 1334–1339.
Sung, C. P., Wiebelhaus, V. D., Jenkins, B. C., Adlercreutz, P., Hirschowitz, B. I., and Sachs, G. (1972). *Am. J. Physiol.* **223,** 648–650.
Sung, C. P., Jenkins, B. C., Burns, L. R., Hackney, V., Spenney, J., Sachs, G., and Wiebelhaus, V. D. (1973). *Am. J. Physiol.* **225,** 1359–1363.
Sutherland, D. J. B., and Singhal, R. L. (1974). *Biochim. Biophys. Acta* **343,** 238–249.
Sutherland, E. W., and Rall, T. W. (1958). *J. Biol. Chem.* **232,** 1077–1091.
Sutherland, E. W., and Robison, G. A. (1966). *Pharmacol. Rev.* **18,** 145–161.
Sutherland, E. W., Rall, T. W., and Menon, T. (1962). *J. Biol. Chem.* **237,** 1220–1227.
Sutherland, E. W., Robison, G. A., and Butcher, R. W. (1968). *Circulation* **37,** 279–306.
Sweat, F. W., and Hupka, A. (1971). *Biochem. Biophys. Res. Commun.* **44,** 1436–1442.
Swislocki, N. I., Tierney, J., and Sonenberg, M. (1973). *Biochem. Biophys. Res. Commun.* **53,** 1109–1114.
Szabo, M., and Burke, G. (1972). *Biochim. Biophys. Acta* **284,** 208–219.
Tao, M., and Lipmann, F. (1969). *Proc. Natl. Acad. Sci. U.S.A.* **63,** 86–92.
Taunton, O. D., Roth, J., and Pastan, I. (1967). *Biochem. Biophys. Res. Commun.* **29,** 1–7.
Taunton, O. D., Roth, J., and Pastan, I. (1969). *J. Biol. Chem.* **244,** 247–253.
Tell, G. P. E., Cuatrecasas, P., Van Wyk, J. J., and Hintz, R. L. (1973). *Science* **180,** 312–315.

Teo, T. S., and Wang, J. H. (1973). *J. Biol. Chem.* **248,** 5950–5955.
Teo, T. S., Wang, T. H., and Wang, J. H. (1973). *J. Biol. Chem.* **248,** 588–595.
Teshima, Y., and Kakiuchi, S. (1974). *Biochem. Biophys. Res. Commun.* **56,** 489–495.
Thanassi, N. M., and Newcombe, D. S. (1974). *Proc. Soc. Exp. Biol. Med.* **147,** 710–714.
Therriault, D. G., and Wingers, V. G. (1970). *Life Sci.* **9,** 421–428.
Therriault, D. G., Morningstar, J. F., Jr., and Winters, V. G. (1969). *Life Sci.* **8,** 1353–1358.
Thomas, J. A., and Singhal, R. L. (1973). *Biochem. Pharmacol.* **22,** 507–511.
Thompson, W. J., and Appleman, M. M. (1971a). *J. Biol. Chem.* **246,** 3145–3150.
Thompson, W. J., and Appleman, M. M. (1971b). *Biochemistry* **10,** 311–316.
Thompson, W. J., and Appleman, M. M. (1971c). *Ann. N.Y. Acad. Sci.* **185,** 36–41.
Thompson, W. J., Williams, R. A., and Little, S. A. (1973a). *Arch. Biochem. Biophys.* **159,** 206–213.
Thompson, W. J., Williams, R. H., and Little, S. A. (1973b). *Biochem. Biophys. Acta* **302,** 329–337.
Thompson, W. J., Little, S. A., and Williams, R. H. (1973c). *Biochemistry* **12,** 1889–1894.
Thompson, W. J., Johnson, D. G., Lavis, V. R., and Williams, R. H. (1974). *Endocrinology* **94,** 276–278.
Tisdale, M. J. (1975). *Biochem. Biophys. Res. Commun.* **62,** 872–882.
Tisdale, M. J., and Phillips, B. J. (1975). *Biochem. Pharmacol.* **24,** 211–217.
Tomasi, V., Koretz, S., Ray, T. K., Dunnick, J., and Marinetti, G. V. (1970). *Biochim. Biophys. Acta* **211,** 31–42.
Toson, G. C., and Carpenedo, F. (1972). *Arch. Pharmacol.* **273,** 168–171.
Trendelenburg, V. (1963). *Pharmacol. Rev.* **15,** 225–276.
Trendelenburg, V. (1966). *Pharmacol. Rev.* **18,** 629–640.
Triner, L., Vulliemoz, Y., Schwartz, I., and Nahas, G. G. (1970). *Biochem. Biophys. Res. Commun.* **40,** 64–69.
Tsung, P-K., and Weissmann, G. (1973). *Biochem. Biophys. Res. Commun.* **51,** 836–842.
Uno, I., and Ishikawa, T. (1973). *J. Bacteriol.* **113,** 1249–1255.
Uzunov, P., and Weiss, B. (1971). *Neuropharmacology* **10,** 697–708.
Uzunov, P., and Weiss, B. (1972a). *Adv. Cyclic Nucleotide Res.* **1,** 435–453.
Uzunov, P., and Weiss, B. (1972b). *Biochim. Biophys. Acta* **284,** 220–226.
Uzunov, P., Shein, H. M., and Weiss, B. (1973). *Science* **180,** 304–306.
Uzunov, P., Shein, H. M., and Weiss. B. (1974). *Neuropharmacology* **13,** 377–391.
Van Inwegen, R. G., Robison, G. A., Thompson, W. J., Armstrong, K. J., and Stouffer, J. E. (1975). *J. Biol. Chem.* **250,** 2452–2456.
Vatner, D. E., and Lefkowitz, R. J. (1974). *Mol. Pharmacol.* **10,** 450–456.
Vaughan, M., and Murad, F. (1969). *Biochemistry* **8,** 3092–3099.
Vaughan, M., and Steinberg, D. (1963). *J. Lipid Res.* **4,** 193–199.
Vernikos-Danellis, J., and Harris, C. G., III. (1968). *Proc. Soc. Exp. Biol. Med.* **128,** 1016–1021.
Vigdahl, R. L., Mongin, J., Jr., and Marquis, N. R. (1971). *Biochem. Biophys. Res. Commun.* **42,** 1088–1094.
von Hungen, K., and Roberts, S. (1973). *Eur. J. Biochem.* **36,** 391–401.
Von Voightlander, P. F., Boukma, S. J., and Johnson, G. A. (1973). *Neuropharmacology* **12,** 1081–1086.
Voorhees, J. J., Duell, E. A., Stawiski, M., Creehan, P., and Harrell, E. R. (1975). *In* "Cyclic Nucleotides in Disease" (B. Weiss, ed.), pp. 79–101. Univ. Park Press, Baltimore, Md.
Walker, J. B., and Walker, J. A. (1973). *Brain Res.* **54,** 391–396.

Walsh, D. A., Ashby, C. D., Gonzales, C., Calkins, D., Fischer, E. H., and Krebs, E. G. (1971). *J. Biol. Chem.* **246,** 1977–1985.
Walter, R., Kirchberger, M. A., and Hruby, V. J. (1972a). *Experientia* **28,** 959–960.
Walter, R., Schwartz, I. L., Hechter, O., Dousa, T., and Hoffman, P. L. (1972b). *Endocrinology* **91,** 39.
Wang, Y. C., Pandey, G. N., Mendels, J., and Frazer, A. (1974). *Biochem. Pharmacol.* **23,** 845–855.
Ward, W. F., and Fain, J. N. (1971). *Biochim. Biophys. Acta* **237,** 387–390.
Webb, D. R., Bourne, H. R., and Levinson, W. (1974). *Biochem. Pharmacol.* **23,** 1663–1667.
Weinryb, I., Chasin, M., Free, C. A., Harris, D. N., Goldenberg, H., Michel, I. M., Paik, V. S., Phillips, M., Samaniego, S., and Hess, S. M. (1972). *J. Pharm. Sci.* **61,** 1556–1567.
Weinryb, I., Michel, I. M., and Hess, S. M. (1973). *Arch. Biochem. Biophys.* **154,** 240–249.
Weis, A. S., Tepperman, H. M., and Tepperman, J. (1973). *Endocrinology* **93,** 504–509.
Weiss, B. (1969a). *J. Pharmacol. Exp. Ther.* **166,** 330–338.
Weiss, B. (1969b). *J. Pharmacol. Exp. Ther.* **168,** 146–152.
Weiss, B. (1970). *In* "Biogenic Amines as Physiological Regulators" (J. J. Blum, ed.), pp. 35–73. Prentice Hall, Englewood Cliffs, N.J.
Weiss, B. (1971a). *Ann. N.Y. Acad. Sci.* **185,** 507–519.
Weiss, B. (1971b). *J. Neurochem.* **18,** 469–477.
Weiss, B. ed. (1975a). "Cyclic Nucleotides in Disease." Univ. Park Press, Baltimore, Md.
Weiss, B. (1975b). Second Int. Comf. Cyclic AMP. *In* "Advances in Cyclic Nucleotide Research" (G. I. Drummond, P. Greenyard, and G. A. Robison, eds.), Vol. 5, pp. 195–211. Raven, New York.
Weiss, B., and Costa, E. (1967). *Science* **156,** 1750–1752.
Weiss, B., and Costa, E. (1968a). *J. Pharmacol. Exp. Ther.* **161,** 310–319.
Weiss, B., and Costa, E. (1968b). *Biochem. Pharmacol.* **17,** 2107–2116.
Weiss, B., and Crayton, J. W. (1970a). *Adv. Biochem. Psychopharmacol.* **3,** 217–239.
Weiss, B., and Crayton, J. (1970b). *Endocrinology* **87,** 527–533.
Weiss, B., and Greenberg, L. H. (1975). *In* "Cyclic Nucleotides in Disease" (B. Weiss, ed.), pp. 269–320. Univ. Park Press, Baltimore, Md.
Weiss, B., and Kidman, A. D. (1969). *Adv. Biochem. Psychopharmacol.* **1,** 131–164.
Weiss, B., and Strada, S. J. (1972). *Adv. Cyclic Nucleotides Res.* **1,** 357–374.
Weiss, B., and Strada, S. J. (1973). *In* "Fetal Pharmacology" (L. Boreus, ed.), pp. 205–232. Raven Press, New York.
Weiss, B., Davies, J. I., and Brodie, B. B. (1966). *Biochem. Pharmacol.* **15,** 1553–1561.
Weiss, B., Shein, H. M., and Snyder, R. (1971). *Life Sci.* **10,** 1253–1260.
Weiss, B., Lehne, R., and Strada, S. J. (1972). *Anal. Biochem.* **45,** 222–235.
Weiss, B., Fertel, R., Figlin, R., and Uzunov, P. (1974). *Mol. Pharmacol.* **10,** 615–625.
White, A. A., and Aurbach, G. D. (1969). *Biochim. Biophys. Acta* **191,** 686–697.
Wickson, D., Bondreau, R. J., and Drummond, G. I. (1975). *Biochemistry* **14,** 669–675.
Williams, R. H., and Thompson, W. J. (1973). *Proc. Soc. Exp. Biol. Med.* **143,** 382–387.
Williams, R. H., Little, S. A., and Ensinck, J. W. (1969). *Am. J. Med. Sci.* **258,** 190–202.
Winchurch, R., Ishizuka, M., Webb, D., and Braun, W. (1971). *J. Immunol.* **106,** 1399–1400.
Wolfe, S. M., and Shulman, N. R. (1969). *Biochem. Biophys. Res. Commun.* **35,** 265–272.

Wolff, D. J., and Brostrom, C. O. (1974). *Arch. Biochem. Biophys.* **163,** 349–358.
Wolff, D. J., and Siegel, F. (1972). *J. Biol. Chem.* **247,** 4180–4185.
Wolff, J., and Cook, G. H. (1973). *J. Biol. Chem.* **248,** 350–355.
Wolff, J., and Jones, A. B. (1970). *Proc. Natl. Acad. Sci. U.S.A.* **65,** 454–459.
Wolff, J., and Jones, A. B. (1971). *J. Biol. Chem.* **12,** 3939–3947.
Wolff, J., Berens, S. C., and Jones, A. B. (1970). *Biochem. Biophys. Res. Commun.* **39,** 77–82.
Wollenberger, A., Schulze, W., and Krause, E. G. (1973). *J. Mol. Cell. Cardiol.* **5,** 427–431.
Woo, Y. T., and Manery, J. F. (1973). *Arch. Biochem. Biophys.* **154,** 510–519.
Wray, H. L., and Harris, A. W. (1973). *Biochem. Biophys. Res. Commun.* **53,** 291–294.
Yamashita, K., and Field, J. B. (1970). *Biochem. Biophys. Res. Commun.* **40,** 171–178.
Yamashita, K., and Field, J. B. (1973). *Biochim. Biophys. Acta* **304,** 686–692.
Zieve, P. D., and Greenough, W. B., III. (1969). *Biochem. Biophys. Res. Commun.* **35,** 462–466.
Zinman, B., and Hollenberg, C. H. (1974). *J. Biol. Chem.* **249,** 2182–2187.
Zor, U., Kaneko, T., Lowe, I. P., Bloom, G., and Field, J. B. (1969). *J. Biol. Chem.* **244,** 5189–5195.

# 5-Azacytidine—A New Anticancer Drug with Significant Activity in Acute Myeloblastic Leukemia

DANIEL D. VON HOFF AND MILAN SLAVIK

*Investigational Drug Branch, Division of Cancer Treatment*
*National Cancer Institute, National Institutes of Health*
*Bethesda, Maryland*

I. Introduction . . . 285
II. Chemical and Physicochemical Properties . . . 286
A. Chemical Properties . . . 286
B. Pharmaceutical Data . . . 288
III. Biological Properties . . . 288
A. Antimicrobial Activity . . . 288
B. Cytotoxic and Antineoplastic Activity . . . 289
C. Abortive Activity . . . 289
D. Mutagenicity . . . 289
E. Leukopenia . . . 290
F. Other Properties . . . 290
IV. Modes of Action and Resistance . . . 291
A. Mechanism of Action . . . 291
B. Resistance . . . 295
V. Experimental Activity . . . 297
A. Antitumor Activity . . . 297
B. Drug Schedule Dependency . . . 299
VI. Animal Toxicity . . . 300
VII. Drug Metabolism and Disposition . . . 303
A. *In Vitro* Studies . . . 303
B. Studies in a Bacterial System . . . 304
C. Studies in Rodents . . . 305
D. Studies in Dogs . . . 306
E. Studies in Man . . . 306
VIII. Clinical Studies . . . 309
A. Phase I Studies . . . 309
B. Antineoplastic Activity by Tumor Type . . . 310
C. Toxicity in Man . . . 317
IX. Summary and Conclusions . . . 322
References . . . 323

## I. Introduction

The Division of Cancer Treatment (DCT) of the National Cancer Institute (NCI) in its drug development function sponsors clinical trials with investigational anticancer drugs. These drugs are gathered from various sources, about two-thirds of them coming from the DCT drug screening program and about one-third from a cooperative drug exchange program conducted throughout the world.

Among the interesting anticancer drugs developed abroad is 5-azacytidine, a ring analog of cytidine originally synthesized by the Czechoslovakian investigators Piskala and Sorm (1964). Two years later, Hanka *et al.* (1966) produced the compound microbiologically in a fermentation broth of *Streptoverticillium ladakanus* (var. *ladakanus*) and it was further characterized by Bergy and Herr (1966).

In the last 10 years, a fair amount of preclinical and clinical data have accumulated. This information requires an updated analysis, particularly in light of the fact that this drug has shown substantial clinical activity in the treatment of acute myelogenous leukemia (AML) previously refractory to other antileukemic drugs.

## II. Chemical and Physicochemical Properties

5-Azacytidine has the empirical formula $C_8H_{12}N_4O_5$ and the structure, in comparison to cytidine, is shown in Fig. 1.

### A. Chemical Properties

Chemical properties (Bergy and Herr, 1966) necessary for identifying the compound are listed in Table I.

The structure–activity relationship of 5-azacytidine has been discussed by Zee-Cheng and Cheng (1970), who found that it has a structural feature in common with some nonalkylating antileukemic agents such as aminopterin, anthramycin, camptothecin, cytosine arabi-

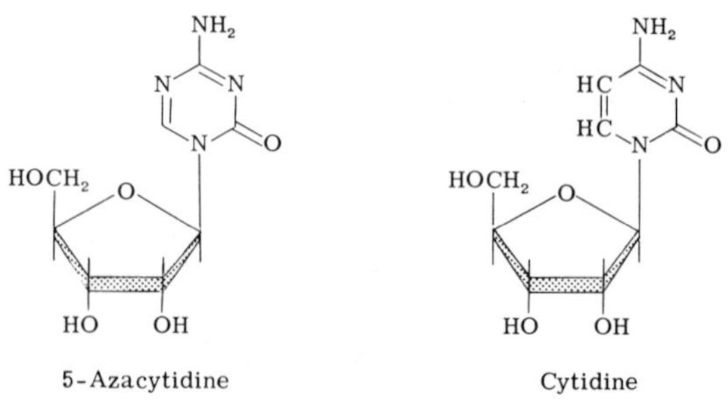


FIG. 1. Structures of 5-azacytidine and cytidine.

TABLE I

CHEMICAL PROPERTIES OF 5-AZACYTIDINE

Description
White crystalline powder, melting point 228–230°C
Molecular weight = 244.2

Solubility
In water = 40 mg/ml
In ethanol = 1 mg/ml
In acetone = 1 mg/ml
In chloroform = 1 mg/ml
In hexane = 1 mg/ml
In dimethylsulfoxide = 1 mg/ml

Specific rotation
$[\alpha]_D^{25}$ + 39 (1% water)

Ultraviolet absorption maxima
In water at 241 m$\mu$, $a$ = 35.9 ($\epsilon$ = 8767)
In 0.01 $N$ HCl at 248 m$\mu$, $a$ = 12.6 ($\epsilon$ = 3077)
In 0.01 $N$ KOH at 223 m$\mu$, $a$ = 99.1 ($\epsilon$ = 24,200);
shoulder at 253 m$\mu$, $a$ = 6.3 ($\epsilon$ = 1538)

Paper chromatography
Paper—Whatman No. 1
Sample—200 (warm water)
Solvent systems:
a. 0.5% $Na_2CO_3$
b. 5% $Na_2HPO_4$
c. $n$-$BuOH^2$/ETOH/$H_2O$ (40:11:19)
Detection:
a. UV
b. Potassium periodatocuprate
c. Aniline citrate spray

noside, daunomycin, emetine, demecolcine, riboside, methotrexate, streptonigrin, vinblastine, and vincristine. This structural feature consists of triangulation between 1 nitrogen and 2 oxygen atoms with rather definite interatomic distances. The pattern of N—O—O triangulation in 5-azacytidine is shown in Fig. 2, with the interatomic distances being N-$O_1$ = 7.05 Å, N-$O_2$ = 8.50 Å, and $O_1$-$O_2$ = 3.30 Å. These values compare favorably with those in the other nonalkylating antileukemic compounds.

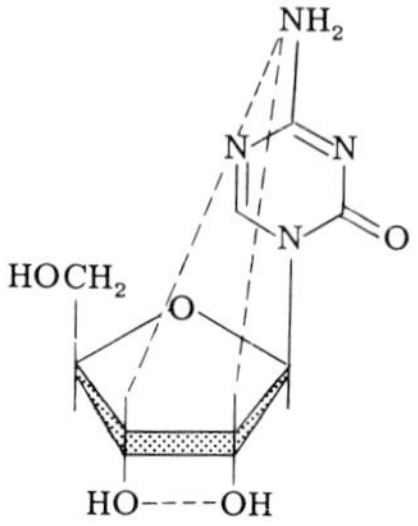

FIG. 2. The N—O—O triangulation pattern for 5-azacytidine. (From Zee-Cheng and Cheng, 1970. Adapted with permission of the copyright owner.)

### B. Pharmaceutical Data

5-Azacytidine for injection can be obtained from the Cancer Therapy Evaluation Program, DCT, NCI, and is supplied in 100-mg vials with 100-mg mannitol (USP). The product is prepared as a white lyophilized powder in 20-ml vials. When reconstituted with 19.9 ml of sterile water for injection (USP), each milliliter of solution contains 5 mg of 5-azacytidine and 5 mg of mannitol at pH 6.0–7.5. The reconstituted solution hydrolyzes at room temperature (Notari and DeYoung, 1975; Pithova *et al.*, 1965) and should be used within 30 minutes.

The reconstituted solution can be further diluted with lactated Ringer's injection (USP), which provides optimum pH for solution stability. The pH of this solution at a concentration of 100 mg/500 ml is approximately 6.37. The reconstituted solution further diluted in this manner should be used within 2 to 3 hours. Over this period of time, 10–15% decomposition occurs based on ultraviolet and nuclear magnetic resonance assay methods (Lim *et al.*, 1974).

## III. Biological Properties

5-Azacytidine became of interest to early investigators because it possessed antimicrobial, cytotoxic, antineoplastic, abortive, leukopenic, and mutagenic activity.

### A. Antimicrobial Activity

Hanka *et al.* (1966) found that 5-azacytidine had no *in vitro* activity against gram-positive organisms but was active against gram-negative bacteria. The minimal inhibitory concentration for *Escherichia coli* in synthetic broth for 24 hours was 0.01 $\mu$g/ml. A drug concentration of about 50 μg/ml was needed for equivalent inhibition of *E. coli* grown in natural broth. This need was attributed to the presence in the natural broth of small amounts of cytidine and uridine which were believed to compete with 5-azacytidine (see below). The inhibition of *E. coli* was bacteriostatic up to the highest concentrations tested (250 μg/ml). *In vivo*, 5-azacytidine was inactive against *E. coli* in mice at subcutaneous doses of 25 mg/kg. The antimicrobial aspects of 5-azacytidine have not been further pursued except to develop an assay system for 5-azacytidine levels. Pittelo and Woolley (1969) have perfected the microbiological assay using *E. coli* type ATCC 9637 (a strain resistant to 6-chloropurine) which has a sensitivity of 0.1 μg/ml. Filter paper is impregnated with a 5-azacytidine control and blood with unknown levels. The level is calculated by the size of the zone of inhibition.

### B. Cytotoxic and Antineoplastic Activity

Hanka *et al.* (1966) also found that 5-azacytidine was moderately cytotoxic to KB cells grown in liquid media. The concentration required for 50% growth inhibition was 0.25 μg/ml, which could be reversed by cytidine or uridine. Antitumor data are discussed in Section V.

### C. Abortive Activity

5-Azacytidine at doses of 2.5 mg/kg/day will interrupt pregnancy in mice during the first week of gestation, with its activity increasing during the first days of pregnancy to an optimum reached between the fourth and sixth days (Svata *et al.*, 1966; Seifertova *et al.*, 1968). During the last 10 days of pregnancy the drug has no discernible effect.

### D. Mutagenicity

5-Azacytidine has been shown to be a potent mutagen of viruses (Halle, 1968; Pringle, 1970) and bacteria (Fucik *et al.*, 1965a). Altanerova and Altaner (1972) investigated the properties of avian sarcoma viruses induced by 5-azacytidine from a hamster cell line transformed with the Schmidt-Ruppin strain of avian sarcoma virus. Results showed the new 5-azacytidine-induced avian viruses were oncogenic for young hamsters. It was the most potent virus in the ability to induce tumors in hamsters. The difference between the control virus and the induced viruses was a higher level of RNA-dependent DNA polymerase in the induced virus. It was concluded that the induction of infectious viruses from virogenic hamster cell lines by 5-azacytidine was leading to mutation of the virus.

## E. Leukopenia

5-Azacytidine causes a decrease in the number of circulating lymphocytes and mature myeloid cells of bone marrow (Sorm and Vesely, 1964).

## F. Other Properties

Other intriguing properties that have been incompletely investigated include the following.

### 1. *Effect on Ultraviolet Damage*

Grunow (1972) has reported that addition of 5-azacytidine to the culture medium decreases the inactivation effects of ultraviolet light on certain strains of *E. coli*.

### 2. *Possible Radioprotective Effect*

The administration of 1.5 mg/kg of 5-azacytidine for 3 days to mice prior to supralethal X-ray doses has reduced mortality from 100 to 40% (Vesely *et al.*, 1969). In the pretreated animals, the number of blood leukocytes and bone marrow nucleated cells was considerably higher than in animals that were only irradiated. The drug was fully effective when given for 3 consecutive days, with the last dose 24 hours prior to irradiation. No clear reversal of the radioprotection effect could be obtained by simultaneous administration of cytidine. The authors proposed that, in view of its potent suppressive effect on leukemia in mice, the radioprotective effect of 5-azacytidine could be used for the combined therapeutic attack of X-ray and chemotherapy.

Different data have been obtained in the broad bean *Vicia faba*, in which pretreatment was without effect on chromosome abberrations induced by X rays (Fucik *et al.*, 1970).

### 3. *Immunosuppression and Antibody Inhibition*

Although Sorm *et al.* (1966) mentioned 5-azacytidine as a strong inhibitor of antibody formation, no data were given to support this claim. Vadlamudi *et al.* (1970a) determined that 5-azacytidine did, indeed, decrease the formation of antibodies against sheep red blood cells (SRBC) in mice when the drug was given after, rather than before, the administration of SRBC. They also showed that simultaneously administered uridine reduced the immunosuppressive effect as measured by hemagglutination tests.

#### 4. *Retention of 5-Azacytidine in Lymphatic Tissue*

Sorm and Vesely (1964) noted pronounced morphological changes and involution of the thymus, spleen, and bone marrow after treatment of mice with 5-azacytidine. Concentrations of 5-azacytidine are highest in the spleen and thymus 24 hours after injection (Raska *et al.*, 1965a).

## IV. Modes of Action and Resistance

### A. Mechanism of Action

Attempts to define the mechanics of 5-azacytidine action have employed many biological systems. Much of the early information pointed to a possible interference with nucleic acid metabolism. Hanka *et al.* (1966) and Cihak and Sorm (1965) noted that cytidine, uridine, and thymidine, but not uracil or cytosine, reversed the antimicrobial effect of 5-azacytidine and suggested that 5-azacytidine may interfere with nucleic acid metabolism prior to the steps involving cytidine and uridine since these pyrimidines could reverse the activity of 5-azacytidine. These results agreed with Sorm *et al.* (1964), who suggested that there was enough cytidine or uridine in the nutrient broth to reverse the antimicrobial effect of the drug. 5-Azacytidine also inhibited growth and produced a high incidence of chromosomal abnormalities in the *V. faba*, but this could be prevented by adding excess cytidine to the 5-azacytidine solution (Fucik *et al.*, 1965b).

More specifically, four mechanisms of action have been proposed for 5-azacytidine interference with nucleic acid metabolism. Each of them is discussed separately in the following.

#### 1. *Incorporation of 5-Azacytidine into DNA*

5-Azacytidine is utilized by the cells of the root system of *V. faba* as a precursor of deoxyribonucleotide in polymeric DNA (Pithova *et al.*, 1964). It is also incorporated into the DNA, where it replaces 52% of the cytosine (Zandrazil *et al.*, 1965, 1972), and into RNA polynucleotides, replacing 20–30% of the cytidine in bacterial enzymes without affecting DNA polymerase (Karon and Benedict, 1970; Paces *et al.*, 1968; Li *et al.*, 1970a).

5-Azacytidine is incorporated into the DNA fractions in L1210 cells in culture (Li *et al.*, 1970a). The 5-azacytidine is phosphorylated in all leukemic cells studies (Li *et al.*, 1970a), with the majority of phosphorylated products existing as a triphosphate (see the proposed sequence model in Fig. 3).

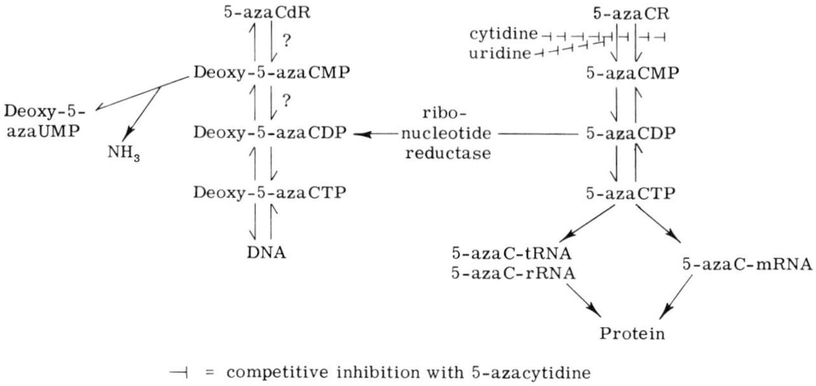

5-azaCdR
?
Deoxy-5-azaCMP
?
Deoxy-5-azaUMP
$NH_3$
Deoxy-5-azaCDP ← ribonucleotide reductase — 5-azaCDP
Deoxy-5-azaCTP
DNA
5-azaCR
cytidine
uridine
5-azaCMP
5-azaCDP
5-azaCTP
5-azaC-tRNA
5-azaC-rRNA
5-azaC-mRNA
Protein

⊣ = competitive inhibition with 5-azacytidine

FIG. 3. Schema for incorporation of 5-azacytidine into DNA and RNA. 5-azaCR = 5-azacytidine, 5-azaCdR = 5-azacytidine deoxyriboside.

There is no unequivocal evidence that 5-azacytidine is incorporated into the DNA of mammalian cells *in vivo* (Heidelberger, 1974). Li *et al.* (1970a) suggested that the inhibition of DNA synthesis by 5-azacytidine is probably the result of its incorporation into DNA and the subsequent prevention of further synthesis since no effect of the 5-azacytidine on thymidine kinase, cytidine kinase, ribonucleotide reductase, and DNA polymerase could be detected. This depression of DNA synthesis by 5-azacytidine has been observed in developing sea urchin embryos (Crkvenjakov *et al.*, 1970), isoproterenol-stimulated mouse salivary glands (Simson and Baserga, 1971), lymphoid and bone marrow tissue (especially mature myeloid elements) of mice (Vesely and Sorm, 1965), rhesus monkey kidney cells in tissue cultures (Sorm *et al.*, 1966), and regenerating rat liver (Cihak and Vesely, 1964). All of these models represent rapidly proliferating systems in which DNA synthesis has been stimulated or induced. Cihak *et al.* (1972a) argue that the rate of thymidine incorporation into the *intact* rat liver is not affected by 5-azacytidine, so it appears that 5-azacytidine does not interfere with the process of DNA synthesis per se but rather at a preceding phase.

In view of the fact that the symmetrical triazine molecule is unstable (Sorm *et al.*, 1964) and readily degrades spontaneously (Cihak *et al.*, 1967a), it is thought that a similar degradation takes place in the nucleic acid molecule. Degradation of 5-azacytidine in nucleic acids has been shown by the decreased denaturation temperature of RNA and DNA with incorporated 5-azacytidine. Perhaps the DNA molecules containing 5-azacytidine are less stable and more liable to disruption of the secondary structure and, therefore, suffer chromosomal breakage (Zandrazil *et al.*, 1965). Local uncoiling (segment extension) of specific chromosome segments and chromatid aberrations have been produced in 5-azacytidine-treated *V. faba* (Fucik *et al.*, 1970). Chromatid breakage was also induced by 5-azacytidine in hamster fibroblast (DON) cells (Karon and Benedict, 1970).

### 2. *Incorporation of 5-Azacytidine into RNA, Producing Interference with Protein Synthesis*

5-Azacytidine causes a breakdown of hepatic polyribosomes to inactive monomers and dimers in the rat (Levitan and Webb, 1969). This effect has been attributed to the incorporation of 5-azacytidine into RNA. 5-Azacytidine has been shown to be incorporated into the RNA of nuclei isolated from cells of calf thymus (Raska *et al.*, 1966b), into the RNA of mouse Ehrlich ascites cells (cytidine decreased this incorporation) (Cihak *et al.*, 1966), and into the RNA fraction of L1210 cells in culture (Li *et al.*, 1970a). After application to mouse cerebral ventricles, 5-azacytidine is phosphorylated and incorporated into the RNA (Raska *et al.*, 1966a).

Evidence of *inhibition of RNA* synthesis is found in studies that showed 5-azacytidine inhibited RNA synthesis in isolated nuclei of calf thymus (Raska *et al.*, 1965b) and in rhesus monkey kidney cells in tissue culture (Sorm *et al.*, 1966). In the bone marrow of AK inbred mice, after a single dose of 5-azacytidine, RNA synthesis is diminished in the myeloid cells (Levitan *et al.*, 1971).

*Protein synthesis inhibition* may also be a mechanism of action. 5-Azacytidine inhibits synthesis of $\beta$-galactoside by *E. coli* (Doskocil *et al.*, 1967), and total protein synthesis in *E. coli* treated with 5-azacytidine is about 6% of the control value. The synthesis of RNA is slightly inhibited, but a general inhibition of RNA synthesis is not observed. Doskocil *et al.* (1967) concluded that 5-azacytidine inhibits protein synthesis by selectively affecting the function of some species or portion of RNA essential for protein synthesis (see Fig. 3).

Raska *et al.* (1966b) found that 5-azacytidine inhibition of protein synthesis takes place in calf thymus nuclei. Cihak *et al.* (1967b) and Sorm *et al.* (1966) observed an inhibition of hormone-induced synthesis of tryptophan pyrrolase, the enzyme catalyzing oxidation of tryptophan to formylkynurenine, in rat liver. The greatest inhibition of hormone induction took place after application of 5-azacytidine either before or with the inducer. The increase in tryptophan pyrrolase synthesis reflects stimulation of RNA synthesis by hormones. Probably the hormonal induction is inhibited due to incorporation of 5-azacytidine into newly synthesized mRNA (Cihak *et al.*, 1967a, b). This incorporation gives defective mRNA that cannot code properly for protein synthesis. The synthesis of serine dehydratase induced by cortisone is also depressed by 5-azacytidine administered simultaneously or after the inducer (Cihak *et al.*, 1972b).

Tyrosine transaminase induction is not inhibited (Vesely and Sorm 1965; Levitan and Webb, 1970) by 5-azacytidine, and two explanations have been proposed. One explanation is that tyrosine transaminase induction by cortisol in the rat takes place by a posttranscriptional mechanism. Perhaps there is an inactive pool of mRNA for tyrosine transaminase residing within the nucleus and hydrocortisone activates it by promoting its transport to the cytoplasm (Vesely and Sorm, 1965). A second explanation is that 5-azacytidine interferes with synthesis of a degradation enzyme for tyrosine transaminase.

Studies with HeLa cells showed that transfer RNA synthesized in the presence of 5-azacytidine is structurally and functionally modified. Such modification may be one of the major actions of 5-azacytidine in inhibiting protein synthesis in mammalian cells (Lee, 1973).

From the foregoing findings it is apparent that 5-azacytidine is capable of inhibiting protein synthesis in diverse biological systems and this inhibition may be responsible for a major part of the cytotoxic effect of this compound.

### 3. *Competition for Uridine Kinase*

The enzyme uridine kinase, which catalyzes the phosphorylation of uridine and cytidine (Cihak and Vesely, 1973), was first isolated from extracts of mammalian liver and Ehrlich ascites tumor cells. It is the first enzyme taking part in the metabolic changes of 5-azacytidine (Vesely *et al.*, 1967) (see Fig. 3). The amount of this enzyme present is generally considered to reflect the relative efficiency with which the system utilizes preformed pyrimidine precursors by the salvage pathway (Cihak and Vesely, 1973). Uridine kinase is regarded as the rate-limiting enzyme in the salvage pathway (Vesely *et al.*, 1968a; Vesely *et al.*, 1970). A possible mechanism of action for 5-azacytidine is competition with uridine and cytidine for uridine kinase since uridine and cytidine will reverse the bacteriostatic effect of 5-azacytidine (Vadlamudi *et al.*, 1970b) (also see Section IV,B).

### 4. *Inhibition of Orotidylic Acid Decarboxylase*

5-Azacytidine blocks *de novo* synthesis of pyrimidines by interfering with orotidylic acid decarboxylase (Vesely *et al.*, 1968b). 5-Azacytidine increases the excretion of orotic acid and orotidine in the case of AKR mice, indicating that one of the sites of action is an interference with the decarboxylation of orotidylic acid (Raska *et al.*, 1965a).

In summary, there are supporting data for four proposed mechanisms of action of 5-azacytidine. 5-Azacytidine probably competes with uridine and cytidine for phosphorylation. It is probably incorporated into DNA and RNA polynucleotides after phosphorylation. The unstable triazine molecule of the 5-azacytidine probably disrupts the secondary structure of the DNA and causes chromosomal breakage. The incorporation of 5-azacytidine into newly synthesized mRNA probably gives a defective mRNA that cannot code properly for protein synthesis and, therefore, protein synthesis is inhibited.

## B. Resistance

Spontaneous mutants of *Bacillus subtilis* resistant to 5-azacytidine have been isolated (Fucik *et al.*, 1972). Genetic transfer by transformation processes was possible. A comparison of the 5-azacytidine sensitive (5-aza-s) and the 5-azacytidine resistant (5-aza-r) strains revealed fundamental differences concerning incorporation of 5-azacytidine-4-$^{14}$C into their nucleic acids (Jurovcik *et al.*, 1972). The transport of the antimetabolite across the cell membrane seemed to be decreased in the resistant strain. The conclusion was that the lack of passage of this compound across the cell membrane of the resistant strain was the mechanism of resistance (Jurovcik *et al.*, 1972).

When studying the changes associated with the development of resistance to 5-azacytidine in mouse leukemia cells, it was found that the specific activity of uridine kinase purified from the resistant mouse leukemic cells was diminished 50–60% in comparison with its nonresistant counterpart from the parental cell line (Vesely *et al.*, 1968a; Vesely *et al.*, 1970; Cihak *et al.*, 1965). The progressive development of resistance to 5-azacytidine in AKR mouse leukemic cells is also associated with a stepwise decrease in uridine kinases (Vesely *et al.*, 1967; Vesely, 1970). With the reduced uridine kinase activity, there was also a drop in the incorporation of 5-azacytidine into the RNA (Cihak *et al.*, 1965). This alteration in enzyme activity is probably a requisite for the development of resistance since uridine kinase is regarded as a rate-limiting enzyme of the salvage pathway (Vesely, 1967).

The 5-azacytidine-resistant leukemic cells are cross-resistant to 5-fluorouracil (5-FU) but more sensitive to aminopterin. The decrease in activity of uridine kinase has also been observed in neoplastic cells during the development of resistance to 5-FU and 6-azacytidine, but the parallelism between the decrease in uridine kinase activity and the development of resistance to a pyrimidine analog is not obligatory (Vesely *et al.*, 1971a). It has been observed that in Ehrlich ascites carcinoma the resistance to 5-FU has been established before the depression of uridine kinase has taken place (Reichard *et al.*, 1961, 1962).

The impaired activity of uridine kinase in the population of cells resistant to 5-azacytidine may be accounted for by reduced synthesis and/or increased degradation of the enzyme (Vesely, 1970). There may also be a change in its properties or conformational or structural changes (Vesely *et al.*, 1971a). This has been investigated by Vesely *et al.*, (1971b) who studied the uridine kinase from 5-aza-s cells and 5-aza-r cells. Elution profiles of both enzymes were similar although the 5-aza-r cells had 50% lower activity than the 5-aza-s cells. The $K_m$ constants were both the same, whereas the $V_{max}$ for the enzyme from the resistant lines was significantly decreased. Inactivation following *p*-chloromercuribenzoate affected the activity from the sensitive cells more than that of the enzyme from the resistant cells. Therefore, there is presumptive evidence that the two enzymes have different properties.

The question arises: Were the 5-aza-r cells preexisting mutants or were they mutants formed under the influence of 5-azacytidine, which possesses marked mutagenic ability (Fucik *et al.*, 1965a)? Resistance to low doses of 5-azacytidine (0.9 mg/kg) was achieved in the third transplant generation of leukemic cells in mice (Vesely, 1967).

It is of interest that in the normal rat liver the activity of uridine kinase is markedly enhanced following intraperitoneal administration of 5-azacytidine by a process independent of adrenal secretion (Cihak and Vesely, 1973). This may be important because the enhanced activity of uridine kinase by the administration of 5-azacytidine could affect the use of 5-azacytidine in combination with uridine and cytidine antimetabolites. The increased uridine kinase could cause increased phosphorylation of the antimetabolites and greater incorporation into nucleic acids, and, hence, an enhancement of their antimetabolic activity (Cihak and Vesely, 1973).

In summary, two possible mechanisms of resistance have been elucidated. Bacteria resistant to 5-azacytidine have an alteration in their cell membrane that does not allow penetration of the drug. Mouse leukemia cells resistant to 5-azacytidine show a decrease in activity of uridine kinase that causes a decrease in phosphorylation of 5-azacytidine and, hence, a drop in the incorporation of the drug into DNA and RNA. The decreased activity of uridine kinase is probably the result of conformational or structural changes in the enzyme.

## V. Experimental Activity

### A. Antitumor Activity

Sorm and Vesely (1964) were the first to report the activity of 5-azacytidine against lymphoid leukemia in AK mice. Vadlamudi and Goldin (1968) found activity of 5-azacytidine against the mouse leukemia L1210. Table II shows the activity of 5-azacytidine against the L1210 at various dosages and dosage schedules. From the data in Table II, one can see the activity in the L1210 system is in both the daily and the intermittent schedules. However, the drug appears to be most active when given parenterally by continuous treatment from days 1 to 9.

Table III summarizes the antitumor activity in other experimental systems. Of note is the inactivity of the drug in the solid tumor systems (Sandberg and Goldin, 1971). However, 5-azacytidine is active in a subline of L1210 resistant to 6-mercaptopurine (6-MP), aminopterin, and

TABLE II

5-Azacytidine Activity against Ascitic L1210 Leukemia in Mice at Various Doses and Dose Schedules

| Route | Schedule[a] | Dose range (mg/kg/day) | Optimal dose (mg/kg/day) | Maximum ILS%[b] |
|---|---|---|---|---|
| | | Single treatment | | |
| I.P. | QD, day 1 | 12–96 | 48 | 82 |
| I.P. | QD, day 1 | 3–384 | 12 | 50 |
| P.O. | QD, day 1 | 32–256 | 156 | 37 |
| P.O. | QD, day 1 | 256–768 | 768 | 57 |
| | | Continuous treatment | | |
| P.O. | Q3H, day 1 | 32–256 | 128 | 94 |
| I.P. | Q3H, day 1 | 12–96 | 24 | 71 |
| I.P. | QD, day 1–5 | 3–48 | 6 | 240 |
| P.O. | QD, day 1–5 | 1–32 | 16 | 133 |
| I.P. | QD, day 1–9 | 3–24 | 12 | 290 |
| P.O. | QD, day 1–9 | 1.1–9 | 9 | 82 |
| I.P. | Q4D, day 1, 5, 9 | 12–96 | 24 | 207 |
| P.O. | Q4D, day 1, 5, 9 | 16–128 | 128 | 141 |
| I.P. | Q3H, Q4D, day 1, 5, 9 | 12–96 | 12 | 201 |
| P.O. | Q3H, Q4D, day 1, 5, 9 | 16–128 | 32 | 73 |

[a] QD, daily; Q3H, every 3 hours; Q4D, every 4 days.

[b] Percent increase in life span of treated L1210-bearing mice over that of untreated L1210-bearing mice.

TABLE III

5-AZACYTIDINE ACTIVITY IN EXPERIMENTAL ANIMAL TUMOR SYSTEMS[a]

| |
|---|
| 5-Azacytidine active in |
| L1210 |
| L1210 subline resistant to 6-MP |
| L1210 subline resistant to DTIC and nitrosoureas |
| L5178Y |
| P815 |
| P815 sublines resistant to Ara-C, 5-FU, 6-MP, and vincristine |
| P388 |
| 5-Azacytidine intermediate activity in |
| MOPC 21 murine myeloma tumor[b] |
| 5-Azacytidine inactive in |
| Walker 256 |
| Spontaneous mammary tumor C3H |
| B16 melanoma |
| Lewis lung |

[a] Ara-C, cytosine arabinoside; 5-FU, 5-fluorouracil; 6-MP, 6-mercaptopurine; DTIC, 5-(3,3-dimethyl-1-triazeno)imidazole-4-carboxamide.

[b] Globulin secreted in presence of 5-azacytidine was still intact but decreased in amounts (Shutt and Krueger, 1972).

cyclophosphamide or a subline resistant to imidazole carboxamide and nitrosoureas (Tyrer *et al.*, 1969). 5-Azacytidine is also active in P815 sublines resistant to cytosine arabinoside (Ara-C), 5-FU, 6-MP, and vincristine (Burchenal *et al.*, 1972).

Combinations of 5-azacytidine with other drugs have been tested in experimental systems. Combination therapy of 5-azacytidine and emetine (NSC 33669) as an every fourth day schedule showed enhanced action against L1210. The therapeutic effect in L1210 leukemic mice of single intraperitoneal doses of Ara-C and 5-azacytidine in combination depends on the time interval between the doses of each agent (Neil *et al.*, 1974). With 5-azacytidine given 10 hours after the Ara-C, a marked enhancement of antileukemic effect was observed. This optimal time interval has been correlated with the time at which L1210 cell DNA synthesis recovered after inhibition by the dose of Ara-C (Neil *et al.*, 1974).

In summary, the animal tumor data would lead one to speculate that 5-azacytidine should have activity in human leukemia but would be less likely to be active in human solid tumors. 5-Azacytidine is active in leukemic cell lines resistant to 6-MP, aminopterin, cyclophosphamide, 5-(3,3-dimethyl-1-triazeno)imidazole-4-carboxamide (DTIC), nitrosoureas, Ara-C, 5-FU, and vincristine, and one could speculate that 5-azacytidine might be active in human leukemia resistant to those drugs. Experimental antitumor data suggest that combination therapy of 5-azacytidine with emetine or Ara-C might be useful in human tumors provided attention is paid to schedules of drug administration.

## B. Drug Schedule Dependency

As noted in the preceding, 5-azacytidine has activity in the L1210 system in both the daily and the intermittent schedules. Venditti (1971) concluded from these data that 5-azacytidine has no important schedule dependency.

When individual DON cells were examined, the effect of the 5-azacytidine seemed to be cell-cycle phase-specific in that it was most toxic to cells in the $S$ phase, especially at low doses (Li *et al.*, 1970b; Tobey, 1972). The percentage of cell kill of an asynchronous DON cell population was minimal during the $M$ and $G_1$ phase. Chinese hamster fibroblast cells were also most sensitive to 5-azacytidine in the $S$ phase. 5-Azacytidine, when added with phytohemagglutinin to cell cultures, can interfere with blastogenesis of lymphocytes (Nitschke, 1974).

Karon and Benedict (1970) showed that 5-azacytidine, like Ara-C, causes chromosome breakage in $S$ and $G_2$ phases. 5-Azacytidine was most cytotoxic to cells in the $S$ phase although high levels of 5-azacytidine (100 $\mu$g/ml) were also lethal to cells in $G_1$, $S_1$, $G_2$, and $M$. Cells in the $S$ phase were the most sensitive.

Kinetics tend to confirm that $S$ phase is the most sensitive. Lloyd *et al.* (1972) showed the kinetics of the reduction in the viability of replicating L1210 cells exposed to the lethal concentrations of 5-azacytidine *deviated from first-order kinetics* and could be described by a Gompertz function. The initial rate of reduction in viability was concentration-dependent, at least for concentrations of 1 to 30 $\mu$g/ml. The maximal degree of cell killing was achieved rapidly (within 360 minutes) at concentrations of 117.1 $\mu$g/ml. Since cell killing was concentration-dependent, this might indicate no important schedule dependency. However, the rapid rates of reduction in the viability of proliferating L1210 cells over the first 180–360 minutes of exposure to 5-azacytidine and the known incorporation of 5-azacytidine into DNA suggest that L1210 cells in $S$ phase are the most sensitive to 5-azacytidine. Lloyd *et al.* (1972) conclude that 5-azacytidine *is a cell-cycle-specific agent* since nonproliferating L1210 cells are relatively insensitive to concentrations of 5-azacytidine that markedly reduce the viability of proliferating cultured L1210 cells.

All of the foregoing data indicate that 5-azacytidine has definite action in the *S* phase, which could be called cell-cycle-specific, but its action is not strictly limited to the *S* phase (and, therefore, not strictly cell-cycle-specific). Lloyd's data do indicate that effective *in vivo* therapy can be enhanced by increasing the dose within the limit of toxicity to normal tissues.

A recent observation by Presant *et al.* (1975) showed that 5-azacytidine given 1 day prior to transplantation of $10^3$ to $10^6$ L1210 cells increased the life-span of the animal by 2 days. The life-span was increased if the 5-azacytidine was given 1 or 2 but not 3 or more days before the cells. Thus, they concluded that the cytotoxicity after high-dose 5-azacytidine persists for several days *after* treatment. They suggest that this delayed cytotoxic effect should be considered when designing combination chemotherapy protocols including 5-azacytidine.

## VI. Animal Toxicity

Toxicity studies have been done in four animal species, i.e., the mouse, hamster, rhesus monkey, and beagle dog. The $LD_{90}$ of the daily × 5 schedule in the mouse was 4.5 mg/kg or 13 mg/m$^2$, with postmortem examination revealing fatty changes in the liver, focal tubular necrosis of the kidney, and congested lungs (Palm and Kensler, 1970). No thromboembolism was noted after application of 5-azacytidine to the everted mucosa of the hamster cheek pouch, but injection of the drug into the jugular vein of the anesthetized hamster did produce reduction of arteriolar and venule blood flow (Palm and Kensler, 1970).

The most sensitive species in the toxicology studies was the beagle dog (Palm and Kensler, 1970). Table IV summarizes and defines the highest nontoxic dose (HNTD), the toxic dose low (TDL), toxic dose high (TDH), and lethal dose in the beagle dog. Of note in Table IV is the fact that the single intravenous HNTD is less toxic than the daily i.v. × 5 dose.

The qualitative toxicity in the dog can be summarized into two areas (Palm and Kensler, 1970). The first area concerns toxic effects on rapidly dividing cells, i.e., the bone marrow, lymphoid organs, and gastrointestinal (GI) cells. 5-Azacytidine is only a moderate panmyelotoxin in the dog, even at its highest dose. The level of circulating leukocytes was not obliterated by the dog. Thrombocytes seemed to be

TABLE IV

5-AZACYTIDINE TOXICITY DATA IN THE BEAGLE DOG

| | Daily, i.v., × 5 | | Single, i.v. | |
|---|---|---|---|---|
| Dose[a] | ($mg/m^2$) | (mg/kg) | ($mg/m^2$) | (mg/kg) |
| HNTD | 5.5 | 0.28 | 81 | 2.2 |
| TDL | 10.0 | 0.55 | — | — |
| TDH | 43.0 | 2.20 | 130 | 3.5 |
| LD | 77.0 | 4.4 | 266 | 7.2 |

[a] *Highest Nontoxic dose* (HNTD): the highest dose at which no hematological, chemical, clinical, or pathological drug-induced alterations occurred; doubling this dose produced the aforementioned alterations.

*Toxic dose low* (TDL): the lowest dose to produce drug-induced pathological alterations in hematological, chemical, clinical, or morphological parameters; doubling this dose produces no lethality.

*Toxic dose high* (TDH): the lowest dose to produce drug-induced pathological alterations in hematological, chemical, clinical, or morphological parameters; doubling this dose produces lethality.

*Lethal dose* (LD): the lowest dose to produce drug-induced death in any animals during the treatment or observation period.

the least and most slowly susceptible of the formed elements. The drug caused widespread necrosis of lymphatic organs in only the highest dose schedule. No detrimental effects were seen in the GI epithelium.

In the second area of concern, the effects on interphase cells of parenchymal organs, moderate single doses and repeated doses of the drug were damaging to the liver. Elevation of serum glutamate pyruvate transaminase (SGPT), alkaline phosphatase, prothrombin time, and occasionally serum glutamic oxalacetic transaminase (SGOT) were noted. Fatty necrotic changes were seen in the hepatocytes. The principal morphological effect on renal tissues was the accumulation of a globular eosinophilic material in the lumen of the renal tubules. Significant elevations of blood urea nitrogen (BUN) were seen in animals receiving toxic doses of the drug.

Rhesus monkey test data showed that, at the level of 2.2 mg/kg/day for 14 days, there was kidney and liver damage marked by elevation in BUN, SGOT, and SGPT values (Palm *et al.*, 1973). Micropathology included cloudy swelling and focal necrosis of kidney tubules, hepatic fatty metamorphosis, bone marrow hypoplasia, and lymphoid hypoplasia of the spleen and lymph nodes. The HNTD in monkeys was set at 0.28 mg/kg/day (4 mg/m$^2$) on the 14-day repeated dose regimen (Palm *et al.*, 1973). Compared with dog data, the monkey is about comparable or slightly less sensitive to the toxic effects of the drug, and the mouse was the least sensitive of all the species tested.

On the basis of the data just cited, the starting dose to be used in Phase I trials in humans could be calculated. This dose is calculated by taking one-third of the TDL in the most sensitive large animal species (Goldsmith *et al.*, 1975), i.e., in this case one-third of 10 mg/m$^2$ on the daily $\times$ 5 schedule (TDL for beagle) or 3.3 mg/m$^2$/day $\times$ 5.

The reversal of toxicity induced by 5-azacytidine has also been explored. As mentioned previously, the complete inhibition of growth of *E. coli* by 5-azacytidine can be reversed by the simultaneous addition of uridine, cytidine, or thymidine but not by uracil or cytosine (Cihak and Sorm, 1965). 6-Azauridine has also been shown to reverse the toxic effects of 5-azacytidine in mice (Sorm and Vesely, 1965). The blocking of 5-azacytidine action by these compounds is probably due to the ability of these nucleosides to compete with 5-azacytidine for phosphorylation and subsequent incorporation into cellular nucleic acid. Mammalian cells do not incorporate 6-azauridine, and for this reason it seems that the reversal effect of 6-azauridine in alleviating toxicity is due to competition of both substances at the level of the kinase system.

Vadlamudi *et al.* (1970b) showed that the simultaneous treatment with 600 or 300 mg/kg of cytidine reversed the antileukemic activity of the optimal dose of 5-azacytidine in the L1210 system. The treatment also reduced the toxicity of higher doses of 5-azacytidine (12–33 mg/kg) to the leukemic mice, permitting the observation of increased survival. Although there was no therapeutic advantage of treatment with a combination of cytidine and 5-azacytidine over treatment with 5-azacytidine alone, the control of toxicity by the cytidine suggests that a temporal administration of cytidine with, before, or after the 5-azacytidine should be explored.

The local perfusion of 5-azacytidine in combination with cytidine as an antidote was investigated in the dog by Hanka and Clark (1975). 5-Azacytidine was infused into the femoral artery of a beagle and cytidine infused into the jugular vein. Blood levels of 20 to 30 $\mu$g/ml of 5-azacytidine in the areas being perfused were noted, and no serious toxic manifestations were observed. The significance of these results for clinical use of 5-azacytidine are being explored.

## VII. Drug Metabolism and Disposition

In an attempt to elucidate the metabolism of 5-azacytidine and to determine if it is 5-azacytidine or perhaps its metabolic products that are cancerostatic, many studies have been performed.

### A. *In Vitro* Studies

The kinetics of the disappearance of 5-azacytidine suggest that there is an intermediate in equilibrium with 5-azacytidine that decomposes irreversibly to products that are nontoxic to *E. coli* (Lloyd *et al.*, 1972). It is possible that the cytotoxic effect and other effects observed for 5-azacytidine are mediated through the formation of this intermediate. These *in vitro* decomposition products have been identified by Pithova *et al.* (1965). The hydrolysis of 5-azacytidine in neutral and basic media produced the following products: (*a*) 1-β-ribofuranosyl-3-guanylurea (substance III in Fig. 4); (*b*) guanidine; (*c*) α-D-ribofuro (1′,2′:4,5)-2-azolidone; (*d*) D-ribose; and, as an intermediate (*e*), the *N*-formyl derivative of compound III in Fig. 4. In acidic media the hydrolysis

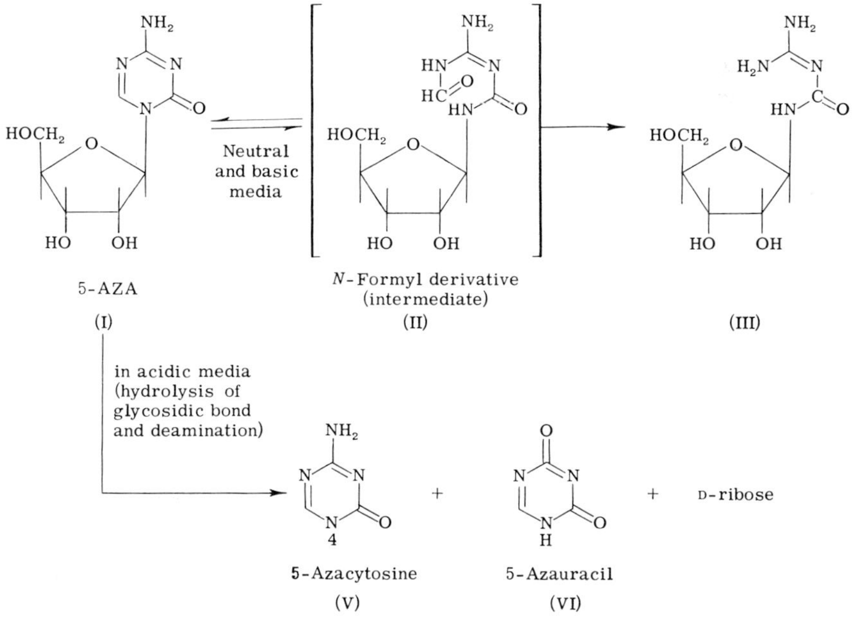

FIG. 4. Hydrolysis products of 5-azacytidine *in vivo*. (From Pithova *et al.*, 1965.)

produces 5-azacytosine (V), 5-azauracil (VI), and D-ribose. These degradation products did not produce as much bacteriostatic activity as did 5-azacytidine. The bioactivity of some of the degradation products have been determined at the national Service Center (NSC). There is no NSC designation for the *N*-formyl derivative of compound III or for 1-$\beta$-D-ribofuranosyl-3-guanylurea. However, the products of acid hydrolysis, 5-azacytosine and 5-azauracil, have been tested in CA 755, Sarcoma 180, and L1210. Activities warranting further studies were not exhibited (NCI, Drug Research and Development Screening Data).

It is of interest that, as reported by Pithova *et al.* (1965), when 5-azacytidine is incubated at 37°C at a pH of 7.2, approximately 25% of the original 5-azacytidine was shown by chemical analysis to remain after 24 hours. There was an initial rapid decline in the concentration of 5-azacytidine. A similar result was obtained (i.e., an initial rapid decline in concentration of 5-azacytidine) by a microbiological assay in buffered saline. However, after 24 hours the solution retained 50% of its original cytotoxicity, as determined by a microbiological assay. The quantitative difference at 24 hours between the chemical analysis and the microbiological assay may be owing to the fact that the microbiological assay detects cytotoxicity *of all* chemical substances. This result also raises the question of possible greater activity of breakdown products of 5-azacytidine, although these did not seem to have increased biological activity individually (Pithova *et al.*, 1965).

### B. Studies in a Bacterial System

Cihak and Sorm (1965) felt that the mechanism of action of 5-azacytidine was polyvalent due to the spontaneous and enzymic transformation of the compound. The conversion of 5-azacytidine to 5-azauridine is accomplished by deamination and the 5-azauridine is transformed to 5-azauracil. However, there is some disagreement as to whether these conversion products have any biological, bacteriostatic, or antitumor activity. Doskocil and Sorm (1970) noted that if 5-azacytidine is rapidly deaminated, producing primarily 5-azauridine, a mutant *E. coli* deficient in cytidine deaminase would permit investigation of the monovalent effects of 5-azacytidine itself. They found that in cultures of *E. coli* deficient in cytidine deaminase, 5-azacytidine is a weak inhibitor of total protein synthesis in spite of being extensively incorporated into RNA. They felt that the strong inhibition of protein synthesis in the wild-type strain was due to the 5-azauridine formed from 5-azacytidine deamination (there is no NSC number for 5-azauridine), whereas strains deficient in cytidine deaminase contain exclusively 5-azacytosine and its open-ring derivative in their RNA (Doskocil and Sorm, 1971).

## C. Studies in Rodents

Mice were given 9.5 and 4.75 mg/kg, i.p. ($LD_{10}$ and 0.5 $LD_{10}$, respectively), of 5-azacytidine (Pittello and Woolley, 1969). Assays on the mice showed that maximal drug concentrations in the blood were obtained slightly before 15 minutes after drug administration, but rapidly diminished. All measurable drug in the blood was gone by 1 hour after the $LD_{10}$ dose and by 30 minutes after injection of the 0.5 $LD_{10}$ dose. No drug was detected in the liver, lung, brain, spleen, or kidneys of the mice at any time after the administration of the drug. Failure to detect 5-azacytidine in the solid tissue of mice may have been due to the possibility that 5-azacytidine, like 6-azacytidine, is deaminated in the mouse.

Raska *et al.* (1965a) examined organs of AKR mice at 2, 8, 16, and 24 hours after administration of 5-azacytidine for 5-azacytidine and its metabolites by using $^{14}C$-labeled 5-azacytidine. This assay was a radioactive assay that may recover metabolites (as opposed to the biological assay of Pitello and Woolley). The radioactivity dropped rapidly in the blood during the first 8 hours after its administration, but the radioactivity could be demonstrated in the blood even after 24 hours [a calculation from the data of Raska *et al.* (1965a) gives a $t_{1/2}$ for 5-azacytidine and its radioactive metabolites of 3.8 hours]. The level of radioactivity in all organs dropped slowly, but its concentration in the spleen and thymus was highest at later time intervals. The radioactivity was greater and the retention longer in lymphatic organs, and this is in agreement with the pronounced morphological changes observed in the thymus, spleen, and bone marrow after treatment with 5-azacytidine (Sorm and Vesely, 1964). The drug penetrated only slightly into the central nervous system and this might account for certain behavioral changes in the mice after administration of the 5-azacytidine. The relatively rapid drop in the concentration of these substances in many of the organs corresponds to their initially rapid excretion in the urine. After treatment with 5-azacytidine, unaltered 5-azacytidine can be found in the urine together with the products of its spontaneous decomposition (i.e., guanylurea ribonucleoside and guanidine, as well as 5-azauracil and its decomposition products biuret and 1-formylbiuret). The longer the interval between the dose of 5-azacytidine and the collection of urine, the greater the appearance in the urine of decomposition products and the smaller the amount of antimetabolite itself.

Other investigators have also examined the urinary metabolites in mice (Coles *et al.*, 1975). Coles *et al.* used a liquid chromatograph assay to analyze 5-azacytidine-$^{14}$C and its metabolites in the urine. They found that six radioactive species could be found (I–VI) in a 0–8 hour urine collection. 5-Azacytidine (IV) was 4% of what was excreted. Three species were derived through deamination (I, II, and V). Tetrahydrouridine given with the 5-azacytidine produced a sixfold increase in the 5-azacytidine found in the urine. The combination of 5-azacytidine, Ara-C, vincristine, and prednisone led to an increased excretion of 5-azacytidine, probably due to competition of Ara-C for cytidine deaminase. Combinations of 5-azacytidine and daunomycin did not alter the metabolic profile (Coles *et al.*, 1975).

### D. Studies in Dogs

Coles *et al.* (1974) studied the plasma and urinary pharmacokinetics of 5-azacytidine-$^{14}$C and its metabolites in the female beagle. Six $^{14}$C peaks were resolved in urine (I–VI). Peak I cochromatographed with 5-azauracil, Peak II corresponded to 5-azacytosine, Peak IV cochromatographed with 5-azacytidine, and Peaks V and VI were degradation products related to urea and guanidine, respectively. They also found that 5-azacytidine is degraded in plasma from dog, rat, and human to a component inactive in inhibiting the growth of L1210 *in vitro* and corresponding to urine Peak VI.

### E. Studies in Man

Elegant studies in man by Troetel *et al.* (1972) showed the pharmacokinetics of 5-azacytidine (radioactively labeled at position 4 with $^{14}$C) after administration by either the intravenous or the subcutaneous route. The dosage in these patients, all of whom had metastatic cancer, was 1.6 mg/kg. Absorption from the subcutaneous site was rapid with peak plasma levels attained as rapidly as within 30 minutes. Within 2 hours, the plasma level of radioactivity was approximately equal to that noted in patients treated with intravenous drug. (In combusted subcutaneous samples in the rat, the drug is shown to be absorbed completely.) The plasma half-life for 5-azacytidine and its radioactive metabolites after intravenous injection was 3.5 hours (close to the $t_{1/2}$ in mice of 3.8 hours obtained by Raska *et al.*, 1965a). After subcutaneous injection the plasma half-life was 4.2 hours. Patients receiving the drug subcutaneously excreted less radioactivity in the urine (50% of total dose) than did those receiving intravenous drug (85% of total dose was found in the urine) (Troetel *et al.*, 1972). The rate of clearance of the radioactivity was less than the average glomerular filtration rate, suggesting that active tubular secretion of the labeled substances probably does not occur. There was no radioactivity in the expired $CO_2$ when the drug was given by either route. Drug uptake into tumor tissue (carcinoma of the colon) was always greater than uptake into the surrounding normal tissue (as high as 1.3–2.5 times the level in surrounding normal tissue), with the highest concentration of radioactivity in tissues achieved when the drug was given intravenously. Traces of radioactivity were noted in tumor tissue as long as 6 days after administration of the drug (Troetel *et al.*, 1972). They also demonstrated incorporation of radioactivity into tumor RNA but not into DNA (at sampling periods of 24 and 48 hours only).

The maximal level of radioactivity in the cerebrospinal fluid was 24 hours after administration and the level of radioactivity detected was equivalent to 0.2 μg/ml of fluid. Radioactivity was detected in ascitic fluid as early as 0.5 hour after the administration of 5-azacytidine, but it did not reach equilibrium with the plasma until 6 hours later (Troetel *et al.*, 1972).

Vogler *et al.* (1974) gave 3 patients radioactive 5-azacytidine as part of a Phase I study at a dose of 200 $mg/m^2$, and plasma levels were followed by radioactivity. Their values agree with those of Troetel *et al.*, with the $t_{1/2}$ of the 5-azacytidine and its radioactive metabolites from 3 to 4.7 hours. Almost all of the plasma radioactivity disappeared by 24 to 48 hours. Approximately 90% of the radioactive label was present in the urine within 24 hours. Significant amounts of radioactivity were not found in vomitus, sputum, or feces.

Israili *et al.* (1974) also studied the disposition of 5-azacytidine-$^{14}C$ in man. Carbon-14 was measured in plasma, red blood cells (RBC), leukemic white cells, white blood cell (WBC) nucleic acids, sputum, vomitus, urine, and feces. The $t_{1/2}$ for $^{14}C$ in plasma was 2.5–5.4 hours. Most of the $^{14}C$ appeared in the urine, whereas small amounts were present in the feces, sputum, and vomitus. Ratios of $^{14}C$ in RBC/plasma = 0.8, WBC/plasma = 1.1–2.3, and WBC–nucleic acid/WBC = 0.3. Thin-layer chromatography of the plasma and urine showed the presence of at least two compounds other than 5-azacytidine. In 2 patients, 5-azacytidine was given by slow intravenous infusion, and plasma levels for $^{14}C$ indicated some accumulation. The spinal fluid-to-plasma ratio of $^{14}C$ was $<0.1$ even though 5-azacytidine *was not bound to human albumin*.

Oliverio (1972) has suggested that perhaps tetrahydrouridine (THU), a pyrimidine nucleoside deaminase inhibitor with no intrinsic antitumor activity, could be used to prevent deamination and this might potentiate the effects of 5-azacytidine. Chabner *et al.* (1973) took leukemic granulocytes from untreated patients with chronic myelogenous leukemia (CML) and demonstrated deamination of 5-azacytidine by an extract of the leukemic leukocytes, which was cytidine deaminase. They demonstrated that 5-azacytidine was a competitive inhibitor of the deamination of both cytidine and Ara-C and that THU also inhibited the deamination of 5-azacytidine by the leukemic cells.

Other investigators (Neil *et al.*, 1975) have stated that with 5-azacytidine the metabolism, including nonenzymic, is very complex, and perhaps simple deamination is not an important factor in the activity of the drug.

Neil *et al.* (1975) have shown that oral administration of THU to mice greatly increases the oral activity of 5-azacytidine in mouse leukemia, but intraperitoneal THU did not increase the intraperitoneal activity of 5-azacytidine. The toxicity of oral 5-azacytidine in the mouse was also increased when THU was employed in oral combination with 5-azacytidine (Neil *et al.*, 1975). The lack of any significant effect of THU on the therapeutic activity of intraperitoneally administered 5-azacytidine is consistent with the rather marginal effect of THU on 5-azacytidine blood levels after intraperitoneal injection.

The possibility of the clinical use of THU to alter the pharmacokinetics of 5-azacytidine in man is currently being explored (Neil *et al.*, 1975).

In summary, the *in vitro* decomposition products of 5-azacytidine have been identified, but the antitumor activity of some of these degradation products has not yet been studied. The question of the bioactivity of the degradation products of 5-azacytidine is an important one in light of its relatively rapid decomposition. Perhaps the products of decomposition have antitumor activity.

The metabolism and disposition of 5-azacytidine seem similar in the mouse, dog, and man. The plasma half-life of 5-azacytidine and/or its radioactive metabolites is 3.8 hours in the mouse which is comparable to the plasma half-life of 3–4.7 hours in man. The administered radioactivity is rapidly excreted in the urine of the mouse, dog, and man. This information should make the clinician exercise care when administering the drug to patients with renal abnormalities.

The relatively low cerebrospinal fluid concentrations of the drug after administration would lead one to expect little activity of 5-azacytidine in CNS tumors or CNS leukemia.

## VIII. Clinical Studies

### A. Phase I Studies

The initial clinical studies using 5-azacytidine were reported by Hrodek and Vesely in 1971. They used the drug on newly diagnosed, childhood leukemia patients with 17 having acute lymphocytic leukemia (ALL), 3 AML, and 1 CML. When 5-azacytidine was used alone during the induction phase there was a decrease in the WBC count, but complete remissions were obtained only with the addition of prednisone. These results were very encouraging, with about an 88% response rate in patients with ALL. Unfortunately, the role of 5-azacytidine could not be well-defined in these remissions.

The first Phase I studies in the United States were started in late 1970. The Phase I study should define the maximally tolerated dosage and explore the clinical pharmacology of the drug. The dog data showed that the initial starting dose in the human should be about 3.3 mg/m²/day × 5 days. Karon *et al.* (1973) started at 2 mg/m²/day and planned to adhere to a modified Fibonachi search scheme (Goldsmith *et al.*, 1975) for dose escalation. They found there was so little response at this dosage that they had to escalate the dose 70–100 times the initial starting dose. The shape of the actual dose escalation curve was similar to the Fibonachi search scheme. Other investigators confirmed Karon's work and modified their dosages upward.

From these investigations it was apparent that, compared with both dogs and rodents, man could tolerate much higher drug doses. The pharmacokinetic studies have shown that excretion patterns are about the same in all three species (Troetel *et al.*, 1972). Perhaps the relative activities of kinases and deaminases in the various species are different and this accounts for the differences in maximally tolerated dosages (Vogler *et al.*, 1974).

Table V summarizes all of the Phase I studies to date involving 207 patients. The starting dose, highest escalated dosages, the maximally tolerated doses (MTD), and the type of cancer treated are also shown in Table V. The dose-limiting toxicities were nausea, vomiting, and leukopenia (see in following). The MTD on a daily × 5 schedule for childhood leukemia seems to be 150–200 mg/m²/day × 5 days with a 14–21 day waiting period before the next course. In adult leukemia the range is from 150–300 mg/m²/day × 5 days every 14–21 days. For solid tumors, the MTD's were 150–225 mg/m²/day i.v. × 5 every 21 days. When continuous infusions were given, the MTD for leukemia and solid

TABLE V

PHASE I 5-AZACYTIDINE STUDIES

| Dose schedule | Cancer | Dose (mg/m²) Starting | Highest escalation | Maximum tolerated | Reference[e] |
|---|---|---|---|---|---|
| Single, i.v., once weekly | Solid tumors | 200 | 633 | 500 | (1) |
| Twice weekly × 5, i.v. | Solid tumors | 50 | 200 | 150 | (2) |
| Daily × 5, i.v., every 14 days | Acute leukemia[c] | 50 | 300 | 150–200 | (3) |
| Daily × 5, i.v., 9 days off | Solid tumors | 50 | 268 | 150 | (1) |
| Daily × 5, i.v., every 21 days | Solid tumors and acute leukemia | 2.2 | 300 | 175–225 | (4) |
| Daily × 5, i.v., every 14 days | Acute leukemia | 400 | 400 | 300 | (5) |
| Daily × 10, i.v. | Solid tumors | 1.11[d] | 89[d] | 59[d] | (6) |
| 5-Day infusion, every 14 days[a] | Solid tumors and acute leukemia | 50 | 400 | 150–200 | (7) |
| 120-Hr infusion, every 28 days[b] | Solid tumors | 150 | 200 | 150 | (8) |

[a] Fresh solution every 3 hours.

[b] Fresh solution every 4 hours.

[c] Children.

[d] Calculated by conversion factor of 37 from milligrams per kilogram to milligrams per square meter.

[e] Key to references: 1—Shnider *et al.* (1975), 2—Vogler *et al.* (1974), 3—Karon *et al.* (1973), 4—K. B. McCredie (personal communication, 1975), 5—McCredie *et al.* (1973), 6—Weiss *et al.* (1972), 7—Vogler *et al.* (1975), 8—Lomen *et al.* (1975).

tumor patients was 150–200 mg/m²/day × 5 every 14–28 days, with the solution being changed every 3–4 hours. The MTD for a single weekly intravenous dose is about 500 mg/m² and for a twice weekly dose, approximately 150 mg/m² biweekly. The MTD for a daily × 10 regimen was 1.5 mg/kg/day × 10 (≃59 mg/m²/day × 10).

## B. ANTINEOPLASTIC ACTIVITY BY TUMOR TYPE

The data in this analysis represent results from fifty-eight protocols involving 829 evaluable patients on file with the Investigational Drug Branch.

### 1. *Acute Myelogenous Leukemia*

This type of leukemia is probably the most widely studied disease in terms of clinical trials for the effectiveness of 5-azacytidine (Table VI). The results on a total of 200 patients treated with 5-azacytidine alone are on file at the Investigational Drug Branch. Sixty-six patients have been treated with 5-azacytidine in combination with one or more other chemotherapeutic agents in Phase III trials (Table VII).

The overall average percentage of complete and partial response (CR + PR) in patients treated with 5-azacytidine alone has been 36%. Twenty percent of these have been complete remissions and 16% partial remissions. Probably the most striking point in these statistics, granted they are taken from many different investigators, is that almost all the patients who responded have been refractory to all conventional therapy.

It is difficult to draw any conclusions as to the most effective dose since approximately equal remission results have been seen with 100–

TABLE VI

5-Azacytidine as Single-Agent Therapy in Acute Myelogenous Leukemia

| Dose (mg/m²) | Dose schedule | No. of evaluable patients | Complete response | | Partial response | | Reference[d] |
|---|---|---|---|---|---|---|---|
| | | | (No.) | (%) | (No.) | (%) | |
| 750 | Single, i.v. | 27 | 11 | 41 | 4 | 15 | (1) |
| 150–200 | Daily × 5, i.v. | 14 | 5 | 36 | 1 | 7 | (2) |
| 150–400 | Daily × 5, i.v. | 18 | 3 | 17 | 4 | 22 | (3) |
| 120–300 | Daily × 5, i.v. | 6 | 0 | — | 1 | 17 | (4) |
| 200 | Daily × 5, i.v.[a] | 18 | 5 | 28 | 1 | 5 | (5) |
| 60 | Every 8 hr × 15 doses | 6 | 0 | — | 0 | — | (6) |
| 100 | Every 8 hr × 15 doses | 26 | 2 | 8 | 7 | 27 | (6) |
| 180 | Daily × 5, i.v. | 8 | 2 | 25 | 0 | — | (6) |
| 300 | Daily × 5, i.v. | 26 | 2 | 8 | 7 | 27 | (6) |
| 150–200 | 5-Day infusion[b] | 22 | 7 | 28 | 3 | 12 | (7) |
| 500 | Daily × 5[c] | 29 | 4 | 14 | 4 | 14 | (1) |

[a] In three divided doses.

[b] Solution changed every 3 hours.

[c] Infusion over 30 minutes.

[d] Key to references: 1—K. B. McCredie (personal communication, 1975), 2—Karon *et al.* (1973), 3—McCredie *et al.* (1973), 4—Tan *et al.* (1973), 5—Levi *et al.* (1975), 6—J. R. Bateman (personal communication, 1975), 7—Vogler *et al.* (1975).

TABLE VII

5-Azacytidine Combined with Other Chemotherapeutic Agents in Therapy of Acute Myelogenous Leukemia

| Drug[a] (plus 5-azacytidine) | No. of evaluable patients | Complete response (No.) | Complete response (%) | Partial response (No.) | Partial response (%) | Reference[d] |
|---|---|---|---|---|---|---|
| Ara-A | 14 | 4 | 29 | 0 | — | (1) |
| Daunomycin | 19 | 11 | 58 | 2 | 10 | (2) |
| Methyl GAG | 8 | 0 | — | 1 | 13 | (3) |
| Adriamycin and bleomycin[b] | 1 | 0 | — | 1 | 100 | (4) |
| Ara-C, prednisone, and vincristine[c] | 24 | 12 | 50 | 4 | 17 | (2) |

[a] Methyl GAG, methylglyoxalbisguanylhydrazone; Ara-C, cytosine arabinoside; Ara-A, adenine arabinoside.

[b] Bleomycin given at nadir of blood counts.

[c] Daunomycin subsequently has been added to this regimen.

[d] Key to references: 1—K. B. McCredie (personal communication, 1975), 2—J. Z. Finklestein and D. Hammond (personal communication, 1975), 3—Levi and Wiernik (1975), 4—C. Tan (personal communication, 1975).

250 mg/m$^2$ biweekly, 150–400 mg/m$^2$/day × 5 days, 750 mg single dose every 3 weeks, and continuous infusions over 5 days. However, as noted in Section VIII, C, there may be some advantages to different dosage schedules so far as toxicity is concerned.

There are five other protocols or pilot studies in progress at this time with preliminary results available (Table VII). The Childrens Cancer Study Group has observed a 68% response (58% CR, 10% PR) with a daunomycin and 5-azacytidine protocol with 19 patients evaluated so far (J. Z. Finklestein and D. Hammond, personal communication, 1975). A Childrens Cancer Study Group pilot study (J. Z. Finklestein and D. Hammond, personal communication, 1975) involving 5-azacytidine, Ara-C, prednisone, and vincristine (called ZAPO) has shown a 67% response rate (50% CR and 17% PR). A pilot study at M.D. Anderson Hospital using adenine arabinoside (Ara-A) and 5-azacytidine via infusion (McCredie, 1975) has shown a 29% response rate (29% CR and 0% PR). Levi and Wiernik (1975) used a methylglyoxalbisguanylhydrazone (methyl GAG) and 5-azacytidine combination, but obtained a disappointing 13% response rate (the methyl GAG was very toxic). C. Tan (personal communcation, 1975) treated 1 patient with 5-azacytidine and Adriamycin with a dose of bleomycin added at the nadir of the blood counts and obtained a partial remission. All of these studies will be continued.

In summary, 5-azacytidine has been effective in inducing remissions in some refractory cases of AML, and further combinations of 5-azacytidine with other drugs are being explored.

## 2. *Acute Lymphocytic Leukemia*

The experience of American investigators has not been as good as the Czechoslovakian investigators (Hrodek and Vesely, 1971), who reported a 88% response rate in children with ALL (all of these patients were newly diagnosed and without prior chemotherapy). Unfortunately, these investigators also gave the patients prednisone, so that it was impossible to sort out what role 5-azacytidine had in these remissions.

Table VIII summarizes the American experience with ALL. Of 49 refractory patients treated with 5-azacytidine alone, there have been 3 complete remissions and 2 partial remissions or an 11% response rate. C. Tan (personal communication, 1975) has obtained a 75% response rate in 4 patients with an Adriamycin and 5-azacytidine combination with bleomycin added at the nadir of the WBC count. However, the overall data indicate that 5-azacytidine does not have a significant effect on ALL.

## 3. *Chronic Myelogenous Leukemia*

Only 9 patients have been treated with 5-azacytidine, and there has been hematologic improvement in 3. No remissions were reported (Table VIII).

## 4. *Myltiple Myeloma*

Nine patients have been evaluated on a 5-azacytidine and prednisone combination. No activity has been seen (J. M. Quagliana and R. Alexanian, personal communication, 1975). (See Table VIII for summary of single-agent activity of 5-azacytidine.)

## 5. *Breast*

Weiss *et al.* (1972) reported 7 of 11 patients with breast cancer responding to 5-azacytidine in early Phase I trials. Most of these patients had either chest wall recurrences or unresectable tumors involving the breast and were treated with 0.55–2.4 mg/kg/day for 10

TABLE VIII

SUMMARY OF U.S. STUDIES ON SINGLE-AGENT ACTIVITY OF 5-AZACYTIDINE IN VARIOUS TUMOR TYPES[a]

| Tumor type | No. evaluable patients | No. patients responding[b] | | % Response | | |
|---|---|---|---|---|---|---|
| | | CR | PR | Total | CR | PR |
| Acute myelogenous leukemia | 200 | 41 | 34 | 36 | 20 | 16 |
| Acute lymphocytic leukemia | 49 | 3 | 2 | 10 | 6 | 4 |
| Chronic myelogenous leukemia | 9[c] | 0 | 0 | 0 | 0 | 0 |
| Multiple myeloma | 9 | 0 | 0 | 0 | 0 | 0 |
| Breast | 75 | 0 | 14 | 19 | 0 | 19 |
| Lung (all cell types) | 45 | 0 | 7 | 16 | 0 | 16 |
| Colorectal | 81 | 0 | 5 | 6 | 0 | 6 |
| Pancreas | 7 | 0 | 1 | 14 | 0 | 14 |
| Esophagus | 2 | 0 | 0 | 0 | 0 | 0 |
| Stomach | 10 | 0 | 1 | 10 | 0 | 10 |
| Melanoma | 44 | 0 | 3 | 7 | 0 | 7 |
| Ovarian | 11 | 0 | 2 | 18 | 0 | 18 |
| Lymphomas (all types) | 7 | 0 | 2 | 29 | 0 | 29 |
| Mesothelioma | 2[d] | 0 | 1 | 50 | 0 | 50 |
| Skin | 1 | 0 | 0 | 0 | 0 | 0 |
| Renal | 17 | 0 | 2 | 12 | 0 | 12 |
| Testicular | 1 | 0 | 1 | 100 | 0 | 100 |
| Prostate | 2 | 0 | 0 | 0 | 0 | 0 |
| Bladder | 1 | 0 | 0 | 0 | 0 | 0 |
| Cervix | 3 | 0 | 0 | 0 | 0 | 0 |
| Endometrium | 3 | 0 | 0 | 0 | 0 | 0 |
| Chordoma | 1 | 0 | 0 | 0 | 0 | 0 |
| Glioblastoma | 2 | 0 | 0 | 0 | 0 | 0 |
| Head and neck | 6[e] | 0 | 0 | 0 | 0 | 0 |
| Sarcomas | 10 | 0 | 0 | 0 | 0 | 0 |
| Hepatoma | 3 | 0 | 0 | 0 | 0 | 0 |
| Adenocarcinoma ? Primary | 11 | 0 | 1 | 9 | 0 | 9 |

[a] Derived from numerous clinical trials by cooperative groups or single investigators.
[b] CR = complete response; PR = partial response.
[c] Three patients had hematological improvement.
[d] One patient treated at two different dose schedules.
[e] Carcinoma of tongue (1); parotid carcinoma (2); larynx carcinoma (1); tonsil carcinoma (1); epiglottis carcinoma (1).

days. One of the remissions did last 6 months. Other investigators have not confirmed these findings. Overall, in all results on file at the Investigational Drug Branch, there have been 75 patients evaluated with a 19% response rate (0% CR and 19% PR). Bellet *et al.* (1974) did notice that remissions, when they occurred, were early and dramatic. From the foregoing results it must be concluded that 5-azacytidine is not a very active agent in breast cancer, although many of these patients had been refractory to other chemotherapy.

### 6. *Lung*

A total of 45 patients have been treated in Phase I and II studies with a total of 7 partial responses. The responses have been in squamous, large cell, and adenocarcinoma.

### 7. *Colon and Rectum*

A total of 81 patients have been treated in Phase I and II trials with a total of 5 partial responses. The drug does not seem to offer much therapeutic benefit in this disease.

### 8. *Pancreas, Islet Cell Tumor, Esophagus, and Stomach*

There has been 1 partial response in 7 patients with cancer of the pancreas. No response was seen in 1 islet cell tumor. There have been no responses in 2 cases of cancer of the esophagus, and 1 partial response in 10 patients with cancer of the stomach.

### 9. *Melanoma*

Forty-four patients with malignant melanoma have been treated with 5-azacytidine. Three patients have had a partial response with 1 remission of 6 months duration.

### 10. *Ovarian Carcinoma*

There have been 11 patients with ovarian cancer treated with 5-azacytidine with 2 patients obtaining partial remissions. Bellet *et al.* (1974) commented that 1 of these remissions was early and dramatic and lasted for 3 months.

### 11. *Lymphoma*

Seven patients have been treated (all refractory to conventional therapy). There have been 2 partial responses. One of them was in a woman with American Burkitt's lymphoma (Lomen *et al.*, 1975).

### 12. *Mesothelioma*

Results reported by Vogler *et al.* (1974) have been encouraging in that 1 patient was treated at two different dose schedules with an objective response both times (relief of intestinal obstruction).

### 13. *Renal, Testicle, Prostate, Bladder*

Seventeen patients with renal carcinoma have received 5-azacytidine, and there have been 2 partial responses. In 1 case of embryonal carcinoma of the testicle, there was a 30-day remission. There have been no responses in the few cases of prostate and bladder cancer in which the drug has been tried.

### 14. *Cervical and Endometrial Cancer*

There have been no responses in 3 cases each of cervical and endometrial carcinoma.

### 15. *Adenocarcinoma (Unknown Primary)*

There was 1 partial remission in 11 cases of adenocarcinoma of unknown primary.

### 16. *Central Nervous System Tumors*

There were no responses in the 2 cases of glioblastoma who were given 5-azacytidine.

### 17. *Head and Neck*

There have been no responses in tumors at various sites of the head and neck in 6 patients.

### 18. *Sarcomas*

Table VIII shows that there have been no responses in 10 patients with soft tissue sarcomas.

### 19. *Hepatomas*

With 5-azacytidine alone, there have been no responses in adult hepatomas. However, C. Tan (personal communication, 1975) has reported 3 responses in 4 patients with childhood hepatomas receiving 5-azacytidine and Adriamycin. One child is still in remission 14 months after therapy.

In summary, 5-azacytidine seems to have its best activity in AML patients who have been refractory to conventional therapy. Its activity in the solid tumors has not been encouraging with the possible exceptions of mesothelioma (number of patients small) and childhood hepatoma (when used in combination with Adriamycin).

## C. Toxicity in Man

The toxicities discovered in the Phase I, II, and III trials can be divided into the several areas summarized in Table IX. This table represents data on file in the Investigational Drug Branch for 748 patients receiving 5-azacytidine alone at various dosage levels. The dose-limiting toxicities have been nausea, vomiting, and leukopenia.

### 1. *Nausea and Vomiting*

This has been a particularly troublesome toxicity with an overall average incidence, regardless of method of administration or dose, of about 73% in 748 patients. The nausea and vomiting begin 1.5–3 hours after the intravenous injection, and usually recur with each subsequent injection (Bellet *et al.*, 1974; Vogler *et al.*, 1974). Analysis of these toxicities suggests a dose–response relationship.

In a Phase II study, Moertel *et al.* (1972) concluded that "the severity of nausea and vomiting induced by 5-azacytidine seriously compromises any hope of clinical usefulness." Because of the nausea and vomiting, some patients have been unwilling to have repeated courses of the drug (Cunningham *et al.*, 1974).

Antiemetics such as chlorpromazine have had a variable effect on these symptoms. Some investigators consider this treatment useful if the patient is given premedication for 24 to 48 hours before the course of 5-azacytidine (Karon *et al.*, 1973). Other investigators feel that the chlorpromazine might be contributing to the abnormal liver function tests and the occasional hypotension seen with 5-azacytidine administration (Moertel *et al.*, 1972; McCredie *et al.*, 1972). Karon *et al.* (1973), Shnider *et al.* (1975), Weiss *et al.* (1972), Tan *et al.* (1973), McCredie *et al.* (1973), and others have noted that there was a slight decrease in the severity of nausea and vomiting if the drug was given in divided doses (b.i.d. or t.i.d.) or by use of a fast drip over 15 minutes.

Two protocols have been designed to give the drug by continuous infusion over a 5-day period (Lomen *et al.*, 1975; Vogler *et al.*, 1975), but there is a difficulty in that the activity of 5-azacytidine (as measured by physicochemical and biological systems) is diminished because of degradation in the infusion solution. The infusion solutions have been in

TABLE IX

SUMMARY OF MAJOR TOXIC EFFECTS OF 5-AZACYTIDINE

| Dose schedule | Dose range (mg/m$^2$) | No. of evaluable patients | Percentage of patients with toxic effects | | | | | | | Reference[f] |
|---|---|---|---|---|---|---|---|---|---|---|
| | | | | | | | | Heptatotoxicity[e] | | |
| | | | Nausea | Vomiting | Diarrhea | Leukopenia (<1500/mm$^3$) | Thrombocytopenia (<$10^5$/mm$^3$) | Abnormal LFT | Coma | |
| Weekly, i.v. | 200–633 | 15 | 94 | 100 | 79 | 35 | 5 | — | — | (1) |
| Twice weekly, i.v. | 50–200 | 88 | 87 | 88 | Occ.[d] | 41 | 0 | — | — | (2) |
| Daily × 5, i.v. | 50–400 | 376 | 71 | 70 | 40 | 24 | 9 | 2 | 0 | (3) |
| Daily × 10, i.v. | 0.5–2.4[c] | 206 | 76 | 93 | 60 | 27 | 29 | 21 | 0.7 | (4) |
| Daily × 10, s.c. | 27–85 | 18 | 44 | 22 | 16 | 22 | 16 | 28 | 16 | (5) |
| 5-Day infusion[a] | 50–200 | 36 | 58 | 58 | Occ.[d] | 76 | 25 | — | — | (6) |
| 120-Hr infusion[b] | 150–200 | 6 | 0 | 0 | 0 | 100 | 33 | — | — | (7) |

[a] Fresh solution prepared every 3 hours.

[b] Fresh solution prepared every 4 hours.

[c] Expressed in milligrams per kilogram.

[d] Occasional.

[e] LFT = liver function tests; (—) no mention of this toxicity.

[f] Key to references: 1—Shnider *et al.* (1975); 2—Vogler *et al.* (1974); 3—Karon *et al.* (1973), Shnider *et al.* (1975), K. B. McCredie (personal communication, 1975), McCredie *et al.* (1973), Levi *et al.* (1975), J. R. Bateman (personal communication, 1975), Quagliana *et al.* (1974), Moertel *et al.* (1972); 4—Cunningham *et al.* (1974), Weiss *et al.* (1972); 5—Bellet *et al.* (1974); 6—Vogler *et al.* (1975); 7—Lomen *et al.* (1975).

Ringer's lactate, and the bottles have been changed with new solutions made up every 3–4 hours (Lomen *et al.*, 1975; Vogler *et al.*, 1975). If one analyzes the nausea and vomiting with the infusion data, there is a 50–70% incidence in Vogler's series (Vogler *et al.*, 1975), and no nausea or vomiting reported in Lomen's series (Lomen *et al.*, 1975) with comparable doses.

Bellet *et al.* (1974) have administered the drug subcutaneously and noted a 44% incidence of nausea and a 22% incidence of vomiting. They noticed that tolerance developed to nausea and vomiting in all patients as additional doses of 5-azacytidine were given over the 10-day loading regimen.

In summary, some data indicate that the incidence of nausea and vomiting accompanying the use of 5-azacytidine may be reduced by using subcutaneous administration over a longer period of time or by using infusions. However, investigators using infusions are cautioned about the relatively rapid decomposition of 5-azacytidine.

### 2. *Diarrhea*

The average reported incidence of diarrhea in all series is 53%. The diarrhea usually occurs with the nausea and vomiting. It has not been a dose-limiting toxicity. Administration via an infusion or subcutaneous route may decrease the incidence slightly.

### 3. *Hematological Toxicities*

Several of the Phase I studies showed leukopenia as a dose-limiting toxicity. The overall incidence of leukopenia (less than 1500 total white count, including all dosage levels) was 34%. This is a dose-related phenomenon.

The mean nadir of the leukopenia has been 25–40 days, with a range of 18–56 days (Moertel *et al.*, 1972; Bellet *et al.*, 1974; Karon *et al.*, 1973 and Vogler *et al.*, 1974). Recovery takes place in 1 to 3 weeks (Vogler *et al.*, 1974; Bellet *et al.*, 1974; Levi *et al.*, 1975), but rigorous support in the leukopenic period has been necessary (McCredie *et al.*, 1973). Subcutaneous administration over 10 days seems to delay the leukopenia somewhat (21–35 days past the start of treatment). Cumulative hematotoxicity with repeated courses has not been observed by Moertel *et al.* (1972).

As pointed out by Karon *et al.* (1973), myelosuppression is not necessarily untoward in leukemia patients. Levi *et al.* (1975) showed that, in 6 patients achieving remission with 5-azacytidine, the degree of leukopenia was definitely more profound (median 660/mm$^3$) after each course than in those patients who failed to respond (median 1700/mm$^3$).

Thrombocytopenia (< 100,000) has been reported in 17% of patients receiving the drug. The dog toxicity data predicted mild thrombocytopenia and only at the largest doses. Thrombocytopenia in the human has been dose-dependent but of surprisingly low incidence. Moertel *et al.* (1972) reported the mean nadir of thrombocytopenia as 18 days with a range of 13 to 21 days. Bellet *et al.* (1974) have noted two deaths directly attributable to thrombocytopenia, and, therefore, platelet support should be available when 5-azacytidine is being given.

Anemia has not been a great problem, with approximately 4% of patients having a greater than 3 gm% drop in hemoglobin.

### 4. *Hepatic Toxicities*

The dog and the monkey predicted a hepatic toxicity for 5-azacytidine (see Section VI).

In August 1971, Dr. Robert Bellet reported 3 deaths secondary to hepatic failure in patients receiving 5-azacytidine. Bellet *et al.* (1973) subsequently did a clinical and pathological study on the hepatotoxicity of 5-azacytidine. In their series of 20 evaluable patients receiving subcutaneous 5-azacytidine, 7 patients experienced liver function tests abnormalities. Four of these patients with significant hepatic tumor burden died of rapidly progressive hepatic coma. When the patients dying in hepatic coma and a surviving group with hepatic metastases were compared, the former had base-line serum albumins less than 2.8 gm% with the latter greater than 3.0 gm% ($p < 0.10$). Serum bilirubin, prothrombin time, SGOT, and alkaline phosphatase did not seem to have this predictive value. Coded liver biopsy specimens in 8 patients without hepatic metastases revealed no significant difference between pre- and post-treatment specimens. They concluded that 5-azacytidine therapy is contraindicated in patients with hepatic metastases and serum albumins of less than 3 gm%. Bellet *et al.* (1973) cite a personal communication from Troetel that preferential hepatic concentration of the labeled drug has been documented in rats and mice, but this does not agree with the published literature (Raska *et al.*, 1965a).

From the limited data on hand, dose schedule or route of administration do not seem to influence hepatic toxicity. In reviewing all of the patients who have received the drug, the hepatotoxicity does not seem to be dose-related. The overall incidence of abnormal liver function tests thought to be secondary to 5-azacytidine is about 7%, with 0.5% of patients receiving the drug developing hepatic coma thought to be secondary to the drug (see Table IX). Some investigators have felt that the antiemetic chlorpromazine might contribute to the abnormal liver function tests (Moertel *et al.*, 1972).

### 5. *Fever*

The overall incidence of fever in all reported trials is 6% and does not seem to be dose-related. McCredie *et al.* (1973) noted temperatures of 104° F 1–4 hours after the administration of the drug with continuation each day for the duration of the course. Body temperatures usually have fallen to normal levels within 24 hours of the completion of the course of 5-azacytidine therapy.

### 6. *Rash*

Two percent of patients receiving the drug have had an accompanying rash, although many of these patients were on multiple drugs. Karon *et al.* (1973) noted the rash to be pruritic, follicular, and transient and did not require any alteration in the drug administration. Other investigators have reported a maculopapular eruption (Shnider *et al.*, 1975).

### 7. *Stomatitis*

Stomatitis occurs in only 5.7% of patients and does not appear to be dose-related.

### 8. *Hypotension*

Hypotension is a relatively rare side effect with an overall incidence of 0.45%. McCredie *et al.* (1973) reported 1 case of a direct relationship between the infusion of 5-azacytidine and the development of hypotension, tachypnea, and cyanosis with eventual death. However, this patient had disseminated *Candida tropicalis* at postmortem examination.

### 9. *Neuromuscular*

Myalgias have been noted by the Western Chemotherapy Group in their coopertive study (J. R. Bateman, personal communication, 1975). Lomen *et al.* (1975) reported 1 female patient who developed somnolence upon receiving the drug. This did not seem to be hepatic coma. Levi *et al.* (1975) noted a peculiar myalgic/asthenic syndrome in 17 of 18 patients receiving 5-azacytidine by intravenous bolus. Onset was day 23 of therapy with generalized muscular tenderness and associated weakness and lethargy. As the syndrome became more severe the patients became confused and somnolent. They reported 1 patient who became comatose on two consecutive occasions after receiving the drug. The particular reason for this toxicity was not established. Multiple laboratory procedures showed no evidence of deterioration in liver function tests, and only a diffuse dysrhythmia consistent with a toxic encephalopathy was seen on electroencephalography in the patient who became comatose after the 5-azacytidine administration. The overall incidence of this neurologic–muscular syndrome in all patients is 0.27%.

### 10. *Miscellaneous*

Phlebitis has been noted occasionally (Levi *et al.*, 1975) in some patients receiving the drug. One patient has been reported by Cunningham *et al.* (1974) to have had cardiac ischemia at postmortem examination, but she was severely ill for days before her death.

Of the 748 patients reported, there were 6 deaths that were felt to be drug-related (0.8%). One was due to hypotension, 3 due to hepatic coma, and 2 secondary to thrombocytopenia.

## IX. Summary and Conclusions

5-Azacytidine has been under study for 11 years and in clinical use for 5 years. The drug is a ring analog of cytidine and possesses cytotoxic, antimicrobial, antineoplastic, leukopenic, abortive, and mutagenic activity in various biological systems. It also has been shown to have a radioprotective effect in mice exposed to lethal irradiation. 5-Azacytidine probably exerts its cytotoxic and antineoplastic properties by incorporation into DNA and RNA after phosphorylation. This incorporation into RNA gives a defective mRNA that cannot code properly for protein synthesis.

The beagle dog and the rhesus monkey were predictive for the bone marrow, hepatic, and cardiovascular (hypotension) toxicity in the human but were overpredictive for renal and lymphoid organ toxicity. These animals were not predictive for GI, neuromuscular, or skin toxicity.

Of particular interest is the fact that man can tolerate much higher doses (20–30 times) of 5-azacytidine than the experimental animals. The pharmacokinetic studies have shown metabolism and excretion patterns that are about the same in rodents, dogs, and man. Perhaps the selective activities of kinases and deaminases in the various species are different and this accounts for the difference in maximally tolerated dosage. Other factors may also be important.

The drug is active in the L1210 and P388 animal leukemia systems, and this correlates well with its promising activity in AML of adults and children that has been refractory to other conventional agents. The mouse L1210 leukemia system predicted activity of 5-azacytidine in both the daily and the intermittent schedules, and this correlates well with the AML experience for whose treatment one schedule does not seem to be more or less efficient than any other schedule.

The activity of 5-azacytidine in animal solid tumor systems has been low, and this also correlates well with the disappointing activity of this drug in human solid tumors.

Further work with this drug will include its use in combination with other effective antileukemic drugs as first-line treatment for patients with AML.

## Acknowledgments

The authors are indebted to Dr. R. Alexanian, Dr. J. R. Bateman, Dr. F. Z. Finklestein, Dr. D. Hammond, Dr. J. A. Levi, Dr. K. B. McCredie, Dr. J. M. Quagliana, Dr. B. Shnider, and Dr. C. Tan for permission to use their previously unpublished data.

## References

Altanerova, V., and Altaner, C. (1972). *Neoplasma* **19,** 405–412.

Bellet, R. E., Mastrangelo, M. J., Engstrom, P. F., and Custer, R. P. (1973). *Neoplasma* **20,** 303–309.

Bellet, R. E., Mastrangelo, M. J., Engstrom, P. F., Strawitz, J. G., Weiss, A. J., and Yarbro, J. W. (1974). *Cancer Chemother. Rep., Part 1* **58,** 217–222.

Bergy, M. E., and Herr, R. R. (1966). *Antimicrob. Agents Chemother.* pp. 625–630.

Burchenal, J. H., Dowling, M. D., Cole, M., Pomeroy, D., and Krakoff, I. H. (1972). *Proc. Am. Assoc. Cancer Res.* **13,** 105.

Chabner, B. A., Drake, J. C., and John, D. G. (1973). *Biochem. Pharmacol.* **22,** 2763–2765.

Cihak, A., and Sorm, F. (1965). *Collect. Czech. Chem. Commun.* **30,** 2091–2102.

Cihak, A., and Vesely, J. (1964). *Collect. Czech. Chem. Commun.* **34,** 910–918.

Cihak, A., and Vesely, J. (1973). *J. Biol. Chem.* **248,** 1307–1313.

Cihak, A., Vesely, J., and Sorm, F. (1965). *Biochim. Biophys. Acta* **108,** 516–518.

Cihak, A., Tykva, R., and Sorm, F. (1966). *Collect. Czech. Chem. Commun.* **31,** 3015–3019.

Cihak, A., Vesely, J., and Sorm, F. (1967a). *Biochim. Biophys. Acta* **134,** 456–489.

Cihak, A., Vesely, J., and Sorm, F. (1967b). *Collect. Czech. Chem. Commun.* **32,** 3427–3436.

Cihak, A., Seifertova, M., Vesely, J., and Şorm, F. (1972a). *Int. J. Cancer* **10,** 20–27.

Cihak, A., Vesely, J., Inoue, H., and Pitot, H. C. (1972b). *Biochem. Pharmacol.* **21,** 2545–2553.

Coles, E., Thayer, P. S., Reinhold, V., Gaudio, L., and Arthur D. Little, Inc. (1974). *Proc. Am. Assoc. Cancer Res.* **15,** 72.

Coles, E., Wodinsky, I., Gaudio, L., and Arthur D. Little, Inc. (1975). *Proc. Am. Assoc. Cancer Res.* **16,** 91.

Crkvenjakov, R., Bajkovic, N., and Glisin, V. (1970). *Biochem. Biophys. Res. Commun.* **39,** 655–660.

Cunningham, T. J., Nemoto, T., Rosner, D., Knight, E., Taylor, S., Rosenbaum, C., Horton, J., and Dao, T. (1974). *Cancer Chemother. Rep., Part 1* **58,** 115–119.

Doskocil, J., and Sorm, F. (1970). *Collect. Czech, Chem. Commun.* **35,** 1880–1891.

Doskocil, J., and Sorm, F. (1971). *FEBS Lett.* **19,** 30–32.

Doskocil, J., Paces, V., and Sorm, F. (1967). *Biochim. Biophys. Acta* **145,** 771–779.

Fucik, V., Zadrazil, S., Sormova, Z., and Sorm, F. (1965a). *Collect. Czech. Chem. Commun.* **30,** 2883–2886.

Fucik, V., Sormova, Z., and Sorm, F. (1965b). *Biol. Plant.* **7,** 58–64.

Fucik, V., Michaelis, A., and Rieger, R. (1970). *Mutat. Res.* **9,** 599–606.

Fucik, V., Zandrazil, S., Jurovcik, M., and Sormova, Z. (1972). *Folia Microbiol. (Prague)* **17,** 517–521.

Goldsmith, M. A., Slavik, M., and Carter, S. K. (1975). *Cancer Res.* **35,** 1354–1364.

Grunow, R. (1972). *Chem. Abst.* **77,** 1158.

Halle, S. (1968). *J. Virol.* **2,** 1228–1229.

Hanka, L. J., and Clark, J. J. (1975). *Proc. Am. Assoc. Cancer Res.* **16,** 113.

Hanka, L. J., Evans, J. S., Mason, D. J., and Dietz, A. (1966). *Antimicrob. Agents Chemother.* pp. 619–624.

Heidelberger, E. (1974). *In* "Cancer Medicine"(J. R. Holland and E. Frei, eds.), p. 785. Lea and Febiger, Philadelphia, Pennsylvania.

Hrodek, O., and Vesely, J. (1971). *Neoplasma* **18,** 493–503.

Israili, Z. H., Vogler, W. R., Mingioli, E. S., Pirkle, J. L., Smithwick, R. W., and Goldstein, J. H. (1974). *Pharmacologist* **16,** 231.

Jurovcik, M., Zandrazil, S., Fucik, V., and Sormova, Z. (1972). *Collect. Czech. Chem. Commun.* **37,** 299–308.

Karon, M., and Benedict, W. F. (1970). *Science* **178,** 62.

Karon, M., Sieger, L., Leimbrock, S., Finklestein, J. Z., Nesbit, M. E., and Swaney, J. J. (1973). *Blood* **42,** 359–365.

Lee, T. (1973). *Proc. Am. Assoc. Cancer Res.* **14,** 94.

Levi, J. A., and Wiernik, P. H. (1975). *Cancer Chemother. Rep., Part 1* **59,** 1043–1045.

Levi, J. A., Wiernik, P. H., Evan, J. J., and Sutherland, J. C. (1975). *Proc. Am. Assoc. Cancer Res.* **16,** 83.

Levitan, I. B., and Webb, T. E. (1969). *Biochim. Biophys. Acta* **182,** 491–500.

Levitan, I. B., and Webb, T. E. (1970). *J. Mol. Biol.* **48,** 339–348.

Levitan, I. B., Morris, H. P., and Webb, T. E. (1971). *Biochim. Biophys. Acta* **240,** 287–295.

Li, L. H., Olin, E. J., Buskirk, H. H., and Reinke, L. M. (1970a). *Cancer Res.* **30,** 2760–2769.

Li, L. H., Olin, E. J., Fraser, T. J., and Bhuyan, B. K. (1970b). *Cancer Res.* **30,** 2770–2775.

Lim, P., Pont, L., and Cheung, A. (1974). NIH Contract I—CM—33723.

Lloyd, H. H., Dulmadge, E. A., and Wilkoff, L. J. (1972). *Cancer Chemother. Rep., Part 1* **56,** 585–591.

Lomen, P. L., Vaitkevicius, K., and Samson, M. K. (1975). *Proc. Am. Assoc. Cancer Res.* **16,** 52.

McCredie, K. B., Bodey, G. P., Burgess, M. A., Rodriguez, V., Sullivan, M. P., and Freireich, E. J. (1972). *Blood* **40,** 975.

McCredie, K. B., Bodey, G. P., Burgess, M. A., Gutterman, J. U., Rodriguez, V.,

Sullivan, M. P., and Freireich, E. J. (1973). *Cancer Chemother. Rep., Part 1* **57,** 319–323.
Moertel, C. G., Shutt, A. J., Reitemeier, R. J., and Hahn, R. G. (1972). *Cancer Chemother. Rep., Part 1* **56,** 649–652.
Neil, G. L., Gray, L. G., and Berger, A. W. (1974). *Pharmacologist* **16,** 209.
Neil, G. L., Moxley, T. E., Kuentzel, S. L., Manak, R. C., and Hanka, L. J. (1975). *Cancer Chemother. Rep., Part 1* **59,** 459–465.
Nitschke, R. (1974). *Proc. Am. Assoc. Cancer Res.* **15,** 127.
Notari, R. E., and DeYoung, J. L. (1975). *J. Pharm. Sci.* **64,** 1148–1156.
Oliverio, V. T. (1972). *Cancer Chemother. Rep., Part 3* **3,** 69–71.
Paces, V., Doskocil, J., and Sorm, F. (1968). *Biochim. Biophys. Acta* **161,** 352–360.
Palm, P. E., and Kensler, C. J. (1970). U.S. Clearinghouse Fed. Sci. Tech. Info. P. B. Rep. No. 194797.
Palm, P. E., Arnold, E. P., Rachwall, P. G., Nick, M. S., and Arthur D. Little, Inc. (1973). *Toxicol. Appl. Pharmacol.* **25,** 492.
Piskala, A., and Sorm, F. (1964). *Collect. Czech. Chem. Commun.* **29,** 2060–2076.
Pithova, P., Fucik, V., Zadrazil, S., Sormova, Z., and Sorm, F. (1964). *Collect. Czech. Chem. Commun.* **30,** 2879–2882.
Pithova, P., Piskala, A., Pitha, J., and Sorm, F. (1965). *Collect. Czech. Chem. Commun.* **30,** 2801–2811.
Pittello, R. F., and Woolley, C. (1969). *Appl. Microbiol.* **18,** 284–286.
Presant, C. A., Vietti, J., and Valeriote, F. (1975). *Proc. Am. Assoc. Cancer Res.* **16,** 62.
Pringle, C. R. (1970). *J. Virol.* **5,** 559–567.
Quagliana, J. M., Costanzi, J., O'Bryan, R., and the Southwest Oncology Group. (1974). *Proc. Am. Assoc. Cancer Res.* **15,** 121.
Raska, K., Jr., Jurovcik, M., Sormova, Z., and Sorm, F. (1965a). *Collect. Czech. Chem. Commun.* **30,** 3001–3006.
Raska, K., Jr., Jurovcik, M., Sormova, Z., and Sorm, F. (1965b). *Collect. Czech. Chem. Commun.* **30,** 3215–3217.
Raska, K., Jr., Jurovcik, M., Sormova, Z., and Sorm, F. (1966a). *Collect. Czech. Chem. Commun.* **31,** 2803–2808.
Raska, K., Jr., Jurovcik, M., Fucik, V., Tykva, R., Sormova, Z., and Sorm, F. (1966b). *Collect. Czech. Chem. Commun.* **31,** 2809–2815.
Reichard, P., Skold, O., Klein, G., Revesz, L., and Magnusson, P. H. (1961). *Cancer Res.* **21,** 110–117.
Reichard, P., Skold, O., Klein, G., Revesz, L., and Magnusson, P. H. (1962). *Cancer Res.* **22,** 235–243.
Sandberg, J., and Goldin, A. (1971). *Cancer Chemother. Rep., Part 1* **55,** 233–238.
Seifertova, M., Vesely, J., and Sorm, F. (1968). *Experientia* **24,** 487–488.
Shnider, B. I., Baig, M., and Colsky, J. (1975). *J. Clin. Pharmacol.* **16,** 205–212.
Shutt, R. H., and Krueger, R. G. (1972). *J. Immunol.* **108,** 819–830.
Simson, J. A. V., and Baserga, R. (1971). *Lab. Invest.* **24,** 464–468.
Sorm, F., and Vesely, J. (1964). *Neoplasma* **11,** 123–130.
Sorm, F., and Vesely, J. (1965). *Experientia* **21,** 581–582.
Sorm, F., Piskala, A., Cihak, A., and Veseley, J. (1964). *Experientia* **20,** 202–203.
Sorm, F., Sormova, Z., Raska, K., Jr., and Jurovcik, M. (1966). *Rev. Roum. Biochim.* **3,** 139–147.
Svata, M., Raska, K., Jr., and Sorm, F. (1966). *Experientia* **22,** 53.
Tan, C., Burchenal, J. H., Clarkson, B., Feinstein, M., Garcia, E., Sidhu, J., and Krakoff, I. H. (1973). *Proc. Am. Assoc. Cancer Res.* **14,** 97.
Tobey, R. (1972). *Cancer Res.* **32,** 2720–2725.

Troetel, W. M., Weiss, A. J., Stambaugh, J. F., Laucius, J., and Manthei, R. W. (1972). *Cancer Chemother. Rep., Part 1* **56,** 405–411.
Tyrer, D. D., Kline, I., Gang, M., Goldin, A., and Venditti, J. M. (1969). *Cancer Chemother. Rep., Part 1* **53,** 229–241.
Vadlamudi, S., and Goldin, A. (1968). *Exp. Hematol. (Oak Ridge, Tenn.)* **17,** 47–51.
Vadlamudi, S., Padarathsingh, M., Bonmassar, E., and Goldin, A. (1970a). *Proc. Soc. Exp. Biol. Med.* **133,** 1232–1238.
Vadlamudi, S., Choudry, J. N., Waravdekar, V. S., and Kline, I. (1970b). *Cancer Res.* **30,** 362–369.
Venditti, J. M. (1971). *Cancer Chemother. Rep., Part 3* **2,** 35–59.
Vesely, J. (1967). *Proc. Int. Congr. Chemother.* **2,** 779–782.
Vesely, J. (1970). *In* "Oncology" (R. L. Clark, R. W. Cumley, J. E. McCay, and M. M. Copeland, eds.), Vol. 2, p. 265–274. Yearbook Publ., Chicago, Illinois.
Vesely, J., and Sorm, F. (1965). *Neoplasma* **12,** 3–9.
Vesely, J., Cihak, A., and Sorm, F. (1967). *Int. J. Cancer* **2,** 639–646.
Vesely, J., Cihak, A., and Sorm, F. (1968a). *Cancer Res.* **28,** 1995–2000.
Vesely, J., Cihak, A., and Sorm, M. F. (1968b). *Biochem. Pharmacol.* **17,** 519–524.
Vesely, J., Gostof, R., Cihak, A., and Sorm, F. (1969). *Z. Naturforsch., Teil B* **24,** 318–320.
Vesely, J., Cihak, A., and Sorm, F. (1970). *Cancer Res.* **30,** 2180–2186.
Vesely, J., Cihak, A., and Sorm, F. (1971a). *Eur. J. Biochem.* **22,** 551–556.
Vesely, J., Dvorak, M., Cihak, A., and Sorm, F. (1971b). *Int. J. Cancer* **8,** 310–319.
Vogler, R., Arkin, S., Velez-Garcia, F. (1974). *Cancer Chemother. Rep., Part 1* **58,** 895–899.
Vogler, W. R., Miller, D., and Keller, J. W. (1975). *Proc. Am. Assoc. Cancer Res.* **16,** 155.
Weiss, A. J., Stambaugh, J. E., Mastrangelo, M. J., Laucius, J. F., and Bellet, R. E. (1972). *Cancer Chemother. Rep., Part 1* **56,** 413–419.
Zandrazil, S., Fucik, V., Bartl, P., Sormova, Z., and Sorm, F. (1965). *Biochim. Biophys. Acta* **108,** 701–703.
Zandrazil, S., Fucik, V., Jurovcik, M., and Sormova, Z. (1972). *Collect. Czech. Chem. Commun.* **37,** 309–318.
Zee-Cheng, K. Y., and Cheng, C. C. (1970). *J. Pharm. Sci.* **59,** 1630–1634.

# Copper in Mammalian Reproduction

GERALD OSTER* AND MIKLOS P. SALGO†‡

I. Introduction . . . 328
II. Copper Intrauterine Device . . . 329
A. Clinical Aspects . . . 329
B. Mode of Contraceptive Action . . . 331
C. Side Effects . . . 345
III. Hormonally Induced Changes in Copper Levels . . . 357
A. Ceruloplasmin . . . 357
B. Other Oxidases . . . 360
C. Taste and Smell . . . 361
IV. Copper Influences on Reproductive Hormones . . . 362
A. Copper-Induced Ovulation and Releasing Hormones . . . 362
B. Sex Steroids . . . 364
C. Prostaglandins . . . 365
D. Thyroid . . . 366
V. Copper in Pregnancy . . . 368
A. Copper Deficiency and Reproductive Failure . . . 368
B. Copper-Chelating Agents and Fetal Resorption . . . 370
C. Teratogenesis of Related Drugs, Environmental Toxins, and Lathyrogenic Agents . . . 371
D. Copper Excess . . . 376
E. Copper in Parturition . . . 378
VI. Copper and Sperm . . . 379
A. Spermicidal Action of Copper and of Chelating Agents . . . 379
B. Sulfhydryl Groups and Sperm Maturation . . . 380
C. Inhibition of Spermatogenesis . . . 381
VII. Copper and the Neonate and Infant . . . 382
A. Copper in Infant Nutrition . . . 382
B. Copper in Inherited Metabolic Diseases . . . 385
VIII. Copper Antagonists . . . 388
A. Zinc and Other Inorganic Antagonists . . . 388
B. Vitamins . . . 389
IX. Copper in the Environment . . . 391
A. Excess Copper . . . 391

* Graduate School of Biological Science, Mount Sinai School of Medicine of the City University of New York, New York, New York.

† Department of Physiology and Biophysics, Mount Sinai School of Medicine of the City University of New York, New York, New York.

‡ Present address: Physiological Laboratory, University of Cambridge, Cambridge, Great Britain.

B. Chelating Agents . . . . . . . . . . . . . . . . . . 392
References . . . . . . . . . . . . . . . . . . . . 393
Notes Added in Proof . . . . . . . . . . . . . . . . . 409

## I. Introduction

Although copper has long been known to be involved in reproductive processes, interest has increased considerably due to the recent clinical application of the copper intrauterine device (Cu-IUD). This device developed in 1969 by Zipper and Tatum (Zipper *et al.,* 1969b), promises to be one of the most important methods of human contraception. It consists of a small plastic T-shaped device or 7-shaped device (Gravigard) the stem of which is wrapped with copper wire. The contraceptive efficacy of the Cu-IUD is far greater than that of the plastic device alone. The nature of the mode of action of the Cu-IUD has been the focus of much research (see Oster and Salgo, 1975).

One of the earliest references to copper in mammalian reproduction is the study by de Quatrefages in 1850 of the effects of cupric ion on human sperm. Another classic example of copper in reproduction is that of Krebs who, in 1928, found that serum copper in women is considerably increased during pregnancy. Dietary copper deficiency causes reproductive failure in pregnant rats, as was demonstrated by Keil and Nelson in 1931. The rats were fed entirely on iron-supplemented milk. Milk is very poor in copper. Copper is a nutritional trace element first shown by Hart *et al.* in 1928 to be required for hemoglobin formation. Indeed, Josephs in 1931 showed that copper, as well as iron, was needed to treat anemia in milk-fed infants. Copper is required for maintaining the health of the embryo, fetus, newborn, and infant. That copper is involved in an earlier process of mammalian reproduction, namely ovulation, is implied from the work of Fevold *et al.* (1936). They showed that injection of copper salts induces ovulation in rabbits.

The Cu-IUD, the spermicidal action of copper, and the copper-induced ovulation are all examples of copper as a pharmacological agent. As will be shown, copper metal has a quite different action than that of cupric salts. The reproductive failure with copper deficiency is a nutritional problem but administering copper-chelating agents, which produce a similar effect (Salgo and Oster, 1974b), is a pharmacological approach. We will cite a number of examples where administration of excess copper has the same end biological result as copper deficiency. Another pharmacological effect related to copper is the rise in serum copper which occurs not only in pregnancy but also with oral contraceptives (von Studnitz and Berezin, 1958).

It has been appreciated for half a century that copper plays a central role in biological autooxidation. The conversion of atmospheric oxygen to water is controlled by enzymes, the majority of which contain copper. The focus of this chapter is on reproductive physiology in which copper is clearly involved. Examples are also given of cases in which copper is implicated. These latter examples suggest the presence of copper-containing enzymes as yet to be well characterized.

## II. Copper Intrauterine Device

### A. Clinical Aspects

Intrauterine devices have certain advantages over other methods of contraception. Unlike other forms of reversible contraception the IUD does not require continuing motivation. Its insertion requires trained personnel. The effect of the IUD is primarily local and the device does not upset the overall hormonal status.

Recent studies of data from women in developed countries indicate that the IUD is as safe if not safer than the pill (Jain, 1975; Tietze *et al.*, 1976). The IUDs have a higher contraceptive failure rate (about 2%) than the pill (about 0.1%) (Jain, 1975). Although information on mortality from use of the IUD is scanty, the mortality rate is thought to be below 1/100,000 per year of use. The total mortality rate including mortalities from pregnancies is below that for the pill (Jain, 1975; Tietze *et al.*, 1976).

The most common side effects of IUDs are pain and bleeding. Bleeding induced by IUDs can be more than twice that of normal menstrual bleeding (see Moyer and Shaw, 1973). This can be particularly serious for women with anemia due to low nutritional status. Pain and bleeding along with spontaneous expulsion and pregnancy are the main reasons for discontinuation of their use (see Tietze, 1973; Huber *et al.*, 1975). Although rare, deaths from the IUD arise primarily from infections and pregnancies (see Huber *et al.*, 1975).

The Cu-IUD was developed in an effort to reduce the pain, bleeding, and spontaneous expulsions in intrauterine contraception as well as to lower the pregnancy rate. The use of copper metal on the IUD arose from the discovery by Zipper *et al.* (1969a) that the metal has a better contraceptive action in the uterus of the rabbit than inert materials. A small piece of plastic has its contraceptive action only immediately adjacent, whereas the copper wire has an effect throughout the uterine horn of the rabbit. In either case, the IUD exerts its effect only in the uterine horn in which it is placed (Zipper *et al.*, 1969a; Chang *et al.*,

1970). Adding copper wire to the IUD permits the use of a small device and, thereby, reduces pain and bleeding while yet retaining, or even improving, the contraceptive efficacy especially for nulliparous or nulligravida women. In parous women, the Cu-IUD and the inert loop have similar low-pregnancy rates. In nulliparous women the copper device also has a low-pregnancy rate and a high continuation rate, but the loop has a higher failure rate as well as a high incidence of side effects.

The most popular Cu-IUDs are polyethylene T-shaped or 7-shaped devices having certain mechanical features. The arms are intended to hold the device high in the uterus. For insertion the device is straightened in an inserter tube. Because of its small size the Cu-IUD inserter tube is smaller than that used for other IUDs and, hence, makes for easier and less painful insertion, especially in nulliparous and nulligravida women (see Huber, 1975).

Adding copper to the inert device seems to lower the expulsion rate (see Zipper *et al.*, 1971; Lippes *et al.*, 1973; see also Huber, 1975) and decreases the bleeding (Zipper *et al.*, 1971; Hefnawi *et al.*, 1974a; Malmqvist *et al.*, 1974; see also Orlans, 1974). Clinical studies show that the continuation rate of the Cu-IUD is generally higher than that for conventional IUDs and the pregnancy rate generally lower. One-year continuation rate for the copper T runs as high as 89% with a pregnancy rate of as low as 1.5% (see Tatum, 1974; Akinla *et al.*, 1975). Statistical clinical comparisons are difficult because of the variables involved, such as the age structure of the population, the ratio of nulliparous to parous women (Jain, 1975), and even the time of insertion during the menstrual cycle (Akinla *et al.*, 1975).

The best time for insertion of an IUD is during menses. This insures that the woman is not pregnant. Often IUDs are inserted postabortum (see for example, Timonen and Luukkainen, 1974). For insertion postpartum, the best time is 6 weeks after birth. Immediate postpartum insertion results in frequent expulsions—up to 6 weeks postpartum the uterus is still soft and perforations could easily take place.

Recently, the Cu-IUD has been used as a postcoital contraceptive (Lippes *et al.*, 1975, 1976; see also Rinehart, 1976). This is based on the idea that the IUD prevents implantation of the blastocyst that occurs 6 days after ovulation. Thus the device can be inserted after coitus but before implantation. The Cu-IUD is chosen because its contraceptive action takes place quickly whereas inert IUDs require several days. An additional advantage of the Cu-IUD is that its small size allows use in nulligravidas, who are often the women who require postcoital contraception.

The pregnancy rate for the T-shaped device is inversely proportional to the surface area of the copper and is 18% with no copper, 5% with 40 $mm^2$, and 1% with 200 $mm^2$ (Tatum, 1974). The copper wire on the most used devices, namely, the Cu-T and the Cu-7, may last for 6 years (Zipper *et al.,* 1976). In a more recent development the wire is replaced with copper sleeves since the wire might fragment with time (Tatum, 1974). The original T-shaped copper device has been further modified by addition of copper to the arms of the device (Tatum, 1974) bringing the metal in closer contact with the fundus of the uterus, where implantation usually occurs. The newest of such devices could last as long as 20 years (Cooper *et al.,* 1976).

With any IUD, there is a hazard of uterine perforation which occurs usually with faulty insertion. An inert open-shaped plastic device in the peritoneal cavity may not be of concern, but with the copper device in the peritoneal cavity inflammation and adhesions have resulted from the metal (Koetsawang, 1973). Here, early surgical removal of the device by laparotomy is indicated.

When pregnancy occurred with a conventional device present, it was often the practice to leave the device in place. With the copper device, however, removal has been advised. A copper wire placed in the uterus of rabbits after implantation can cause fetal resorption (Chang and Tatum, 1975). Injection of copper salts in pregnant laboratory animals can cause teratologies (Ferm and Hanlon, 1974). The question of human teratologies with the Cu-IUD in place during pregnancy is considered in Section II, C, 4.

### B. Mode of Contraceptive Action

It is not clear how inert IUDs exert their contraceptive effect. With the Cu-IUD it is not simply an inert foreign body reaction in the uterus. Reactions taking place at the surface of the metal can have profound effects on the nearby tissue. The copper ions released from the metal could affect the sperm as well as all the tissues of the female genital tract. Most studies on the effect of copper have dealt with the biochemical changes taking place at the lining of the uterus, the endometrium. Also of interest, not only for the problem of the action of the Cu-IUD but also for understanding smooth muscle contraction generally, is the effect of copper ions on the myometrium.

One opinion widely held at the present time is that IUDs, including the Cu-IUD, act to prevent implantation of the blastocyst (Moyer and Shaw, 1973). With the Cu-IUD so many effects can take place that it may turn out that a combination of factors are involved acting in sequence or in concert to bring about contraception.

### 1. *Action on Sperm*

It has been suggested that the Cu-IUD has its principal contraceptive effect by inactivation of sperm (Ullman and Hammerstein, 1972; Elstein and Ferrer, 1973; Hefnawi *et al.,* 1975). Although about $10^{-4}$ *M* cupric ion will render sperm nonmotile (Mann, 1964; White, 1955b), the concentration in the endometrium of copper ions, namely, $3 \times 10^{-5}$ *M* (Hagenfeldt, 1972a,b) is too low to be spermicidal. The available copper is still lower because the ions are mainly in the complexed form in association with the mucoids and some other components of the endometrium. Ovulatory cervical mucus from women with the Cu-IUD inactivates sperm after standing 3–4 hours but this is probably irrelevant to the contraceptive action of the Cu-IUD (Jecht and Bernstein, 1973). Sperm is known to travel from the vagina to the oviducts in a matter of minutes.

Intrauterine devices cause a reduction in sperm found in the fallopian tubes (Tredway *et al.,* 1975). Women undergoing at midcycle tubal ligation and who were wearing an IUD (including a Cu-IUD) were artificially inseminated 15–30 minutes before the operation. No sperm were found in the oviducts. Uterine aspirants from women with IUDs show no sperm with the Cu-IUD (Kesserü *et al.,* 1974), an effect that is less striking with inert IUDs (Moyer and Shaw, 1973). This loss of sperm is generally attributed to the phagocytotic action of leukocytes present in abundance with IUDs, especially the Cu-IUD (see Section II, B, 6).

### 2. *Fertilization and Ovulation*

The Cu-IUD does not seem to affect fertilization, although copper salts will inhibit fertilization for sea urchins (Lillie, 1921). If a rat with a copper wire *in utero* is mated and then the copper wire is removed within 4 days, i.e., the time after fertilization but before implantation, there is no contraceptive effect (Chang and Tatum, 1972). Fertilized eggs can be recovered from rabbits with intrauterine copper wire (Polidoro and Black, 1970). Fertilized eggs from rats with intrauterine copper develop normally on transplantation to recipient control animals (Chang and Tatum, 1970). The use of the Cu-IUD as a postcoital contraceptive (Lippes *et al.,* 1975, 1976) demonstrates that for humans, as well, the action cannot be exclusively at the fertilization stage.

For women the Cu-IUD does not alter the duration of the menstrual or the ovulatory pattern of hormone secretion (Nygren and Johansson, 1973; Johansson and Nygren, 1974). This together with the postcoital effectiveness of the Cu-IUD strongly suggest that ovulation in humans is not affected. The estrous cycle of rats is somewhat altered by intrauterine copper, but only after 2 months. The number of eggs ovulated from the adjacent ovary is somewhat reduced (Peppler, 1975).

### 3. *Time of the Contraceptive Action*

The foregoing considerations indicate that the contraceptive action of the Cu-IUD takes place around the time of implantation. This argument is further strengthened by the following experiment (Chang and Tatum, 1970): when blastocysts are transferred from a donor rat to a rat at the proper stage from which the intrauterine copper had just been removed, then implantation does not occur. If the uterine copper in the mated rat is removed within 4 days after mating, pregnancy will continue but removal on the evening of the fourth day or on the fifth day gives no implantation (Webb, 1973). Inserting a copper wire in the uterus of a pregnant rat 5 days after mating has no contraceptive effect (Chang and Tatum, 1972).

These experiments show that the copper has its effect during a definite time. What has not, however, been answered is the question as to whether the contraceptive action is due to (*a*) a destruction of the blastocyst, (*b*) an inhibition of its ability to implant, (*c*) inhibition of the ability of the endometrium to allow implantation or, finally, (*d*) a rendering of the blastocyst–endometrium interaction to be inappropriate (e.g., a loss of stickiness). The successful use of the Cu-IUD for postcoital contraception in women (Lippes *et al.*, 1975, 1976) implies that the action occurs around the time of implantation. In addition, as Gräfenberg originally observed, removal of an IUD at midcycle with no further intercourse can still result in pregnancy (see Lehfeldt, 1975a).

### 4. *Blastocysts*

Copper is toxic to blastocysts. *In vitro* incubation of preimplantation rabbit blastocysts with $10^{-4}$–$10^{-5}$ *M* cupric salt produces a decrease in membrane ion transport (Cross, 1973). In studies on the *in vitro* killing of mouse blastocysts, it was found that copper wire was more effective than the addition of cupric ions alone, at a concentration equal to that which the metal would produce over the same time (Brinster and Cross, 1972). In either case, serum albumin has somewhat of a protective effect (see also Noeslund, 1972).

For laboratory animals with intrauterine copper wire, no blastocysts have been recovered just prior to when implantation would be expected (Chang *et al.*, 1970; Nutting and Mueller, 1975a). Blastocysts recovered from a rabbit on day 6 of gestation show numerous copper-containing lysosomes in those from the uterine horn containing the copper wire (Abraham *et al.*, 1974). The disappearance of blastocysts after this time was attributed to autolysis. Copper causes release of lytic enzymes from lysosomes (Lindquist, 1968; see also Chvapil *et al.*, 1972). Copper lysis of mucins (Oster, 1972) could disrupt the immunological protection of the trophoblast (see Section II,B,6). Toxic products from IUD-associated inflammatory reactions could also kill the blastocyst, or blastocysts might disappear as a result of leukocyte phagocytosis (see Section II, B, 6).

5. *Endometrium*

Because of its accessibility via uterine aspirants, changes in the endometrium caused by the Cu-IUD have been extensively studied notably by Hagenfeldt (see summary, 1972b). The release of copper from the device (of 200 $mm^2$ area of copper) is about 100 $\mu g$/day for the first 2 months of use and drops to a constant rate of 50 $\mu g$/day thereafter. For the first half-year, there is an increase of copper in the endometrium in the proliferative and especially the secretory phase, and after a year the increase is significant only in the secretory phase (Hagenfeldt, 1972b). Half the released copper appears in the menstrual blood (G. K. Oster, G. Oster, and H. Lehfeldt, unpublished observations, 1972; see also Moo-Young, *et al.*, 1974; Laufe *et al.*, 1976).

The zinc enzyme carbonic anhydrase, because it causes a rise in pH of tissue and thereby renders the acidic mucoids more sticky, is thought to play a crucial role in implantation (see Boving and Larsen, 1975). For this reason the level of zinc in the endometrium was followed (Hagenfeldt, 1972a, b). The Cu-IUD causes a gradual loss in endometrial zinc. There is an associated decrease in the zinc enzymes carbonic anhydrase and alkaline phosphatase despite the overall increase in protein synthesis. Progesterone stimulation of carbonic anhydrase is blocked by the Cu-IUD (Nutting and Mueller, 1975b). Zipper *et al.* (1971) had earlier suggested that the contraceptive action of copper is its antagonism with zinc in crucial enzymes.

The released copper can be seen in structures of the endometrium. Staining with rubeanic acid the uterus of monkeys that have the Cu-IUD reveals particulate localizations of copper in the endometrial epithelium (Ranney *et al.*, 1975). In endometrial biopsies of women with the Cu-IUD, copper has been found concentrated in secretory vacuoles of the endometrial epithelium during the secretory phase (Salverry *et al.*, 1973). Others have not found localizations of copper, perhaps because of sampling problems (Gonzalez-Angulo and Aznar-Ramos, 1976).

Some ultrastructural changes have been seen in endometrial biopsies of women with the Cu-IUD. Among these are mitochondrial changes and an increase in the number of mitochondria and lysosomes (Gonzalez-Angulo and Aznar-Ramos, 1976). Normal secretory endometrium possesses apical protrusions containing glycogen. With the Cu-IUD these structures are no longer seen in the scanning electron microscope (Nilsson and Hagenfeldt, 1973). Another manifestation of this altered carbohydrate metabolism is the depression of $\alpha$-amylase activity (de la Osa *et al.,* 1972). The normal cyclic increase in glycogen synthetase in the endometrium is altered by the Cu-IUD (de la Osa *et al.,* 1972). Suppression of glucose metabolism in the endometrium could deprive the blastocyst of its nutrition. Blastokinin, an endometrial protein that stimulates growth of the blastocyst and increases before implantation is greatly reduced with the Cu-IUD (Johnson, 1972). The changes in endometrial enzyme levels in both the proliferative and secretory phases of conventional and copper devices have been reviewed in detail (Middleton and Kennedy, 1975). Copper salts, even at low concentrations, inhibit several proteinases, including plasma fibrinolysin (Kowalski *et al.,* 1956) (see Section II, C, 2) and the enzyme that liquefies the semen coagulum (Syner and Moghissi, 1972). Proteinase activity is associated with implantation (see Pinsker *et al.,* 1974). The possibility that copper inhibits a proteolytic enzyme necessary for implantation is worthy of consideration.

*In vitro,* cupric salts are inhibitors of certain enzymes but only at high concentrations, greater than about $10^{-4}$ $M$ cupric ions. At these high concentrations, the cupric ion causes precipitation of many proteins, but with the low concentrations associated with the device, namely $3 \times 10^{-5}$ $M$ or less, inhibition of activity for most enzymes does not occur. Although the cupric ions produced by the metal may not be able to inhibit the enzyme, the reactions associated with the dissolution of the metal, i.e., copper corrosion, may, as shown in the following, inactivate the enzymes.

Proliferation of the endometrium of rats is seen around the copper wire (Zipper *et al.,* 1969a) suggestive of inflammation or of an estrogenic effect. Estrogen uptake, presumably by specific estrogen-binding proteins, is greater than in the rat uterus containing nylon or nothing (Adadevoh and Dada, 1973; Aedo and Zipper, 1973). This qualitative difference in uptake occurs 1 week after insertion of the copper wire (Adadevoh and Dada, 1973), but the contraceptive effect occurs in 12 hours (Webb, 1973). In monkeys, an inert or a copper T decreases progesterone uptake, and the inert but not the Cu-IUD increases estrogen binding (Ghosh and Roy, 1976). Steroid receptor binding sites are destroyed by copper salts even at micromolar concentrations (Tamaya *et al.,* 1976) presumably by cleavage of the disulfide bonds in the receptor protein. In rabbits, copper inhibits endometrial maturation and prevents the normal response to estradiol (Grundsell *et al.,* 1976). In women, no endometrial proliferation has been observed with the copper device (Hagenfeldt, 1972b; Hagenfeldt *et al.,* 1972). Decidualization has been seen in a few women with the Cu-IUD (Salverry *et al.,* 1973) and in rabbits (Tobert, 1975) but is inhibited in rats (Chang *et al.,* 1970; Webb, 1973; see Tobert, 1975).

For women there seems to be no influence of the copper device on endometrial DNA (Hagenfeldt, 1972b) although RNA levels are decreased (Hicks *et al.,* 1975). The incorporation of labeled thymidine into endometrial DNA is inhibited by intrauterine copper wire in rats (Prager, 1969) and in rabbits (Grundsell, 1975). Copper salts also dissociate endometrial polysomes *in vitro* (Hernandez *et al.,* 1974).

In the rat endometrium, inert plastic causes a decrease in the incorporation of sulfate into mucoproteins, but with copper wire the effect is much more pronounced (Prager, 1969). This loss of mucoproteins could account for the inhibition of implantation (Prager, 1969). It is of interest that vitamin A deficiency likewise decreases the incorporation of sulfates into mucoproteins (Wolf and Varandani, 1960; for review, see Roels, 1967) and that vitamin A-deficient animals are sterile (for review, see Moore, 1967; Moustgaard, 1971; Wasserman and Corradino, 1971). It has long been known that one of the earliest signs of vitamin A deficiency in rats is the continuous keratinization, i.e., dryness of the uterus and vagina (Evans and Bishop, 1922). The incorporation of hexoses into endometrial mucoids in women is altered with the Cu-IUD (Hicks *et al.*, 1975).

### 6. *Inflammation*

The sterile inflammatory reaction seen with IUDs is thought to be a likely cause of the contraceptive effect (Moyer and Shaw, 1973). This inflammation reaction is characterized by an infiltration of polymorphonuclear leukocytes, plasma cells, and lymphocytes that can act phagocytically against sperm as well as the blastocyst. The inflammatory reaction can also produce toxins that can kill blastocysts. Inflammatory reactions are associated with prostaglandin synthesis, which could affect uterine blood circulation or uterine motility (see Section II, B, 7). Intrauterine devices removed from women and then placed in incubation media show an extensive production of prostaglandins (Myatt *et al.,* 1975).

Endometrial aspirants from women with IUDs also show an increase in prostaglandin (PG) synthesis (Hillier and Kasonde, 1976) (see Sections, II, B, 7 and IV, C). Prostaglandin production from incubating the just removed IUDs showed more $PGF_{2\alpha}$ than $PGE_2$. The PG production was correlated with the number of macrophages adhering to the IUD (Myatt *et al.*, 1975). Neutrophiles were also seen but were thought not to be associated with PG production. The Cu-IUDs showed a particularly high production of $PGF_{2\alpha}$ (Myatt *et al.*, 1975). As pointed out (Myatt *et al.*, 1975) this finding is consistent with the known effects of copper on PG biosynthesis (see Sections II, B, 7 and IV, C). In endometrial aspirants from women with IUDs only an increase in $PGE_2$ was seen, and the results seemed similar for the Cu-IUD. The data, however, showed large variations, perhaps because of differences in the site from which aspirant was taken in relation to the IUD (Hillier and Kasonde, 1976).

The Cu-IUD causes a considerable increase in leukocytic infiltration as compared with the inert IUD (Cuadros and Hirsch, 1972). Others have not found such an increase (Salverry *et al.*, 1973). Endometrial biopsies of a large number of women show a difference in the inflammatory reaction for the Cu-IUD as compared to inert IUDs. With the Cu-IUD, there is a predominance of polymorphonuclear leukocytes, whereas with the inert IUD there are more plasma cells (H. Lehfeldt, personal communication, 1976). It is known that cupric salts increase the inflammatory infiltrate around a scratch in the skin (Stone and Willis, 1958). Intraperitoneal implantation of copper rods results in a greater exudation of neutrophiles and mononuclear cells than with glass rods (McGarry, 1975). On the other hand, copper salts can inhibit the erythema and edema of inflammation in some bioassays. They are also highly irritant (Bonta, 1969; see also Sorenson, 1974; Whitehouse *et al.*, 1975). These facts favor the hypothesis that the contraceptive action of IUDs is a result of a sterile inflammation that is enhanced by copper. It is of interest that when indomethacin, an anti-inflammatory agent, is given to animals with IUDs, at least in some cases the contraceptive action of the device is lost (Saksena and Harper, 1974). This problem is considered in more detail in Section II, B, 7.

The mucolytic action of copper (Oster, 1971, 1972; Elstein and Ferrer, 1973) could remove the protective mucopolysaccharides of the trophoblast. This action, similar to the use of neuraminidase to expose the covert antigens of tumor cells in cancer immunotherapy (see Bekesi *et al.*, 1976), could lead to an immunological attack on the trophoblast. Neuraminidase treatment of the uterus or blastocyst blocks implantation in mice (Porter, 1975). The copper might, thus, destroy the immunologically protected status of the trophoblast (for review of trophoblast immune protection, see Beer and Billingham, 1971; Boving and Larsen, 1973). Such an immunological reaction might be the cause for the alterations in serum immunoglobulins seen in women with IUDs (see Section II, C, 6).

7. *Myometrium*

Clinical as well as animal studies with the copper device indicate that copper has an effect on the uterine smooth muscle, the myometrium. Thus in the preliminary clinical trials of Zipper *et al.* (1971) the T-shaped Cu-IUD showed a lower initial expulsion rate (0.6%) than the same device without copper (5.9%). Similarly, addition of copper to the Lippes loop device reduced the expulsion rate from 14.6 to 2.9% (Lippes *et al.,* 1973). Zipper *et al.* (1975) have found that IUDs with copper also modify uterine activity. In rabbits there is a lower expulsion rate for a copper wire than for a thin piece of polyethylene inserted in the control uterine horn (Medel *et al.,* 1972).

The effect of copper ions and of copper metal on the rat uterus *in vitro* has been studied (Salgo and Oster, 1974a; see also Formanek and Höller, 1959; Shen, 1960; Daniel, 1964; Daniel *et al.,* 1970). Essentially similar results to those of Salgo and Oster (1974a) have been found with human fallopian tube smooth muscle (Larsson *et al.,* 1976; see also Salgo and Oster, 1977). Cupric ions at low concentrations ($10^{-6}$–$10^{-5}$ $M$) cause the uterus to contract, whereas at higher concentrations ($>10^{-4}$ $M$) and with prolonged exposure cupric ions cause a decrease in contractile force (Salgo and Oster, 1974a). The stimulating action of low concentrations of cupric ions can exceed the maximum response achieved with the naturally occurring uterine stimulant, oxytocin. Copper-induced contractions are more sustained than those induced by oxytocin and are harder to reverse by rinsing of the uterus. Copper wire placed in the lumen of the *in vitro* uterus initially causes stimulation. Although the control horn after 6 hours still responds to oxytocin stimulation the same degree that it had initially, the horn containing the bare copper wire could not be stimulated with oxytocin to more than 50% of the tension that it initially had (Salgo and Oster, 1974a). Copper salts at $10^{-4}$ $M$ depress electrically induced *in vitro* rabbit uterine contractions after 2 hours (Salgo and Csapo, 1972).

*In vitro* experiments have immediate relevance to the effect of copper on the expulsion of the device. The *in vitro* experiment just described suggests why a copper device might have a lower expulsion rate than a similar device without copper. After prolonged exposure to copper metal the uterus has lost much of its ability to contract. On the other hand, the initial stimulatory effect of copper could cause an early expulsion, but if the device were retained initially its chances of being expelled later would be diminished. Copper ion concentrations as high as $3 \times 10^{-5}$ *M* have been found in the cervical mucus and uterine aspirants of women wearing the copper device (Hagenfeldt, 1972a,b). This concentration is probably sufficient to affect the uterus if this level is achieved in the extracellular fluid of the myometrium. Some workers attribute low expulsion of the copper device to mechanical factors rather than to the copper metal per se (Lippes *et al.,* 1973; Kamal *et al.,* 1973). These authors, however, did not consider the effect of copper on uterine contractions (Salgo and Oster, 1974a). Large doses of copper salts injected into the uterus of rats or rabbits increase uterine contractions (see Section V,E).

Copper may be acting to stimulate the uterus in a variety of ways. Mechanisms of action for copper-induced uterine contraction involving mercaptyl groups, cyclic AMP, or sodium–potassium ATPase have been considered by us (Salgo and Oster, 1974a). These interactions of copper with cellular processes have broader implications for the action of copper on cell membranes and ion fluxes, particularly for erythrocytes, nerves, and smooth muscle generally.

Cyclic AMP might be involved in copper-induced uterine contraction. Theophylline, a phosphodiesterase inhibitor that causes buildup of cyclic AMP, suppresses copper-induced activity (Salgo and Oster, 1974a). Copper has an effect on cyclic AMP-mediated oxytocin-induced water permeability in the toad bladder (Parisi and Piccinni, 1972). In both the uterus and bladder, copper could be related to a decrease in cyclic AMP (see Salgo and Oster, 1974a).

It has been suggested that copper stimulates the uterus by inhibiting $Na^+$–$K^+$ ATPase (Daniel, 1964; Daniel *et al.,* 1970). On the other hand, the ATPase inhibitor, ouabain, only induces small contractions of the uterus at high concentrations ($10^{-3}$ *M*) (Daniel, 1964; Salgo and Oster, 1974a), as compared to the strong copper-induced contractions. This comparison of ouabain to copper tends to weaken the $Na^+$–$K^+$ ATPase argument. Others have found copper inhibition of membrane ATPase in other systems (Peters *et al.,* 1966; Epstein and McIlwain 1966; Bowler and Duncan, 1970; Ting-Beall *et al.,* 1973; Cross, 1973).

Copper ions cause a profound loss in chloride transport in frog skin (Ussing and Zerahn, 1951; Koefoed-Johnson *et al.,* 1973). If this also occurred in the uterus, one would expect depolarization of the smooth muscle membrane and subsequent contraction. The loss in chloride transport could arise from copper-induced membrane lipid peroxidation (see Section II, C, 1). Lipid peroxidation has been found on incubating erythrocytes in the presence of copper sulfate (Moroff *et al.,* 1974). Prior incubation with cupric ions causes red cells to be more susceptible to isotonic lysis by progesterone (Moroff *et al.,* 1974). Copper also causes peroxidation and leakiness of lysosomal membranes (Lindquist, 1968). Metal salts including copper prolong the action potential and potentiate contractions in skeletal muscle (Sandow and Isaacson, 1966).

The action of copper with the Cu-IUD could be through prostaglandin synthesis (Salgo and Oster, 1972a; Forder, 1974). Copper salts have been shown to increase the biosynthesis of $PGF_2$ in sheep vesicular gland preparations at copper concentrations in the range found to stimulate the uterus—around $10^{-5}$ *M* (Lands *et al.,* 1971; Lee and Lands, 1972; Maddox, 1973; see also Nugteren *et al.* 1966) (see Section IV, C).

Particularly high $PGF_{2\alpha}$ production is seen in incubating copper devices with adhering macrophages just removed from women (Myatt *et al.,* 1975) (see Section II, B, 6). Prostaglandin $F_{2\alpha}$ causes pronounced uterine contractions (Caton, 1971). The endogenous production of PGs is probably critical for normal uterine activity (Aiken, 1972; Vane and Williams, 1972; Csapo and Csapo, 1974), and hence, administration of copper could stimulate the uterus by causing the production of $PGF_{2\alpha}$. High concentrations of cupric salts ($10^{-3}$ *M*), on the other hand, inhibit the production of $PGF_{2\alpha}$ (Maddox, 1973). This inhibition could be the origin of the suppressive effect of high concentrations of copper on uterine contractions. Dithiols, which can chelate copper, inhibit the biosynthesis of PGs (Lee and Lands, 1972). Diethyldithiocarbamate irreversibly inhibits uterine activity (Daniel, 1964) and this cannot be reversed with copper (Salgo and Oster, 1974a). The inhibitory action of diethyldithiocarbamate on uterine contraction may be by inhibiting the production of PGs. Zinc inhibits the copper-induced contraction of the rat uterine muscle (Verdugo and Medel, 1974, quoted by Zipper *et al.,* 1976). This is a manifestation of copper–zinc antagonism (see Section VIII, A).

The possible role of copper in PG biosynthesis with the Cu-IUD could be related in several ways to its contraceptive effect. Inflammatory reactions are mediated by means of PGs (Vane, 1971). Thus, if the copper causes increased PG production, this effect could account for the increased inflammatory reaction seen with the copper device (Cuadros and Hirsch, 1972), as mentioned in Section II, B, 6. Anti-inflammatory drugs inhibit the production of PGs (Vane, 1971; Fereira and Vane,

1974). Some anti-inflammatory drugs, notably aspirin, are copper-chelating agents, and it has been proposed that their action depends on this property (Reid *et al.*, 1951; Schubert, 1966). The anti-inflammatory drug indomethacin counteracts the contraceptive action of inert IUDs in the rabbit (Saksena and Harper, 1974) but apparently not in the mouse (Lau *et al.*, 1974) or the rat (Chaudhuri, 1973, 1975). Alkylating agent immunosuppressants reduce the contraceptive effect of IUDs in rats, however (Holub, 1972).

Copper-induced PG production might also exert a contraceptive effect through increased uterine motility. This action has been hypothesized to explain the decrease in the number of ova that can be recovered from rabbits with intrauterine copper (Polidoro *et al.*, 1975). Measurements of uterine electrical activity in rabbits show an increase with intrauterine copper metal (Yoshida and Wagner, 1974). There seem to be some differences in uterine activity in women wearing the copper device (Hagenfeldt, 1971). With inert devices, abnormal prelabor-like contractions have been observed around the time of implantation (Bengtsson and Moawad, 1967; Moawad and Bengtsson, 1970). Presumably, these contractions are induced by the increased production of PGs probably occurring with intrauterine devices (Chaudhuri, 1971, 1974; Johansson and Nygren, 1974).

The reduced bleeding for the copper device (Orlans, 1974; Hefnawi *et al.*, 1974a; Malmqvist *et al.*, 1974) as compared with inert devices suggests that copper is affecting the vascular system of the endometrium. Copper salts cause the contraction not only of uterine muscle but also of a wide variety of other smooth muscles (Shen, 1960), probably including those of the arterioles of the uterus. The copper device could exert its contraceptive action by inducing uterine production of PGs, which, in turn, would cause uterine vasoconstriction thereby suppressing the blood supply necessary for successful implantation (A. I. Csapo, personal communication, 1975).

### 8. *Corrosion Chemistry of Copper and Its Biochemical Effects*

To understand the biological action of the Cu-IUD, one must be aware not only of the chemistry of copper ions in solution but also of the corrosion chemistry of metallic copper. The chemical reactions at the surface of copper metal may have effects more profound than, or even qualitatively different from, the reactions of cupric ions finally produced in the dissolution of the metal. For example, cupric sulfate at $10^{-3}$ *M* added to semen has only a slight effect on sperm motility after an incubation of 6 hours. Incubation with metallic copper is spermicidal after 4 hours even though the copper ions produced by the metal are less than $10^{-3}$ $M$ (Jecht and Bernstein, 1973). Similarly, as mentioned earlier, blastocysts are more easily killed by metallic copper than by the produced cupric salt alone (Brinster and Cross, 1972). It would appear that the contraceptive action of the Cu-IUD is derived from the direct corrosion action or at least from the action of products produced at the surface of the metal during its dissolution in the saline environment of the endometrium.

The corrosion chemistry of pure copper metal is a poorly developed area of science despite the widespread use of copper over the millennia. Studies on the corrosive action of seawater on copper have been confined to its alloys, namely bronzes and brasses (for review, see Leidheiser, 1971), but do not extend to pure copper which is well known to be unstable in contact with saline solutions. With copper cooking pots the usual practice is to clad the interior with tin. Copper tubing as in plumbing is never pure copper. A principal use of pure copper is as an electrical conductor, but here the wire is coated to provide not only electrical insulation but also as a protection against corrosion by moisture and salts. In our laboratory, we undertook a study of the corrosion chemistry of electrolytically pure copper under conditions intended to simulate the conditions in the uterus (Oster, 1971, 1972; Oster and Oster, 1974).

A strip of copper 200 $mm^2$ will dissolve in physiological saline (0.9% NaCl) at a rate comparable with that of the Cu-IUD in women. Although amino acids, notably glycine and histidine, and proteins, such as serum albumin, complex with copper ions and increase the rate of dissolution of the metal, the presence of saline is a prime factor. In distilled water, no measurable cupric ions are produced. The dissolution of copper metal in saline requires oxygen; the system rendered oxygen-free during the incubation (by purging with nitrogen) shows no detectable ions in solution. Although Cu(II) salts are the end product in the dissolution of copper metal in saline, Cu(I) is formed as an intermediate. This is shown by the red color produced by overlaying with an amyl alcohol solution, 2,2′-biquinoline. Biquinoline forms a red complex with Cu(I) but not with Cu(II) (Guest, 1953). In the absence of oxygen and/or saline no cuprous ions are formed from metallic copper.

The action of chloride ion and molecular oxygen on the dissolution of copper metal probably arises from the well-known stabilization of cuprous by chloride ion, Cu(I) being produced by the oxidation of Cu(0) at the metal–liquid interface as seen by the pink patina. The cuprous chloride complex is autooxidizable to yield cupric ions. Cupric ions form stable complexes with histidine and with glycine and this would account for the increased rate of dissolution of Cu(0) induced by these two amino acids. It has recently been found that a transient species of half-life of 2 hours with copper of valence 3 is formed when Cu(II) is complexed with glycine in the presence of air (Margerum *et al.*, 1976).

Copper metal incubated with a saline solution of a disulfide will cleave the S—S bond when oxygen is present (Oster, 1972; Oster and Oster, 1974). The mercaptans formed are detected by the Ellman's sulfhydryl test with $Na_2EDTA$ present to chelate the copper that interferes with the test. Serum albumin in saline when incubated with metallic copper undergoes a conformational change as indicated by alteration in its solubility and the availability of sulfhydryl groups (Oster, 1972). Similarly, ovalbumin undergoes denaturation with copper metal and, indeed, French chefs recommend using an unlined copper bowl when whipping egg white (see, for example, Beck *et al.*, 1961). Carbonic anhydrase and alkaline phosphatase, enzymes thought to be important in the implantation process are inactivated on incubation with copper metal in saline (Oster, 1972). Cupric ion at a concentration produced by the dissolution of the metal during the incubation period does not inhibit these enzymes.

Cuprous salts freshly prepared and stabilized by chloride ions will cleave disulfide bonds as well as produce all the aforementioned biochemical changes due to the metal (Oster and Oster, 1974). It is known that Cu(I) reduces disulfide groups to give the mercaptan stabilized by copper (see, for example, Swan, 1959; also Williamson, 1970). Copper (I) can be prepared from a cupric chloride solution by adding mild reducing agents, such as hydrazine hydrochloride, ascorbic acid, or ferrous sulfate. The autooxidation of Cu(I) is prevented by stabilization of Cu(I) by addition of cyanide or azide. Carbon monoxide, on the other hand, accelerates the autooxidation of Cu(I) to Cu(II). Autooxidation of Cu(I) has peroxidase action—the conversion of iodide ion to iodine, for example (see Sections IV, D and VII, B). All this is relevant not only to an understanding of the nature of the action of the Cu-IUD but also in helping to explain a wide variety of biological autooxidations which are particularly important in reproduction (see, especially, Sections IV, D and VII, B).

Copper metal incubated in saline in the presence of oxygen produces free radicals (Oster and Oster, 1974). This system initiates the free-radical polymerization of acrylamide. The polymerization of acrylamide is inhibited by cupric ions and, hence, will proceed only when $Na_2EDTA$ is added to chelate the cupric ions that are produced. The presence of polymer is easily demonstrated by the fact that a drop of the reacting solution produces a voluminous precipitate in methanol, whereas the unreacted monomer is soluble in methanol. The polymerization reaction is very rapid, especially when using copper powder that presents a large surface, and, indeed, the system rises quickly in temperature due to the exothermic nature of the reaction. The copper-initiated polymerization requires chloride ion and also oxygen, but oxygen causes the usual induction period present in vinyl polymerization when the oxygen concentration is high.

The free radicals produced on the dissolution of metallic copper will convert benzene into phenol. By using benzene-saturated saline solutions, one may determine the rate of free-radical production by the rate of formation of phenol. Since cupric ions interfere with the Folin-Ciocalteau phenol reagent (Lowry *et al.*, 1951), the determination should be carried out in the presence of $Na_2EDTA$. Here again, the reaction does not proceed in the absence of saline or of oxygen. For a 200-$mm^2$ sheet of copper metal 28 $\mu$mole of phenol are produced in the first hour.

The polymerization of acrylamide and the conversion of benzene to phenol can also be carried out with freshly prepared cuprous chloride (Oster and Oster, 1974). Cuprous ions are formed in the dissolution of the metal and are complexed with chloride ions. Free radicals are formed in the autooxidation of cuprous ions. A similar hydroxylation of a synthetic substrate occurs with the free radicals produced when cupric salts are combined with ascorbic acid (Staudinger *et al.*, 1964). Our overall picture is that, on the surface of pure copper metal in the presence of oxygen, a layer of cuprous oxide is formed; the reducing action of the metal keeps the oxide as cuprous. In contact with saline the well-known water-soluble cuprous chloride complex ($CuCl_2^-$) is formed and diffuses away from the metal. The oxygen dissolved in this aqueous medium rapidly oxidizes the cuprous complex to yield cupric ion and free radicals. The free radicals may be hydroxyl radicals or, as has been recently proposed for many biological autooxidations, superoxide free radicals (Fridovich, 1972, 1974). If there is a paucity of substrate with which the radicals can react, the radicals will combine with each other, especially in the presence of superoxide dismutase, to form hydrogen peroxide. The hydrogen peroxide will not accumulate, however, because of the presence of cupric ions. When cupric ions are added to hydrogen peroxide, cuprous ions are formed and oxygen is evolved. From these considerations it appears that copper metal in saline is an efficient source of free radicals. We postulate that the free radicals produced by the metal are the primary inhibitors of implantation. Ultimately, it is probably the free radicals formed by the metal that are responsible for the contraceptive action of the Cu-IUD (Oster and Salgo, 1975).

## C. Side Effects

### 1. *The Question of Cancer and the IUD*

The rate of production of free radicals by 200 $mm^2$ of copper metal in saline is prodigious (see Section II, B, 8). It is equivalent to that produced by 14,000 rads of X rays per hour (Oster and Oster, 1974). The implications of this high initial rate of free-radical production by metallic copper for the long-term safety of the copper device are unclear. Many substances—notably, naturally occurring reducing compounds—in the endometrial fluid could consume free radicals without deleterious effect. In addition, intrauterine copper stimulates the activity of catalase in the rat endometrium in excess of that produced by a nylon thread (Dasgupta *et al.,* 1972). A direct comparison of the copper production of free radicals with that for ionizing radiation may not be justified since in the latter free radicals can be generated intracellularly, whereas with the copper device one might expect the free radicals to be produced extracellularly. On the other hand, fine copper metal fragments have been found around the device in the endometrial fluid (Tatum, 1973) and could conceivably enter cells. Still further, the cuprous chloride produced might diffuse into cells, and, likewise, on autooxidation form free radicals intracellularly. Cupric salts reacting with reducing agents such as ascorbic acid generate free radicals (see Staudinger *et al.,* 1964). Cupric mixed with ascorbic acid is mutagenic as determined by bacterial tests and damages DNA in cultured human fibroblasts (Stich *et al.,* 1976).

Copper could produce carcinogens. Copper ions cause milk and edible oils to become rancid by the peroxidation of the unsaturated fatty acids present (Oser, 1965). One of the products of lipid peroxidation is malonaldehyde. Indeed, the presence of this dialdehyde, as detected by color formation with thiobarbituric acid (Kohn and Liversedge, 1944), is used as a measure of polyunsaturated fat autooxidation. Malonaldehyde is carcinogenic in mice (Shamberger *et al.,* 1974). It is also mutagenic, as determined with bacteria (Mukai and Goldstein, 1976). The mutations are thought to arise by cross-linking of DNA. We found that malonaldehyde is produced when human erythrocytes are incubated with cupric ions (Moroff *et al.,* 1974). Incubation of erythrocytes with cupric ions also causes the formation of Heinz bodies (Metz, 1969) which we now feel are hemoglobin cross-linked by malonaldehyde. Copper loading in rats leads to increased liver lysomal lipid peroxidation, as does cupric treatment of isolated lysosomes or emulsions of fatty acids *in vitro* (Lindquist, 1968; see also Chvapil *et al.,* 1972). Further indication of copper-catalyzed lipid peroxidation is the formation of lipofuscin seen in the livers of animals with chronic copper poisoning (Mallory and Parker, 1931).

Malonaldehyde might well be produced in the uterus by the Cu-IUD. It could be argued that this would not lead to cancer formation because most of the endometrium is sloughed off every month. For a woman with the Cu-IUD who is approaching menopause or who is amenorrhoic for some other reason, the accumulation of this carcinogen could be serious. Copper buildup in the myometrium or elsewhere in the body (see Section II, C, 6) may lead to a dangerous cumulation of this carcinogen.

Newer Cu-IUDs are being developed that contain more copper than the regular 7- or T-type devices so as to still further reduce the pregnancy rate and side effects (Tatum, 1974; Cooper *et al.,* 1976). If there is copper on the arms of the device, this might result in constant contact of the metal with the myometrium which, of course, is not renewed each month. With the present devices, the plastic arms often embed into the wall of the uterus (Timonen *et al.,* 1972; Kamal *et al.,* 1973) or the arms or tip penetrate the cervical canal (Lehfeldt and Wan, 1971; Khatamee and Lehfeldt, 1975; Cedarqvist *et al.,* 1975).

Copper buildup in the myometrium or elsewhere in the body (see Section II, C, 6) could lead to an accumulation of malonaldehyde in various tissues. In addition, copper-induced production of malonaldehyde might be mutagenic to an embryo developing in pregnancies where the Cu-IUD is *in situ*.

Copper salts have not proved carcinogenic in some animal models (Gilman, 1962; see also Sunderman, 1971) but intratesticular injection of copper sulfate in chickens has led to teratomas (Faline and Anissimova, 1940; see also Furst and Haro, 1969). This carcinogenic action could, however, be a result of tissue necrosis which the copper injection produces (Faline and Anissimova, 1940).

So far, there is no evidence linking cancer, at least endometrial or cervical cancer with use of the copper device (Tatum, 1973, 1974) or, for that matter, any type of IUD (Tietze, 1973). The question of malformations is treated in Section II, C, 4.

### 2. *Bleeding*

Excess uterine bleeding is one of the major reasons for removal of the IUD, another being pain (Tietze, 1973; see also Huber *et al.,* 1975; Mischell, 1975). Bleeding induced by inert IUDs averages, in the first few months, twice the amount of that of normal bleeding (Moyer and

Shaw, 1973). Typically there is a premature onset of menstruation (Nygren and Johansson, 1973; Johansson and Nygren, 1974). Such blood losses can lead to anemia. Losses of 80 ml are common with IUDs. A loss of this much menstrual blood is associated with a high incidence of anemia (Hallberg *et al.,* 1966). In industrial countries, anemia can be 4–5 times more common in IUD users than nonusers (Guttorm, 1971). The increased blood loss would be particularly serious for women who have a tendency toward anemia. Those who have marginal nutritional iron or are subject to parasitic infection are particularly vulnerable. In certain societies (e.g., orthodox Jewish or Moslem communities), a woman when menstruating is considered "unclean" and is not even allowed to prepare food. Any prolongation and/or increase of bleeding would be unacceptable and, indeed, this is a principal factor in the choice of the method of contraception (see Whelan, 1975).

The Cu-IUD causes less excess bleeding than does the inert IUD (Orlans, 1974; Hefnawi *et al.,* 1974a; Malmquist *et al.,* 1974; Israel *et al.,* 1974; see also Huber *et al.,* 1975). In some studies, bleeding with the Cu-IUD was found to be measurably greater than in women not wearing any device (Liedholm *et al.,* 1975), whereas in other studies (Hefnawi *et al.,* 1974a) the loss of blood with the Cu-IUD approached that of normal menstruation.

Why the commonly used inert IUDs cause excess bleeding is not known. Indeed, little is understood per se about menstruation, a phenomenon peculiar to primates. Among the possible reasons for more bleeding with IUDs may be erosions of blood vessels in the endometrium caused by abrasion or pressure of the device. The commonly used Cu-IUDs, the T or the 7, are smaller than the commonly used inert IUD, notably the Lippes loop. When the Lippes loop is clad with copper sleeves, the incidence of bleeding was found to be increased (Lippes *et al.,* 1973). This was attributed to the increased stiffness imparted by the sleeves. Although with inert IUDs the incidence of excess bleeding decreases with decreasing size (Tietze, 1973; Huber *et al.,* 1975), with the Cu-IUD other mechanisms could be acting as well. In the early studies with the T-shaped IUD, a comparison was made of the T with varying amounts of copper (Zipper *et al.,* 1971). With no copper, removals due to bleeding and spotting were 1.8%, whereas with 120 $mm^2$ copper there were no such removals. Evidently the size of the device is the main factor in excess bleeding but the presence of copper itself lowers the incidence.

The direct effect of copper on suppression of the excess bleeding with IUDs is still not demonstrated definitively. One suggested study (A. Southam, personal communication, 1976) would be to compare the menstrual blood losses over a few cycles from women with a plain T as compared with the same women at a different time with a copper IUD of the same size and shape. The women volunteers would either be women with tubal ligations or be protected from pregnancy by other means while using the plain T device.

It is possible that copper, as the metal or the ions, inhibits fibrinolysin in the endometrium. The nonclotting quality of menstrual blood has long been ascribed to the fibrinolytic action of plasmin (for review, see Fearnley, 1965). Plasminogen, a normal constituent of blood is converted to plasmin, a trypsin-like enzyme, by an activator. The amount of activator in the endometrium increases before the onset of menstruation (Rybø, 1966a,b). In monkeys, there is an increase in the endometrium of proteolysis and activator concentration with the inert IUD (Shaw *et al.*, 1973). Women who have IUDs, including Cu-IUDs, removed because of excess bleeding have higher endometrial fibrinolytic activity than women who have the device removed for other reasons. The increase is due to an increase in fibrinogen activator (Bonnar *et al.*, 1976; Kasonde and Bonnar, 1976). Endometrial biopsies of women with the Cu-IUD show increased fibrinolysis over that before insertion of the device (Larsson *et al.*, 1974, 1975a). In a comparison of the Lippes loop to the copper T, fibrinolytic activity of menstrual blood was greatest with the loop. With the copper T, fibrinolytic activity approached that of normal menstrual blood (Hefnawi *et al.*, 1974c). In rats, fibrinolytic activity seems more widespread in the endometrium with a copper device than with a plastic one (Larsson *et al.*, 1975b). The increased inflammatory reaction seen with the Cu-IUD over that of inert IUDs (Cuadros and Hirsch, 1972) or the difference in the type of inflammatory reaction (H. Lehfeldt, personal communication, 1976) (see Section II, B, 6) may be the cause for the suppressed fibrinolysis (cf. Chapter 12 of Fearnley, 1965).

Perhaps the clearest *in vitro* demonstration that copper itself could decrease excess uterine bleeding is the work of Kowalski *et al.* (1956). They showed that copper sulfate at concentrations as low as $10^{-5}$ $M$ will inhibit the fibrinolytic activity of plasmin. Work is in progress in our laboratory to ascertain whether the copper inhibition of fibrinolysin is inhibition of the activator, direct inhibition of plasmin, or protection of the substrate from proteolysis. Also of interest is the question of whether the copper metal is a more powerful inhibitor of fibrinolysin than the ions produced during the dissolution of the metal. Other inhibitors of fibrinolysis such as $\epsilon$-aminocaproic acid differ from copper in that they are competitive inhibitors by providing an alternative substrate for the action of plasmin (for recent review, see Shapiro,

1973). $\epsilon$-Aminocaproic acid is used in cases of excess uterine bleeding including that associated with IUDs (Westrom and Bengtsson, 1970; Nilsson and Rybø, 1971). The disadvantage of this drug is that one runs the risk of thromboemboli, whereas with the copper IUD the inhibitor of fibrinolysis would presumably be confined to the uterus.

Copper-induced alterations in PG synthesis could be the cause for decreased bleeding with the Cu-IUD. Such PG changes could influence uterine pain (Halbert *et al.*, 1976). Inflammation can influence bleeding without involving fibrinolysis. The inflammatory reaction of IUDs is thought to be mediated by prostaglandins (see Section II, B, 7). Since the addition of copper to an IUD may alter PG synthesis (see Sections II, B, 7 and IV, C) and since PGs are powerful vasoconstricting agents (especially $PGF_{2\alpha}$) less bleeding should result. Thus, copper-induced PG synthesis could influence both the smooth muscle of the myometrium to suppress spontaneous expulsion of the Cu-IUD as well as the smooth muscles of the endometrial vasculature to decrease bleeding. Possibly an IUD with slow-releasing PG would make an effective contraceptive.

### 3. *Infection*

A side effect of IUDs of increasing concern is infection. There does not seem to be greater incidence of pelvic inflammatory disease in women wearing an IUD than in those without the device (Lippes, 1975; see also Huber *et al.*, 1975) although only a large-scale prospective study can give a definite answer. On the other hand, the course of the disease in infected women wearing an IUD can be different (H. Lehfeldt, personal communication, 1975). Unusually rapid onset of symptoms sometimes with development of a tubo-ovarian abscess, and culminating in sepsis and death have been seen in women wearing IUDs (Christian, 1974; Taylor *et al.*, 1975; see also the discussion following Taylor's article). Infections were particularly severe with the Dalkon shield, an IUD with a relatively poor contraceptive efficacy (Tatum *et al.*, 1975; see Mischell, 1975). This, coupled with the fact that the multifilament trailing thread of the device acts as a wick for transporting bacteria into the uterus, contributed to cases of fatal septic abortion (Tatum *et al.*, 1975). Both the Cu-IUD and the Lippes loop have monofilament trailing threads, and the safety record as regards infection with these devices is good (Jain, 1975). In one isolated community, septic abortion was related, in 9 out of 10 cases, to use of the Dalkon shield, but gynecological infections were associated with the use of a variety of devices, including the Cu-IUD (Mead *et al.*, 1976).

It had been thought that the Cu-IUD would have a protective effect in gonorrheal infections. This was based on the observation that metallic copper or low concentrations of Cu(II) ion inhibit the growth of gonococci *in vitro* (Fiscina *et al.,* 1973). These *in vitro* findings have been confirmed by others (Spence *et al.,* 1975). It is of theoretical interest that gonococci are killed by copper despite their high content of the copper-containing oxidase that causes the oxidation of *p*-phenylenediamine, the classic staining reaction for identifying the anaerobe, *Neisseria gonorrhoeae*. Of practical interest is that gonococci are so sensitive to copper that even tap water suppresses their growth (Fiscina *et al.,* 1973). Despite the high sensitivity of the microorganism to copper, the Cu-IUD does not protect women from gonorrhea (Spellacy, 1974) nor does it prevent pelvic inflammatory disease due to gonorrhea (H. Lehfeldt, 1975b; personal communication, 1976).

### 4. *Contraceptive Failures*

Ectopic pregnancies occur occasionally with the Cu-IUD (Beral, 1975). This further demonstrates that the contraceptive effect of copper is localized within the uterine cavity. For IUDs generally, it is estimated that uterine implantations are inhibited by 99.5%, tubal implantations by 95%, and ovarian pregnancies are not inhibited at all (Lehfeldt *et al.,* 1970). Because of the serious consequences of ectopic pregnancies, a missed menstrual period by a woman wearing an IUD should be promptly dealt with to rule out ectopic pregnancy.

When pregnancy occurred with the conventional inert IUD present, it was often the practice to leave the device in place. Copper introduced after implantation in animals can produce fetal resorption or teratologies (see Section V, D). Because of this, removal of the Cu-IUD in cases of pregnancy with the device has been advised. Some cases of births have been reported for women who retained the Cu-IUD throughout pregnancy, and these babies appear normal (Tatum, 1974; Snowden, 1976)

Limb reduction malformations were seen in infants from two women who became pregnant with an IUD in place (Barrie, 1976). The IUDs in these two cases, namely the Gräfenberg ring of "German silver," and the Dalkon shield, contain small amounts of copper (less than 0.5%). One woman with a true Cu-IUD (copper 7) in place through most of gestation delivered a child with more severe limb reduction malformations (Leighton *et al.,* 1976). In one study of 317 pregnancies in women with a variety of IUDs in place during gestation, although 33% of the pregnancies ended in spontaneous abortion, no congenital malformations were seen in the 21% of the pregnancies that reached term (Snowden,

1976). In a study with the copper 7 device, 714 pregnancies occurred with the device in place and 167 of these pregnancies went to term. Five babies had various malformations, one resulting in neonatal death. None of them had limb reduction malformations, however. Including three doubtful cases, the incidence of malformations was 4.8%, close to the expected rate for the general population (Guilleband, 1976).

In one case of an infant born with a Cu-IUD in place the serum copper of the chord blood was 2 to 5.5 times higher, and ceruloplasmin 3.5 to 8 times higher than normal (Alderman, 1976a,b). Although the infant appeared normal he died shortly after birth, presumably because of prematurity.

### 5. *Injurious Effects*

One hazard characteristic of an IUD is perforation of the uterus, most commonly the result of faulty insertion. The presence in the peritoneal cavity of an inert open (i.e., linear) plastic device may not be of concern but with copper, inflammation occurs and adhesions may form around the metal (Koetsawang, 1973). Here, early surgical removal of the device is indicated. Because of the adhesions, removal under direct visualization has been recommended (Tatum, 1973, 1974).

There is an extensive literature on the eye injuries produced by copper fragments (for review, see Grant, 1974). Initially the metal causes liquefaction of the vitreous humor. This effect is followed by leukocyte infiltration and inflammation finally resulting in fibrosis. The liquefaction of mucoids and the inflammation are similar to the reactions produced by the Cu-IUD as described earlier. The introduction of copper metal into the eye of a laboratory animal could lead to a further understanding of the action of the Cu-IUD. This could be combined with the classic experiment of Markee (1940) in which changes in the endometrium were studied by observation of a piece of endometrial tissue from a monkey and implanted into the anterior chamber of its eye.

The fibrosis seen as a result of injury by copper metal in the eye suggests that fibrosis might also occur with the copper device. This possibility could be of particular importance for women whose endometrium is not replaced monthly because they are approaching menopause or because they are amenorrhoic for other reasons. Cervicitis has been found in some women with the Cu-IUD in whom the cervical epithelial response to estrogen was thought to be low (Rubinstein, 1974; 1976).

### 6. *Systemic Effects*

The toxicity of copper has long been appreciated (see, for example, Mallory and Parker, 1931). With the Cu-IUD the metal is dissolved at a rate of 50 μg/day (Hagenfeldt, 1972a). The copper levels in the endometrium as well as in the endometrial aspirants and in cervical mucus are increased with the copper device and are of the order of $10^{-5}$ *M* cupric ion (Hagenfeldt, 1972a,b) (see also Section II, B, 5). Menstrual blood collected by means of a Tassaway menstrual cup from women wearing the copper device contains about half the total copper lost from the device during 1 month (G. K. Oster, G. Oster, and H. Lehfeldt, unpublished observations, 1972; cf. Laufe *et al.*, 1976). Tracer studies in rats show that a certain amount of copper from the wire inserted *in utero* becomes systemic and appears throughout the body (Okereke *et al.*, 1972).

The possible toxicity of this systemic copper from the Cu-IUD must be viewed in terms of normal copper metabolism and homeostatic mechanisms and experimental and clinical studies of copper toxicology. Of the 2–5 mg of copper normally taken in the diet each day, only between 0.6 and 1.6 mg is absorbed by the intestine (Cartwright and Wintrobe, 1964). The copper absorption system is an energy-dependent transport with copper being bound to the specific binding protein, metallothionein. Upon release from metallothionein, copper enters the blood either free or complexed to free amino acids or especially to serum albumin (for review of copper metabolism, see Evans, 1973). This loosely bound copper is also called "direct reacting" because it can be chelated by the copper-chelating agent, diethyldithiocarbonate. The direct reacting copper makes up about 7% of the copper in the serum, the rest being tightly bound to the copper protein ceruloplasmin. The loosely bound copper complexed to serum albumin is the source of copper to the liver, bone marrow, and other tissues (Cartwright and Wintrobe, 1964). In the liver, ceruloplasmin is synthesized and secreted into the blood. The copper in ceruloplasmin does not exchange with the copper loosely bound to serum albumin or amino acids in the serum (Cartwright and Wintrobe, 1964). Copper is excreted mainly through the biliary system, although some is lost directly to the intestines and a small part via the urine (Cartwright and Wintrobe, 1964).

Experimental copper toxicology and clinical cases of copper poisoning, although they usually involve larger quantities of copper than can be expected to become systemic from the Cu-IUD, are revelant to the IUD in that they show how excess copper is handled and where one would expect to find copper accumulation or toxic effects.

Human poisoning by oral intake of copper salts is rare because of the metallic taste and the emesis that it causes. The emetic action of copper salts, which may be related to the smooth muscle-stimulating action of cupric ions discussed in Section II, B, 7, is used medically (Gleason *et al.*, 1969). Limited intestinal absorption of copper provides an additional protective effect for oral copper poisoning, but human acute oral copper poisoning occasionally occurs (for example, Chuttani *et al.*, 1965). Chronic oral poisoning, although rare, has been reported (Salmon and Wright, 1971; see also Holtzman *et al.*, 1966). Oral poisoning, both acute and chronic, is common in ruminants (see Underwood, 1971).

The route of administration is particularly important in copper toxicity. Parenteral administration bypasses the emesis that would occur with oral administration as well as bypassing the limiting copper absorption of the intestines (Beliles, 1975). Intravenous copper has recently been responsible for an epidemic of sometimes fatal copper poisonings among patients on hemodialysis machines (for review, see Barbour *et al.*, 1971). The dialysis membrane in these cases was a cuprammonium cellophane, Cuprofam. Copper intoxication has also been seen when copper salts have been applied to the skin to debride burned areas (Holtzman *et al.*, 1966). Parenteral metallic copper can be toxic as well, especially if the surface area is large. The extreme case of enormous surface area is fine copper powder. Intraperitoneal injection of copper powder into mice can be lethal—a 25-mg dose causes death after 5 days (see Oster and Salgo, 1976). Death is preceded by hemolytic anemia and with higher doses (100 mg), hemolysis is seen within 1 day after injection. Even subcutaneous injection of powdered copper can cause chronic toxicity and be lethal if the dosage is high. Monthly injection of 80 mg of copper powder was not toxic to a monkey over 7 months of treatment, but when the monthly dose was increased to 1000 mg the monkey died after 9 months (Mallory and Parker, 1931). Sheep are particularly sensitive to copper poisoning and die with much smaller amounts (Mallory and Parker, 1931; see Underwood, 1971). In humans, chronic copper poisoning can occur from inhalation of copper dust (for references, see Holtzman *et al.*, 1966).

With acute copper poisoning in animals and man, the symptoms usually include vomiting, diarrhea, jaundice, and hemolysis (Chuttani *et al.*, 1965; Barbour *et al.*, 1971; see Underwood, 1971). With chronic copper poisoning, however, the symptoms are different and tend to be similar to those of the slow copper intoxication of Wilson's disease (Owen and Hazelrig, 1968). This inherited metabolic disease, also called hepatolentricular degeneration, is a disorder of copper homeostasis. Although the precise nature of the metabolic defect is not known, copper accumulates in tissue, particularly in the liver, brain, kidneys, and the cornea. The classic symptoms of Wilson's disease are neurological disturbances, liver disease, renal problems, and Kayser-Fleischer rings zones of green-brown copper deposition in the cornea. Often only some of these symptoms occur; children presenting with the disease usually only have liver disease. Some patients develop the disease in their thirties and present primarily with neurological or psychiatric problems (for reviews on Wilson's disease, see Scheinberg and Sternlieb, 1965; Walshe, 1966; Sass-Kortsak, 1975).

In copper intoxication and in Wilson's disease, there is accumulation of copper in various tissues. The primary site of accumulation is the liver. Chronic hemodialysis with copper-containing dialysis membranes can lead to liver copper levels twice that of normals (Barbour *et al.*, 1971). Animals given excess copper can have liver accumulation of copper 20 times the normal value (see Underwood 1971; Owen and Hazelrig, 1968). Wilson's disease patients can have liver copper levels a hundredfold higher than normal (Scheinberg and Sternlieb, 1965).

Ceruloplasmin levels in patients with Wilson's disease are much lower than normals and this is often used in diagnosis of the disease. In some patients, however, the liver symptoms of Wilson's disease are found with ceruloplasmin levels within the normal range (Scheinberg and Sternlieb, 1965; Saas-Kortsak, 1975). In copper-loaded animals, ceruloplasmin production as measured by label studies was sharply reduced although ceruloplasmin levels were slightly increased (Owen and Hazelrig, 1968). Ceruloplasmin levels are not increased in cases of copper poisoning in hemodialysis (Barbour *et al.*, 1971). In acute copper poisoning, the "free reacting" or nonceruloplasmin serum copper increases initially but decreases again within hours in mice (Gubler *et al.*, 1953) and within a day in humans (Chutani *er al.*, 1965). In human copper poisoning, the total blood copper rather than total serum copper is correlated with the severity of symptoms (Chuttani *et al.*, 1965). Copper administration to mice also causes an accumulation of copper in the red blood cells rather than in serum (Gubler *et al.*, 1953).

Returning to the Cu-IUD, clinical studies have shown that use of the copper device does not lead to an increase in serum copper. Hagenfeldt (1972a,b) found no increase in serum copper compared to non-IUD controls. Hefnawi *et al.* (1974b) found an increase in serum copper in women with either a Cu-IUD or an inert Lippes loop compared to non-IUD controls and attributed the increase to a generalized reaction to intrauterine foreign bodies (see in following). As already mentioned, red blood cells are more likely to show an increase in copper during copper poisoning than does serum. Hagenfeldt (1972b) found that erythrocyte copper remains unchanged even after a year of use of the device.

Copper accumulation would be most likely to occur in the liver and kidneys if the Cu-IUD produces copper toxicity. Although no measurements of liver or kidney copper levels have been done with women on the Cu-IUD, tissue copper levels have been measured in rabbits (Moo-Young and Tatum, 1974) and monkeys (Moo-Young *et al.*, 1973; Ranney *et al.*, 1975) with intrauterine copper. In the rabbits, the copper wire was inserted into the uterus after implantation and maternal as well as fetal copper levels were measured just before term. There was no maternal accumulation of copper in any tissue other than the uterus (Moo-Young and Tatum, 1974). In monkeys, no increase in tissue copper was seen other than in the uterus after 1 month with the Cu-IUD *in situ* (Ranney *et al.*, 1975). After 1 year, however, there is a small accumulation of copper in the kidneys of monkeys with intrauterine or intra-abdominal Cu-IUDs (Moo-Young *et al.*, 1973). The kidney copper levels of 28 $\mu$g/gm dry tissue compared to 23.5 $\mu$g/gm for the controls was significant ($p < 0.05$). Other tissues showed very slight increases, but none were significantly higher than controls. Highly localized copper deposits, as seen histologically with rubeanic acid, have been detected in livers and kidneys of monkeys with Cu-IUDs but are also found in controls (Ranney *et al.*, 1975). In no case was any pathology seen in monkeys in nonuterine tissue that could be attributed to the Cu-IUD (Moo-Young *et al.*, 1973; Ranney *et al.*, 1975; Nutting and Mueller 1975a,b).

The small but significant increase in tissue copper in kidneys of monkeys with Cu-IUDs raises the question of recondite toxicity of copper from the Cu-IUD. *Recondite toxicity* is defined as the slow accumulation over time of a potentially hazardous substance that eventually has a toxic effect (Schroeder, 1973). Oral copper administration is thought not to have recondite toxicity (Schroeder, 1973). Copper injection has induced tumors in chickens (see Beliles, 1975) (see Section II, C, 1) and can be teratological (see Section V, D).

Recently, recondite copper toxicity has been alleged to occur in man (Pfeiffer and Iliev, 1972). Copper and zinc are known to antagonize each other in a variety of systems. Zinc deficiencies cause severe consequences in animals (Hurley, 1976a,b) and may be involved in psychiatric disorders in humans (Pfeiffer and Iliev, 1972). In some cases zinc deficiency is thought to be manifested by white spots on the fingernails (Pfeiffer, 1975). It is also thought that excess copper may bring about zinc deficiency (Pfeiffer and Iliev, 1972). Copper excess or copper imbalance has been suggested as a cause for various mental illnesses over the years (for review, see Pfeiffer and Iliev, 1972). The psychiatric symptoms due to copper accumulation in Wilson's disease are well known (for review, see Scheinberg and Sternlieb, 1965).

There has been particular concern that the Cu-IUD by its parenteral administration of copper could alter the copper balance of the body (I.

H. Scheinberg, personal communication, 1975; Okereke *et al.,* 1972). Any slight accumulation of copper could become serious if the device is to be used for 10–20 years, as is planned for some of the newer copper-sleeved IUDs. Slight alterations in the balance of copper may cause increased peroxidation of lipids in various tissues, and the products of this peroxidation may also be harmful (see Section II, C, 1). Copper-induced lipid peroxidation is thought by some to be a factor in aging (Harman, 1965; see also Harman, 1972).

The Cu-IUD has systemic effects unrelated to systemic accumulation of copper (see Oster and Salgo, 1976). Copper wires in mice cause severe rouleau formation (Davis *et al.,* 1976). This rouleau formation might well be related to serum immunoglobulin changes seen in women (Holub *et al.,* 1971; Gump *et al.,* 1973; Chandra *et al.,* 1974; Shulman *et al.,* 1974; Mountrose *et al.,* 1975) as well as in animals (Holub, 1972) with IUDs. The workers just cited found various increases in immunoglobulin G (IgG), immunoglobulin M (IgM), and immunoglobulin A (IgA) although the alterations are not consistent from one study to another. These changes in immunoglobulins imply that an immunological reaction is part of the IUD action. Increased levels of immunoglobulins are a prime factor causing high sedimentation rate, which, in turn, is associated with rouleau formation (Wintrobe *et al.,* 1974). Thus women with IUDs might be expected to have a high sedimentation rate. An increased level of plasma copper has been seen with copper as well as with inert IUDs (Hefnawi *et al.,* 1974b). This rise in ceruloplasmin is probably a generalized foreign body reaction (Hefnawi *et al.,* 1974b) since serum copper is known to increase in response to inflammation (Pekarek *et al.,* 1972; Evans, 1973) or stress (Evans, 1973).

A related systemic effect of IUDs is an increase in most leukocyte types in blood of women with IUDs (Săgiroğlu and Săgiroğlu, 1970). There does not appear to be any change in the leukocyte distribution in mice with intraabdominal copper wires (Davis *et al.,* 1976). Bone marrow myelopoiesis is increased, however, in mice with copper intraperitoneal implants (McGarry, 1975).

In some animals, especially heifers, an inert intravaginal contraceptive device is being used to cause an increased weight gain. It probably acts via a hypothalamic pathway (see Maugh, 1976).

The systemic effects seen with inert devices may be more pronounced with copper IUDs since copper causes an increased (Cuadros and Hirsch, 1972) or a different type of inflammatory response (H. Lehfeldt, personal communication, 1976). Indeed, copper devices cause an increase in IgM within 4 weeks after insertion in women (Holub *et al.,* 1971). Metallic copper denatures proteins (Oster, 1971, 1972), presumably via a free-radical reaction (Oster and Oster, 1974). These altered proteins could be the antigens that bring about the rise in immunoglobulins (Holub, 1972). In this way, IUDs might cause autoimmune reactions (Holub *et al.*, 1971).

A case of eczematous dermatitis caused by the Cu-IUD has been reported (Barranco, 1972). Two weeks after insertion of the Cu-IUD, the woman developed dermatitis on the arms and trunk which later covered most of her body. The condition cleared up 4 days after removal of the Cu-IUD, and the only positive patch test was that to copper sulfate. We feel that this allergic dermatitis is an autoimmune reaction of the kind already described.

## III. Hormonally Induced Changes in Copper Levels

### A. Ceruloplasmin

So far we have been considering the pharmacology of copper as it applies to the Cu-IUD. There are significant changes in copper metabolism related to reproduction when no exogenous copper is given. Serum copper rises dramatically during pregnancy (Krebs, 1928; for additional references, see Evans, 1973; Fisher,1975). The characteristic greenish color of serum from pregnant women is due to copper in the form of the blue copper-containing protein ceruloplasmin. Serum copper increases throughout gestation, the rate of increase being particularly high in the first trimester. Near term serum copper is almost threefold higher than the nonpregnant value. The serum copper level decreases at term and during delivery and then slowly during the postpartum period (for additional references, see Schenker *et al.*, 1969, 1971).

A drop in the copper level during pregnancy has been proposed as an index of placental insufficiency as it has been seen in cases of postmaturity, premature rupture of the membranes, and spontaneous abortion (Schenker *et al.*, 1969). It has also been suggested as an indicator of impending fetal death (O'Leary, 1969). For a normal pregnancy, serum copper may rise at 30 weeks of gestation from 270 $\mu$g/100 cc to a value near term of 350 $\mu$g/100 cc. In a case of fetal death *in utero*, the serum copper levels did not rise after the thirtieth week but remained stationary and actually decreased 2 weeks before the death of the fetus. A rise in serum copper levels above the normal pregnancy levels is found in toxemia of pregnancy and the copper levels are correlated with the severity of the clinical symptoms (Schenker *et al.*, 1969).

When contraceptive steroids are administered to nonpregnant women the serum copper level rises about 50% above normal (Schenker *et al.*,

1971). The rise in serum copper is due primarily to the estrogens that cause a *de novo* synthesis of ceruloplasmin (see Evans, 1973) and this is why the rise is particularly dramatic during pregnancy. An estrogen-binding protein has been found in the liver (Eisenfeld *et al.,* 1976). This may be involved in the liver's response. Progesterone causes a less drastic increase in serum copper (Sato and Henkin, 1973), and cortisol causes a decrease (see Evans, 1973). Diurnal fluctuations in ACTH and corticosteroids are reflected in diurnal variations in ceruloplasmin levels, and ceruloplasmin is also increased during stress (see Evans, 1973). Urinary copper levels have a circadian rhythm and are decreased with estrogens (Weinmann *et al.,* 1976). In the normal menstrual cycle, serum copper levels change only by about 10–20 μg% (Sarata, 1935; Schenker *et al.,* 1969; von Studnitz and Berezin, 1958; Dokumov, 1968; see also Southam and Gonzaga, 1965). Average serum copper for man is about 100 μg%, and, for nonpregnant women in the fertile age, is about 130 μg% (Schenker *et al.,* 1969). Apparently androgens can also effect a rise in serum copper. Administration of either testosterone or estradiol to elderly men or postmenopausal women increases serum copper significantly (von Studnitz and Berezin, 1958; Johnson *et al.,* 1959). In schizophrenic women, ceruloplasmin levels increase much more with birth control pills than in normal women (Pfeiffer and Iliev, 1972).

About 93% of serum copper is complexed as ceruloplasmin, and the other 7% bound to serum albumin (Cartwright and Wintrobe, 1964). Serum albumin reversibly binds cupric ions (Klotz and Curme, 1948), whereas the copper in ceruloplasmin is tightly complexed and cannot be removed by diethyldithiocarbamate except after strong acid treatment (Cartwright and Wintrobe, 1964). Thus, the copper that is available to cells comes from serum albumin and there is no transfer from ceruloplasmin (Cartwright and Wintrobe, 1964; for additional references, see Evans, 1973; see also Scheinberg and Morell, 1973).

The affinity of copper ions for serum albumin has been attributed in part to the complexation of copper to the histidyl residue of the amino terminal sequence of the protein (Dixon and Sarkar, 1972, 1974). Copper forms a strong complex with the histidyl nitrogen. The decreased copper binding of dog serum albumin is said to be owing to the fact that dogs lack histidine at position 3 as compared to most other species (Dixon and Sarker, 1972, 1974).

Ceruloplasmin is an oxidase; for example, it will oxidize phenylenediamine (see Scheinberg and Morell, 1973; Malmström *et al.,* 1975). Ceruloplasmin has recently been called ferroxidase I because of its role in iron metabolism (Curzon and O'Reilly, 1960; Osaki *et al.,* 1966; Frieden, 1971, 1973; Frieden and Osaki, 1974; Seelig, 1972). Ceruloplasmin oxidizes ferrous to ferric and, thereby, allows ferric to be incorporated into the iron-transporting protein, transferrin, making iron available to the blood-forming tissues. The increase in ceruloplasmin accompanying increases in estrogen affects iron metabolism. Thus, with roosters, it was shown that estrogen administration first causes an increase in ferroxidase and subsequently an increase in total serum iron (Planas and Frieden, 1973). Transferrin mobilizes iron for erythropoiesis. Thus, the high estrogen levels of pregnancy that induce production of ceruloplasmin increase iron mobilization needed for red cell production in the mother and fetus.

The oxidative actions of ceruloplasmin are similar to those of copper ions *in vitro*. Cupric ions oxidize ferrous to ferric. Cupric ions will cause the oxidation of hemoglobin to the ferric form, namely methemoglobin. The reaction is slow, however. The production of methemoglobin by copper is enormously accelerated if a weak reducing agent, such as phenylhydrazine or ascorbic acid, is also present. By itself phenylhydrazine has a lesser effect: it reduces the cupric to cuprous, which, on autooxidation, produces powerful oxidizing free radicals. The paradoxical classic oxidation of hemoglobin to form methemoglobin by reducing agents (e.g., phenylhydrazine and hydroxylamine) may well involve autooxidation of the copper that is normally present in the blood cells.

Ceruloplasmin has ascorbic acid oxidase activity *in vitro* (Frieden *et al.*, 1965) which may be related to the pronounced changes in urinary ascorbic acid over the menstrual cycle. Women were given 200 mg of vitamin C in the evening, and the morning urine was tested for ascorbic acid (Pillay, 1946; Neuweiler, 1948; Schafroth, 1956; Loh and Wilson, 1971). As much as a tenfold decrease in urinary ascorbic acid was seen at midcycle. Since ceruloplasmin undergoes only slight changes in concentration during the menstrual cycle (von Studnitz and Berezin, 1958; Dukumov, 1968; Schenker *et al.*, 1969; Hagenfeldt, 1972b), other causes for the changes in ascorbic acid metabolism must be considered. The ascorbic acid oxidase activity of ceruloplasmin is inhibited by citrate (Frieden *et al.*, 1965). Serum citrate is a minimum at midcycle (Goldsmith *et al.*, 1970), implying greater ascorbic acid oxidase activity of ceruloplasmin at that time and, hence, lowered urinary vitamin C. Vitamin C deficiency is often encountered in pregnancy (Mason and Rivers, 1971) and when oral contraceptives are administered (Theuer, 1972; Rivers, and Devine, 1972, 1975; Briggs and Briggs, 1972; see Wynn, 1975), especially in women with marginal nutritional status (see also Section VIII, B). The vitamin deficiency may be attributed to the increased ceruloplasmin either directly, with ceruloplasmin oxidizing the ascorbic acid, or indirectly, with increased iron metabolism. Oxidation of ascorbic acid has been implicated in iron metabolism in the reduction of ferric to ferrous, thereby, releasing iron from transferrin for use in erythropoiesis (Heilmeyer, 1958) (see Section VIII, B).

Whatever the mechanism of the decrease in urinary ascorbic acid in the menstrual cycle may be, the vitamin C test could serve as a convenient indicator of ovulation. The woman would apply the test herself using the vitamin C molybdate test paper.* Ceruloplasmin is also elevated in certain types of cancer, notably leukemia and Hodgkin's disease, and declines as successful treatment of the disease proceeds (Tessmer *et al.*, 1973; Delves *et al.*, 1973; Ray *et al.*, 1973; Jelliffe, 1973). It would be interesting to follow urinary vitamin C in such patients. Other glycoproteins are also increased in cancer (see Winzler and Bekesi, 1967).

## B. Other Oxidases

Another oxidase that is influenced by estrogens is glutathione peroxidase. The oxidation of glutathione catalyzed primarily by glutathione peroxidase is 80% higher in female rat liver than in male or female castrate liver (Pinto and Bartley, 1969a,b). In addition, the enzyme activity varies over the estrous cycle, being highest at estrus. It also increases in pregnancy and with estrogen administration to the castrated animal (Pinto and Bartley, 1969a,b). Also, it was found that glutathione peroxidase activity was correlated with aerobic glutathione oxidation. This suggests to us the presence of a copper enzyme. Copper is known to be the most powerful catalyst for the autoxidation of glutathione *in vitro* (Tsen and Tappel, 1958; see also Michaelis and Barrón, 1929).

Lipid peroxidation, which is related to glutathione oxidation, is much greater in female rat liver than in males; the rate is 15–30-fold greater than that for males or ovariectomized females (Pinto and Bartley, 1969b). A product of this lipid peroxidation is malonaldehyde (see Section II, C, 1). With addition of exogenous reduced glutathione to liver homogenates the formation of malonaldehyde was completely suppressed (Pinto and Bartley, 1969b).

Chloasma, a darkening of the skin, ultimately produced by a copper-containing enzyme, is often a manifestation of high estrogen levels. This phenomenon, sometimes called "the mask of pregnancy," appears as dark splotches on the face. Chloasma is noted not only in pregnancy but also with women taking high estrogen oral contraceptives; the splotches

* "C-Stix," Ames Company, Miles Laboratories, Inc., Elkhart, Indiana 46514.

are enhanced by sunlight (Esoda, 1963). Topical application of estrogens on the nipple will cause a darkening of the nipple and areolae (Lorincz, 1954). Skin pigmentation is a result of oxidation of tyrosine to melanin by tyrosinase, a copper-containing enzyme (see McGuire, 1972; Okun *et al.,* 1972). Chloasma, thus, can be regarded as another manifestation of the interrelation of estrogens and copper.

### C. Taste and Smell

Copper is involved in the physiology of taste and smell. The olfactory and gustatory sensations may be critical in a variety of reproductive functions in man as well as in animals.

Oral administration of the copper-chelating agent, penicillamine, in some human cases causes a loss in taste and smell, and copper sulfate reverses this reaction (Henkin and Bradley, 1969). In rats, there is severe anorexia when high levels of the copper-chelating agent, disulfiram, are given, and this drug also causes fetal resorption (Salgo and Oster, 1974b) (see Section V, B). There is a condition, found in both men and women, of anosmia together with gonadal hypoplasia, which is usually associated with gross anatomical abnormalities of the olfactory regions of the brain (for review, see Marshall and Henkin, 1971; see also de Morisier and Gautier, 1963; Muller, 1963). Menstrual abnormalities have been correlated with various types of decreases in olfactory activity (Marshall and Henkin, 1971). In men various types of hyposmia are also found with gonadotropin deficiencies and infertility (Hamilton *et al.,* 1973). Zinc is also important for proper sensation of taste and smell (Henkin and Bradley, 1969; Schechter *et al.,* 1972). Zinc deficiency in young men leads to hypogonadism and small stature (Prasad, 1967, 1972; see also Anonymous, 1975). Decreased or altered sensations of taste and smell are also seen in thyroid disorders (McConnell *et al.,* 1975). Since copper seems to play such a critical role in the sensation of taste and smell (Henkin and Bradley, 1969) as well as in reproductive status, one wonders if copper could be the connecting link. The interaction of copper with hypothalamic-releasing factors (see Section IV, A) or with the thyroid (see Section IV, D) might be of particular importance. Some antithyroid compounds are copper-chelating agents. The thyroid is, of course, important for proper reproductive function (see Section, IV, D).

Sex steroids also can influence the perception of taste and smell. Thus a woman's ability to detect the odor of the synthetic musk, Exaltolide, is greatest at midcycle (Le Magnen, 1953; Vierling and Rock, 1967). A related phenomenon is the change in salivary mucoids over the menstrual cycle; the sialic acid content of the saliva being a minimum around midcycle (Oster and Yang, 1972). Pheromones, substances that are put out by one individual and affect another, are critical to reproductive function in animals (for review, see Whitten, 1966; Bronson, 1968; Bruce, 1970) and seems to play a role in normal human sexual function (see Comfort, 1971; McClintock, 1971; Doty *et al.,* 1975). Copper-chelating agents or antagonists that can cause a loss of smell could obviously interfere with pheromone-mediated reproductive processes.

## IV. Copper Influences on Reproductive Hormones

### A. Copper-Induced Ovulation and Releasing Hormones

Copper can also cause changes in levels of gonadotropic hormones. It has long been known that intravenous injection of copper salts will cause ovulation and pseudopregnancy in the rabbit (Fevold *et al.,* 1936). The rabbit is an induced ovulator, i.e., vaginal stimulation provokes the release of luteinizing hormone (LH) and follicle-stimulating hormone (FSH) causing ovulation as well as pseudopregnancy, a state of prolonged life of the corpus luteum (see Everett, 1964). In order to produce ovulation in the rabbit by intravenous injection of cupric salts, high doses of copper (3 mg/kg) must be used (Hiroi *et al.,* 1965). When cupric sulfate is applied directly into the hypothalamus of rabbits, only 0.76 $\mu$g/kg or 1/4000 of the intravenous dose of copper is required (Hiroi *et al.,* 1965). Copper administration has been shown to produce an increase in LH and FSH (Suzuki *et al.,* 1970) resulting in ovulation. Hypothalamic extracts are rich in metal ion, particularly in copper. Inorganic ash residues from these extracts cause a release of various pituitary hormones including LH when added to pituitary preparations *in vitro* (LaBella *et al.,* 1973). Cupric salts alone at concentrations less than 1 $\mu$g/ml (i.e., $>10^{-5}$ *M*) will also cause this release of LH (LaBella *et al.,* 1973). Copper salts potentiate the uterotropic activity of estradiol (Kar and Sarkar, 1960).

Copper complexes with many amino acids (for review, see Greenstein and Winitz, 1961) and peptides (for review, see Breslow, 1973). The copper-catalyzed hydrolysis of amino acid esters is believed to proceed via the copper-coordinated ester linkage (Nakon *et al.,* 1974). The NMR spectra of copper octapeptide complexes show that peptide bonds removed from the site of binding are affected (Walter *et al.,* 1971), suggesting a change in conformation has occurred. Chelates of copper are generally more lipid-soluble than either the parent ligand or the copper ion. The hypothalamic LH-FSH-releasing hormone is a decapeptide containing histidyl and arginyl residues (Arimura *et al.,* 1971). These are particularly strong copper-complexing groups. In the form of a copper complex, the decapeptide would be more lipid-soluble. In this way copper might act synergistically with the releasing hormone to cause the release of LH and FSH (see also Fevold *et al.,* 1936; Suzuki *et al.,* 1970; LaBella *et al.,* 1973). Inhibitory analogs of LH-releasing hormone have been synthesized and these are rich in phenylalanine (de la Cruz *et al.,* 1976). It is possible that the lipophilic nature of these groups is important in their action.

Copper administration leads to gonadotropin changes in the rat as well as in the rabbit. In the rat, in contrast to the case for the rabbit, intravenous injection of copper at estrus causes pseudopregnancy (Dury and Bradbury, 1941). The rat is a spontaneous ovulator, and after ovulation, vaginal stimulation causes pseudopregnancy. This condition is brought about in the rat by the release of prolactin. This substance is the principal luteotropic hormone in the rat, and with its release there is a consequent inhibition of the release of LH and FSH (see Everett, 1964). To produce pseudopregnancy in the rat by intravenous injection of copper salts, doses of 16 mg/kg must be used (Hiroi *et al.,* 1969); these approach the lethal dose of 18 mg/kg (Hiroi *et al.,* 1969). Similarly, to the induction of ovulation in the rabbit, when cupric sulfate is applied directly into the hypothalamus of rats, much lower doses of copper are required to induce pseudopregnancy (Kato, 1969). An increase in prolactin and a decrease in LH and FSH have been shown with copper-induced pseudopregnancy (Suzuki *et al.,* 1969). Luteinizing hormone is the main luteotropic hormone in the rabbit, and prolactin serves this function in the rat (see Everett, 1964). In both species, copper administration causes the release of hormones that maintain the corpus luteum. It is perhaps significant that during early pregnancy, when maintenance of the corpus luteum is crucial for the continuation of the pregnancy, serum copper levels are increasing (see Section III, A).

Dopamine treatment causes the release of LH-releasing hormone (LHRH) in pituitary stalk plasma and is thought to be the normal mediator of LHRH release (Kamberi *et al.,* 1969). Administration of the copper-chelating agent, disulfiram, to rats reduces the activity of the copper-containing enzyme, dopamine $\beta$-hydroxylase, in the brain (Goldstein and Nakajima, 1967). This enzyme converts dopamine to norepinephrine. Changes in the activity of the enzyme influence the ratio of these neurotransmitters and hence, perhaps, the liberation of hypothalamic releasing factors. *In vitro,* addition of excess copper inhibits dopamine $\beta$-hydroxylase activity (Goldstein *et al.,* 1965). In Wilson's disease, a disorder of copper metabolism characterized by low levels of serum ceruloplasmin and high levels of copper in tissues (see Goldfisher and Sternlieb, 1968; Scheinberg and Sternlieb, 1965) (also see

Sections II, C, 6 and VII, B), dopamine β-hydroxylase may be inhibited by the high level of copper in the brain.

### B. Sex Steroids

Copper plays a role in liver microsomal hydroxylation. Copper deficiency in rats leads to a decrease in liver microsomal hydroxylating enzymes as measured by an increase in hexobarbitone sleeping time and a decreased aniline hydroxylase and hexobarbital oxidase activity (Moffitt and Murphy, 1972). Adding large amounts of copper salts to normal liver microsomal preparations causes a decrease in aniline hydroxylating activity. Similarly, giving rats excess copper in their drinking water for several weeks reduces the microsomal aniline hydroxylase activity (Moffitt and Murphy, 1972). All of these changes in microsomal hydroxylation strongly suggest that the microsomal enzyme responsible, presumably one of the P-450 enzymes, contains copper.

Among the substrates of liver microsomal hydroxylation are the steroids, including estrogen (see Cooney, 1967). Severe copper deficiencies or excess could, thus, interfere with steroid metabolism. The abnormalities in the estrous cycle of copper-deficient animals (see Section V, A) could be a result of changes in liver hydroxylation of steroids.

Copper is present in microsomes and has been proposed as a participant in microsomal hydroxylation (Mason *et al.*, 1965). The paramagnetic species Cu(II) may not appear in the electron-paramagnetic spectrum of the P-450 cytochromes (for review, see Ullrich and Duppel, 1975) since the copper may be present in the reduced state, Cu(I), or even the trivalent oxidized state, Cu(III), neither of which is paramagnetic. There is evidence that the copper in galactose oxidase is in the Cu(III) state, and this may also be the case for tyrosinase (Dyrkacz *et al.*, 1976; Gutteridge and Robb, 1975). The oxidative reactions of these enzymes may arise from autooxidation of Cu(I). In any case, free radicals are generated by microsomal enzymes as was demonstrated by the initiation of vinyl polymerization with rat liver microsomes (Oster, 1975).

The level of microsomal enzymes in the liver is often increased upon administration of drugs that are metabolized by this system—a process termed enzyme induction (for review, see Cooney, 1967). Microsomal enzyme induction, usually brought about by administration of barbiturates, has been shown to cause a concomitant increase in the copper concentrations in rat liver microsomes (Moffitt *et al.*, 1972; Moffitt and Murphy, 1972). Copper deficiency does not prevent the enzyme induction. Since microsomal copper levels are increased in livers of normal or copper-deficient rats upon enzyme induction by phenobarbital, it seems that copper is still available for this induction (Moffitt and Murphy, 1972). Copper deficiency delays the normal increases with age seen in liver hydroxylating enzymes, however (Moffitt and Murphy, 1972).

Among the compounds hydroxylated by the liver microsomal system, which may also cause positive or negative induction, are the sex steroids (Quinn *et al.*, 1958; Cooney, 1967; for a recent review, see Goble, 1975). The naturally occurring steroids lead to male–female differences in hydroxylating enzymes, at least in the rat, but perhaps not in man (see Goble, 1975). Of 200 common drugs studied (Cooney, 1967), most of them increase the activity of liver microsomal enzymes, some have no effect, and only 2, namely morphine and estradiol, decrease enzyme activity. It may be significant that these two are the only compounds on the list that contain phenolic groups. One would expect that steroids affecting microsomal enzymes could also alter the level of microsomal copper.

Copper might conceivably also be involved in steroid metabolism in the aromatization of androgens to estrogens in the ovaries and placenta. This process is hydroxylation by a microsomal cytochrome of the P-450 type (Thompson and Siiteri, 1973). The rate-determining step is believed to be a hydroxylation of the carbon-19 methyl group (Wilcox and Engel, 1965). One might expect ovarian or placental microsomes also to be capable of generating free radicals.

Copper may also influence the sulfonation of steroids. *In vitro* copper salts are catalysts of sulfite oxidation to sulfate (G. Oster, unpublished observations, 1976). The normal sulfite oxidase is a molybdenum- and heme-containing enzyme (see Bray, 1975), but excess copper *in vivo* may also catalyze the reaction (see also Section VIII, B). Sulfination renders estrogens water-soluble, and estrogen sulfates are thought to be the major source of available estrogens in the body (Tseng *et al.*, 1972).

### C. Prostaglandins

Prostaglandins as they occur naturally in the body are believed to be important mediators in a wide variety of reproductive processes (for review, see Karim, 1975). These bio-active compounds are synthesized in the body from arachidonic acid. Of particular importance in reproductive biology are the E and F series of PGs. In the biosynthetic pathways, there is a route leading to the E compounds and another to the F series. Copper inhibits the biosynthesis of PGE, (Nugteren *et al.*, 1966) and causes a shift in the biosynthesis away from $PGE_2$ toward

$PGF_{2\alpha}$ (Lands *et al.*, 1971). Thiols are important in the biosynthesis, and it has been postulated that copper stabilizes a diradical endoperoxide allowing reduction of the carbonyl group in E series to the F series (Lands *et al.*, 1971; Lee and Lands, 1972). Copper salts at $10^{-5}$ *M* in sheep vesicular gland homogenates with added arachidonic acid inhibit $PGE_2$ synthesis and stimulate $PGF_{2\alpha}$ synthesis (Maddox, 1973). Copper in excess of $10^{-3}$ *M* inhibits the reaction. Chelating agents that remove all of the copper likewise stop the reaction (Maddox, 1973; see also Rome *et al.*, 1976). Glutathione peroxidase (see Section II, B) may also be a regulatory factor in PG biosynthesis (Cook and Lands, 1976).

These concentrations of copper and chelating agents are the same as those seen to cause changes in myometrial activity (see Section II, B, 7), supporting our hypothesis that copper acts on the uterus by altering PG metabolism. The Cu-IUD could alter PG biosynthesis and this could account for the effect of the device on uterine motility (see Section II, B, 7), uterine bleeding (see Section II, C, 2), and inflammation (see Sections II, B, 6 and 7). Anti-inflammatory agents are inhibitors of PG biosynthesis (Vane, 1971; for review, see Ferreira and Vane, 1974). These agents have been used effectively in animal models to delay the onset of labor with a view toward preventing premature births (for review, see Karim and Hillier, 1975). Some of these agents, notably aspirin, are strong copper chelators and may thereby prevent the production of the endogenous uterine stimulant, $PGF_{2\alpha}$.

## D. Thyroid

Copper could influence reproductive function via its probable role in thyroid metabolism. Thyroid function is well known to interrelate with many aspects of reproduction (for review, see Leathem, 1972; Botella-Llusía, 1973; Ingbar and Woeber, 1974; Burrow, 1972). Proper thyroid functioning is required for normal pubertal development in males and females, spermatogenesis, ovarian follicular development, ovulation, implantation, normal pregnancy, and milk production. Hypothyroidism in children leads to sexual immaturity in adulthood or a delay in the onset of puberty. In adults, hypothyroidism is associated with conditions such as diminished libido, failure of ovulation, impotence, and oligospermia. Hypothyroidism also alters the metabolism of androgens and estrogens. If conception takes place in hypothyroid women, it often ends in abortion, stillbirths, or births of malformed babies (Botella-Llusía, 1973, p. 925), and of course, goiter leads to cretinism (for review, see Warkany, 1971). The incidence of thyroid disease is higher in women who had children with spina bifida than in women with normal babies (P. Stanway, personal communication, 1976).

Hyperthyroidism can also lead to delayed sexual development. In adulthood, thyrotoxicosis can cause menstrual irregularities, amenorrhea, or anovulatory cycles. Again, if conception does occur it may end in abortion. Hyperthyroidism sometimes is associated with an increase in libido in either sex. With increased thyroid function, there is an increase in steroid-binding globulin with a resulting increase in total estradiol or testosterone in the blood, although the fraction of free steroid is decreased. Hyperthyroidism can often lead to gynecomastia (Botella-Llusía, 1973; Ingbar-Woeber, 1974). Increased thyroid hormones cause an increase in ceruloplasmin (see Evans, 1973).

In addition to the requirement of proper thyroid metabolism for normal reproductive function, reproductive steroids have an effect on thyroid metabolism. Estrogens or androgens stimulate thyroid function, whereas progesterone or cortisone decrease it (Botella-Llusía, 1973). The increase is particularly dramatic during pregnancy when the thyroid is enlarged and iodine uptake is increased. There is also an increase in renal iodine clearance. Serum $T_3$ and $T_4$ levels increase substantially in pregnancy. The increase is due to an increase of thyroid-binding globulin, and the amount of free thyroxine is thought to remain unchanged (Ingbar and Woeber, 1974). This is similar to the increase in serum copper seen in pregnancy, increase being due to increased ceruloplasmin, the copper-binding globulin (see Section II, A).

There is strong suggestive evidence that copper is involved in the synthesis of thyroid hormones. *In vitro* cell-free thyroid homogenates will incorporate iodine into organically bound form if cupric is added (Weiss, 1953). An enzyme, tyrosine iodinase, that will effect the incorporation of iodine to tyrosine when cupric is supplemented has been characterized (Fawcett and Kirkwood, 1954). The peroxidation, which is thought to be required for oxidation and iodination, is considered by some to be caused by an iron protein (Alexander, 1959) since addition of ferrous ion has a stimulating effect. However, ferrous could be acting to reduce cupric to cuprous. The autooxidation of cuprous is a peroxidation which, as can be demonstrated, will oxidize iodide to iodine via a free-radical mechanism (see Section II, B, 8). That the peroxidation that takes place in the thyroid is due to the action of copper is strengthened by the fact that the classic antithyroid agents, such as thiocyanate or thiouracil, are copper-complexing agents. Thus, thiouracil added to a precipitate of cupric hydroxide will produce a water-soluble yellow complex (G. Oster, unpublished observations, 1976). The effect of these antithyroid drugs in interfering with various reproductive processes could be produced by inhibiting necessary thyroid hormone production. This is thought to be the case in the blockage of implantation in rats by thiouracil in that thyroidectomy has the same effect (Holland *et al.,* 1967, 1968). Thiouracil may also have effects by chelating copper in nonthyroid tissues. This may be the case in thiouracil-induced teratologies (Warkany, 1971, p. 126) (see Section V, C). Hypothyroidism results in the interference of the conversion of carotene to vitamin A (Claussen and McCord, 1938). This suggests that agents which inhibit iodide peroxidase also inhibit the enzyme for carotene oxidative cleavage (see Section VIII, B).

Copper, aside from its involvement in the peroxidation of iodide, might play a role in thyroid function via hypothalamic releasing hormones. As mentioned earlier, copper can cause the release of FSH and LH from the pituitary, and various metal salts including copper are found in hypothalamic extracts that have hormone-releasing activity (see Section IV, A). These metal salts also cause the release of thyroid-stimulating hormone from the pituitary (LaBella *et al.,* 1973). As with the releasing hormones for FSH and LH, copper may be complexing with the thyroid-stimulating releasing hormone *in situ* with a resulting increase in the lipid solubility of the peptide.

## V. Copper in Pregnancy

### A. Copper Deficiency and Reproductive Failure

Copper deficiency in animals has long been known to cause reproductive failure or abnormal offspring (for review, see Underwood, 1971). Aside from being required for hemoglobin regeneration, copper is also necessary for proper reproduction in rats (Keil and Nelson, 1931). Lambs born in certain pastures have a neonatal ataxia called swayback. The pastures in these cases are low in copper, and the ewes and lambs are copper-deficient (Bennetts and Chapman, 1937). Supplying additional copper to the ewes during pregnancy prevents the disease (Bennetts and Beck, 1942). Cattle have reproductive disturbances and low fertility on copper-deficient pastures (Bennetts and Hall, 1939). The deficiency is thought to cause delayed or depressed estrus (Underwood, 1971, p. 90). Other dietary factors, notably molybdenum, zinc sulfate, and vitamin C, can influence the severity of copper deficiency, as discussed in Section VIII, A. Zinc deficiency can also lead to teratologies (see Section V, C).

Rats fed on a copper-deficient diet have normal estrous cycles and conceive, but the pregnancy ends in fetal death and resorption (Dutt and Mill, 1960). When a copper-deficient diet is started 6 weeks before mating, ovulation and implantation occur during the 22-day gestation, but fetal necrosis is seen by day 13 and placental necrosis by day 15 after mating. If copper is supplemented, the fetuses develop normally (Hall and Howell, 1969; Howell and Hall, 1969). Copper deficiency also induces similar infertility in guinea pigs and sheep (Howell and Hall, 1970). With less severe copper deficiency, the young are born anemic and nonviable and/or have teratologies. Many are edematous and have subcutaneous hemorrhagic lesions and abdominal hernias (O'Dell *et al.*, 1961). Neural lesions are also seen if the live babies are kept on a copper-deficient diet (Carlton and Kelly, 1968). The hemorrhages seen with copper deficiency are probably a result of defective collagen synthesis. Chick embryos from hens receiving a copper-deficient diet show similar hemorrhages, as well as anemia and skeletal deformities (for review, see Levene, 1973). The hemorrhages are the result of defective collagen formation. Copper deficiency in growing animals or adults causes anemia. In addition, there are several other symptoms that can be attributed to defective collagen synthesis. These include bone deformities, cardiovascular disorders, and, especially in poultry, rupture of the aorta (O'Dell *et al.*, 1961; Carnes *et al.*, 1961; Lalich *et al.*, 1965; for review, see Underwood, 1971). The defect in collagen synthesis with copper deficiency is now understood to be a deficiency of the amine oxidase called peptidyl lysyl oxidase (Hill 1969; Pinnell and Martin, 1968). This copper enzyme oxidizes lysine after it has been incorporated into the polypeptide. The aldehydes thus produced form collagen cross-links by aldol condensation (Pinnell and Martin, 1968; Harris *et al.*, 1974; Harris, 1976) (see also Section V, C). If copper is deficient or withdrawn by chelating agents, the resulting defectively formed collagen has fewer cross-links and is structually weaker.

Another way that copper deficiency leads to fetal death could be because of a decline in protein synthesis. Rats fed on a copper-deficient diet have a lower rate of protein synthesis and this is attributed to a decrease in mRNA formation (Halbreich and Weissenberg, 1967). Iron deficiency does not produce this.

For humans, copper deficiency in adults as contrasted with infants (see Section VII, A) is unknown. The diet for adults in most cases far exceeds the daily requirement for copper (Cartwright and Wintrobe, 1964).

Low copper levels in drinking water are correlated with a high incidence of neural tube congenital malformations in Wales (Morton *et al.*, 1976). Many other factors may, however, be involved in the causation of anencephaly and spina bifida (see Morton *et al.*, 1976; Leck, 1974; Carter, 1974; Smithells, 1976). Low zinc levels may also be a factor (see Leck, 1974; cf. Morton *et al.*, 1976).

### B. Copper-Chelating Agents and Fetal Resorption

The diet in the copper deficiency studies on rats is milk treated with hydrogen sulfide to remove the last traces of copper. Perhaps a simple approach to the removal of copper from rats during pregnancy would be to feed the animals a copper-chelating agent. Disulfiram given orally to rats at a dose of 100 mg/day from day 3 of pregnancy causes fetal resorption (Salgo and Oster, 1974b). Just as in the case with the copper-deficient diet, implantation occurs for the disulfiram-tested rats and by day 13 most of the implants were resorbed. Disulfiram itself is not, strictly speaking, a chelating agent but is reduced *in vivo* to form the diethyldithiocarbamate (Ströme, 1965).

The carbamate is a well-known chelating agent specific for copper with much less chelation for zinc (Sandell, 1959, pp. 191–194). The water-soluble sodium salt becomes soluble in nonaqueous solvents when complexed with copper. The disulfide, disulfiram, is lipid-soluble. For rats, the copper-containing enzyme, dopamine $\beta$-hydrolase, is inhibited *in vivo* with a dosage of disulfiram of about 100 mg/day (Goldstein and Nakajima, 1967). Disulfiram is called Antabuse because of the alcohol-intolerance it induces in humans. This effect is thought to be primarily due to the buildup of aldehydes brought about by the inhibition by disulfiram of aldehyde dehydrogenase (for review, see Ritchie, 1974). Inhibition of dopamine $\beta$-hydrolylase and acetaldehyde-induced release of norepinephrine are also involved (see Truitt and Walsh, 1971; Morgan and Cagan, 1974).

For fetal resorption in rats, the dosages of disulfiram required cause toxic reactions in the mother (Salgo and Oster, 1974b). A striking characteristic of the treated animals was their almost total loss of appetite. This anorexia produced by copper-chelating agents is attributed to the loss of taste and smell (see Section III, C). Additional toxic reactions occurred ranging from lethargy to coma and death. Autopsies of the rats revealed discoloration of the liver. The cause of fetal death may be damage to the liver of the fetus by disulfiram. Disulfiram-induced copper deficiency could disrupt fetal development in a variety of ways. Copper deficiencies less severe than those that produce fetal resorption cause internal hemorrhage in the rat fetus as a result of elastin disorders (O'Dell *et al.*, 1961). Lysyl oxidase, a copper enzyme, is required for elastin synthesis (see Section V, A). Copper deficiencies can also cause disorders in erythropoiesis and in bone development (for a review, see Scheinberg and Sternlieb, 1960), both of which might also explain the disulfiram results. Disulfiram in smaller amounts than we used has produced occasional teratologies when given to animals in combination with other agents (Faure-Tissot and Delatour, 1965; Robens, 1969).

### C. Teratogenesis of Related Drugs, Environmental Toxins, and Lathyrogenic Agents

In our further search for oral abortifacients, we tried the experimental drug, *N,N′*-bis(dichloracetyl)-1,8-octamethylenediamine (Win 18,446, Sterling-Winthrop). This bis(dichloracetyl)diamine has many pharmacological properties similar to disulfiram. Both compounds cause alcohol intolerance (Dietrich and Hellerman, 1963) and both inhibit mitochrondrial oxidation and electron transport in similar ways (Merola and Brierley, 1970). Win 18,446 may be a copper-chelating agent. The interaction of the dichloracetylamine group with copper in lipids is suggested by our observation that compounds containing this group enhance the cuprous biquinoline color formation in chloroform.

When Win 18,446 is administered to rats at the appropriate dosage and time of gestation, it produces the resorption of 100% of the embryos with no toxic effect to the mother (Oster *et al.*, 1974). The optimal regimen for embryocidal action is 200 mg daily given at days 10 and 11 of pregnancy. Days 8 through 14 in the rat, corresponding in humans to weeks 3 through 6 after conception, is the period of organogenesis.

When the total dose is less than optimal for fetal resorption and when applied during the period of organogenesis, teratologies appear (Taleporos *et al.*, 1977). Day 11 is the most sensitive time. The teratologies are of high incidence, often occurring in 100% of the offspring of mothers with a certain regimen. Thus, with dosages of Win 18,446 between 50 and 200 mg daily and if the treatment includes day 11, then 100% of the fetuses show persistent truncus arteriosus, a septal heart defect. Other teratologies of high incidence found in this study include bilateral cleft lip, blunt snout, diaphragmatic hernia, cytochemism, and tracheoesophageal abnormalities. From these and other observations it was concluded that Win 18,446 inhibits the proliferation and/or spread of embryonic mesenchyme. It is postulated (Taleporos *et al.*, 1977) that the immediate action of the drug is to inhibit the production of the embryonic ground substance, namely the mucopolysaccharides, that provides the necessary framework for the proliferation and movement of the mesenchyme cells. It was further noted (Taleporos *et al.*, 1977) that the teratologies produced by Win 18,446 have certain similarities to those produced by vitamin A deficiency (Warkany, 1971, pp. 32–33) Vitamin A is required for the synthesis of mucopolysaccharides (Wolf and Varandani, 1960), and Win 18,446 probably inhibits the synthesis of the mucopolysaccharide ground substance (Taleporos *et al.*, 1977). The only obvious adverse effect of prolonged administration of Win 18,446 to the mother rat is xerophthalmia (Oster *et al.*, 1974), the first obvious sign of vitamin A deficiency (for review, see Moore, 1957). We have also found that a large dose of Win 18,446 (200 mg/day) given for several weeks causes in nonpregnant rats persistent cornification of vaginal cells (G. Oster and M. P. Salgo, unpublished observations, 1976). Vitamin A deficiency is known to produce this keratinization and indeed is used as a bioassay for the vitamin (Moore, 1967).

Organogenesis is characterized by periods of intense cell replication followed by differentiation. These periods require not only considerable energy derived from mitochondrial metabolism but, in addition, require the replication of mitochondria themselves. We have tested three drugs, namely disulfiram, Win 18,446, and chloramphenicol, for their effects on rat liver mitochondria (G. Oster, M. P. Salgo, D. S. Beattie, and N. G. Ibraham, unpublished observations, 1973). Chloramphenicol, which, like Win 18,446, is a dichloroacetylamine, is usually considered the most powerful inhibitor of mitochondrial protein synthesis (de Vries and Kroon, 1970; for reviews, see Beattie, 1971). It also inhibits mitochondrial reproduction (Oerter and Merker, 1972). We found that isolated mitochondria are effected by Win 18,446 more than by chloramphenicol. To inhibit tritiated leucine incorporation into mitochondrial protein by two-thirds requires 150 $\mu M$ chloramphenicol but only 25 $\mu M$ Win 18,446. We further found that Win 18,446 and disulfiram are inhibitors of cytochrome oxidase production in the mitochondria of regenerating rat liver. Partially hepatectomized male rats were fed the drugs for 3 days and sacrificed. Aside from the enormous increase in liver fat in the treated rats, the cytochrome oxidase content was markedly depressed. These drugs may be acting directly to withhold copper from cytochrome oxidase synthesis. Copper is considered an essential constituent of cytochrome oxidase and undergoes valence changes in its action in the last step of electron transfer to molecular oxygen (for reviews, see Wharton, 1973; Nicholls and Chance, 1974). One of the first indicators of copper deficiency is a decrease in cytochrome oxidase (Cohen and Elvehjem, 1934; Howell and Davison, 1959). In extreme cases of copper deficiency the oxidative capacity of mitochondria is lost due to a decrease in cytochrome oxidase (Gallagher and Reeve, 1971).

We have confirmed the unpublished findings of others (A. R. Surrey, personal communication, 1974; D. J. Patanelli, personal communication, 1976) that Win 18,446 at doses considerably below those that cause obvious teratologies cause death of the newborn rats within 4 days after birth.

There are a variety of chelating agents that induce abortion, teratologies, fetal death, or obstetrical complications. Dithizone (diphenylthiocarbazone) prevents implantation in rats and reduces fertility in monkeys when given after mating (H. A. Nash, personal communication, 1975, on the work of R. Hertz, L. E. Atkinson, A. Brinson, R. Sanchez, and H. A. Nash). It is not considered a useful postcoital contraceptive agent because of its toxicity. The mode of action of the drug was attributed to probable inhibition of the zinc enzyme carbonic anhydrase, but dithizone binds a variety of other elements including copper (Sandell, 1959, pp. 141 and 453), which can, in fact, displace zinc from dithizone under certain conditions.

Dietary zinc deficiency leads to well-characterized teratologies in rats. The malformations seen include anencephaly and other severe central nervous system and skeletal malformations (Hurley, 1966; for reviews, see Hurley and Shrader, 1972; Warkany and Petering, 1972; Hurley, 1976a,b). In humans there is a potentially fatal disease, acrodermatitis enteropathica in which the skin lesions and bowel problems are a result of zinc deficiency probably due to malabsorption (Moynahan, 1974; see also Anonymous, 1975). Several women with this disease have had spontaneous abortions or delivered babies who were grossly malformed. Some of these malformations resembled those seen in animals with zinc deficiency (Hambridge *et al.,* 1975). Ethylenediaminetetraacetic acid (EDTA) administration to rats also causes deformities, and these can be prevented by concomitant administration of zinc (Swenerton and Hurley, 1971). As discussed in Section VIII, A, sometimes an excess of copper produces the biological effects of zinc deficiency.

Salicylic acid and its derivative salicylamide form strong complexes with metals, particularly with cupric ions (Reid *et al.,* 1951; see Schubert, 1964, pp. 13,63, and 67; Schubert, 1966; Martell and Calvin, 1952). Copper aspirin and copper salicylate are more effective than the parent drug when given parenterally (Sorenson, 1974, 1976). The advantages of the complex when given orally are not as striking (Rainford and Whitehouse, 1976). Aspirin is known to be teratological in rats (Eriksson, 1971) and metal chelation may be a mechanism for this action (Kimmel *et al.,* 1974). Aspirin teratogenicity has been suspected in retrospective studies of mothers who had malformed children (Richards, 1969; Nelson and Forfar, 1971). A recent prospective study of women taking salicylates during pregnancy did not show any teratogenicity.

They did, however, show an increase in anemia, hemorrhages, complicated deliveries, prenatal deaths, and stillbirths in women who took large amounts of salicylates (Collins and Turner, 1975; Turner and Collins, 1975). Large doses of vitamin C can retard the excretion of aspirin, possibly because of the acidification of urine by ascorbic acid. This could increase the aspirin-induced complications in pregnant women taking both aspirin and large doses of vitamin C for a cold. Aspirin also alters the metabolism of vitamin C, changing the tissue–blood distributions in health and diseased states (Wilson, 1976).

There has been concern about the effects of the copper-chelating agent, penicillamine, given during pregnancy (Mjølnerød *et al.,* 1971; Scheinberg and Sternlieb, 1975). Penicillamine is teratological in animals (see in the following). Treatment of Wilson's disease with penicillamine relieves the amenorrhea and spontaneous abortions frequently found in women with the disease (see Section V, D), as well as the other symptoms allowing a normal reproductive life (see Scheinberg and Sternlieb, 1975). There seems to be no adverse effects on either the mother or the child of taking penicillamine in the quantities, usually 1 gm/day, used in the treatment of Wilson's disease. Eighteen women treated for the disease took penicillamine before and throughout pregnancy. A total of twenty-nine offspring were born with no defects (Scheinberg and Sternlieb, 1975). One woman treated with penicillamine through pregnancy had two children with mannosidosis (Arbisser *et al.,* 1976), an inherited metabolic disorder of lysosomal storage (Davis *et al.,* 1972). A third child died with similar symptoms. The association of mannosidosis and penicillamine in pregnancy was thought to be fortuitous since both parents had low mannosidase levels (Arbisser *et al.,* 1976). If higher doses of penicillamine are given, however, there seems to be toxic effects on the fetus. One woman given 2 gm/day for treatment of cystinuria delivered an infant with connective tissue disorders (Mjølnerød *et al.,* 1971; see also Scheinberg and Sternlieb, 1975). Such disorders are not unexpected as penicillamine is known to interfere with collagen synthesis, presumably by withdrawing copper from lysine oxidase (see Section V, A).

The collagen disorders seen with penicillamine are similar to those seen in lathyrism, a toxicity induced by substances in some types of peas. If weanling rats are fed a diet high in seeds of sweet pea, *Lathyrus odoratus,* they develop skeletal abnormalities. Their growth is suppressed and many have hernias (Geiger *et al.,* 1933; for review, see Levene, 1973). The lathyrism seen in animals with *L. odoratus* is also referred to as osteolathyrism to differentiate it from the human neural disease, neurolathyrism, which is seen particularly in India when drought forces people to subsist almost entirely on chick peas, *Lathyrus sativa* (see Levene, 1973).

Lathyrogenic agents are teratological to a variety of animals. Feeding rats a diet of 50% ground sweet pea seeds from day 10 to 20 of pregnancy results in a high incidence of fetal resorption and various malformations in the surviving offspring including edema, severely bent spinal columns, small jaws, and cleft palate (Stamler, 1955; Steffek *et al.*, 1972). Ingestion of plants of the genus *Lathyrus* by grazing animals also results in teratogenesis (see Keeler, 1972). Lathyrogens are also teratological to chicks (see Levene, 1973).

The toxic factor of lathyrism is β-aminopropionitrile (BAPN), at least for osteolathyrism (see Levene, 1971, 1973). A variety of other substances have lathyrogenic activity as measured by inhibition of collagen synthesis in chick eggs (see Levene, 1973). These include organic nitriles, semicarbazides, hydrazides, and hydrazines (Levene, 1971, 1973). Penicillamine is also considered a lathyrogenic agent. Treating rats with high doses of penicillamine during pregnancy resulted in fetal resorption or malformed offspring similar to treatment with the lathyrogens, aminoacetonitrile and semicarbazide. In some penicillamine regimens, 80% of the surviving offspring had cleft palate (Steffek *et al.*, 1972).

The symptoms of osteolathyrism resemble those seen in copper deficiency (Savage *et al.*, 1962; see Levene, 1973). One of the principal theories of the mode of action of lathyrogenic agents is that they are copper-chelating agents (Dasler and Stoner, 1959; see also Levene, 1973). In a comparison of the lathyrogenic activity of homologous compounds, only those that could form 5 or 6-membered chelate rings are lathyrogenic (Dasler and Stoner, 1959; see also Levene, 1973). Some chelating agents such as Versene (EDTA) and alizarin are not lathyrogenic (Levene, 1961, 1973), but these two chelating agents are not particularly specific. Although copper forms strong complexes with EDTA, the presence in higher concentrations of calcium or iron could diminish the effect (see Martell and Calvin, 1952, pp. 537–538).

Another related teratogenic agent is a breakdown product of copper-chelating agent fungicides (Khera, 1973; Ruddick and Khera, 1975). The fungicides themselves are teratological only at high doses (see Section IX, B, 1). Cooking of vegetables sprayed with ethylenebis(dithiocarbamate) fungicides results in the production of the much more potent teratogen, ethylene thiourea (Newsome and Laver, 1973; Watts *et al.*, 1974). This compound causes teratologies in rats even with a single oral dose during days 10–21 of pregnancy. A large variety of teratologies are produced, some in 100% of the offspring. The teratologies found include cleft lip, cleft palate, hydrocephalus, hydranencephaly, edema, and spina bifida. The type of teratology found depends on the day of pregnancy on which ethylene thiourea is administered (Ruddick and Khera, 1975). Aside from being carcinogenic (for references, see Ruddick and Khera, 1975), ethylene thiourea also causes enlargement of the thyroid in rats (Graham and Hansen, 1972), but this is thought to be independent of its teratogenic action (Lu and Staples, 1976). There are naturally occurring goitrogenic substances called goitrins found in some vegetables including cabbage, rutabagas, and turnips. These are thiocyanate and thiooxazolidone (Kingsbury, 1975) and are obviously related to ethylene thiourea. Although many factors may be involved in the causation of neural tube malformations in man (see Leck, 1974; Carter, 1974; Smithells, 1976), the naturally occurring goitrins (P. Stanway, personal communications, 1976) and ethylene thiourea (Aylett, 1974) have been hypothesized as a possible cause of anencephaly and spina bifida. Recently, however, goitrin has been found to be nonteratogenic, at least for rats (Khera, 1976). Ethylene thiourea is used in the rubber industry. An alarmingly high incidence of spina bifida in one town may be related to the rubber or plastic industry there (Aylett, 1973). The ability to taste bitter compounds such as the copper-chelating agents, phenylthiocarbamide, propylthiouracil, and goitrin, is inherited (see Weinstein and Kitchin, 1971). The proportion of nontasters in women who have had children with spina bifida is presently being measured compared to the population generally (P. Stanway, personal communication, 1976). Nontasters do not find vegetables bitter and thus might eat more goitrin-containing vegetables than tasters. This may be one factor in the incidence of goiter (McConnell *et al.,* 1975). (In Section III, C other aspects of copper in taste and smell are considered.)

### D. Copper Excess

Placing a small copper wire loop through the uterine lumen after implantation in rats, hamsters, and rabbits has no effect on the offspring (Chang and Tatum, 1973). The wire loops, thought to release about 2.75 mg of copper a day for the rats and hamsters and about 5.5 mg of copper a day for the rabbits, had no demonstrable effect on gestation, parturition, or lactation except for a decrease in the number of offspring seen. The offspring ($F_1$) and their subsequent offspring ($F_2$) all appeared normal (Chang and Tatum, 1973).

The decrease in the number of pups born to rats with copper wires inserted into the uterus after implantation is attributable to an increase in fetal resorption, as seen by sacrificing the rats at different stages of gestation (Chang and Tatum, 1975). The incidence of fetal resorption increased the longer the copper was left *in utero*, with the highest incidence (59.6%) when the wire was left in place until day 18. No teratologies were noted under these conditions (Chang and Tatum, 1975). Placing Cu-IUDs into the uteri of sheep so that they come into contact with the embryonic membranes of the developing embryo seems to have no greater detrimental effect on embryo survival than inert IUDs (Hawk *et al.*, 1974) (see also Section II, C, 4).

Intravenous or subcutaneous injection of copper salts during pregnancy has serious effects, however. In rats, subcutaneous injection of copper acetate from day 7 to 10 of pregnancy interrupts pregnancy in 50% of the cases. Progesterone has a protective effect (Marois and Buvet, 1972). Intravenous injection of cupric salts in pregnant rabbits on days 8, 9, and 10 had no effect, even though doses used were the same high doses used to induce ovulation in rabbits (Marois and Buvet, 1972) (see Section IV, A). The action of copper on the rat, but not on the rabbit, and the protection in the rat by progesterone suggests that copper interrupts pregnancy by acting on the hypothalamus (Marois and Buvet, 1972).

Copper salts injected into pregnant hamsters are teratological (Ferm and Hanlon, 1974). Injection on day 8 of pregnancy causes an increase in resorptions and incidence of malformations in surviving fetuses. Malformations of the heart were especially evident, but others including thoracic wall hernias, spina bifida, and even complete nonclosure of the spinal cord and brain were also seen (Fern and Hanlon, 1974). Injection of copper salts into chicken eggs is also teratological and embryocidal (King and Hsu, 1976). Endogenous copper is thought to participate in normal genetic information transfer *via* interaction with chromatin (Bryan *et al.,* 1976) and hence copper excess might be expected to interfere with genetic regulation.

Women having Wilson's disease, an inherited disorder of copper accumulation (see Section VII, B), are frequently amenorrheic (Scheinberg and Sternlieb, 1965, 1975). This might be a result of copper interference with the hypothalamus or pituitary (see Section IV, A). Pregnancy that occurs in women with untreated Wilson's disease often ends in spontaneous abortion (Sternlieb and Scheinberg, 1964; Scheinberg and Sternlieb, 1965, 1975). These changes are thought to be secondary to liver damage, but the copper might be acting on steroid metabolism in the liver, on the hypothalamus, or the excess copper could be affecting the uterus (see Sections IV, B; II, A, 7; and V, E). Treatment of women with Wilson's disease with penicillamine allows normal reproduction (Scheinberg and Sternlieb, 1975) (see also Section V, C).

Copper and zinc are antagonists, and an excess of one can cause a relative deficiency of the other (Van Campen, 1969; Murthy *et al.*, 1975) (see Section VIII, A). Copper excess may contribute to zinc deficiency in humans (see, for example, Pfeiffer and Iliev, 1972). Zinc deficiency, which can be induced in a few days in animals, leads to teratologies in a variety of species (see Section V, C) (for recent reviews, see Hurley, 1976a,b). Partial zinc deficiency prenatally results in increased aggressive behavior in rats (Halas *et al.*, 1975). Women with acrodermatitis enteropathica, a disease of aberrant zinc metabolism, have given birth to grossly malformed children (Hambridge *et al.*, 1975) (see also Section V, C). Zinc deficiency in otherwise healthy women has been suggested as a contributing factor to human teratologies (Hurley and Shrader, 1972; Warkany and Petering, 1972; for additional references, see Hambridge *et al.*, 1975; Hurley, 1976a).

### E. Copper in Parturition

There are reports from the Soviet literature of relations of copper with labor. In cases of spontaneous abortion, blood copper levels are lower than in women with normal deliveries (Khodak, 1971). This is another example of ceruloplasmin changes during normal and abnormal pregnancies discussed in Section III, A. Placentas from cases of spontaneous abortion bind more copper than placentas from normal pregnancies (Fogel, 1971). Copper salts have been used to speed up labor. Injection of 0.2% $CuSO_4$ i.m. is said to shorten parturition and lower the incidence of obstetrical complications (see, for example, Shaimanov, 1970). These findings are compatible with the effects of copper on the rat myometrium *in vitro* (Salgo and Oster, 1974a) (see Section II, B, 7). Intrauterine copper sulfate administration has been used in attempts to induce abortion in animals (M. P. Salgo and A. I. Csapo, unpublished observations, 1972). Large doses of cupric salts injected into the uterus resulted in slight increases in intrauterine pressure, but no abortion.

The Soviet work in humans described above may be related to the effects of copper on PG biosynthesis (see Sections II, B, 7 and IV, C). Inhibitors of PG synthesis delay parturition (Aiken, 1972; see also Karim and Hillier, 1975). One such inhibitor, aspirin, used in the animal study, chelates copper (Martell and Calvin, 1952) (see also Section V, C). Women taking large quantities of salicylates have an increased incidence of prolonged gestation and of complications during delivery (Collins and Turner, 1975).

In rats, a dietary deficiency of copper has a limited effect on labor (Apgar, 1968b). The length of parturition was slightly but not significantly increased in rats kept on a copper-deficient diet for 2 months prior to mating. Perinatal mortality was higher for offspring from copper-deficient mothers. Some of the copper-deficient mother rats had difficulty in parturition. The young of these rats had lower liver copper levels than those born from copper-deficient mothers that did not have difficulty in labor. This suggests that copper may be required for parturition (Apgar, 1968b). Compatible with this result is that rats given disulfiram for the 2 days prior to expected delivery (day 22) seem to have a delayed and difficult labor in addition to a high incidence of stillbirths (M. P. Salgo and G. Oster, unpublished observations, 1973). Zinc deficiency in rats results in severe difficulties in parturition (Apgar, 1968a,b). Rats put on a zinc-deficient diet on day 1 of pregnancy develop zinc deficiency, as evidenced by anorexia by day 11. At delivery, the zinc-deficient rats had severe problems in parturition not seen in control or pair fed control rats (Apgar, 1968a). In view of the antagonism between copper and zinc (Section VIII, A), one might expect an excess of copper to produce the same effect.

## VI. Copper and Sperm

### A. Spermicidal Action of Copper and of Chelating Agents

By far the most effective spermicidal agent yet found is diethyldithiocarbamate; a $10^{-5}$ $M$ solution produces complete sperm immobilization (Holzaepfel *et al.*, 1959; see also White, 1955a; Rice, 1964; Saito *et al.*, 1967a,b). In a comparison of spermicidal action of chelating agents, those that are characteristic for copper were effective (White, 1955a) but many of the agents (e.g., cupferron, dithizone, 8-hydroxylquinoline, and *o*-phenanthroline) also chelate other transition metal ions (Phillips and Williams, 1966). Diethyldithiocarbamate strongly chelates Cu(II), less strongly Zn(II), but Fe(II) practically not at all (see Sandell, 1959).

An excess of cupric ion, of the order of $10^{-4}$ $M$ is likewise spermicidal (see Section II, B, 1) (see also White, 1955b; Saito *et al.*, 1967a,b). The action of copper may be to cause the conversion of essential sulfhydryl groups to disulfides. Copper(II) is a powerful catalyst for the autooxidation of glutathione (Tsen and Tappel, 1958). It may be reduced by SH and the Cu(I) thereby formed reacts with oxygen to generate oxidizing free radicals and to re-form Cu(II). The addition of a chelating agent with copper can have diverse effects. For example, the oxidation of glutathione can be enhanced by addition of *o*-phenanthroline so that as little as $10^{-9}$ *M* Cu(II) is effective (Kobashi, 1968), whereas other chelating agents (e.g., EDTA) can inhibit the effect. The chemistry of disulfide formation and cleavage involves intermediates (Rosenthal and Oster, 1954), many of which could complex with either Cu(I) or Cu(II). The addition of chelating agent further complicates the picture. Still another complication, at least in bull sperm, is the presence of sulfite (Mann, 1964, p. 96) which, as is practiced in standard protein chemistry (see, for example, Bailey, 1967) interchanges with disulfide bonds when catalyzed by copper ions.

The survival of sperm can be limited by the action of spermine oxidase, a copper-containing enzyme (for review, see Malmström *et al.*, 1975). The characteristic odor of human semen is due to the action of this enzyme on spermine, a polyamine normally found in the seminal plasma. These volatile breakdown products are toxic to spermatozoa (Tabor and Rosenthal, 1956).

Copper wires implanted into the seminal vesicles of animals have a limited effect on subsequent fertility (Gilmore *et al.*, 1973). The copper seminal vesical implants resulted in a 91% decrease in conception rate in rats, a 25% decrease for hamsters, and no decrease for rabbits. Copper wires in rats were more effective than Silastic implant. The copper showed only slight restoration of fertility on removal. Surgical removal of the seminal vesicles causes a decrease in fertility in rats but not in hamsters or rabbits (Gilmore *et al.*, 1973). The semen of the treated rabbits did show an occasional increase in copper but apparently not regularly enough or in great enough amounts to alter fertility (Gilmore *et al.*, 1973).

### B. Sulfhydryl Groups and Sperm Maturation

It has long been appreciated that spermatozoa are rich in sulfur. The histones of mammalian sperm nucleoproteins are difficult to extract because of the large amount of disulfide bonds presumably formed during extraction. The tail proteins are rich in cysteine and the importance of sulfhydryl compounds, such as glutathione, in the semen for maintenance of sperm motility is appreciated (Mann, 1964, p. 284).

It can be shown that S—S bonds are important for the structural stability of sperm since reduction of these bonds with dithiothreitol followed by detergent (SDS) causes the head to swell and the tail to dissolve (Calvin and Bedford, 1971; see also Calvin *et al.*, 1976). In this sense, the structural proteins of spermatozoa resemble the keratin of hair. As the spermatozoa mature in the epididymis, there is an increasing amount of disulfide bond formation. This leads to increased stability, but, if oxidation is carried too far, as occurs with cupric ion, the tail may be too stiff for proper motility. Rigidification of the head by normal disulfide formation could play a crucial role in the fertilization process (Bedford and Calvin, 1974).

The high concentration of zinc in the prostate gland and hence in the semen has long been considered remarkable (Mann, 1964, pp. 25 and 44). Zinc ions form complexes with sulfhydryl groups as shown by the decrease in reaction with indoacetamide (Calvin *et al.*, 1973). Zinc protects the sulfhydryl groups from oxidation by copper (Calvin *et al.*, 1973). Although copper ions as well as zinc ions bind strongly to SH, only the former can undergo valence changes leading to oxidation of the substrate. Thus, copper and zinc work in opposite ways to maintain the appropriate SH to SS ratio as the sperm matures.

### C. Inhibition of Spermatogenesis

Cadmium salts cause testicular damage in laboratory animals (for review, see Patanelli, 1975). The effect of cadmium is ultimately on the vasculature of the testes resulting in ischemia and necrosis. Zinc ions or added mercaptans will block this action of cadmium implying that in the capillaries cadmium binds strongly to sulfhydryl groups. Because cadmium has widespread toxicity, especially in inducing high blood pressure (for review, see Beliles, 1975), it is not seriously considered as a male contraceptive.

Copper ions injected into laboratory animals produce testicular damage which is histologically similar to that produced by cadmium, but to a lesser degree (Hoey, 1966). Copper and cadmium differ, however, in that copper does not produce the ultimate necrosis characteristic of cadmium although there is some necrosis at the head of the epididymis caused by copper. Apparently the action of copper is not as specifically directed to the vasculature as it is for cadmium (Hoey, 1966). Intratesticular injection of copper sulfate has caused teratomas in chickens (see Section II, C, 1).

There seems to be no evidence of male sterility in cases of copper deficiency in animals (see Underwood, 1971). Zinc deficiency, however, leads to testicular atrophy (Prasad, 1967). Gross zinc deficiency has been seen in young men in Iran and Egypt, probably due to poor diet and perhaps to malabsorption from eating clay. The resulting symptoms include dwarfism, hypogonadism and lack of secondary sex characteristics, which all respond to zinc treatment. Similar symptoms are seen in zinc-deficient animals (Prasad, 1967, 1972; see also Anonymous, 1975) (see Section III, C).

The monoamine oxidase inhibitor, pargyline, has been shown to interfere with spermatogenesis in rats (Urry and Dougherty, 1975). Brain monoamine oxidases, which is inhibited by pargyline and related agents, may not be a copper enzyme (see Bright and Porter, 1975; Malmström *et al.,* 1975). Long-term oral administration of the copper-chelating agent sodium diethyldithiocarbamate to dogs led, at least in some cases, to partial testicular atrophy (Sunderman *et al.,* 1967). A low sperm count was seen in 2 men taking Antabuse (Rice, 1964). Loss of libido is one side effect sometimes seen with Antabuse (see Ritchie, 1965). A far more definitive finding is the suppression of spermatogenesis in rats by bis(dichloracetyl)diamines (Coulston *et al.,* 1960). The most effective of this class of drugs is Win 18,446, which causes a complete arrest of spermatogenesis (Beyler *et al.,* 1961). Leydig cell morphology was not altered nor was the production of androgens. This drug does not suppress the production of gonadotropins. It acts at a very early stage of spermatogenesis. At maximal dosage, only Sertoli cells and a few spermatogonia are seen in the seminiferous tubules (Beyler *et al.,* 1961). Win 18,446 was shown to be successful in the suppression of spermatogenesis in man (Heller *et al.,* 1961), but, because of the alcohol intolerance it produces, similar to that of the copper-chelating agent disulfiram, this use was abandoned (see Patanelli, 1975).

The mode of action of Win 18,446 in the suppression of spermatogenesis is unclear but our findings of its effect on the embryo (see Section V, C) strongly suggest that copper chelation is involved, and the ultimate biochemical action may involve inhibition of mitochondrial cytochrome oxidase assembly and/or mucopolysaccharide synthesis. Vitamin A deficiency causes male sterility (for review, see Moore, 1967; Wasserman and Corradino, 1971) with testicular injury as well as effects on accessory male organs. Vitamin A is required for mucopolysaccharide production, and its deficiency results in decreased incorporation of sulfonic acid groups into mucopolysaccharides (Wolf and Varandani, 1960; see also Wasserman and Corradino, 1971). Our finding that prolonged administration of high doses of Win 18,446 to rats leads to xerophthalmia further implicates some common pathway for the actions of the drug and of vitamin A (Oster *et al.,* 1974).

## VII. Copper and the Neonate and Infant

### A. Copper in Infant Nutrition

The nursing infant depends almost entirely on its liver reserves for copper. Milk has copper in only trace amounts, about $1.5 \times 10^{-6}$ *M* for human milk and less for cow milk (Silver *et al.*, 1973). Indeed, if the copper level in milk were much higher there would be considerable autooxidation of unsaturated lipids, including vitamin A, and of vitamin C (Oser, 1965, p. 378). Cupric-catalyzed autooxidation of vitamin C is dependent on chloride ion but not sulfate or phosphate (Abel, 1956; Géro and le Gallic, 1952). This strongly suggests the involvement of Cu(I) since cuprous ion forms a complex with chloride ion (see also Section II, B, 8).

Most newborn mammals have higher liver copper concentrations than do adults (see Underwood, 1971, Table 9). For man the liver of the newborn infant has about 7 times the copper concentration of that of the adult (Kleinman and Klinke, 1930; Morrison and Nash, 1930). In marked contrast, the serum levels are low—one-tenth of the adult (Friis-Hansen, 1971). The peak in liver copper occurs at, or shortly after, birth and declines during the suckling period. The neonatal liver copper is found predominantly in the mitochondrial fraction (Porter *et al.*, 1962). The copper content of subcellular fractions of the liver as the animal ages has been studied for the rat (Gregoriadis and Sorukes, 1967). Whereas at birth most of the copper is in the mitochondrial fraction and only one-fifth in the soluble (supernatant) fraction, in the adult rat half the copper is in this fraction. A specific copper-binding protein has been found in the heavy lysosomes of the mitochondrial fraction of liver homogenates (Porter, 1974). The protein is very rich in cysteine similar to the copper-binding protein metallothionein (see Evans, 1973). The protein is particularly characteristic of the neonate and probably serves a specific storage and detoxifying function for copper (Porter, 1974). The high copper levels in the neonate liver are not damaging as they are in cases of copper accumulation in the adult liver (see Section II, C, 6) perhaps because of the protective action of this neonatal liver protein.

On the basis of the foregoing, one would expect copper deficiency in infants to occur either (*a*) in premature babies when the liver copper did not rise to the normal high level or (*b*) when the infant is kept exclusively on milk for too long. Copper is required for erythropoiesis (Hart *et al.*, 1928; Frieden, 1973) and, hence, copper deficiency is manifested as hypochromic anemia. There is a classic rat nutrition experiment demonstrating the relief of anemia with supplemental copper (Oser, 1965, p. 572). It has long been appreciated that milk-fed infants with anemia respond to iron supplemented with copper (Josephs, 1931). Copper deficiency is part of a multiple deficiency associated with diets consisting mainly of milk (Sturgeon and Brubaker, 1956).

Pure copper deficiency as a true clinical entity has now been confirmed. In premature infants fed on unsupplemented milk diet, the hypochromic anemia that developed was unresponsive to iron alone but responded immediately to added copper (Al-Rashid and Spangler, 1971; Seely *et al.*, 1972; Ashkenazi *et al.* 1973; see also Graham, 1971; Griscom *et al.*, 1971). Symptoms include, aside from the anemia, a failure to thrive, leukopenia, bone changes, depigmentation of the skin, dermatitis, and psychomotor and visual problems (see especially Ashkenazi *et al.*, 1973). A copper-deficiency anemia in a full-term baby arising from prolonged parenteral feeding was likewise responsive to additional copper (Karpel and Peden, 1972). In most infant copper deficiencies, accompanying the anemia that is resistant to iron therapy are neutropenia, bone changes similar to those of vitamin C deficiency, neurological symptoms, and hair changes (see in the following). The necessity of copper in infant diet has prompted the American Academy of Pediatrics to consider addition of copper to formulas for low-birth-weight infants (Holliday, 1974; see also Cordano, 1974).

The severe protein deficiency, kwashiorkor, refers in an African language to the deposed child who is no longer suckled. Some of the manifestations of the disease, notably the poor quality of the hair and its loss of pigmentation are also seen in animals whose diet is deficient in copper. Thus, sheep raised on copper-deficient soil develop poor quality wool and, for black-wooled sheep, the hair is not pigmented (see Underwood, 1971, pp. 87–90). When copper is restored to the diet, the quality and normal color of the wool returns (see remarkable photographs in Underwood 1971, pp. 88 and 89). This same type of phenomenon can be demonstrated in a variety of domestic animals. These are manifestations of the requirement of copper for the autooxidation of sulfhydryl groups in keratin formation (see Section, VI, B) and of the well-known melanin reactions of tyrosinase to cause pigmentation (for reviews, see Montagna and Hu, 1967; cf. Okun *et al.*, 1972). For the case of kwashiorkor, there is not necessarily an overall loss of copper content in the hair (Lea and Luttrell, 1965). Copper deficiency is associated with iron deficiency in hypoproteinemia (Sturgeon and Brubaker, 1956), and the anemia accompanying the disease responds best if copper is added with the iron (Zipursky *et al.*, 1958; Schubert and Lahey, 1959). Treatment of severely malnourished infants with high-calorie diet can lead to a full blown copper-deficiency anemia with some resemblance to a vitamin C deficiency (Cordano *et al.*, 1964). Vitamin A deficiency usually accompanies kwashiorkor even when carotenes are supplied in the diet, but copper may be required for oxidative cleavage of $\beta$-carotene to yield vitamin A. Copper deficiency has likewise been found in the severe protein–calorie infant malnutrition, marasmus (Graham and Cordano, 1969; Lehmann *et al.*, 1971). The copper deficiency encountered in these severely protein-deficient diseases may be a result of the lack of chelating amino acids which are important for copper transport across the intestines. Amino acids are important in the transport of copper across membranes (Kirchgessner and Grassmann, 1970; see also Evans, 1973). Some symptoms of kwashiorkor, particularly the mental depression, are similar to symptoms seen with zinc deficiency (Moynahan, 1976).

Supplemental copper in the diet of young pigs has been shown to increase their rate of growth (Evvard *et al.*, 1928; Barber *et al.*, 1955; Braude and Ryder, 1973). Thus, giving copper salts in the feed to early weaned piglets may cause a rate of growth as much as 20% higher than that of the controls. The treated pigs require less feed. Under some circumstances, the usually recommended highest dose, namely 250 ppm Cu in the pig ration, may be toxic, in which case zinc salt added to the rations counteracts the copper toxicity (Suttle and Mills, 1966). One effect of copper supplementation is the change in quality of the fat; the copper diet produces a softer adipose tissue (Castell and Bowland, 1968). The fat is lower in melting point due to the increased unsaturation in the fatty acids and to alteration of the triglyceride structure (Christie and Moore, 1969; Elliott and Bowland, 1970). Despite the obvious economic importance of enhanced growth rate and more efficient utilization of feed by copper supplementation, the biochemical basis for the phenomenon is not understood (for bibliographies, see Underwood, 1971; Braude, 1975).

### B. Copper in Inherited Metabolic Diseases

One inherited disorder of copper metabolism is Menkes's kinky hair syndrome (Menkes *et al.*, 1962; for recent review, see Danks, 1975). This rare X-linked recessive disease, fatal before the child is 3 years old, is characterized by slow growth, cerebral degeneration, and peculiar stubby pale hair called kinky or steely hair. There are low levels of serum copper and ceruloplasmin. The defect lies in decreased intestinal absorption of copper (Danks *et al.*, 1972a,b). Duodenal mucosa from patients with the disease showed abnormally high concentrations of copper due to failure to transport copper across the serosal cell membrane (Danks *et al.*, 1973). Treatment by parenteral copper administration gives increased plasma and liver copper levels but, when treatment was started at 3 months of age, no clinical improvement occurred (Danks *et al.*, 1972a; Bucknall *et al.*, 1973). Parenteral copper treatment started at an earlier age seems effective (Grover and Scrutton,

1975). Defective placental transport does not seem to be a cause for the disease (Horn *et al.*, 1975).

Two inherited diseases of young mice show symptoms similar to those of human babies suffering from the Menkes's kinky hair syndrome (Hunt, 1974; Hurley and Bell, 1975). Both mice mutants show crinkled hair and pale coloration. One disease, the mottled syndrome (Hunt, 1974), is an X-linked recessive with neurological disturbances and high fatalities similar to Menkes's kinky hair syndrome. Intestinal absorption of copper is impaired in the mottled syndrome mice, and tissue levels are less than those of normals. The other disease, crinkled mutant, is an autosomal recessive mutant with thin skin and high infant mortality (Hurley and Bell, 1975). The appearance of the hair is exactly like that of Menkes's kinky syndrome. When extra dietary copper is given to the mother during pregnancy and lactation, the offspring become darker in color, their skin is thicker, the hair improves, and there is higher survival.

A third mouse mutant, called quaking, is similar to some of the neurological signs of copper-deficient animals. Copper supplementation to the diet of homozygous quaking mice decreases their tremors, indicating that copper metabolism is involved in the expression of the gene (Keen and Hurley, 1976).

There are other inherited metabolic diseases characterized by poor pigmentation and/or low quality hair suggesting that biochemical pathways involving copper enzymes are impaired. The metabolic defects in the varieties of albinism are in the pathways from tyrosine to melanin, and some forms of the disease involve differences of the copper enzyme, tryosinase (for reviews, see Fitzpatrick and Quevedo, 1972; Witkop *et al.*, 1974). Phenylketonuria is a disease in which a deficiency in phenylalanine hydroxylase is believed to be the cause of the observed buildup of phenylalanine, some 50 times the normal plasma level. These children have light-colored hair because the excess phenylalanine can act as a competitive inhibitor for tyrosinase, and administration of tyrosine causes the hair to grow dark (see Knox, 1972). The added tyrosine does not, however, reverse the brain damage resulting from some by-product, probably phenylethylamine, of the excess phenylalanine (G. Jervis, personal communication).

It is difficult to isolate the enzymes whose deficiency causes the metabolic disorder. To establish which metal, if any, is acting as a cofactor is a problem of extreme subtlety. Often it is especially difficult to decide whether an oxidase is a copper or an iron (or both) enzyme. For example, to demonstrate that *p*-hydroxypyruvate oxidase, an important enzyme in the catabolic pathway of tyrosine, was a copper enzyme required testing for inhibition with a variety of chelating agents (Goodwin, 1972). Phenylalanine hydroxylase is believed to be a heme enzyme, but the demonstration for this (Fisher *et al.*, 1972; see also Kaufman and Fisher, 1974) does not rule out the possibility that it is a copper oxidase. The inhibiting chelating agents not only chelate iron but also copper. There are a number of chelating agents that specifically inhibit copper enzymes (see, for example, Nara and Yasunoba, 1966) and added copper may not restore the activity. Activation by addition of Fe(II) could serve to reduce Cu(II) to Cu(I) (see Goodwin, 1972, p. 23) which, on autooxidation, would produce oxidizing free radicals. Incidentally, most samples of commercially available iron salts, even the analytically pure grades, contain appreciable amounts of copper as an impurity. The fact that an enzyme is inhibited by excess copper does not exclude it from being a copper enzyme. For example, ceruloplasmin shows this property (I. H. Scheinberg, personal communication, 1975), as do dopamine hydroxylase, tyrosinase, and other enzymes. As described in Section II, B, 8, copper can cause the autooxidation of benzene to produce phenol. Whatever the phenylalanine hydroxylase enzyme is, its deficiency in phenylketonuria might conceivably be circumvented by administration of an artificial oxidase, such as copper in appropriate form. The present method of treating the disease involves the costly procedure of supplying a phenylalanine-free diet from birth until 4 years of age.

The disorder of copper metabolism in humans that has been most studied is Wilson's disease (for reviews, see, for example, Scheinberg and Sternlieb, 1965; Walshe, 1966; and for emphasis on pediatric aspects, see Sass-Kortsak, 1975). This is a rare disease inherited as an autosomal recessive, in which copper accumulates in the tissue, particularly in the liver, kidney, and brain. Copper accumulation is often visible as Kayser-Fleisher rings: zones of green-brown deposition in the cornea. The classic finding in children is hepatic degeneration similar to liver damage seen in animals with copper poisoning (see Section II, C, 6). Adult onset of the disease is characterized primarily by neurological disturbances.

The metabolic lesion that results in the tissue accumulation of copper is not known. In practically all cases, ceruloplasmin levels are low. Ceruloplasmin is a glycoprotein. If rabbit ceruloplasmin is treated with neuraminidase and injected into the animal, it disappears from the circulation and the copper is found in the liver (Morell *et al.*, 1968). There are other important glycoproteins including FSH, LH, and human chorionic gonadotropin (HCG) whose maintenance in the bloodstream is dependent on its sialic acid content, since the glycoproteins disappear from the circulation after treatment with neuraminidase (for review, see Ashwell and Morell, 1974).

Untreated Wilson's disease eventually leads to death. The similarity of Wilson's disease to copper poisoning suggests the use of zinc salts, which have a protective effect in copper toxicity (see Sections VII, A and VIII, A). So far as we are aware, zinc therapy for this disease has not been tried. The disease can be controlled by the copper-chelating agent penicillamine ($\beta$-dimethylcysteine) (Walshe, 1956). More recently, another oral copper-chelating agent, triethylenetetramine, has been successfully used for patients who cannot, primarily because of allergic reactions, tolerate penicillamine (Walshe, 1969; Dixon *et al.*, 1972). Only the D-isomer of penicillamine is used; the L-isomer is poisonous (for review, see Jocelyn, 1972). This toxicity is due to a depletion of pyridoxal phosphate (vitamin $B_6$); pyridoxal administration can prevent the toxicity (Kuchinsas and Du Vigneaud, 1957). Thiols react with the aldehyde of pyridoxal, and the pyridoxal can thus no longer interact as a cofactor; the excretion of pyridoxal is increased (Jocelyn, 1972, p. 346). It should be recalled that added copper enhances transamination and other pyridoxal-catalyzed reactions (for review, see Holm, 1973), suggesting that copper chelation by penicillamine may also play a role in altering pyridoxal-related functions. D-Penicillamine, aside from acting as a metal chelator, can also cause cystine excretion. Penicillamine undergoes disulfide interchange with cystine to give the mixed disulfide, which is more water-soluble than cystine itself (see Jocelyn, 1972, p. 344). This increased excretion of cysteinyl residues is the basis for its use in cystinuria, another inherited disease (Hartley and Walshe, 1963; see also Jocelyn, 1972, p. 344). D-Penicillamine also interferes with the synthesis of collagen (Hartley and Walshe, 1963; see also Jocelyn, 1972, p. 345). This could arise by disulfide interchange or other mechanisms (Jocelyn, 1972, p. 345) but, in our opinion, is more likely to be due to chelation of copper which removes it from the copper enzyme, lysyl oxidase. This enzyme oxidizes lysine after it has been incorporated into the peptide (Harris, 1976). The oxidation forms aldehydes. The cross-linking is believed to occur by subsequent aldol condensation of the aldehyde groups (for review, see Rojkind and Zeichner, 1973).

## VIII. Copper Antagonists

### A. Zinc and Other Inorganic Antagonists

Zinc, like copper, effects practically all phases of mammalian reproductive process for both male and female (for review, see Underwood,

1971, pp. 226–230). Copper and zinc are often antagonists in reproductive physiology and in metabolism generally. They are nutritional antagonists (Van Campen, 1969; Murthy *et al.*, 1975; see Underwood, 1974, p. 218). In sperm maturation (Section VI, B) we discussed another level of antagonism. The anemia and reproductive failure of zinc toxicity in animals is thought to be due to the induced copper deficiency (Li and Vallee, 1973). It is reversed if copper is added (see also Underwood, 1971, pp. 243–244). Conversely, copper toxicity can be alleviated with added zinc (see Underwood 1971, p. 102). Indeed, one hypothesis of the mode of action of copper metal in the Cu-IUD is that copper replaces zinc in carbonic anhydrase, an enzyme thought to by crucial for implantation (Zipper *et al.*, 1971) (see Section II, B, 5).

Zinc ions and cupric ions compete for mercaptan-binding sites in metallothionein (Evans *et al.*, 1970) and this may also occur for ceruloplasmin (Frieden and Osaki, 1970). Cadmium ions as well as zinc ions compete with copper ions for binding sites on duodenal protein (Starcher, 1969). The toxic action of cadmium as in testicular damage is probably due to the particularly strong ability of cadmium to precipitate proteins, whereas copper is less damaging (see Section VI, C). Zinc is required for the activity of large numbers of enzymes (Vallee, 1959; Parisi and Vallee, 1969; Li and Vallee, 1973) and in most cases acts by maintaining the conformation of the protein. Zinc and cadmium differ from copper in that copper ions may undergo valence changes, whereas zinc and cadmium ions do not. Thus only copper can produce autooxidations.

Molybdenum–copper interactions, an important factor in animal nutrition, is complicated and depends on other factors, notably sulfate (for review, see Underwood, 1971, pp. 132–135; see also Anonymous, 1970; Suttle, 1973). Molybdenum can, like copper, undergo valence changes. Eight valence states are common and some of these play a role in such molybdenum-containing enzymes as xanthine oxidase and sulfite oxidase (for review, see Bray, 1975). Copper also seems to be important for *in vivo* oxidation of sulfur (Siegel and Monty, 1961). It seems that high dietary copper can compensate for the decreased oxidation of sulfur encountered with very high levels of molybdenum. This may be an example of copper serving as an *in vivo* source of oxidase activity.

### B. Vitamins

Vitamin A deficiency leads to many reproductive problems (see Sections II, B, 5; V, C; and VI, C). Vitamin A is required for the incorporation of sulfate into mucopolysaccharides (Wolf and Varandini,

1960; cf., however, Silbert, 1973) and, as seen in the foregoing, copper can play a role in availability of sulfate. Win 18,446, which we believe to be a copper-chelating agent active in lipid media, produces biological effects similar to those encountered with vitamin A deficiency (see Section V, C). A condition in cattle known as X-disease which has the appearance of vitamin A deficiency can be induced by spraying the animals with thiocyanate derivative insecticides (Hoekstra, *et al.*, 1954; Roels, 1967, p. 166). Presumably here too, copper-catalyzed oxidation is inhibited. One of the early vitamin A deficiency symptoms is an incoordination of bulls with a resulting inability to mount a receptive cow (for review, see Salisbury and Van Demark, 1961). This incoordination has the aspect of a vestibular disorder and may be due to a shortage of the crucial mucopolysaccharide in which the hair cells of the otolith are embedded.

There is some relationship between plasma vitamin A levels and plasma copper (for review, see Moore *et al.*, 1972). In experimental copper poisoning in sheep with greatly increased copper levels, there is a drastic reduction in plasma vitamin A. For humans during pregnancy when ceruloplasmin levels are high, plasma levels of vitamin A are low. Just as women have higher ceruloplasmin levels than men, they have lower vitamin A levels than men (see Moore *et al.*, 1972). Zinc is essential for vitamin A metabolism (Smith *et al.*, 1973). The inverse relation between vitamin A and copper may be a consequence of the antagonism between zinc and copper. Both copper (Lindquist, 1968) and vitamin A (see Wasserman and Corradino, 1971; Roels and Lui, 1973) have profound effects on lysosomal membranes. Copper ions labilize isolated liver lysosomes and this is reversed by chelating agents (Chvapil *et al.*, 1972).

The link between the metabolism of copper and vitamin A could be through the conversion of carotene to vitamin A. This is suggested by the fact that chelating agents inhibit the enzymic conversion of carotene to vitamin A (Goodman *et al.*, 1967; see also Olson, 1969). Carotene peroxidase is obtained from rat intestinal mucosa and the reaction requires oxygen, The inhibitors are strong chelating agents for copper as well as for iron, It is possible that Win 18,446, which mimics vitamin A deficiency in rats, may also be an inhibitor for carotene peroxidase.

The fact that copper is the most powerful catalyst for the autooxidation of ascorbic acid has implications in reproductive physiology, some examples of which we have already discussed (see Sections III, A and VII, A). The cupric ion-catalyzed autooxidation of ascorbic acid generates free radicals (see Staudinger *et al.*, 1964; also Section II, B, 8), and this combination can induce mutations and damage DNA (Stich *et al.*,

1976). This has a practical implication in terms of vitamin C deficiency for women taking oral contraceptives. Increased ceruloplasmin associated with exogenous estrogens is accompanied by reduced plasma levels of ascorbic acid (see Section III, A). A woman taking oral contraceptives must take about 500 mg vitamin C per day, i.e., 10 times the normal recommended daily level, to compensate for the increased loss (see Wynn, 1975; Rivers and Devine, 1975).

Vitamin C also has effects on copper metabolism. In copper-deficient animals, additional vitamin C makes the deficiency more severe. On the other hand, in copper toxicity, the vitamin has a protective effect (Spivey Fox, 1975; see also Hunt *et al.,* 1970). Both vitamin C and copper are required for collagen synthesis, but for different stages. Vitamin C is required for hydroxylation of peptidyl proline, and is also known to be required for hydroxylation of peptidyl lysine in collagen fiber formation (Barnes, 1975). Lysyl oxidase, required for the cross-linking of the collagen fibers, is a copper enzyme (see Sections V, A–C).

Copper could play an important role in reproduction via its destructive action on vitamin E. Vitamin E deficiency causes fetal resorption in female rats and inhibition of spermatogenesis in male rats (for review, see Horawitt, 1973). The hemolytic anemia often seen in premature infants has been ascribed to a deficiency of vitamin E (for review, see Anderson and Fomon, 1974; Dallman, 1974). Vitamin E, a mixture of tocopherols, is an antioxidant found in nature in conjunction with unsaturated lipids. With oxygen, copper ions destroy the vitamin and then peroxidize the lipid. The hemolytic anemia encountered in severe copper poisoning (see, for example, Chuttani *et al.,* 1965; for additional references, see Moroff *et al.,* 1974) is probably a result of the peroxidation of the unsaturated lipids of the erythrocyte membrane. Vitamin E may be required in the body to protect the organism from autooxidation by copper. The richest source of vitamin E are seed oils; of all the plant parts, seeds are the richest in copper. Incidentally, the reproductive phase in higher plants is more affected by copper deficiency than is the vegetative phase (see Graham, 1975).

## IX. Copper in the Environment

### A. Excess Copper

Copper and its more common salts are not considered particularly poisonous (see Section II, C, 6). Bordeaux Mixture, a basic copper salt introduced into vineyards in 1866 as a fungicide, apparently causes no toxicity to animals that eat the leaves. Copper metal in continuous contact with the skin, as with a copper bracelet, usually shows only a browning of the skin especially with sweating. Some copper is lost, typically 13 mg per day for a bracelet 18 $cm^2$ in area (Walker and Keats, 1976). This is practically the same rate of copper loss per unit area as with the Cu-IUD, namely 1.5 mg/month for an area of 2 $cm^2$. Copper bracelets are frequently worn for the treatment of arthritis (Walker and Griffin, 1975). Copper in the drinking water, however, may be a serious matter. Copper salts may be added as a molluscicide or as an algicide. In recent years with the introduction of copper plumbing, excessive copper levels may exceed by 10 times the U.S. Public Health Service upper safety limit of 1 ppm (see, for example, Pfeiffer and Iliev, 1972). At least 1 case of overt copper poisoning from drinking was an infant who was fed formulas made from hot tap water (Salmon and Wright, 1971). Copper excess is considered by some to play a role in certain psychiatric disorders in addition to those of Wilson's disease (see Pfeiffer and Iliev, 1972). On the other hand, a demographic study of teratologies in Wales has indicated a significant negative correlation of incidence of neural tube defects with copper levels of tap water (Morton *et al.*, 1976; see Section V, A).

## B. Chelating Agents

### 1. *Fungicides*

Just as excess copper, as with Bordeaux Mixture, is fungicidal so a withdrawal of copper, as with chelates, kills fungi. Fungi are generally rich in the copper-containing oxidases. Diethyldithiocarbamate and other strong copper chelators are effective fungicides (for review, see Lukens, 1971). Some of the fungicides are chelated metal ion salts (Norton, 1975). Another class of fungicides, Captan and Folpet, are structurally related to Thalidomide and, indeed, are teratological (Murphy, 1975). Judging from the NCO arrangement of the phthalimide group in these compounds, one might expect them to be copper chelators.

There are a group of widely used fungicides, the metal salts of ethylenebis(dithiocarbamates), Maneb, Zineb, Ziram, etc., whose breakdown products, on cooking the sprayed vegetables, produce a known teratological agent (see Section V, C). Although the parent fungicides are only teratological in large doses (in excess of 500 mg/kg) (Petrova-Vergieva and Ivanova-Tchemishanska, 1973), the thermal breakdown product ethylenethiourea is teratological at much lower doses (in excess of 10 mg/kg) (Khera, 1973; Ruddick and Khera, 1975).

### 2. *Antiprooxidants*

Antiprooxidants are generally copper chelators. In order to preserve foods, particularly those containing fatty acids, copper should be removed since the presence of the element leads to rancidity and oxidation of vitamins (see Section VIII, B). Chelating agents such as EDTA also help to preserve the original color of vegetables and are widely used prior to freezing in the frozen food industry. Chelating agents are so extensively used in processed foods that it would be difficult to ascribe some birth defect to a particular chelating agent. Such is not the case, however, when the chelating agent is in abundance in a work situation. For example, disulfiram is extensively used as a rubber stabilizer. Indeed, its Antabuse activity was first noted among workers in the rubber industry (for review, see Jacobsen, 1950). The teratogen ethylenethiourea is also used in the rubber industry (see Section V,C). Admittedly, copper-chelating agents have great utility in the home (e.g., the Versene cleaners), in agriculture, in the food industry, and in plastic stabilization, but one should be aware that they could produce reproductive disorders in man and animals.

## Acknowledgments

This work was supported by the Ford Foundation on Grant No. 690-0106. We wish to thank Dr. Hans Lehfeldt for his critical evaluation of the clinical aspects of Section II.

## References

Abel, E. (1956). *Monatsh. Chem.* **87,** 328.
Abraham, R., Mankes, R., Fulfs, J., Goldberg, L., and Coulston, F. (1974). *J. Reprod. Fertil.* **36,** 59.
Adadevoh, B. K., and Dada, O. A. (1973). *Fertil. Steril.* **24,** 54.
Aedo, A. R., and Zipper, J. (1973) *Fertil. Steril.* **24,** 345.
Aiken, J. W. (1972). *Nature (London)* **240,** 21.
Akinla, O., Luukkainen, T., and Timonen, H. (1975). *Contraception* **12,** 697.
Al-Rashid, R. A., and Spangler, J. (1971). *N. Engl. Med.* **285,** 841.
Alderman, B. (1976a). *Brit. Med. J.* **1,** 770.
Alderman, B. (1976b). *Proc. Roy. Soc. Med.* (in press.)
Alexander, N. M. (1959). *J. Biol. Chem.* **234,** 1530.
Anderson, T. A., and Fomon, S. J. (1974). *In* "Infant Nutrition" (S. J. Fomon, ed.), 2nd ed., Chapter 9, pp. 218–221. Saunders, Philadelphia, Pennsylvania.
Anonymous (1970). *Nutr. Rev.* **28,** 82.
Anonymous (1975). *Lancet* **2,** 351.
Apgar, J. (1968a). *Am. J. Physiol.* **215,** 160.
Apgar, J. (1968b). *Am. J. Physiol.* **215,** 1478.
Arbisser, A. I., Scott, C. I., Jr., and Howell, R. R. (1976). *Lancet* **1,** 312.
Arimura, A., Matsuo, H., Baba, Y., and Shally, A. V. (1971). *Science* **174,** 511.

Ashkenazi, A., Levin, S., Djaldetti, M., Fishel, E., and Benvenisti, D. (1973). *Pediatrics* **52,** 525.
Ashwell, G., and Morell, A. G. (1974). *Adv. Enzymol.* **41,** 99.
Aylett, M. J. (1973). *Practitioner* **211,** 75.
Aylett, M. J. (1974). *Update* Nov., p. 1177.
Bailey, J. L. (1967). "Techniques in Protein Chemistry," 2nd ed., Chapter 4. Am. Elsevier, New York.
Barber, R. S., Braude, R., Mitchell, K. G., and Cassidy, J. (1955). *Chem. Ind. (London)* **21,** 601.
Barbour, B. H., Bischel, M., and Abrams, D. E. (1971). *Nephron* **8,** 455.
Barnes, M. J. (1975). *Ann. N.Y. Acad. Sci.* **258,** 264.
Barranco, V. P. (1972). *Arch. Dermatol.* **106,** 386.
Barrie, H. (1976). *Brit. Med. J.* **1,** 488.
Beattie, D. S. (1971). *Sub-Cell. Biochem.* **1,** 1.
Beck, S., Bertholle, L., and Childs, J. (1961). "Mastering the Art of French Cooking," p. 159. Knopf, New York.
Bedford, J. M., and Calvin, H. I. (1974). *J. Exp. Zool.* **188,** 137.
Beer, A. N., and Billingham, R. E. (1971). *Adv. Immunol.* **14,** 1.
Bekesi, J. G., Roboz, J. P., and Holland, J. F. (1976). *Ann. N.Y. Acad. Sci.* **277,** 313.
Beliles, R. P. (1975). *In* "Toxicology" (L. J. Casarett and J. Doull, eds.), Chapter 18. Macmillan, New York.
Bengtsson, L. P., and Moawad, A. H. (1967). *Am. J. Obstet. Gynecol.* **98,** 957.
Bennetts, H. W., and Beck, A. B. (1942). *Aust., C. S. I. R. O., Bull.* **147.**
Bennetts, H. W., and Chapman, F. E. (1937). *Aust. Vet. J.* **13,** 138.
Bennetts, H. W., and Hall, H. T. B. (1939). *Aust. Vet. J.* **15,** 52.
Beral, V. (1975). *Br. J. Obstet. Gynaecol.* **82,** 775.
Beyler, A. L., Potts, G. O., Coulston, F., and Surrey, A. R. (1961). *Endocrinology* **69,** 819.
Bonnar, J., Kasonde, K., Haddon, M., Hassanein, M. K., and Allington, M. J. (1976). *Br. J. Obstet. Gynaecol.* **83,** 160.
Bonta, I. L. (1969). *Acta Physiol. Pharmacol. Neerl.* **15,** 188.
Botella-Llusía, J. (1973). "Endocrinology of Woman," pp. 187–194 and 425–426. Saunders, Philadelphia, Pennsylvania.
Boving, B. G., and Larsen, J. F. (1973). *In* "Human Reproduction" (E. S. E. Hafez and T. N. Evans, eds.), Chapter 7. Harper, New York.
Bowler, K., and Duncan, C. J. (1970). *Biochim. Biophys. Acta* **196,** 116.
Braude, R. (1975). Presented at "Copper in Agriculture," London, October 1975, sponsored by the Copper Development Association.
Braude, R., and Ryder, K. (1973). *J. Agric. Sci.* **80,** 489.
Bray, R. C. (1975). *In* "The Enzymes" (P. D. Boyer, ed.), 3rd ed., Vol. 12, Part B, Chapter, 6. Academic Press, New York.
Breslow, E. (1973). *In* "Inorganic Biochemistry" (G. L. Eichhorn, ed.), Chapter 7. Am. Elsevier, New York.
Briggs, M., and Briggs, M. (1972). *Nature (London)* **238,** 277.
Bright, H. J., and Porter, D. J. T. (1975). *In* "The Enzymes" (P. D. Boyer, ed.), 3rd ed., Vol. 12, Part B, Chapter 7. Academic Press, New York.
Brinster, R. L., and Cross, P. C. (1972). *Nature (London)* **238,** 398.
Bronson, F. H. (1968). *In* "Perspectives in Reproduction and Sexual Behavior" (M. Diamond, ed.), p. 341. Indiana Univ. Press, Bloomington.
Bruce, H. M. (1970). *Br. Med. Bull.* **26,** 10.

Bryan, S. E., Simons, S. J., Vizard, D. L., and Hardy, K. J. (1976). *Biochemistry* **15,** 1667.
Bucknall, W. E., Haslam, R. H. A., and Holtzman, N. A. (1973). *Pediatrics* **52,** 653.
Burrow, G. N. (1972). "The Thyroid Gland in Pregnancy." Saunders, Philadelphia, Pennsylvania.
Calvin, H. I., and Bedford, J. M. (1971). *J. Reprod. Fertil., Suppl.* **13,** 65.
Calvin, H. I., Yu, C. C., and Bedford, J. M. (1973). *Exp. Cell Res.* **81,** 333.
Calvin, H. I., Hwang, F. H. -F., and Wohlrab, H. (1975). *Biol. Reprod.* **13,** 228.
Carlton, W. W., and Kelly, W. A. (1968). *J. Nutr.* **97,** 42.
Carnes, W. H., Shields, G. S., Cartwright, G. E., and Wintrobe, M. M. (1961). *Fed. Proc., Fed. Am. Soc. Exp. Biol.* **20,** 118.
Carter, C. O. (1974). *Dev. Med. Child Neurol.* **16,** Suppl. 32, 3.
Cartwright, G. E., and Wintrobe, M. M. (1964). *Am. J. Clin. Nutr.* **14,** 224.
Castell, A. G., and Bowland, J. P. (1968). *Can. J. Anim. Sci.* **48,** 403.
Caton, M. P. L. (1971). *Prog. Med. Chem.* **8,** 317.
Cedarqvist, L. L., Lindhe, B. -A., and Fuchs, F. (1975). *Acta Obstet. Gynecol. Scand.* **54,** 183.
Chandra, R. K., Malkani, P. K., and Bhasin, K. (1974). *J. Reprod. Fertil* **37,** 1.
Chang, C. C., and Tatum, H. J. (1970). *Contraception* **1,** 265.
Chang, C. C., and Tatum, H. J. (1972). *Fertil. Steril.* **23,** 191.
Chang, C. C., and Tatum, H. J. (1973). *Contraception* **7,** 413.
Chang, C. C., and Tatum, H. J. 1975). *Contraception* **11,** 79.
Chang, C. C., Tatum, H. J., and Kincl, F. A. (1970). *Fertil. Steril* **21,** 274.
Chaudhuri, G. (1971). *Lancet* **1,** 480.
Chaudhuri, G. (1973). *Prostaglandins* **3,** 773.
Chaudhuri, G. (1974). *In* "Third International Conference on Intrauterine Contraception," Abstracts, p. 39. The Population Council, New York.
Chaudhury, M. R. (1975). *J. Reprod. Fertil.* **42,** 571.
Christian, C. D. (1974). *Am. J. Obstet. Gynecol.* **119,** 441.
Christie, W. W., and Moore, J. H. (1969). *Lipids* **4,** 345.
Chuttani, H. K., Gupta, P. S., Gulati, S., and Gupta, D. N. (1965). *Am. J. Med.* **39,** 849.
Chvapil, M., Ryan, J. N., and Brada, Z. (1972). *Biochem. Pharmacol.* **21,** 1097.
Claussen, S. W. and McCord, A. B. (1938). *J. Pediat.* **13,** 635.
Cohen, E., and Elvehjem, C. A. (1934). *J. Biol. Chem.* **107,** 97.
Collins, E., and Turner, G. (1975). *Lancet* **2,** 335.
Comfort, A. (1971). *Nature (London)* **230,** 432.
Conney, A. H. (1967). *Pharmacol. Rev.* **19,** 317.
Cook, H. W., and Lands, W. E. M. (1976). *Nature (London)* **260,** 630.
Cooper, D. L., Millen, A. K., and Mishell, D. R. (1976). *Am. J. Obstet. Gynecol.* **124,** 121.
Cordano, A. (1974). *Pediatrics* **54,** 524.
Cordano, A., Beartl, J. M., and Graham, G. G. (1964). *Pediatrics* **34,** 324.
Coulston, F., Beyler, A. L., and Drobeck, H. P. (1960). *Toxicol. Appl. Pharmacol.* **2,** 715.
Cross, M. H., (1973) *J. Reprod. Fertil.* **32,** 485.
Csapo, A. I., and Csapo, E. E. (1974). *Life Sci.* **14,** 719.
Cuadros, A., and Hirsch, J. G. (1972). *Science* **175,** 175.
Curzon, G., and O'Reilly, S. O. (1960). *Biochem. Biophys. Res. Commun.* **2,** 284.
Dallman, P. R. (1974). *In* "Hematology of Infancy and Childhood" (D. G. Nathan and F. A. Oski, eds.), Chapter 4. Saunders, Philadelphia, Pennsylvania.

Daniel, E. E. (1964). *Can. J. Physiol. Pharmacol.* **42,** 497.
Daniel, E. E., Massingham, R., and Nasmyth, P. A. (1970). *J. Pharmacol. Exp. Ther.* **173,** 293.
Danks, D. M. (1975). *N. Engl. J. Med.* **293,** 1147.
Danks, D. M., Campbell, P. E., Stevens, B. J., Mayne, V., and Cartwright, E. (1972a). *Pediatrics* **50,** 188.
Danks, D. M., Stevens, B. J., Campbell, P. E., Gillespie, J. M., Walker-Smith, J., Bloomfield, J., and Turner, B. (1972b). *Lancet* **1,** 1100.
Danks, D. M., Cartwright, E., Stevens, B. J., and Townley, R. R. W. (1973). *Science* **179,** 1140.
Dasgupta, P. R., Pande, J. K., Garg, R., Srivastava, K., and Kar, A. B. (1972). *Contraception* **6,** 459.
Dasler, W., and Stoner, R. E. (1959). *Experientia* **15,** 112.
Davis, R. H., Kramer, D. L., and Sackman, J. W. (1976). *N. Engl. J. Med.* **294,** 279.
Davis, W. M., Madden, J. W., and Peacock, E. E., Jr. (1972). *Ann. Surg.* **176,** 469.
de la Cruz, A., Coy, D. H., Vilchez-Martinez, J. A., Arimura, A., and Shally, A. V. (1976). *Science* **191,** 195.
de la Osa, E. L., Hagenfeldt, K., and Diczfalusy, E. (1972). *Contraception* **6,** 449.
Delves, H. T., Alexander, F. W., and Lay, H. (1973). *Br. J. Haematol.* **24,** 525.
de Morisier, C., and Gautier, G. (1963). *Pathol. Biol.* **11,** 1267.
de Quatrefages, A. (1850). *Ann. Sci. Nat.* **13,** 111.
de Vries, H., and Kroon, A. M. (1970). *Biochim. Biophys. Acta* **204,** 531.
Dietrich, R. A., and Hellerman, L. (1963). *J. Biol. Chem.* **238,** 1683.
Dixon, H. B. F., Gibbs, K., and Walshe, J. M. (1972). *Lancet* **1,** 853.
Dixon, J. W., and Sarkar, B. (1972). *Biochem. Biophys. Res. Commun.* **48,** 197.
Dixon, J. W., and Sarkar, B. (1974). *J. Biol. Chem.* **249,** 5872.
Dokumov, S. (1968). *Rev. Fr. Gynecol. Obstet.* **63,** 37.
Doty, R. L., Ford, M., Preti, G., and Huggins, G. R. (1975). *Science* **190,** 1316.
Dury, A., and Bradbury, J. T. (1941). *Am. J. Physiol.* **135,** 587.
Dutt, B., and Mills, C. F. (1960). *J. Comp. Pathol.* **70,** 120.
Dyrkacz, G. R., Libby, R. D., and Hamilton, G. A. (1976). *J. Am. Chem. Soc.* **98,** 626.
Eisenfeld, A. J., Atens, R., Weinberger, M., Haselbacher, G., Halpern, K., and Krakoff, L. (1976). *Science* **191,** 862.
Elliot, J. I., and Bowland, J. P. (1970). *J. Anim. Sci.* **30,** 923.
Elstein, M., and Ferrer, K. (1973). *J. Reprod. Fertil.* **32,** 109.
Epstein, P. S., and McIlwain, M. (1966). *Proc. R. Soc. London, Ser. B* **166,** 295.
Eriksson, M. (1971). *Acta Paediat. Scand., Suppl.* **211,** 5.
Esoda, E. C. J. (1963). *Arch. Dermatol.* **87,** 486.
Evans, G. W. (1973). *Physiol. Rev.* **53,** 535.
Evans, G. W., Majors, P. F., and Cornatzer, W. E. (1970). *Biochem. Biophys. Res. Commun.* **40,** 1142.
Evans, H. M., and Bishop, K. S. (1922). *Anat. Rec.* **23,** 17.
Everett, J. W. (1964). *Physiol. Rev.* **44,** 373.
Evvard, J. M., Nelson, V. E., and Sewell, W. E. (1928). *Proc. Iowa Acad. Sci.* **35,** 487.
Faline, L., and Anissimova, V. (1940). *Bull. Biol. Med. Exp. URSS* **9,** 519.
Faure-Tissot, M., and Delatour, P. (1965). *Ann. Med.-Psychol.* **1,** No. 5, 735.
Fawcett, D. M., and Kirkwood, S. (1954). *J. Biol. Chem.* **209,** 249.
Fearnley, G. R. (1965). "Fibrinolysis." Williams & Wilkins, Baltimore, Maryland.
Ferm, V. H., and Hanlon, D. P. (1974). *Biol. Reprod.* **11,** 97.

Ferreira, S. H., and Vane, J. R. (1974). *In* "The Prostaglandins" (P. W. Ramwell, ed.), Vol. 2, Chapter 1. Plenum, New York.

Fevold, H. L., Shiaw, F. L., and Greep, R. O. (1936). *Am. J. Physiol.* **117,** 68.

Fiscina, B., Oster, G., Oster, G. K., and Swanson, J. (1973). *Am. J. Obstet. Gynecol.* **116,**86.

Fisher, D. B., Kirkwood, R., and Kaufman, S. (1972). *J. Biol. Chem.* **247,** 5161.

Fisher, G. L. (1975). *Sci. Total Environ.* **4,** 373.

Fitzpatrick, T. B., and Quevedo, W. C., Jr. (1972). *In* "The Metabolic Basis of Inherited Disease" (J. B. Stanbury, J. B. Wyngaarden, and D. S. Fredrickson, eds.), 3rd ed., Chapter 14. McGraw-Hill, New York.

Fogel, P. I. (1971). *Akush. Ginekol. (Moscow)* **47,** No. 8, 45.

Forder, J. V. H. (1974). *Lancet* **2,** 1009.

Formanek, K., and Höller, H. (1959). *Arch. Int. Pharmacodyn. Ther.* **120,** 17.

Fridovich, I. (1972). *Acc. Chem. Res.* **5,** 321.

Fridovich, I. (1974). *Adv. Enzymol.* **41,** 35.

Frieden, E. (1971). *In* "Advances in Chemistry Series, Bioinorganic Chemistry" (R. F. Gould, ed.), p. 292. Am. Chem. Soc., Washington, D. C.

Frieden, E. (1973). *Nutr. Rev.* **31,** 41.

Frieden, E., and Osaki, S. (1970). *In* "Effects of Metals on Cells, Subcellular Elements and Macromolecules" (J. Maniloff, J. Coleman, Jr., and M. W. Miller, eds.), p. 34. Thomas, Springfield, Illinois.

Frieden, E., and Osaki, S. (1974). *In* "Protein-Metal Interactions" (M. Friedman, ed.), Plenum, New York.

Frieden, E., Osaki, S., and Kobayashi, H. (1965). *J. Gen. Physiol.* **49,** 213.

Friis-Hansen, B. (1971). *Pediatrics* **47,** 264.

Furst, A., and Haro, R. T. (1969). *Prog. Exp. Tumor Res.* **12,** 102.

Gallagher, C. H., and Reeve, V. E. (1971). *Aust. J. Exp. Biol. Med. Sci.* **49,** 21.

Geiger, B. J., Steenbock, J., and Parsons, H. T. (1933). *J. Nutr.* **6,** 427.

Géro, E., and le Gallic, P. (1952). *Bull. Soc. Chim. Biol.* **34,** 557.

Ghosh, M., and Roy, S. K. (1976). *Contraception* **13,** 355.

Gilmore, D. P., Hooker, R. H., and Davis, B. K. (1973). *Fertil. Steril.* **24,** 60.

Gleason, M. N., Gosselin, R. E., Hodge, H. C., and Smith, R. P. (1969). "Clinical Toxicology of Commercial Products," p. 72. Williams & Wilkins, Baltimore, Maryland.

Goble, F. C. (1975). *Adv. Pharmacol. Chemother.* **13,** 174.

Goldfischer, S., and Sternlieb, I. (1968). *Am. J. Pathol.* **53,** 883.

Goldsmith, N. F., Pace, N., Baumberger, J. P., and Ury, H. (1970). *Fertil. Steril.* **21,** 292.

Goldstein, M., and Nakajima, K. (1967). *J. Pharmacol. Exp. Ther.* **157,** 96.

Goldstein, M., Lauber, E., and McKereghan, M. R. (1965). *J. Biol. Chem.* **240,** 2066.

González-Angulo, A., and Aznar-Ramos, R. (1976). *Am. J. Obstet. Gynecol.* **125,** 170.

Goodman, D. S., Huang, H. S., Kanai, M., and Shiratori, T. (1967). *J. Biol. Chem.* **242,** 3543.

Goodwin, B. L. (1972). "Tyrosine Catabolism." Oxford Univ. Press, London and New York.

Graham, G. G. (1971). *N. Engl. J. Med.* **285,** 857.

Graham, G. G., and Cordano, A. (1969). *Johns Hopkins Med. J.* **124,** 139.

Graham, R. D. (1975). *Nature (London)* **254,** 514.

Graham, S. L., and Hansen, W. H. (1972). *Bull. Environ. Contam. Toxicol.* **7,** 19.

Grant, W. M. (1974). "Toxicology of the Eye," 2nd ed., pp. 312–319. Thomas, Springfield, Illinois.

Greenstein, J. P., and Winitz, M. (1961). "Chemistry of the Amino Acids," Vol. 1, Chapter 6. Wiley, New York.
Gregoriadis, G. and Sorukes, T. L. (1967). *Can. J. Biochem.* **45,** 1841.
Griscom, N. T., Craig, J. N., and Neuhauser, E. R. D. (1971). *Pediatrics* **48,** 883.
Grover, W. D., and Scrutton, M. C. (1975). *J. Pediat.* **86,** 216.
Grundsell, H. (1975). *J. Reprod. Fertil.* **42,** 447.
Grundsell, H., Håkansson, L., and Hägerstrand, I. (1976). *Acta Obstet. Gynecol. Scand.* **55,** 155.
Gubler, C. J., Lahey, M. E., Cartwright, G. E., and Wintrobe, M. M. (1953). *J. Lab. Clin. Invest.* **32,** 405.
Guest, R. J. (1953). *Anal. Chem.* **25,** 1484.
Guillebaud, J. (1976). *Br. Med. J.* **1,** 1016.
Gump, D. W., Mead, P. B., Horton, E. L., Lamborn, K. R., and Forsyth, B. R. (1973). *Obstet. Gynecol.* **41,** 259.
Gutteridge, S., and Robb, D. (1975). *Eur. J. Biochem.* **54,** 107.
Guttorm, E. (1971). *Acta Obstet. Gynecol. Scand.* **50,** 9.
Hagenfeldt, K. (1971). *Control Hum. Fertil., Proc. Nobel Symp.,* 15th, 1970, p. 214.
Hagenfeldt, K. (1972a). *Contraception* **6,** 37.
Hagenfeldt, K. (1972b). *Acta Endocrinol. (Copenhagen), Suppl.* **169,** 3.
Hagenfeldt, K., Johannisson, E., and Brenner, P. (1972). *Contraception* **6,** 207.
Halas, E. S., Hanlon, M. J., and Sandstead, H. H. (1975). *Nature (London)* **257,** 221.
Halbert, D. R., Demers, L. M., and Jones, D. E. D. (1976). *Obstet. Gynecol. Surv.* **31,** 77.
Halbreich, A., and Weissenberg, E. (1967). *Isr. J. Chem.* **5,** 118.
Hall, G. A., and Howell, J. McC. (1969). *Br. J. Nutr.* **23,** 41.
Hallberg, L., Högdahl, A. M., Nilsson, L., and Rybø, G. (1966). *Acta Obstet. Gynecol. Scand.* **45,** 320.
Hambridge, K. M., Neldner, K. H., and Walravens, P. A. (1975). *Lancet* **1,** 577.
Hamilton, C. R., Jr., Henkin, R. I., Weir, G., and Kliman, B., (1973). *Ann. Intern. Med.* **78,** 47.
Harman, D. (1965). *J. Gerontol.* **20,** 151.
Harman, D. (1972). *Am. J. Clin. Nutr.* **25,** 839.
Harris, E. D. (1976). *Proc. Natl. Acad. Sci. U.S.A.* **73,** 371.
Harris, E. D., Gonnerman, W. A., Savage, J. E., and O'Dell, B. L. (1974). *Biochim. Biophys. Acta* **341,** 332.
Hart, E. B., Steenbock, H., Waddell, J., and Elvehjem, C. A. (1928). *J. Biol. Chem.* **77,** 797.
Hartley, B. S., and Walshe, J. M. (1963). *Lancet* **2,** 434.
Hawk, H. W., Cooper, B. S., and Conley, H. H. (1974). *Am. J. Obstet. Gynecol.* **118,** 480.
Hefnawi, F., Askalani, H., and Zaki, K. (1974a). *Contraception* **9,** 133.
Hefnawi, F., Kandil, O., Askalani, H., Zaki, K., Nasr, F., and Mousa, M. (1974b). *Fertil. Steril.* **25,** 556.
Hefnawi, F., Saleh, A. A., and Kandil, O. (1974c). *In* "Third International Conference on Intrauterine Contraception," Abstracts, p. 28. The Population Council, New York.
Hefnawi, F., Kandil, O., Askalani, H., and Serour, G. (1975). *Contraception* **11,** 541.
Heilmeyer, L. (1958). *In* "Iron in Clinical Medicine" (R. O. Wallerstein and S. R. Mettier, eds.), p. 24. Univ. of California Press, Berkeley,
Heller, C. G., Moore, D. J., and Paulsen, C. A. (1961). *Toxicol. Appl. Pharmacol.* **3,** 1.
Henkin, R. I., and Bradley, D. F. (1969). *Proc. Natl. Acad. Sci. U.S.A.* **62,** 30.

Hernandez, O., Ballesteros, L. M., Mendez, J. D., and Rosado, A. (1974). *Fertil. Steril.* **25,** 108.
Hicks, J. J., Hernandez-Perez, O., Aznar, R., Mendez, J. D., and Rosado, A. (1975). *Am. J. Obstet. Gynecol.* **121,** 981.
Hill, H. C. (1969). *Nutr. Rev.* **27,** 99.
Hillier, K., and Kasonde, J. M. (1976). *Lancet* **1,** 15.
Hiroi, M., Sugita, S., and Suzuki, M. (1965). *Endocrinology* **77,** 963.
Hiroi, M., Stevens, K., and Gorski, R. (1969). *J. Reprod. Fertil.* **18,** 439.
Hoekstra, W. G., Dicke, R. J., and Phillips, P. H. (1954). *Am. J. Vet. Res* **15,** 47.
Hoey, M. J. (1966). *J. Reprod. Fertil.* **12,** 461.
Holland, J. P., Dorsey, J. M., Harris, N. N., and Johnson, F. L. (1967). *J. Reprod. Fertil.* **14,** 81.
Holland, J. P., Calhoun, F. J., Farris, F. J., and Walton, N. W. (1968). *Acta Endocrinol. (Copenhagen)* **59,** 335.
Holliday, M. A. (1974). *Pediatrics* **54,** 524.
Holm, R. H. (1973). *In* "Inorganic Biochemistry" (G. L. Eichhorn, ed.), Chapter 31. Am. Elsevier, New York.
Holtzman, N. A., Elliott, D. A., and Heller, R. H. (1966). *N. Engl. J. Med.* **275,** 347.
Holub, W. R. (1972). *Am. J. Obstet. Gynecol.* **114,** 492.
Holub, W. R., Reyner, F. C., and Forman, G. H. (1971). *Am. J. Obstet. Gynecol.* **110,** 362.
Holzaepfel, J. H., Greenlee, R. W., Wyant, R. E., and Ellis, W. C., Jr. (1959). *Fertil. Steril.* **10,** 272.
Horawitt, M. K. (1973). *In* "Modern Nutrition in Health and Disease" (R. S. Goodhart and M. E. Shils, eds.), 5th ed., Chapter 5D. Lea & Febiger, Philadelphia, Pennsylvania.
Horn, N., Mikkelsen, M., Heydorn, K., Damsgaard, H. K., and Tygstrup, I. (1975). *Lancet* **1,** 1236.
Howell, J. McC., and Davison, A. N. (1959). *Biochem. J.* **72,** 365.
Howell, J. McC., and Hall, G. A. (1969). *Br. J. Nutr.* **23,** 47.
Howell, J. McC., and Hall, G. A. (1970). *Trace Elem. Metab. Anim., Proc. WAAP/IBP Int. Symp., 1969.*
Huber, S. C., Piotrow, P. T., Orlans, F. B., and Kommer, G. (1975). *Popul. Rep., Ser. B* p. B21.
Hunt, C. E., Landesman, J., and Newberne, P. M. (1970). *Br. J. Nutr.* **24,** 607.
Hunt, D. M. (1974). *Nature (London)* **249,** 852.
Hurley, L. S. (1966). *Proc. Soc. Exp. Biol. Med.* **123,** 692.
Hurley, L. S. (1976a). *In* "Trace Elements and Human Disease" (A. Prasad, ed.), Vol. 2, pp. 301–314. Academic Press, New York.
Hurley, L. S. (1976b). *Med. Clin. North Am.* (in press).
Hurley, L. S., and Bell, L. T. (1975). *Proc. Soc. Exp. Biol. Med.* **149,** 830.
Hurley, L. S., and Shrader, R. E. (1972). *Int. Rev. Neurobiol., Suppl.* **1,** 7.
Ingbar, S. H., and Woeber, K. A. (1974). *In* "Textbook of Endocrinology" (R. H. Williams, ed.), 5th ed., pp. 95–232. Saunders, Philadelphia, Pennsylvania.
Israel, R., Shaw, S. T., and Martin, M. A. (1974). *Contraception* **10,** 63.
Jacobsen, E. (1950). *Br. J. Addict.* **47,** 26.
Jain, A. K. (1975). *Contraception* **11,** 243.
Jecht, E. W., and Bernstein, G. S. (1973). *Contraception* **7,** 381.
Jelliffe, A. M. (1973). *Natl. Cancer Inst., Monogr.* **36,** 325.
Jocelyn, P. C., ed. (1972). "Biochemistry of the SH Group," Chapter 16. Academic Press, New York.

Johansson, E. D. B., and Nygren, K.-G. (1974). *In* "Third International Conference on Intrauterine Contraception," Abstracts, p. 24. The Population Council, New York.
Johnson, M. H. (1972). *Fertil. Steril.* **23,** 123.
Johnson, N. C., Kheim, T., and Kountz, W. B. (1959). *Proc. Soc. Exp. Biol. Med.* **102,** 98.
Josephs, H. W. (1931). *Bull. Johns Hopkins Hosp.* **49,** 246.
Kamal, I., Ghoneim, M., Talaat, M., and Mallawani, A. (1973). *Fertil. Steril.* **24,** 165.
Kamberi, I. A., Mical, R. S., and Porter, J. C. (1969). *Science* **166,** 388.
Kar, A. B., and Sarkar, S. L. (1960). *J. Sci. Ind. Res. (India)* **19C,** 241.
Karim, S. M. M., ed. (1975). "Prostaglandins and Reproduction." Univ. Park Press, Baltimore, Maryland.
Karim, S. M. M., and Hillier, K. (1975). *In* "Prostaglandins and Reproduction" (S. M. M. Karim, ed.), Chapter 2. Univ. Park Press, Baltimore, Maryland.
Karpel, J. T., and Peden, V. H. (1972). *J. Pediatr.* **80,** 32.
Kasonde, J. M., and Bonnar, J. (1976). *Br. J. Obstet. Gynecol.* **83,** 315.
Kato, T. (1969). *Acta Obstet. Gynaecol. Jpn.* **16,** No. 4, 303.
Kaufman, S., and Fisher, D. B. (1974). *In* "Molecular Mechanisms of Oxygen Activation" (O. Hayaishi, ed.), Chapter 8. Academic Press, New York.
Keeler, R. F. (1972). *Clin. Toxicol.* **5,** 529.
Keen, C. L., and Hurley, L. S. (1976). *Science* **193,** 244.
Keil, H. L., and Nelson, V. E. (1931). *J. Biol. Chem.* **93,** 49.
Kesserü, E., Hurtado, H., and Mühe, B. (1974). *Contraception* **9,** 141.
Khatamee, M. A., and Lehfeldt, H. (1975). *Adv. Planned Parent.* **10,** 90.
Khera, K. S. (1973). *Teratology* **7,** 243.
Khera, K. S. (1976). *Experientia* (in press).
Khodak, A. A. (1971). *Akush. Ginekol. (Moscow)* **47,** No. 5, 69.
Kimmel, C. A., Butcher, R. E., Vorhees, C. V., and Schumacher, J. J. (1974). *Teratology* **10,** 293.
King, D. W., and Hsu, J. L. (1976). *Teratology* **13,** 28A.
Kingsbury, J. M. (1975). *In* "Toxicology" (L. J. Casarett and J. Doull, eds.), Chapter 23. Macmillan, New York.
Kirchgessner, M., and Grassmann, E. (1970). *In* "Trace Element Metabolism in Animals" (C. F. Mills, ed.), p. 277. Livingstone, Edinburgh.
Kleinmann, H., and Klinke, J. (1930). *Virchows Arch. Pathol. Anat. Physiol. 122* **275,** 422.
Klotz, I. M., and Curme, H. G. (1948). *J. Am. Chem. Soc.* **70,** 939.
Knox, W. E. (1972). *In* "The Metabolic Basis of Inherited Diseases" (J. B. Stanbury, J. B. Wyngaarden, and D. S. Fredrickson, eds.), 3rd ed., Chapter 11. McGraw-Hill, New York.
Kobashi, K. (1968). *Biochim. Biophys. Acta* **158,** 239.
Koefoed-Johnsen, V., Lyon, I., and Ussing, H. H. (1973). *Acta Physiol. Scand., Suppl.* **396,** 102.
Koetsawang, S. (1973). *Contraception* **7,** 327.
Kohn, H. I., and Liversedge, M. (1944). *J. Pharmacol.* **83,** 292.
Kowalski, E., Latallo, Z., and Niewiarowski, S. (1956). *Sang* **27,** 466.
Krebs, H. A. (1928). *Klin. Wochenschr.* **7,** 584.
Kuchinsas, E. J., and Du Vigneaud, V. (1957). *Arch. Biochem. Biophys.* **66,** 1.
LaBella, F.,, Dunlar, R., Vivian, S., and Queen, G. (1973). *Biochem. Biophys. Res. Commun.* **52,** 786.
Lalich, J. J., Groupner, K., and Jolin, J. (1965). *Lab. Invest.* **14,** 1482.
Lands, W., Lee, R., and Smith, W. (1971). *Ann. N.Y. Acad. Sci.* **180,** 107.

Larsson, B., Liedholm, P., Sjöberg, N. O., and Åstedt, B. (1974). *Contraception* **9,** 531.
Larsson, B., Liedholm, P., and Åstedt, B. (1975a). *Int. J. Fertil.* **20,** 77.
Larsson, B., Liedholm, P., and Åstedt, B. (1975b). *Int. J. Fertil.* **20,** 145.
Larsson, B., Ljung, B., and Hamberger, L. (1976). *Am. J. Obstet. Gynecol.* **125,** 682.
Lau, I. F., Saksena, S. K., and Chang, M. C. (1974). *J. Reprod. Fertil.* **37,** 429.
Laufe, L. E., Gibor, Y., McClanahan, B. J., and Wheeler, R. F. (1976). *Adv. Planned Parent.* **11,** 38.
Lea, C. M. and Luttrell, V. A. (1965). *Nature (London)* **206,** 413.
Leathem, J. H. (1972). *In* "Reproductive Biology" (H. Balin and S. Glasser, eds.), Chapter 23. Excerpta Med. Found., Amsterdam.
Leck, I. (1974). *Br. Med. Bull.* **30,** 158.
Lee, R. E., and Lands, W. E. M. (1972). *Biochim. Biophys. Acta* **260,** 203.
Lehfeldt, H. (1975a). *Mt. Sinai J. Med., N.Y.* **42,** 345.
Lehfeldt, H. (1975b). *In* "Familien Planung, 1975," p. 127. Osterreichische Gesellschaft für Familienplanung, c/o 11. Universitäts-Frauenklinik, Vienna, Austria.
Lehfeldt, H., and Wan, L. S. (1971). *Obstet. Gynecol.* **37,** 826.
Lehfeldt, H., Tietze, C., and Gorstein, F. (1970). *Am. J. Obstet. Gynecol.* **108,** 1005.
Lehmann, B. H., Hansen, J. D. L., and Warren, P. J. (1971). *Br. J. Nutr.* **26,** 197.
Leidheiser, H., Jr. (1971). "The Corrosion of Copper, Tin and Their Alloys." Wiley, New York.
Leighton, P. C., Evans, D. G., and Wallis, S. M. (1976). *Br. Med. J.* **1,** 959.
Le Magnen, J. (1953). *J. Physiol. (Paris)* **45,** 285.
Levene, C. I. (1961). *J. Exp. Med.* **114,** 295.
Levene, C. I. (1971). *In* "A Symposium on Mechanisms of Toxicity" (W. N. Aldridge, ed.), p. 67. St. Martins Press, New York.
Levene, C. I. (1973). *In* "Molecular Pathology of Connective Tissues" (R. Pèrez-Tamayo and M. Rojkind, eds.), p. 175. Dekker, New York.
Li, T. -K., and Vallee, B. L. (1973). *In* "Modern Nutrition in Health and Disease" (R. S. Goodhart and M. E. Shils, eds.) 5th ed., Chapter 8B. Lea & Febiger, Philadelphia, Pennsylvania.
Liedholm, P., Rybø, G., Sjöberg, N. -O., and Sölvell, L. (1975). *Contraception* **12,** 317.
Lillie, F. R. (1921). *Biol. Bull. (Woods Hole, Mass.)* **41,** 125.
Lindquist, R. R. (1968). *Am. J. Pathol.* **53,** 903.
Lippes, J. (1975). *Contraception* **12,** 103.
Lippes, J., Zielezny, M., and Sultz, H. (1973). *J. Reprod. Med.* **10,** 166.
Lippes, J., Malik, T., and Tatum, H. J. (1975). *13th Annu. Meet. Assoc. Planned Parenthood Physicians, 1975* pp. 1–8.
Lippes, J., Malik, T., and Tatum, H. J. (1976). *Adv. Planned Parent.* **11,** 24.
Loh, H. S., and Wilson, C. W. M. (1971). *Lancet* **1,** 110.
Lorincz, A. L. (1954). *In* "Physiology and Biochemistry of the Skin" (S. Rothman, ed), p. 547. Univ. of Chicago Press, Chicago, Illinois.
Lowry, O. H., Rosenbrough, N. J., Farr, A. L., and Randall, R. J. (1951). *J. Biol. Chem.* **193,** 265.
Lu, M. -H., and Staples, R. E. (1976). *Teratology* **13,** 29A.
Lukens, R. J. (1971). "Chemistry of Fungicidal Action." Springer-Verlag, Berlin and New York.
McClintock, M. K. (1971). *Nature (London)* **229,** 244.
McConnell, R. J., Menendez, C. E., Smith, F. R., Henkin, R. I., and Rivlin, R. S. (1975). *Am. J. Med.* **59,** 354.
McGarry, M. P. (1975). *Cell Tissue Kinet.* **8,** 355.

McGuire, J. (1972). *In* "Pharmacology and the Skin" (W. Montagna, E. J. van Scott, and R. B. Stoughton, eds.), p. 421. Appleton, New York.

Maddox, I. S. (1973). *Biochim. Biophys. Acta* **306,** 74.

Mallory, F. B., and Parker, F., Jr. (1931). *Am. J. Pathol.* **7,** 351.

Malmqvist, R., Petersohn, L., and Bengtsson, L. P. (1974). *Contraception* **9,** 627.

Malström, B. G., Andreasson, L. -E., and Reinhammer, B. (1975). *In* "The Enzymes" (P. D. Boyer, ed.), 3rd ed., Vol. 12, Part B, Chapter 8. Academic Press, New York.

Mann, T. (1964). "The Biochemistry of Semen and of the Male Reproductive Tract." Barnes & Noble, New York.

Margerum, D. W., Chellappa, K. L., Bossu, F. P., and Bruce, G. L. (1976). *J. Am. Chem. Soc.* **97,** 6894.

Markee, J. E. (1940). *Contrib. Embryol. Carnegie Inst.* **28,** 219.

Marois, M., and Buvet, M. (1972). *C. R. Seances Soc. Biol. (Paris)* **166,** 1237.

Marshall, J. R., and Henkin, R. I. (1971). *Ann. Intern. Med.* **75,** 207.

Martell, A. E., and Calvin, M. (1952). "Chemistry of the Metal Chelate Compounds," p. 543. Prentice-Hall, Englewood Cliffs, New Jersey.

Mason, H. S., Yamana, T., North, J. -C., Hashimato, Y., and Sakagishi, P. (1965). *In* "Oxidases and Related Redox Systems" (T. E. King, H. S. Mason, and M. Morrison, eds.), Vol. 2, p. 879. Wiley, New York.

Mason, M., and Rivers, J. M. (1971). *Am. J. Obstet. Gynecol.* **109,** 960.

Maugh, T. H. (1976). *Science* **191,** 453.

Mead, P. B., Beecham, J. B., and Maeck, J. V. S. (1976). *Am. J. Obstet. Gynecol.* **125,** 79.

Medel, M., Espinoza, C., Zipper. J., and Prager, R. (1972). *Contraception* **5,** 203.

Menkes, J. H., Atter, M., Steigleder, G. K., Weakley, D. R., and Sung, J. H. (1962). *Pediatrics* **29,** 764.

Merola, A. J., and Brierley, G. P. (1970). *Biochem. Pharmacol.* **19,** 1429.

Metz, E. N. (1969). *Clin. Res.* **17,** 32.

Michaelis, L., and Barrón, E. S. G. (1929). *J. Biol. Chem.* **81,** 29.

Middleton, J. C., and Kennedy, M. (1975). *Contraception* **11,** 209.

Mischell, D. J. (1975). *Fam. Plan. Perspect.* **7,** 103.

Mjølnerød, O. K., Rasmussen, K., Dommerud, S. A., and Gjeruldsen, S. T. (1971). *Lancet* **1,** 673.

Moawad, A. H., and Bengtsson, L. P. (1970). *Acta Obstet. Gynecol. Scand.* **49,** Suppl. 6, 31.

Moffitt, A. E., Jr., and Murphy, S. D. (1972). *Biochem. Pharmacol.* **22,** 1463.

Moffitt, A. E., Jr., Dixon, J. R., Phipps, F. C., and Stokinger, H. E. (1972). *Cancer Res.* **32,** 1148.

Montagna, W., and Hu, F., eds. (1966). "Advances in Biology of Skin," Vol. VIII. Pergamon, Oxford.

Moore, T. (1957). "Vitamin A," Chapter 5. Am. Elsevier, New York.

Moore, T. (1967). *In* "The Vitamins" (W. H. Sebrell, Jr. and R. S. Harris, eds.), 2nd ed., Vol. 1, Chapters 9A and 11A. Academic Press, New York.

Moore, T., Sharman, I. M., Todd, J. R., and Thompson, R. H. (1972). *Br. J. Nutr.* **28,** 23.

Moo-Young, A. J., and Tatum, H. J. (1974). *Contraception* **9,** 487.

Moo-Young, A. J., Tatum, H. J., Brinson, A. O., and Hood, W. (1973). *Fertil. Steril.* **24,** 848.

Moo-Young, A. J., Tatum, H. J., Wan, L. S., and Lane, M. E. (1974). *In* "Third International Conference on Intrauterine Contraception." Abstracts, p. 35. The Population Council, New York.

Morell, A. G., Irvine, R. A., Sternlieb, I., Scheinberg, I. H., and Ashwell, G. J. (1968). *J. Biol. Chem.* **243,** 155.
Morgan, R., and Cagan, E. J. (1974). *In* "The Biology of Alcoholism" (B. Kissin and H. Begleiter, eds.), Vol. 3, Chapter 5, Plenum, New York.
Moroff, G., Poster, J., and Oster, G. (1974). *J. Steroid Biochem.* **5,** 601.
Morrison, D. B., and Nash, T. P., Jr. (1930). *J. Biol. Chem.* **88,** 479.
Morton, M. S., Elwood, P. C., and Abernethy, M. (1976). *Br. J. Prev. Soc. Med.* **30,** 36.
Mountrose, U. E., Whitehouse, W. L., and Slater, L. (1975). *Br. J. Obstet. Gynaecol.* **83,** 992.
Moustgaard, J. (1971). *J. Reprod. Med.* **7,** 275.
Moyer, D. L., and Shaw, S. T., Jr. (1973). *In* "Human Reproduction" (E. S. E. Hafez and T. N. Evans, eds.), Chapter 14. Harper, New York.
Moynahan, E. J. (1974). *Lancet* **2,** 399.
Moynahan, E. J. (1976). *Lancet* **1,** 91.
Mukai, F. H., and Goldstein, B. D. (1976). *Science* **191,** 868.
Muller, P. (1963). *Pathol. Biol.* **11,** 1273.
Murphy, S. D. (1975). *In* "Toxicology" (L. J. Casarett and J. Doull, eds.), p. 441. Macmillan, New York.
Murthy, L., Klevag, L. M., and Petring, H. G. (1975). *J. Nutr.* **104,** 1458.
Myatt, L., Bray, M. A., Gordon, D., and Morley, J. (1975). *Nature (London)* **257,** 227.
Nakon, R., Rechani, P. R., and Angelici, R. J. (1974). *J. Am. Chem. Soc.* **96,** 2117.
Nara, S., and Yasunoba, K. T. (1966). *In* "Biochemistry of Copper" (J. Peisach, P. Aisen, and W. E. Blumberg, eds.), pp. 243–441. Academic Press, New York.
Nelson, M. M., and Forfar, J. P. (1971). *Br. Med. J.* **1,** 523.
Neuweiler, W. (1948). *Gynaecologia* **125,** 227.
Newsome, W. H., and Laver, G. W. (1973). *Bull. Environ. Contam. Toxicol.* **10,** 151.
Nicholls, P., and Chance, B. (1974). *In* "Molecular Mechanisms of Oxygen Activation" (O. Hayashi, ed.), p. 479. Academic Press, New York.
Nilsson, I. M., and Rybø, G. (1971). *Am. J. Obstet. Gynecol.* **110,** 713.
Nilsson, O., and Hagenfeldt, K. (1973). *Am. J. Obstet. Gynecol.* **117,** 469.
Noeslund, G. (1972). *Contraception* **6,** 281.
Norton, S. (1975). *In* "Toxicology" (L. J. Casarett and J. Doull, eds.), p. 114. Macmillan, New York.
Nugteren, D. H., Beerthuis, R. K., and van Dorp, D. A. (1966). *Rec. Trav. Chim. Pays-Bas* **85,** 405.
Nutting, E. F., and Mueller, M. R. (1975a). *Fertil. Steril.* **26,** 838.
Nutting, E. F., and Mueller, M. R. (1975b). *Fertil. Steril.* **26,** 845.
Nygren, K.-G., and Johansson, E. D. B. (1973). *Am. J. Obstet. Gynecol.* **117,** 971.
O'Dell, B. L., Hardwick, B. C., and Reynolds, G. (1961). *J. Nutr.* **73,** 151.
Oerter, D. and Merker, H. J. (1972). *In* "Drugs and Fetal Development" (M. A. Klingberg, A. Abramovici, and J. Chemke, eds.), p. 291. Plenum, New York.
Okereke, T., Sternlieb, J., Morell, A. G., and Scheinberg, I. H. (1972). *Science* **177,** 358.
Okun, M. R., Edelstein, L. M., Hamada, O. N., Blumenthal, G., Donnellan, B., and Burnett, J. (1972). *In* "Pigmentation: Its Genesis and Biological Controls" (V. Riley, ed.). Appleton, New York.
O'Leary, J. A. (1969). *Am. J. Obstet. Gynecol.* **105,** 636.
Olson, J. A. (1969). *Am. J. Clin. Nutr.* **22,** 953.
Orlans, E. B. (1974). *Contraception* **10,** 543.
Osaki, S., Johnson, D. A., and Frieden, E. (1966). *J. Biol. Chem.* **241,** 2746.

Oser, B. L., ed. (1965). "Hawk's Physiological Chemistry," 14th ed., Chapters 3 and 13. McGraw-Hill, New York.
Oster, G. (1975). *Ann. N.Y. Acad. Sci.* **246,** 149.
Oster, G., and Oster, G. K. (1974). *Contraception* **10,** 273.
Oster, G., and Salgo, M. P. (1975). *N. Engl. J. Med.* **293,** 432.
Oster, G., and Salgo, M. P. (1976). *N. Engl. J. Med.* **294,** 279.
Oster, G., and Yang, S. -L. (1972). *Am. J. Obstet. Gynecol.* **114,** 190.
Oster, G., Salgo, M. P., and Taleporos, P. (1974). *Am. J. Obstet. Gynecol.* **119,** 538.
Oster, G. K (1971). *Nature (London)* **234,** 153.
Oster, G. K. (1972). *Fertil Steril.* **23,** 18.
Owen, C. A., and Hazelrig, J. B. (1968). *Am. J. Physiol.* **215,** 334.
Parisi, A. F., and Vallee, B. L. (1969). *Am. J. Clin. Nutr.* **22,** 1222.
Parisi, M., and Piccinni, Z. F. (1972). *J. Endocrinol.* **55,** 1.
Patanelli, D. L. (1975). *In* "Handbook of Physiology" (Am. Physiol. Soc., J. Field, ed.), Sect. 7, Vol. V, Chapter 12. Williams & Wilkins, Baltimore, Maryland.
Pekarek, R. S., Powanda, M. C., and Wannemacher, R. W., Jr. (1972). *Proc. Soc. Exp. Biol. Med.* **141,** 1029.
Peppler, R. D. (1975). *Contraception* **12,** 327.
Peters, R., Shorthouse, M., and Walshe, J. M. (1966). *Proc. R. Soc. London, Ser. B* **166,** 285.
Petrova-Vergieva, T., and Ivanova-Tchemishanska, L. (1973). *Food Cosmet. Toxicol.* **11,** 239.
Pfeiffer, C. (1975). *J. Am. Med. Assoc.* **228,** 157.
Pfeiffer, C. C., and Iliev, V. (1972). *Int. Rev. Neurobiol., Suppl.* **1,** 141.
Phillips, C. S. G., and Williams, R. J. P. (1966). "Inorganic Chemistry," Vol. II, p. 602. Oxford Univ. Press, New York and Oxford.
Pillay, A. P. (1946). *Hum. Fertil.* **11,** 109.
Pinnell, S. R., and Martin, G. R. (1968). *Proc. Natl. Acad. Sci. U.S.A.* **61,** 708.
Pinsker, M. C., Sacco, A. G., and Mintz, B. (1974). *Dev. Biol.* **38,** 285.
Pinto, R. E., and Bartley, W. (1969a). *Biochem. J.* **112,** 109.
Pinto, R. E., and Bartley, W. (1969b). *Biochem. J.* **115,** 449.
Planas, J., and Frieden, E. (1973). *Am. J. Physiol.* **225,** 423.
Polidoro, J. P., and Black, D. L. (1970). *J. Reprod. Fertil.* **23,** 151.
Polidoro, J. P., Culver, R. M., and Thomas, S. (1975). *Contraception* **10,** 481.
Porter, C. W. (1975). *Int. J. Fertil.* **20,** 194.
Porter, H. (1974). *Biochem. Biophys. Res. Commun.* **56,** 661.
Porter, H., Johnston, J., and Porter, E. M. (1962). *Biochim. Biophys. Acta* **65,** 66.
Prager, R. (1969). *Fertil. Steril.* **20,** 944.
Prasad, A. S. (1967). *Fed. Proc., Fed. Am. Soc. Exp. Biol.* **26,** 172.
Prasad, A. S. (1972). *Int. Rev. Neurobiol., Suppl.* **1,** 1.
Quinn, G. P., Axelrod, J., and Brodie, B. B. (1958). *Biochem. Pharmacol.* **1,** 152.
Rainsford, K. D., and Whitehouse, M. W. (1976). *J. Pharm. Pharmacol.* **28,** 83.
Ranney, R. E., Nutting, E. F., Hackett, P. L., Rancitelli, L. A., Daniel, J. L., Clarke, W. J., and Wheeler, R. G. (1975). *Fertil. Steril.* **26,** 80.
Ray, G. R., Wolf, P. H., and Kaplan, H. S. (1973). *Natl. Cancer Inst. Monogr.* **36,** 315.
Reid, J., Watson, R. D., Cochtar, J. B., and Sproull, D. H. (1951). *Br. Med. J.* **2,** 321.
Rice, E. W. (1964). *Exp. Cell Res.* **34,** 186.
Richards, I. D. G. (1969). *Br. J. Prev. Soc. Med.* **23,** 218.
Rinehart, W. (1976). *Popul. Rep. Ser. J.* No. 9, p. 141.

Ritchie, J. M. (1965). *In* "The Pharmacological Basis of Therapeutics" (L. S. Goodman and A. Gilman, eds.), 3rd ed., Chapter 11. Macmillan, New York.
Ritchie, J. M. (1974). *In* "The Pharmaceutical Basis of Therapeutics" (L. S. Goodman and A. Gilman, eds.), 4th ed., Chapter 11. Macmillan, New York.
Rivers, J. M., and Devine, M. M. (1972). *Am. J. Clin. Nutr.* **25,** 684.
Rivers, J. M., and Devine, M. M. (1975). *Ann. N. Y. Acad. Sci.* **258,** 465.
Robens, J. F. (1969). *Toxicol. Appl. Pharmacol.* **15,** 152.
Roels, O. A. (1967). *In* "The Vitamins" (W. H. Sebrell, Jr. and R. S. Harris, eds.), 2nd ed., Vol. 1, Chapters 7 and 8. Academic Press, New York.
Roels, O. A., and Lui, N. S. T. (1973). *In* "Modern Nutrition in Health and Disease" (R. S. Goodhart and M. E. Shils, eds.) 5th ed., Chapter 5. Lea & Febiger, Philadelphia, Pennsylvania.
Rojkind, M., and Zeichner, M. (1973). *In* "Molecular Pathology of Connective Tissue" (R. Pérez-Tamayo and M. Rojkind, eds.), p. 135. Dekker, New York.
Rome, L. H., Lands, W. E. M., Roth, G. J., and Marjerns, P. W. (1976). *Prostaglandins* **11,** 23.
Rosenthal, N. A., and Oster, G. (1954). *J. Soc. Cosmet. Chem.* **5,** 286.
Rubinstein, E. (1974). *Contraception* **10,** 673.
Rubinstein, E. (1976). *Am. J. Obstet. Gynecol.* **125,** 277.
Ruddick, J. A., and Khera, K. S. (1975). *Teratology* **12,** 277.
Rybø, G. (1966a). *Acta Obstet. Gynecol. Scand.* **45,** 97.
Rybø, G. (1966b). *Acta Obstet. Gynecol. Scand.* **45,** 429.
Săgiroğlu, N., and Săgiroğlu, E. (1970). *Am. J. Obstet. Gynecol.* **106,** 506.
Saito, S., Bush, I. M., and Whitmore, W. F. (1967a). *Invest. Urol.* **4,** 546.
Saito, S., Bush, I. M., and Whitmore, W. F. (1967b). *Fertil. Steril.* **18,** 517.
Saksena, S. K., and Harper, M. J. (1974). *Fertil. Steril.* **25,** 121.
Salgo, M. P., and Oster, G. (1974a). *Fertil. Steril.* **25,** 113.
Salgo, M. P., and Oster, G. (1974b). *J. Reprod. Fertil.* **39,** 375.
Salgo, M. P. and Oster, G. (1977). *Am. J. Obstet. Gynecol.* (in press).
Salin, M. L., and McCord, J. M. (1975). *J. Clin. Invest.* **56,** 1319.
Salisbury, G. W., and Van Demark, N. L. (1961). "Physiology of Reproduction and Artificial Insemination of Cattle" p. 619. Freeman, San Francisco, California.
Salmon, M. A., and Wright, T. (1971). *Arch. Dis. Child.* **46,** 108.
Salverry, G., Méndez, M. del C., Zipper, J., and Medel, M. (1973). *Am. J. Obstet. Gynecol.* **115,** 163.
Sandell, E. B. (1959). "Colorimetric Determination of Trace Metals," 3rd. ed., Chapter 16. Wiley, New York.
Sandow, A., and Isaacson, A. (1966). *J. Gen. Physiol.* **49,** 937.
Sarata, U. (1935). *Jpn. J. Med. Sci. Biol.* **3,** 1.
Sass-Kortsak, A. (1975). *Pediatr. Clin. North Am.* **22,** 963.
Sato, N., and Henkin, R. I. (1973). *Am. J. Physiol.* **225,** 508.
Savage, J. E., Ross, D. A., and Reynolds, G. (1962). *Fed. Proc., Fed. Am. Soc. Exp. Biol.* **21,** 311.
Schafroth, H. J. (1956). *Arch. Gynaekol.* **188,** 142.
Schechter, P. J., Friedewald, W. T., Bronzert, D. A., Raff, M. S., and Henkin, R. I. (1972). *Int. Rev. Neurobiol., Suppl.* **1,** 125.
Scheinberg, I. H., and Morell, A. G. (1973). *In* "Inorganic Biochemistry" (G. L. Eichhorn, ed.), Chapter 10. Am. Elsevier, New York.
Scheinberg, I. H., and Sternlieb, I. (1960). *Pharmacol. Rev.* **12,** 355.

Scheinberg, I. H., and Sternlieb, I. (1965). *Annu. Rev. Med.* **16,** 119.
Scheinberg, I. H., and Sternlieb, I. (1975). *N. Engl. J. Med.* **293,** 1300.
Schenker, J. G., Jungreis, E., and Polishuk, W. Z. (1969). *Am. J. Obstet. Gynecol.* **105,** 933.
Schenker, J. G., Hellerstein, S., Jungreis, E., and Polishuk, W. Z. (1971). *Fertil. Steril.* **22,** 229.
Schroeder, H. A. (1973). *Essays Toxicol.* **4,** 107.
Schubert, J. (1964). "Copper and Peroxides in Radiobiology and Medicine." Thomas, Springfield, Illinois.
Schubert, J. (1966). *Sci. Am.* **214,** 40.
Schubert, W. K., and Lahey, M. E. (1959). *Pediatrics* **24,** 710.
Seelig, M. S. (1972). *Am. J. Clin. Nutr.* **25,** 1022.
Seely, J. R., Humphrey, G. B., and Matter, B. H. (1972). *N. Engl. J. Med.* **286,** 109.
Shaimanov, O. K. (1970). *Med. Zh. Uzb.* **8,** 66.
Shamberger, R. J., Andreone, T. L., and Willis, C. E. (1974). *J. Natl. Cancer Inst.* **53,** 1771.
Shapiro, S. S. (1973). *In* "Drugs and Hematologic Reactions" (E. V. Dimitrov and J. H. Nodine, eds.), Chapter 26. Grune & Stratton, New York.
Shaw, S. T., Jr., Jimenez, J. M., Moyer, D. L. and Cihak, R. W., (1973). *Am. J. Obstet. Gynecol.* **115,** 983.
Shen, T. C. R. (1960). *Sci. Sin.* **9,** 481.
Shulman, G., Polakow, E. S., and Bauer, H. D. (1974). *J. Obstet. Gynaecol. Br. Commonw.* **81,** 155.
Siegel, L. M., and Monty, K. J. (1961). *J. Nutr.* **74,** 167.
Silbert, J. H. (1973). *In* "Molecular Pathology of Connective Tissues" (R. Perez-Tomayo and M. Rojkind, eds.), p. 323. Dekker, New York.
Silver, H. K., Kempe, C. H., and Bruyn, H. B. (1973). "Handbook of Pediatrics," 10th ed., p. 45. Lange Med. Publ., Los Altos, California.
Smith, J. C., Jr., McDaniel, E. G., Fan, F. F., and Halstead, J. A. (1973). *Science* **181,** 954.
Smithells, R. W. (1976). *Br. Med. Bull.* **32,** 27.
Snowden, R. (1976) *Br. Med. J.* **1,** 770.
Sorenson, J. R. J. (1974). *Trace Subst. Environ. Health—8, Proc. Univ. Mo. Annu. Conf., 8th, 1973* pp. 305–311.
Sorenson, J. R. J. (1976). *J. Med. Chem.* (in press).
Southam, A. L., and Gonzaga, F. P. (1965). *Am. J. Obstet. Gynecol.* **91,** 142.
Spellacy, W. N., Hiser, B. J., and Birk, S. A. (1974). *Fertil. Steril.* **25,** 772.
Spence, M. R., Stuta, D. R., and Paniom, W. (1975). *Am. J. Obstet. Gynecol.* **122,** 783.
Spivey Fox, M. R. (1975). *Ann. N. Y. Acad. Sci.* **258,** 144.
Stamler, F. W. (1955). *Proc. Soc. Exp. Biol. Med.* **90,** 294.
Starcher, B. C. (1969). *J. Nutr.* **97,** 321.
Staudinger, H. J., Kerekjárto, B., Ullrich, V., and Zubrzycki, Z. (1964). *In* "Oxidases and Related Redox Systems" (T. E. King, H. S. Mason, and M. Morrison, eds.), Vol. 2, p. 815. Wiley, New York.
Steffek, A. J., Verrusio, A. C., and Watkins, C. A. (1972). *Teratology* **5,** 33.
Sternlieb, I., and Scheinberg, I. H. (1964). *J. Am. Med. Assoc.* **189,** 748.
Stich, H. F., Karim, J., Koropatrick, J., and Lo, L. (1976). *Nature (London)* **260,** 722.
Stone, O. J., and Willis, C. J. (1958). *Dermatol. Int.* **8,** 28.
Strömme, J. H. (1965). *Biochem. Pharmacol.* **14,** 393.
Sturgeon, P., and Brubaker, C. B. (1956). *AMA J. Dis. Child.* **92,** 254.

Sunderman, F. W., Paynter, O. E., and George, R. B. (1967). *Am. J. Med. Sci.* **254,** 24.
Sunderman, F. W., Jr. (1971). *Food Cosmet. Toxicol.* **9,** 105.
Suttle, N. F. (1973). *Proc. Nutr. Soc.* **32,** 69A.
Suttle, N. F., and Mills, C. F. (1966). *Br. J. Nutr.* **20,** 135.
Suzuki, M., Hiroi, M., Nagamatsu, M. *et al.* (1969). *Acta Med. Biol. (Niigata)* **17,** 243.
Suzuki, M., Murai, A., Hiroi, M., Nagamatsu, M., Seike, H., Ueno, T., Hojyo, T., Otake, S., Takahashi, T., Nonokawo, O., Terajima, T., and Yanemoto, Y. (1970). *Acta Obstet. Gynaecol. Jpn.* **17,** No. 2, 94.
Swan, J. M. (1957). *Nature (London)* **180,** 643.
Swenerton, H., and Hurley, L. S. (1971). *Science* **173,** 62.
Syner, F. N., and Moghissi, K. S. (1972). *In* "Biology of Mammalian Fertilization and Implantation" (K. S. Moghissi and E. S. E. Hafez, eds.), p. 11. Thomas, Springfield, Illinois.
Tabor, C. W., and Rosenthal, S. M. (1956). *J. Pharmacol. Exp. Ther.* **116,** 139.
Taleporos, P., Salgo, M. P., and Oster, G. (1977). Submitted.
Tamaya, T., Nakata, Y., Ohno, Y., Nioka, S., Furuta, N., and Okada, H. (1976). *Fertil. Steril.* **27,** 767.
Tatum, H. J. (1973). *Am. J. Obstet. Gynecol.* **117,** 602.
Tatum, H. J. (1974). *Clin. Obstet. Gynecol.* **17,** 93.
Tatum, H. J., Schmidt, F. H., Phillips, D., McCarty, M., and O'Leary, W. M. (1975). *J. Am. Med. Assoc.* **231,** 711.
Taylor, E. S., McMillan, J. H., Greer, B. E., Droegemueller, W., and Thompson, H. E. (1975). *Am. J. Obstet. Gynecol.* **123,** 338.
Tessmer, C. F., Hrgovic, M., and Wilbur, J. (1973). *Cancer (Philadelphia)* **31,** 303.
Theuer, R. C. (1972). *J. Reprod. Med.* **8,** 13.
Thompson, E. A., and Siiteri, P. K. (1973). *Ann. N.Y. Acad. Sci.* **212,** 378.
Tietze, C. (1973). *In* "Human Reproduction" (E. S. E. Hafez and T. N. Evans, eds.), pp. 293–308. Harper, New York.
Tietze, C., Bongaarts, J., and Schearer, B. (1976). *Fam. Plan. Perspect.* **8,** 6.
Timonen, H., and Luukkainen, T. (1974). *Contraception* **9,** 153.
Timonen, H., Luukkainen, T., Rainio, J., and Tatum, H. J. (1972). *Contraception* **6,** 513.
Ting-Beall, H. P., Clark, D. A., Suelter, C. H., and Wells, W. W. (1973). *Biochim. Biophys. Acta* **291,** 229.
Tobert, J. A. (1975). *J. Reprod. Fertil.* **45,** 197.
Tredway, D. R., Umezaki, C. U., Mishell, D. R., Jr., and Settlage, D. S. F. (1975) *Am. J. Obstet. Gynecol.* **123,** 734.
Truitt, E. B., Jr., and Walsh, M. J. (1971). *In* "The Biology of Alcoholism" (B. Kissin and H. Begleiter, eds.), Vol. 1, Chapter 5. Plenum, New York.
Tsen, C. C., and Tappel, A. L. (1958). *J. Biol. Chem.* **233,** 1230.
Tseng, L., Stolee, A., and Gurpide, E. (1972). *Endocrinology* **90,** 390.
Turner, G., and Collins, E. (1975). *Lancet* **2,** 338.
Ullman, G., and Hammerstein, J. (1972). *Contraception* **6,** 71.
Ullrich, V., and Duppel, W. (1975). *In* "The Enzymes" (P. D. Boyer, ed.), 3rd ed., Vol. 12, p. 253. Academic Press, New York.
Underwood, E. J. (1971). "Trace Elements in Human and Animal Nutrition," 3rd ed., Chapter 3. Academic Press, New York.
Urry, R. L., and Dougherty, K. A. (1975). *Fertil. Steril.* **26,** 232.
Ussing, H. H., and Zerahn, K. (1951). *Acta Physiol. Scand.* **23,** 110.
Vallee, B. L. (1959). *Physiol. Rev.* **39,** 443.
Van Campen, D. R. (1969). *J. Nutr.* **97,** 104.

Vane, J. R. (1971). *Nature (London), New Biol.* **231,** 232.
Vane, J. R., and Williams, K. I. (1972). *Br. J. Pharmacol.* **45,** 146P.
Vierling, J. S., and Rock, J. (1967). *J. Appl. Physiol.* **22,** 311.
von Studnitz, W., and Berezin, D. (1958). *Acta Endocrinol. (Copenhagen)* **27,** 245.
Walker, W. R., and Griffin, B. J. (1975). *Search* **6,** No. 11.
Walker, W. R., and Keats, D. M. (1976). *Agents Actions* **6,** 454.
Walshe, J. M. (1956). *Am. J. Med.* **21,** 487.
Walshe, J. M. (1966). *In* "The Biochemistry of Copper" (K. Peisach, P. Aisen, and W. E. Blumberg, eds.), pp. 475–502. Academic Press, New York.
Walshe, J. M. (1969). *Lancet* **2,** 1401.
Walter, R., Havran, R. T., Schwartz, I. L., and Johnson, L. F. (1971). *In* "Peptides, 1969" (E. Scoffone, ed.), p. 255. North-Holland Publ., Amsterdam.
Warkany, J. (1971). "Congenital Malformations," pp. 102–124. Yearbook Publ., Chicago, Illinois.
Warkany, J., and Petering, H. G. (1972). *Teratology* **5,** 319.
Wasserman, R. H., and Corradino, R. A. (1971). *Annu. Rev. Biochem.* **40,** 501.
Watts, R. R., Storherr, R. W., and Onley, J. H. (1974). *Bull. Environ. Contam. Toxicol.* **12,** 224.
Webb, F. T. G. (1973). *J. Reprod. Fertil.* **32,** 429.
Weinmann, S., Dawson, E. B., Smolensky, M. H., and Weisberg, R. F. (1976). *Am. J. Obstet. Gynecol.* **124,** 719.
Weinstein, I. B., and Kitchin, F. D. (1971). *In* "The Thyroid" (S. C. Werner and S. H. Ingbar, eds.), 3rd ed., p. 384. Harper, New York.
Weiss, B. (1953). *J. Biol. Chem.* **201,** 31.
Westrom, L., and Bengtsson, I. P. (1970). *J. Reprod. Med.* **5,** 154.
Wharton, D. C. (1973). *In* "Inorganic Biochemistry" (G. I. Eichhorn, ed.), Chapter 27. Am. Elsevier, New York.
Whelan, E. M. (1975). *Studies Fam. Plann.* **6,** 106.
White, I. G. (1955a). *Aust. J. Biol. Sci.* **8**; 387.
White, I. G. (1955b). *Aust. J. Exp. Biol.* **33,** 359.
Whitehouse, M. W., Field, L., Denko, C. W., and Ryall, R. G. (1975). *Scand. J. Rheumatol.* **4,** Suppl. 8, Abstract 183.
Whitten, W. K. (1966). *Adv. Reprod. Physiol.* **1,** 155.
Wilcox, B. R., and Engel, I. L. (1965). *Steroids, Suppl.* **1,** 49.
Williamson, M. B. (1970). *Biochem. Biophys. Res. Commun.* **39**,379.
Wilson, C. W. M. (1976). *Ann. N. Y. Acad. Sci.* **258,** 355.
Wintrobe, M. M., Lee, G. R., Bogg, D. R., Bithell, T. C., Athens, J. W., and Forester, J., eds. (1974). "Clinical Hematology," 7th ed., pp. 124–127. Lea & Febiger, Philadelphia, Pennsylvania.
Winzler, R. J., and Bekesi, J. G. (1967). *Methods Cancer Res.* **2,** 159.
Witkop, C. J., Jr., White, J. G., and King, R. A. (1974). *In* "Heritable Disorders of Amino Acid Metabolism" (W. L. Nyhan, ed.), Chapter 11. Wiley, New York.
Wolf, G., and Varandani, P. T. (1960). *Biochim. Biophys. Acta* **43,** 501.
Wynn, V. (1975). *Lancet* **1,** 561.
Yoshida, T., and Wagner, G. (1974). *J. Reprod. Fertil.* **41,** 231.
Zipper, J. A., Medel, M., and Prager, R. (1969a). *Am. J. Obstet. Gynecol.* **105,** 529.
Zipper, J. A., Tatum, H. J., Pastene, L., Medel, M., and Rivers, M. (1969b). *Am. J. Obstet. Gynecol.* **105,** 1274.
Zipper, J. A., Medel, M., Pastene, L., Rivera, M., and Tatum, H. J. (1971). *Control Hum. Fertil., Proc. Nobel Symp., 15th, 1970* pp. 199–218.

Zipper, J. A., Medel, M., Pastene, L., Torres, L., Osorio, A., Rivera, M., and Toscanini, C. (1975). *Contraception* **12,** 1.
Zipper, J. A., Medel, M., Pastene, L., Rivera, M., Torres, L., Osorio, A., and Toscanini, C. (1976). *Contraception* **13,** 7.
Zipursky, A., Dempsey, H., Markowitz, H., Cartwright, G., and Wintrobe, M. M. (1958). *AMA Am. J. Dis. Child.* **96,** 148.

## Notes Added in Proof

Since the writing of this review some new applications of copper in contraception have been proposed: Ahsan *et al.* (1976) (see also Zbuzkova and Kincl, 1971) have demonstrated that copper wires inserted into the vas deferens of rats lead to a complete contraceptive effect for as long as 4 months. Davis (1976) has shown that a copper coil placed at the oviduct of the rabbit can block fertility, and fertility is restored when the coil is removed.

The papers cited from "Third International Conference on Intrauterine Contraception" (Abstracts, 1974) have now been published in book form (Hefnawi and Segal, 1975).

A comprehensive review of the effects of copper on the endometrium has appeared recently (Hagenfeldt, 1976).

## References for Notes Added in Proof

Ahsan, R. K., Faroog, A., Kapur, M. M., and Laumas, K. R. (1976). *J. Reprod. Fertil.* **48,** 271.
Davis, B. K. (1976). *Int. J. Fertil.* **21,** 123.
Hagenfeldt, K. (1976). *J. Reprod. Fertil. Suppl.* **25,** 117.
Hefnawi, F., and Segal, S. J., eds. (1975). "Analysis of Intrauterine Contraception." Am. Elsevier, New York.
Zbuzkova, V., and Kincl, K. A. (1971). *Acta Endocrinol (Copenhagen)* **66,** 379.

# SUBJECT INDEX

## A


A-16,612, antischistosomal activity of, 51
2-Acetylaminofluorene, effect on adenylate cyclase, 220
ACTA scanner, in pancreatic cancer diagnosis, 110
ACTH, secretion by islet cell tumors, 131
ACTH analog, effect on adenylate cyclase, 210
Acute lymphocytic leukemia, 5-azacytidine therapy of, 313
Acute myeloblastic leukemia
  5-azacytidine in therapy of, 285–326
    clinical studies, 311–313, 317
Adenocarcinoma
  5-azacytidine effects on, 316
  of pancreas, 108–127
Adenosine, effect on adenylate cyclase, 210
Adenylate cyclase
  cellular location of, 193–194
  chemistry of, 191–193
  chronic factors influencing activity of, 209–220
  distribution and properties of, 191–194
  endogenous activators of, 194–206
  endogenous inhibitors of, 206–207
  exogenous activators of, 207
  exogenous inhibitors of, 208–209
  hormonal effects on, 218
  modulation of, 194–209
  neuronal effects on, 219–220
  species and tissue distribution of, 193
  subcellular distribution of, 194
Adipose tissue, adenylate cyclase activation in, 196
Adrenal cortex, adenylate cyclase activation in, 196
β-Adrenergic agonists, effect on adenylase cyclase, 211
α-Adrenergic blockers, effect on adenylate cyclase, 210
β-Adrenergic blockers, effect on adenylate cyclase, 211
Alkylating agents
  as cyclic nucleotide phosphodiesterase inhibitors, 256
  in pancreatic cancer chemotherapy, 116–117
Alkylenebisbenzylamines, use in schistosomiasis chemotherapy, 4
Alloxan, effect on adenylate cyclase, 210
Aminoglutethimide, in islet cell tumor therapy, 131
*p*-Aminophenoxyalkanes, use is schistosomiasis therapy, 4, 11, 52–53
Amphetamine, effect on adenylate cyclase, 210
*d*-Amphetamine, behavioral toxicity of, comparison with MAO-inhibiting drugs, 96
Amphotericin B, antischistosomal activity of, 50–51
Amphothalide, antischistosomal activity of, 52
Angiography, in pancreatic cancer diagnosis, 111–112
Anorexia, from pancreatic cancer, 109
Antibiotics, effect on adenylate cyclase, 210
Antidepressants, behavioral toxicity of, 73
Antifertility agents, antischistosomal activity of, 54
Anti-inflammatory agents, as cyclic nucleotide phosphodiesterase inhibitors, 256–257
Antimonials, for schistosomiasis therapy, 2, 4, 11, 21–31
Antiprooxidants, as copper chelators, 393
Apomorphine, effect on adenylate cyclase, 210
Aristolochic acid, as phagocytosis activator, 183, 184
Arylazonaphthylamine derivatives, antischistosomal activity of, 48
Asbestos fibers, persorption of, 186
Ascorbic acid, as cyclic nucleotide phosphodiesterase inhibitor, 254

L-Asparaginase, in palliation of islet cell tumors, 130
Atropine, effects on persorption rate, 176
5-Azacytidine, 285–326
  abortive activity of, 289
  animal toxicity of, 300–302
  antimicrobial activity of, 288–289
  antitumor activity of, 297–299, 310–317
  biological properties of, 288–291
  chemical properties of, 286–288
  clinical studies on, 309–317
  cytotoxicity of, 289
  drug schedule dependency of, 299–300
  effects on, UV damage, 290
  immunosuppression by, 290
  incorporation into DNA, 291–293
  incorporation into RNA, 293–294
  in leukopenia, 290
  metabolism and disposition of, 303–308
  modes of action and resistance, 291–296
  mutagenicity of, 289
  as orotidylic acid decarboxylase inhibitor, 294–295
  pharmaceutical data on, 288
  possible radioprotective effect of, 290
  retention in lymphatic tissue, 291
  structure of, 286
  toxicity of, in man, 317–322
  triangulation pattern of, 288
  as uridine kinase competitor, 294

## B

Bacillus Calmette-Guérin (BCG), as immunopotentiator in cancer chemotherapy, 144–146
Bacteria
  as antischistosomal agents, 55
  5-azacytidine metabolism in, 304–305
  as immunopotentiators in cancer chemotherapy, 144–147
Barbituric acid, effects on persorption rate, 176
Bax 439, effect on adenylate cyclase, 211
Behavioral toxicity
  definition of, 72
  of MAO-inhibiting drugs, 71–105
Benzodiazepines, as cyclic nucleotide phosphodiesterase inhibitors, 252
Benzopyran derivatives, as cyclic nucleotide phosphodiesterase inhibitor, 255
*Besnoitia jellisoni*, as immunopotentiating factor in cancer chemotherapy, 149
Betazole, effect on adenylate cyclase, 211
Bile, persorbed particle excretion in, 181, 182
*Biophalaria glabrata*
  infection of, 6–8
  use in schistosomiasis chemotherapy tests, 5–6
Biological stimulators, as immunopotentiators in cancer therapy, 144–151
Biopsy, pancreatic, in cancer diagnosis, 113
1,2-Bis(2-chloroethyl)-1-nitrosourea (BCNU), in pancreatic cancer chemotherapy, 116, 118–120
Bitter taste stimuli, as cyclic nucleotide phosphodiesterase inhibitors, 256
Bladder
  adenylate cyclase activation in, 197
  cancer of, 5-azacytidine effects on, 316
Blastocysts, Cu-IUD effect on, 333–334
Blood, persorbed particles in, 170–172
Brain, adenylate cyclase activation in, 197
Breast cancer, 5-azacytidine effects on, 313–315
Breast milk, persorbed particle excretion by, 181
Butaclamol chelators, effect on adenylate cyclase, 200

## C

Caffeine, effects on persorption rate, 175, 181
Cancer
  Cu-IUD and, 345–346
  immunopotentiating agents in, therapy of, 143–187
  phosphodiesterase inhibition in control of, 265
Carcinoembryonic antigen (CEA), in pancreatic cancer diagnosis, 111, 112
Carcinoid syndrome, from islet cell tumors, 129, 131
Cardiac glycosides, as cyclic nucleotide phosphodiesterase inhibitors, 253
Castor oil, effects on persorption rate, 176

Caudate nucleus, adenylate cyclase activation in, 197
*Cebus* sp., *Schistosoma mansoni* infection of, 9–10, 15
Central nervous system tumors, 5-azacytidine effects on, 316
*Cercopithecus* sp., *Schistosoma mansoni* infection of, 9
Cerebrospinal fluid
  persorbed particle breakdown by, 183
  persorbed particle excretion by, 181
Ceruloplasmin, in reproduction, 357–360
Cervical cancer, 5-azacytidine effects on, 316
Chemical carcinogens, pancreatic cancer and, 107
Chemosterilants, antischistosomal activity of, 54–55
Chemotherapy
  of islet cell tumors, 129–136
  of pancreatic cancer, 114–127
Chickens, persorption rate in, 168–169
Chloasma, copper and, 360–361
Chlorambucil, in pancreatic cancer chemotherapy, 117
2-Chloroadenosine, effect on adenylate cyclase, 210
1-(2-Chloroethyl)-3-(4-methylcyclohexyl)-1-nitrosourea, in pancreatic cancer chemotherapy, 117, 125
*p*-Chlorophenylalanine, in islet cell tumor therapy, 132
Cholera toxin, effect on adenylate cyclase, 220
Cholesterol, in diet, pancreatic cancer and, 107
Cholinomimetics, effect on adenylate cyclase, 210
Chronic myelogenous leukemia, 5-azacytidine effects on, 313
Chyle, persorbed particle transport by, 166, 185
Cigarette smoking, pancreatic cancer and, 107
Cinchonine, antischistosomal activity of, 53
C-norprednisone acetate, antischistosomal activity of, 53
Cornstarch, in studies of persorption, 168–174
Coffee
  caffeine-free, effect on persorption rate, 177
  effect on persorption rate, 177
Colon cancer, 5-azacytidine effects on, 315
Computerized axial tomography, in pancreatic cancer diagnosis, 110
Copper, 327–409
  antagonists of, 388–391
  chelating agents for, 392
  contraceptive failures from, 350–351
  corrosion chemistry of, biochemical effects of, 341–344
  effects on reproductive hormones, 362–368
  in the environment, 391–393
  excess of, 376–379, 391–392
  fetal resorption and, 370–371
  hormonally induced changes in levels of, 357–368
  in infant nutrition, 382–385
  in inherited metabolic diseases, 385–388
  in intrauterine device, 327–409
  in mammalian reproduction, 327–409
  ovulation induced by, 362–364
  in parturition, 378–379
  in pregnancy, 368–379
  reproductive failure from deficiency of, 368–370
  spermicidal action of, 379–380
  teratogenesis of, 344, 369–376
Corpus luteum, adenylate cyclase activation in, 197
Cortisone, antischistosomal activity of, 53
*Corynebacterium parvum*, as immunopotentiating agent in cancer chemotherapy, 146–147
Courvoisier's sign, in pancreatic cancer, 109
Cushing's syndrome, from islet cell tumors, 129, 131
Cyclic AMP
  clinical applications of, 264–265
  effects of, 190
  inhibition of, 262
  transport of, 262
Cyclic nucleotide(s)
  as cyclic nucleotide phosphodiesterase activator, 239–240

as cyclic nucleotide phosphodiesterase inhibitor, 245–246
pharmacological control of synthesis and metabolism of, 189–283
Cyclic nucleotide phosphodiesterases
discovery and characterization of, 226
distribution of, 226–227
inhibition of, 241–255
ion dependence of, 228
multiple forms of, 228–233
pharmacological agent effect on, 257–261
properties, 230–233
tissue and cellular distribution, 229–230
pH dependence of, 227–228
properties of, 227–228
regulation of, 233–257
stimulation by exogenous activators, 241
substrate specificity of, 228
Cyclophosphamide, in pancreatic cancer chemotherapy, 117, 119

## D

Dapsone, antischistosomal activity of, 54–55
Dehydroascorbic acid, as cyclic nucleotide phosphodiesterase inhibitor, 254
Dehydroemetine, antischistosomal activity of, 53
Depression, MAO-inhibiting drug therapy of, behavioral toxicity of, 71–105
Detergents, effects on persorption rate, 176
Dexamethasone, antischistosomal activity of, 53
Dextrans, as immunopotentiators in cancer chemotherapy, 153
Diaminodiphenoxyalkanes, use in schistosomiasis chemotherapy, 4
Diazoxide, in therapy of islet cell tumors, 129
Dibenzazepines, as cyclic nucleotide phosphodiesterase inhibitors, 252
Dibutyryl cyclic AMP, as cyclic nucleotide phosphodiesterase inhibitor, 246–247
Dihydrotestosterone, effect on adenylate cyclase, 212
Diphenylhydantoin, in palliation of islet cell tumors, 129–130
Di-*N*-propylnitrosamine, pancreatic cancer from, 108
Disodium cromoglycate, as cyclic nucleotide, phosphodiesterase inhibitor, 253–254
Diuretics
as cyclic nucleotide phosphodiesterase inhibitors, 255
effect on persorption, 181
Dogs, 5-azacytidine metabolism in, 306
L-Dopa, behavioral changes from, comparison with MAO-inhibiting drugs, 95–96, 100

## E

Ecdysterone, effect on adenylate cyclase, 212
Ectopic pregnancies, in IUD wearers, 350
Egg suppressants, antischistosomal activity of, 54–55
Endometrial cancer, 5-azacytidine effects on, 316
Endometrium, Cu-IUD effects on, 334–336
Endoscopic cholangiopancreatography (ERCP), in pancreatic cancer diagnosis, 110–111
Endotoxin
effect on adenylate cyclase, 212
as immunopotentiating factor in cancer chemotherapy, 147–148
Enzymes
breakdown of persorbed particles by, 182–183
of schistosomes, use in chemotherapy, 3
Epidermis, adenylate cyclase activation in, 197
Ergot alkaloids, as cyclic nucleotide phosphodiesterase inhibitors, 251
Eritadenine, as cyclic nucleotide phosphodiesterase inhibitor, 254
Erythrocytes
adenylate cyclase activation in, 198
of monkey, disrupted membranes of, antischistosomal activity of, 55
*Escherichia coli*, adenylate cyclase activation in, 197

Esophageal cancer, 5-azacytidine effects on, 315
Ethanol, effect on adenylate cyclase, 212, 220
Ethylene 1,2-dimethanesulfonate, antischistosomal activity of, 54
*N,N*-Ethyleneurea, antischistosomal activity of, 54
α-Ethyl tryptamine, behavioral toxicity of, 90

## F

Fertilization, Cu-IUD effect on, 332–333
α-Fetoglobulin, in pancreatic cancer diagnosis, 112
Fibroblasts, adenylate cyclase activation in, 198
Flavoxate, as cyclic nucleotide phosphodiesterase inhibitor, 255
5-Fluorouracil (5-FU)
 in islet cell tumor therapy, 132
 in pancreatic cancer chemotherapy, 114–127
Fungal products, as immunopotentiating factors in cancer chemotherapy, 148
Fungicides
 copper in, 392
  breakdown and teratogenicity of, 375–376
Furosemide, effect on persorption, 181

## G

Ganglia, adenylate cyclase activation in, 198
Gastric mucosa, adenylate cyclase activation in, 198
Gastrin, secretion by islet cell tumors, 130–131
Gerbils, *Schistosoma mansoni* infection of, 10
Glial cells, adenylate cyclase activation in, 198
Glioblastoma, 5-azacytidine effects on, 316
Glucagon, as cyclic nucleotide phosphodiesterase activator, 239
Glucagon analog, effect on adenylate cyclase, 212
Glucosamine, use in schistosomiasis chemotherapy, 4
Glutathione peroxidase, estrogen effects on, 360–361
Guanylate cyclase, 221–226
 activation of, 224–225
 cellular and subcellular distribution of, 221–222
 inhibition of, 225
 ion effects on, 222–224
 multiple forms of, 222
 pH optimum of, 224
 tissue distribution of, 221

## H

Hair follicles, adenylate cyclase activation in, 198
Haloperidol, effect on adenylate cyclase, 210
Hamster, *Schistosoma mansoni* infection of, 9
Head tumors, 5-azacytidine effects on, 316
Heart, adenylate cyclase activation in, 198–199
HeLa cells, adenylate cyclase activation in, 199
Hemolymph, of snail, antischistosomal activity of, 55
Hepatomas
 adenylate cyclase activation in, 199
 5-azacytidine effects on, 316
Hexachloro-*p*-xylene, antischistosomal activity of, 53
Hexamethylphosphoramide, antischistosomal activity of, 54
Hormones, effects on adenylate cyclase, 218
Hybrid cells, adenylate cyclase activation in, 199
Hycanthone
 for schistosomiasis therapy, 2, 4, 11, 36–42
 structure of, 36
Hydantoins, antischistosomal activity of, 53
Hydrochlorothiazide, effect on persorption, 181
Hypoglycemia, from islet cell tumors, 127

Hypotonic duodenography, in pancreatic cancer diagnosis, 110

## I

Imidazolidinone derivatives, as cyclic nucleotide phosphodiesterase inhibitor, 249
Imidazoline derivatives, as cyclic nucleotide phosphodiesterase inhibitors, 250
Imidazopyrazines, as cyclic nucleotide phosphodiesterase inhibitors, 250
Immunopotentiating agents, 143–162
  biological type, 144–151
  in cancer therapy, 143–187
  chemical type, 151–154
Immunoreactive insulin (IRI), in islet cell tumors, 127
Infant nutrition, copper in, 382–385
Insecticides, effect on adenylate cyclase, 210
Insulin
  as cyclic nucleotide phosphodiesterase activator, 239
  effect on adenylate cyclase, 212
  secretion by islet-cell tumors, 129–130
Intrauterine device (copper), 329–357
  bleeding from, 346–349
  cancer and, 345–346
  clinical aspects of, 329–331
  effect on pregnancy, 331
  infection from, 349–350
  inflammatory effects of, 336–338
  injurious effects of, 351
  mode of contraceptive action, 331–344
  systemic effects of, 351–357
  teratology of, 344, 350
Iproniazid
  adverse behavior changes from, 76–83
    incidence, 76–79
    patient differences, 77–80
    specific types, 80–83
Islet cell tumors
  ACTH-secreting type, 131–132
  chemotherapy of, 129–136
  gastrin-secreting type, 130–131
  insulin-secreting type, 129–130
  serotonin-secreting type, 131–132
  symptoms of, 127–128
Isocarboxazid, behavioral toxicity of, 90, 92–93

## J

Jaundice, from pancreatic cancer, 109

## K

Kidney
  adenylate cyclase activation in, 199–200
  of guinea pig, Forssman-positive extract of, antischistosomal activity of, 55

## L

Lathyrism, 374–375
Lentinan, as immunopotentiating agent in cancer chemotherapy, 150–151
Leucovorin, in pancreatic cancer chemotherapy, 118
Leukocytes, adenylate cyclase activation in, 200
Levamisole, as immunopotentiator in cancer chemotherapy, 154
Lipids, as cyclic nucleotide phosphodiesterase activator, 240
Lipopolysaccharides, as immunopotentiating factors in cancer chemotherapy, 147–148
Lithium, effect on adenylate cyclase, 210
Lithium antimony thiomalate
  as antischistosomal agent, 29
  structure of, 29
Lithium carbonate, behavioral changes from, comparison with MAO-inhibiting drugs, 96
Liver
  adenylate cyclase activation in, 200–201
  phagocytosis in, 183
Lucanthone, as antischistosomal agent, 36–42
*Ludwiga palustris*, use for snail culture, 5
Lung
  adenylate cyclase activation in, 201
  cancer of, 5-azacytidine effects on, 315
Lymphocytes, adenylate cyclase activation in, 202
Lymphoma, 5-azacytidine effects on, 315

Lysergic acid derivatives, as cyclic nucleotide phosphodiesterase inhibitors, 251

## M

*Macaca mulatta, Schistosoma mansoni* infection of, 9
Macrophages, tumoricidal activity of, 144
Malabsorption, from pancreatic cancer, 109
Mechlorethimine, in pancreatic cancer chemotherapy, 117
Melanoma
  adenylate cyclase activation in, 202
  5-azacytidine effects on, 315
Melphalan, in pancreatic cancer chemotherapy, 125
Menkes' kinky hair syndrome, copper metabolic disorder in, 385–386
Mesothelioma, 5-azacytidine effects on, 316
Metabolic inhibitors, of cyclic nucleotide phosphodiesterases, 255–256
Methotrexate, in pancreatic cancer chemotherapy, 117–119
Methylene dimethanesulfonate, antischistosomal activity of, 54
1-Methyl-1-nitrosourea, pancreatic cancer from, 108
Metiamide, in islet cell tumor therapy, 130–131
Metoclopramide, effects on persorption rate, 175
Miracil D, antischistosomal activity of, 3
Mirasans, use in schistosomiasis therapy, 3, 4
Mitoclomine, antischistosomal activity of, 54
Mitomycin C, in pancreatic cancer chemotherapy, 115–116, 118
Monkeys, *Schistosoma mansoni* infection of, 9–10
Monoamine oxidase, forms of, 73
Monoamine oxidase-inhibiting drugs
  behavioral toxicity of, 71–105
    in animals, 97–98
    comparison with other drugs, 95–96
    iproniazid, 76–83
    methods for study, 75–76
    miscellaneous drugs, 90–94
    phenelzine, 83–90
    tranylcypromane, 90, 91
  biochemical effects of, 97–98
  classes and uses of, 74
Morphine, effect on adenylate cyclase, 213, 220
Mouse, *Schistosoma mansoni* infection of, 8–9
Mucopolysaccharides, as cyclic nucleotide phosphodiesterase inhibitor, 254–255
Multiple myeloma, 5-azacytidine effects on, 313
*Mycobacterium bovis*, as immunopotentiator in cancer chemotherapy, 144–146
Myometrium, Cu-IUD effects on, 338–341

## N

Naphthoquinones, use in schistosomiasis chemotherapy, 4
Neck tumors, 5-azacytidine effects on, 316
Neocarzinostatin, in pancreatic cancer chemotherapy, 118
Neostigmine, effects on persorption rate, 175
Neuronal factors, effect on adenylate cyclase, 218–220
Nialamide, behavioral toxicity of, 90, 94
Nicarbazin, antischistosomal activity of, 54
Nicotine, effect on persorption rate, 177
Nicotinic acid, effect on adenylate cyclase, 213
Niridazole
  for schistosomiasis therapy, 2, 4, 11, 31–35
  structure of, 31
Nitrofurans, antischistosomal activity of, 46–47
Nitrosoureas, in pancreatic cancer chemotherapy, 116
Nitrothiazolines, antischistosomal activity of, 47–48

## O

Oncofetal antigen, in pancreatic cancer diagnosis, 112
Organophosphorus compounds, antischistosomal activity of, 49–50

Orotidylic acid decarboxylase, 5-azacytidine as inhibitor of, 294–295
Ouabain, effect on adenyclate cyclase, 213
Ovary
adenylate cyclase activation in, 202
carcinoma of, 5-azacytidine effects on, 315
Oviduct, adenylate cyclase activation in, 202
Ovulation
copper-induced, 362–364
Cu-IUD effect on, 332–333
Oxamniquine
for schistosomiasis therapy, 2, 11, 42–46
structure of, 42
Oxytocin analogs, effect on adenylate cyclase, 213

## P

Pain, from pancreatic carcinoma, 109
Pancreas
adenylate cyclase activation in, 202
cancer of, 5-azacytidine effects on, 315
Pancreatic cancer, 107–142
chemotherapy of, 114–127
combinations, 118–127
single agent, 114–118
diagnosis of, 109–114
islet cell tumors, 127–136
symptoms of, 108–109
"Pancreatic cholera" from islet cell tumors, 128–129
Papaverine
as cyclic nucleotide phosphodiesterase inhibitor, 244–245
effects on persorption rate, 175
*Papio* sp., *Schistosoma mansoni* infection of, 9
Parathyroid, adenylate cyclase activation in, 202
Pargyline, behavioral toxicity of, 90, 92
Parotid gland, adenylate cyclase activation in, 202
Parturition, copper role in, 378–379
Penicillamine, as teratogen, 374
Peritoneal cavity, persorbed particle breakdown in, 182
Peritoneoscopy, in pancreatic cancer diagnosis, 113
Persorption, 163–187
absorption and, 163–164
drug effects on, 175–176
mechanism of, 165–167
modification of, 175–177
of particles
breakdown of, 182–183
excretion of, 178–182
rate, determination of, 167–175, 185
age differences, 173–174
in animals, 168–170
during sleep, 174
in man, 170–175
methods, 167
Persorption ratio, definition of, 186
Phagocytosis, of persorbed particles, 183
Phenelzine, behavioral toxicity of, 83–90, 97
incidence, 83–87
patient differences, 87–88
specific changes, 88–90
Phenethylamines, as cyclic nucleotide phosphodiesterase inhibitors, 250–251
Pheniprazine, behavioral toxicity of, 94
Phenothiazines
as cyclic nucleotide phosphodiesterase inhibitors, 251–252
effect on adenylate cyclase, 213
L-Phenylalanine mustard, in pancreatic cancer chemotherapy, 116–117
Pineal gland, adenylate cyclase activation in, 202
Pituitary, adenylate cyclase activation in, 202
Placenta, adenylate cyclase activation in, 202
Platelets, adenylate cyclase activation in, 202
Polygalacturonic acid, effects on persorption rate, 176
Polymers, as immunopotentiators in cancer chemotherapy, 151–154
Polynucleotides, as immunopotentiators in cancer chemotherapy, 151–152
Portal transport, of persorbed particles, 166, 185
Potassium antimonyltartrate
as antischistosomal agent, 26–28
structure of, 27
Pregnancy, copper effects on, 368–379

Procarbazine, behavioral toxicity of, 90, 93
Proinsulin-like component (PLC) islet cell tumors and, 127–128
Prostaglandins, copper effects on, 365–366
Prostate
  adenylate cyclase activation in, 202
  cancer of, 5-azacytidine effects on, 316
Protozoa, as immunopotentiating factor in cancer chemotherapy, 149
Purine analogs, effect on adenylate cyclase, 213
PVC particles, persorption of, 186
Pyran copolymer, as immunopotentiator in cancer chemotherapy, 152–153
Pyrazolo and pyridine derivatives, as cyclic nucleotide phosphodiesterase inhibitors, 249–251
Pyrophosphate, effect on adenylate cyclase, 213
3-Pyridylacetic acid, effect on adenylate cyclase, 213
Pyrroles, as cyclic nucleotide phosphodiesterase inhibitors, 250

## Q

Quinazolones, as cyclic nucleotide phosphodiesterase inhibitors, 250
Quinidine, antischistosomal activity of, 53
Quinine, antischistosomal activity of, 53

## R

Radiation therapy, of pancreatic cancer, 121–122
Rats, *Schistosoma mansoni* infection of, 10
RD-12,869, antischistosomal activity of, 51–52
Rectal cancer, 5-azacytidine effects on, 315
REM sleep, MAO-inhibitor effects on, 98, 100
Renal cancer, 5-azacytidine effects on, 316
Reproduction, copper in, 327–409
Reserpine, as cyclic nucleotide phosphodiesterase inhibitors, 251
Reticulocytes, adenylate cyclase activation in, 202
Retina, adenylate cyclase activation in, 203
Rhesus hemolysate, antischistosomal activity of, 55
Rhodanines, antischistosomal activity of, 53
Rice starch, persorption tests on, 183, 184
RNA, as immunopotentiating agent in cancer chemotherapy, 149–150
Rodents, 5-azacytidine metabolism in, 305–306

## S

S-201, antischistosomal activity of, 51
Salicylates, as teratogens, 373–374
Sarcomas, 5-azacytidine effects on, 316
Schistomide, antischistosomal activity of, 52
*Schistosoma mansoni*
  egg suppressants for 54–55
  laboratory maintenance of, 5–10
Schistosomiasis mansoni chemotherapy, 1–70
  A-16,612 in, 51
  *p*-aminophenoxyalkanes in, 4, 52–53
  amphotericin B in, 50–51
  antimonials for, 21–46
  arylazonaphthylamines in, 48
  biochemical approach to, 3
  biological agents in, 55
  chemosterilants in, 54–55
  clinical trials of, 16–21
    in field, 18–21
    in hospital, 16–18
    in outpatient clinic, 18
  criteria for, 13–15
  egg suppressants in, 54–55
  empirical approach to, 3
  *in vitro* testing of, 10–11
  *in vivo* testing, 11–15
  mechanism of, 11
  nitrofuran derivatives for, 46–47
  nitrothiazolines for, 47–48
  organophosphorus compounds in, 49–50
  prerequisites for, 2
  preclinical trials of, 15–16
  S-201 in, 51
  selective approach to, 3
  SN 10,275 in, 50
  thiazolines in, 47–48
  thiophene derivatives in, 48–49
  tris(*p*-aminophenyl)carbonium salts in, 52
  tubercidin in, 50

Selenomethionine-$^{75}$Se scanning, in pancreatic cancer diagnosis, 110
Semicarbazones, as cyclic nucleotide phosphodiesterase inhibitors, 250
Serotonin
  effect on adenylate cyclase, 214
  secretion by islet cell tumors, 131–132
Sex steroids, copper effects on, 364–365
Skeletal muscle, adenylate cyclase activation in, 203
Sleep, persorption during, 174
Small intestine, adenylate cyclase activation in, 203
Smell, copper role in physiology of, 361–362
SN 10,275, antischistosomal activity of, 50
Snail, as vector of *Schistosoma mansoni,* 5–6
Sodium antimony gluconate, use in schistosomiasis therapy, 29
Somatomedin, effect on adenylate cyclase, 214
Sperm
  adenylate cyclase activation in, 204
  copper effects on, 379–382
  Cu-IUD effect on, 332
Spermatogenesis, copper inhibition of, 381–382
Spironolactone, in pancreatic cancer chemotherapy, 124, 125
Spleen
  adenylate cyclase activation in, 204
  phagocytosis in, 183
Starch, in studies of persorption, 165–175
Statolon, as immunopotentiating factor in cancer chemotherapy, 148
Steroids, as cyclic nucleotide phosphodiesterase inhibitors, 253
Stibocaptate
  as antischistosomal agent, 29–31
  structure of, 30
Stibophen
  as antischistosomal agent, 28
  chemical structure of, 28
Stomach
  adenylate cyclase activation in, 204
  cancer of, 5-azacytidine effects on, 315
Streptozoticin
  in islet cell tumor therapy, 133–136
  in pancreatic cancer chemotherapy, 116–117, 124, 126
Submaxillary gland, adenylate cyclase activation in, 204
Sulfhydryl groups, sperm maturation and, 380–381
Sulfhydryl reagents, effect on adenylate cyclase, 214
Sulfonylureas, as cyclic nucleotide phosphodiesterase inhibitors, 252–253
Synovial membrane, adenylate cyclase activation in, 204

## T

T lymphocytes, in cancer cell destruction, 143
Tartar emetic, as antischistosomal agent, 26–28
Taste, copper role in physiology of, 361–362
Teratology, of Cu-IUDs, 344
Testes, adenylate cyclase activation in, 204
Testicular cancer, 5-azacytidine effects on, 316
Testolactone, in pancreatic cancer chemotherapy, 120–121, 124
Thiamine antimetabolite, antischistosomal activity of, 53
Thiazolines, antischistosomal activity of, 47–48
Thin-needle cytological aspirate, use in pancreatic cancer diagnosis, 113–114
Thiophene derivatives, antischistosomal activity of, 48–49
Thiosinamine, antischistosomal activity of, 54
Thioxanthones, use in schistosomiasis chemotherapy, 4
Thymus, adenylate cyclase activation in, 204
Thyroid
  adenylate cyclase activation in, 205
  copper effects on, 366–368
Thyroxine, as cyclic nucleotide phosphodiesterase inhibitor, 254
Tilorones, as immunopotentiators in cancer chemotherapy, 153–154

α-Tocopherol, as cyclic nucleotide phosphodiesterase inhibitors, 253
Tolbutamide, effect on adenylate cyclase, 214
*Toxoplasma gondii*, as immunopotentiating factor in cancer chemotherapy, 149
Transfer factor, as immunopotentiating agent, 149–150
Transhepatic cholangiography, in pancreatic cancer diagnosis, 111
Tranylcypromine, behavioral toxicity of, 90, 97
Trehalose-6,6-dimycolic acid, as immunopotentiating factor, 146
Triazines, as cyclic nucleotide phosphodiesterase inhibitors, 250
Tricyclic antidepressants, behavioral changes from, comparison with MAO-inhibiting drugs, 95
Triiodothyronine
  as cyclic nucleotide phosphodiesterase inhibitor, 254
  effect on adenylate cyclase, 214
Tris(*p*-aminophenyl)carbonium chloride, antischistosomal activity of, 52
L-Tryptophan, behavioral changes from, comparison with MAO-inhibiting drugs, 95–96
Tubercidin
  antischistosomal activity of, 50
  in islet cell tumor therapy, 132–133
  in pancreatic cancer chemotherapy, 124

**U**

Ultrasonography, in pancreatic cancer diagnosis, 110
Upper gastrointestinal (UGI) series, in pancreatic cancer diagnosis, 109–110
Uridine kinase, 5-azacytidine competition for, 294
Urine, persorbed particle excretion in, 178–181
Uterus, adenylate cyclase activation in, 205

**V**

Vitamins, in copper metabolism, 389–391

**W**

Weight loss from pancreatic cancer, 109
Wilson's disease, copper accumulation in, 377–378, 387–388

**X**

Xanthine analogs, as cyclic nucleotide phosphodiesterase inhibitor, 243–244

**Z**

Zinc, as copper antagonist, 388–389
Zollinger-Ellison syndrome, from islet cell tumors, 128